Statistical Issues
in Drug Development

Statistics in Practice

Advisory Editor

Stephen Senn
University of Glasgow, UK

Founding Editor

Vic Barnett
Nottingham Trent University, UK

Statistics in Practice is an important international series of texts which provide detailed coverage of statistical concepts, methods and worked case studies in specific fields of investigation and study.

With sound motivation and many worked practical examples, the books show in down-to-earth terms how to select and use an appropriate range of statistical techniques in a particular practical field within each title's special topic area.

The books provide statistical support for professionals and research workers across a range of employment fields and research environments. Subject areas covered include medicine and pharmaceutics; industry, finance and commerce; public services; the earth and environmental sciences, and so on.

The books also provide support to students studying statistical courses applied to the above areas. The demand for graduates to be equipped for the work environment has led to such courses becoming increasingly prevalent at universities and colleges.

It is our aim to present judiciously chosen and well-written workbooks to meet everyday practical needs. Feedback of views from readers will be most valuable to monitor the success of this aim.

A complete list of titles in this series appears at the end of the volume.

Statistical Issues in Drug Development

Second Edition

Stephen Senn

Department of Statistics
University of Glasgow, UK

John Wiley & Sons, Ltd

Other Wiley Editorial Offices

John Wiley & Sons Inc., 111 River Street, Hoboken, NJ 07030, USA

Jossey-Bass, 989 Market Street, San Francisco, CA 94103-1741, USA

Wiley-VCH Verlag GmbH, Boschstr. 12, D-69469 Weinheim, Germany

John Wiley & Sons Australia Ltd, 42 McDougall Street, Milton, Queensland 4064, Australia

John Wiley & Sons (Asia) Pte Ltd, 2 Clementi Loop #02-01, Jin Xing Distripark, Singapore 129809

John Wiley & Sons Canada Ltd, 6045 Freemont Blvd, Mississauga, Ontario, L5R 4J3

Wiley also publishes its books in a variety of electronic formats. Some content that appears in print may not
be available in electronic books.

Anniversary Logo Design: Richard J. Pacifico

British Library Cataloguing in Publication Data

A catalogue record for this book is available from the British Library

ISBN 978-0-470-01877-4

Typeset in 10/12pt Times by Integra Software Services Pvt. Ltd, Pondicherry, India
Printed and bound in Great Britain by Antony Rowe Ltd, Chippenham, Wiltshire
This book is printed on acid-free paper responsibly manufactured from sustainable forestry in which at least
two trees are planted for each one used for paper production.

To Victoria, Helen and Mark

Contents

Preface to the Second Edition

There have been many developments since the first edition of this book and it was high time for a second. My own period working in the pharmaceutical industry is now a distant memory but the ten years working as an academic since the first edition has had its compensations. I have been fortunate enough to be able to consult for many pharmaceutical companies during this time and this has certainly widened my appreciation of the work that statisticians do within the industry and the problems they face.

Alas, this appreciation is not shared by all. Many take it as almost axiomatic that statistical analysis carried out within the pharmaceutical industry is necessarily inferior to that carried out elsewhere. Indeed, one medical journal has even gone so far as to make it a requirement for publication that analyses from the pharmaceutical industry should be confirmed by an academic statistician, a policy which is as impractical as it is illogical.

Two related developments since the first edition, one of which is personal, are highly relevant. The first is that I have been honoured to succeed Vic Barnett as an editor for Wiley's *Statistics in Practice* series, in which this book appears. The second is that the series itself, so ably founded by Vic and Helen Ramsey, has been growing steadily and since the first edition now has attracted a number of further volumes that are highly relevant to this one. The chapters that have particularly benefited are listed with the relevant references as follows.

Chapter 6   Allocating treatments to patients in clinical trials (Berger, 2005)
Chapter 7   Baselines and covariate information (Berger, 2005)
Chapter 11   Intention to treat, missing data and related matters (Molenberghs and Kenward, 2007)
Chapter 16   Meta-analysis (Whitehead, 2002)
Chapter 19   Sequential trials (Ellenberg, et al., 2003)
Chapter 20   Dose-finding (Chevret, 2006)
Chapter 22   Bioequivalence studies (Hauschke, et al., 2007)
Chapter 23   Safety data, harms, drug-monitoring and pharmacoepidemiology (Lui, 2004)
Chapter 24   Pharmacoeconomics and portfolio management (Parmigiani, 2002, Willan and Briggs, 2006)

Also extremely useful are two books on Bayesian methods (O'Hagan *et al.*, 2006, Spiegelhalter *et al.*, 2003) and Brown and Prescott's book on mixed models (Brown and Prescott, 2006), which is already in a second edition. The books on survival analysis and

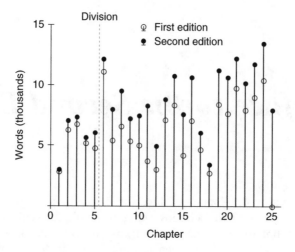

Figure P.1   Comparison of the first and second editions in length.

sequential analysis by Marubini and Valsecchi (1995) and Whitehead (1997) remain highly relevant, of course, as does my own on cross-over trials, (Senn, 2002), also now in a second edition.

All chapters have been brought up to date in the new edition and in particular, there is extensive reference to various guidelines of the International Conference of Harmonization that have been issued since the first edition, in particular ICH E9, *Statistical Principles for Clinical Trials*. A new chapter on pharmaco-genetics has been added. For the reader in possession of a first edition who wishes to know whether to splash out on a second, Figure P.1 may be helpful. (This is partly so that I can underline the fact that nothing in life, not even an author's preface, should be exempt from statistics!) This compares the two editions chapter by chapter in terms of their length in thousands of words.

The major division of the book occurs after Chapter 5, when material introducing statistics in drug development from historical, philosophical, technical and professional perspectives is succeeded by single-issue chapters. Figure P.2 shows even more clearly that much of the additional material has gone into chapters in Part 2. Apart from the wholly new chapter on pharmacogenetics in particular, chapters on baselines, measuring effects, intention to treat and missing data, equivalence, meta-analysis, sequential analysis, dose-finding, pharmaco-epidemiology and pharmaco-economics have had extensive additions.

It is appropriate for me to repeat a general warning about the book that Carl-Fredrik Burman has drawn to my attention. A number of the section headings contain statements of position. For example, Chapter 7 has a section, 'The propensity score is a superior alternative to adjusting for confounders than analysis of covariance'. You will get a very misleading impression of the message of the book if you take these as being *my* position. This is a book about issues and where such statements are made it is nearly always because, as is the case with this one, I wish to take issue with them.

I am grateful to Frank Bretz, Diane Elbourne, Paul Gallo, Oliver Keene, Dieter Hauschke, Nick Holford, Paul Johnson, Vincent Macaulay, Helmut Schütz, Helen Senn and John Sorkin for comments, and to Mateo Aboy, Nick Holford, Jerry Nedelman,

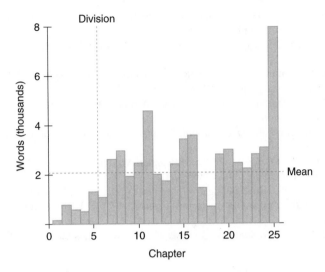

Figure P.2 Additional length (in thousand of words) of the second edition compared to the first. The mean increase (excluding chapter 25) is 2000 words.

Luis Pereira and Michael Talias for providing copies of their papers. Since the first edition, I have acquired several new co-authors whose work is reflected in this edition: my PhD students Dimitris Lambrou and Sally Lee and also, Pina D'Angelo, Frank Bretz, Carl-Fredrik Burman, Angelika Caputo, Farkad Ezzett, Erika Graf, Emmanuel Lesaffre, Frank Harrell, Hans van Houwelingen, William Mezanotte, Christopher Miller, Diane Potvin, Peter Regan and Nicoletta Rosati, whom I thank. I am also extremely grateful to Andy Grieve, for continued collaboration and to my PhD students Steven Julious, Andy Garrett for their work. I thank Kathryn Sharples, Susan Barclay, Beth Dufour and Simon Lightfoot at Wiley and also Len Cegielka and Cherline Daniel for work on preparing the book.

I continue to hope, of course, that this book will aid dialogue between statisticians and life-scientists within the pharmaceutical industry but also hope that it will contribute to a wider appreciation of the interesting challenges that statisticians within the pharmaceutical industry face and the seriousness with which they are met. I hope that the reader finds both stimulation and enjoyment in encountering these challenges.

References

Berger VW (2005) *Selection Bias and Covariate Imbalances in Randomized Clinical Trials*. John Wiley & Sons, Ltd, Chichester.

Brown H, Prescott R (2006) *Applied Mixed Models in Medicine*. John Wiley & Sons, Ltd, Chichester.

Chevret S (ed.) (2006) *Statistical Methods for Dose-Finding Experiments*. John Wiley & Sons, Ltd, Chichester.

Ellenberg S, Fleming T, DeMets D (2003) *Data Monitoring Committees in Clinical Trials: A Practical Perspective*. John Wiley & Sons, Ltd, Chichester.

Hauschke D, Steinijans V, Pigeot I (2007) *Bioequivalence Studies in Drug Development: Methods and Applications*. John Wiley & Sons, Ltd, Chichester.

Lui K-J (2004) *Statistical Estimation of Epidemiological Risk*. John Wiley & Sons, Inc., Hoboken.

Marubini E, Valsecchi MG (1995) *Analysing Survival Data from Clinical Trials and Observational Studies*. John Wiley & Sons, Ltd, Chichester.

Molenberghs G, Kenward MG (2007) *Missing Data in Clinical Studies*. John Wiley & Sons, Ltd, Chichester.

O'Hagan A, Buck CE, Daneshkah A, Eiser JR, Garthwaite PH, Jenkinson DJ, Oakley JE, Rakpw T (2006) *Uncertain Judgements*. John Wiley & Sons, Ltd, Chichester.

Parmigiani G (2002) *Modeling in Medical Decision Making: A Bayesian Approach*. John Wiley & Sons, Ltd, Chichester.

Senn SJ (2002) *Cross-over Trials in Clinical Research* (2nd edition). John Wiley & Sons, Ltd, Chichester.

Spiegelhalter DJ, Abrams KR, Myles JP (2003) *Bayesian Approaches to Clinical Trials and Health-Care Evaluation*. John Wiley & Sons, Ltd, Chichester.

Whitehead A (2002) *Meta-analysis of Controlled Clinical Trials*. John Wiley & Sons, Ltd, Chichester.

Whitehead J (1997) *The Design and Analysis of Sequential Trials*, revised 2nd edn. John Wiley & Sons, Ltd, Chichester.

Willan AR, Briggs AH (2006) *Statistical Analysis of Cost-effectiveness Data*. John Wiley & Sons, Ltd, Chichester.

Preface to the First Edition

The conscientious mathematician acts in this respect like the lady who is a conscientious shopper. Wishing to satisfy herself of the quality of a fabric, she wants to see it and to touch it. Intuitive insight and formal proof are two different ways of perceiving the truth, comparable to the perception of a material object through two different senses, sight and touch.

Polya, *How to Solve It*

When I first started work in the Swiss pharmaceutical industry in 1987, I had already been working as a statistician for twelve years: three years in the National Health Service in England and then nine years lecturing in Scotland. What struck me then was how much I still had to learn, not only about medicine, pharmacology and drug development in general, but also about my own subject, statistics. Working with other professionals, many of them experts in fields of which I knew nothing, called for a different approach to statistics in at least four ways. First, I had to examine what I 'knew' in order to establish what was useful and what was not. Second, I had to supplement it with knowledge of many fields of statistical theory which were new to me (design and analysis of cross-over trials was an example). Third, I had to pay attention to the scientific fields of my colleagues, in particular pharmacology, and try to work out the implications in statistical terms. Fourth, I had to repay my colleagues' willingness to explain their sciences to me by making my statistical points in terms that were clear to them.

In doing the latter, it became clear to me that there were many things which I myself had taken for granted which were debatable. I also came to the conclusion that many of the difficulties with statistical ideas lie deeper than statistics itself (an example would be notions of causality). Furthermore, I became convinced that statisticians pay their non-statistical colleagues a disservice if they try to gloss over genuine disagreements. This book is an attempt to present many of the statistical issues in drug development in a way which is comprehensible to life scientists working in drug development whilst avoiding false consensus. The emphasis will be on the intuition which Polya, although himself a distinguished mathematician, valued so highly. Although addressed to the life-scientist it is my hope that many statisticians, in particular those studying medical statistics or embarking on a career in drug development, will also find it useful. Above all I hope that it will help communication between the disciplines: a process by which the statistician stands to benefit as much as any other professional in drug development. I cannot pretend, however, to be objective on all issues and am not even sure of what such objectivity might consist. In my defence, however, I think that I may justly claim, that if all viewpoints are not given equal care and consideration, the reader will at least come away with a wider awareness that other views exist, than would have been the case in a more conventional approach.

The book is in two sections. The first, and by far the shorter section, is based on a statistics appreciation course which I gave a number of times to my colleagues at Ciba-Geigy. In addition to a brief introduction it consists of four chapters, each of which takes a different view, of statistics in drug development: historical, 'philosophical', technical and professional. I recommend that every reader will either read these chapters or satisfy her or himself that the material is familiar. The second and larger section is loosely based on a course (but less technical than that course) which I give to students on the Postgraduate Diploma in Statistics at Neuchatel University and consists of nineteen chapters of varying length which may be read in almost any order and consulted as considered desirable. Each chapter consists of a brief background statement and then a second section split into a number of issues. These are sometimes presented as true open issues and sometimes as positions which one might take on an issue. (Where the latter is the case, the reader should be warned that I usually *disagree* with the position taken.) At the end of each chapter are a number of references. Sometimes these will have been referred to explicitly but in some cases they are merely listed because they are useful additional reading.

When it comes to handling statistics, the life-scientist in drug development has two particular advantages over his or her colleagues elsewhere. First, (s)he will, through the nature of the work, come into frequent contact with statistical problems. Consequently, a basic familiarity with some essential concepts will be obtained. Second, technical statistical matters will be handled as a matter of course by the statisticians assigned to the various drug development projects. Life scientists working elsewhere will not always be so fortunate as to have resident experts whom they may consult. This provides a further justification for my decision to concentrate on issues rather than technicalities.

I find the subject matter fascinating, of course, but am aware that the reader will not always share my enthusiasm. I have tried to leaven the mix by adding chapter quotations and even the occasional joke or anecdote, ignoring Sterne's warning that: *Tis no extravagant arithmetic to say, that for every ten jokes, - thou has got an hundred enemies; and till thou hast gone on, and raised a swarm of wasps about thine ears, and art half stung to death by them, thou wilt never be convinced it is so.*

This book would have been impossible to write without the help of many statisticians and life scientists from whom I received my education at Ciba-Geigy (now merged with Sandoz to form Novartis). In particular, amongst statisticians, I have to thank my former colleagues Farkad Ezzet, Hans-Peter Graf, Andy Grieve, Walter Kremers, Gunther Mehring, Amy Racine and Jakob Schenker for many helpful discussions during my time at Ciba-Geigy, as well as the various members of my own group, Bernhard Bablok, Nathalie Ezzet, Friedhelm Hornig, Rolf Meinert, Erhard Quebe-Fehling, Peter Sacares, Denise Till, Elizabeth Wehrle and Albert Widmer for shared work over the years, and also others in Switzerland, the USA and elsewhere, too numerous to mention. I also learned a great deal from the life scientists with whom I collaborated and I would particularly like to thank Reto Brambilla, Giovanni Della Cioppa, Brigitte Franke, Francesco Patalano and Bill Richardson for sharing the joys and pains of drug development with me. I also owe a particular thank you to William Jenkins who, in introducing me to the problem of portfolio management, led me to a wider appreciation of the role of statistics in drug development, and to Anders Hove, Keith Widdowson, Marc Cohen, Bill Huebner, Ronald Steele of CIBA-Geigy and Peter Regan, formerly of Strategic Decisions Group for working on this problem with me. My UCL colleagues, Vern Farewell and Rebecca Hardy made helpful comments on various chapters as did Leon Aarons, Peter Bauer, Michael

Budde, Stephen Evans, Farkad Ezzet, Dieter Hauschke, Oliver Keene, Walter Kremers, John Lewis, Bill Richardson, Joachim Röhmel, Mark Sculpher and John Whitehead. I thank Lew Sheiner for permission to reproduce figure 22.1 from one of his papers. I am also grateful to Peter Bauer, Roger Berger, Michael Dewey, Farkad Ezzet, Nancy Geller, Andy Grieve, Miranda Mugford and Wendy Ungar for giving me access to (as yet) unpublished work of theirs and to Yadolah Dodge, professor of statistics at the University of Neuchatel and the students on the postgraduate diploma there for the opportunity to expound this subject. Thanks are also due to Guernsey McPearson for contributing quotations and other material.

Acknowledgements

With thanks to the following copyright holders for their kind permission to reproduce quotations from their publications:

Chapter 1
Brazzaville Beach, by William Boyd, published by Sinclair-Stevenson. Reprinted by permission of The Random House Group.

Chapter 6
The Lottery in Babylon, by Jorge Luis Borges, Translated by John M. Fein from Labyrinths, copyright © 1962, 1964, by New Directions Publishing Corp. Reprinted by permission of New Directions Publishing Corp.

Chapter 9
Roots Schmoots: Journey Among Jews, by Howard Jacobson. Reproduced with permission from Peters Fraser & Dunlop Group Ltd.

Chapter 22
Enderby Outside, by Anthony Burgess. © Estate of Anthony Burgess from Enderby Outside (1968), reproduced with permission.

Chapter 24
The Bear, Wodwo (1967), by Ted Hughes. Reproduced with permission from Faber & Faber.

1

Introduction

Ye maun understand I found my remarks on figures, whilk . . . is the only true demonstrable root of human knowledge.

Sir Walter Scott, *Rob Roy*

Statisticians know that words are important to statistics, yet surely their importance is not fully recognized.

William Kruskal

Opinions are made to be changed – or how is truth to be got at? We don't arrive at it by standing on one leg.

Lord Byron, *letter to Murray*

1.1 DRUG DEVELOPMENT

Drug development is the process not only of finding and producing therapeutically useful pharmaceuticals and of turning them into high-quality formulations of usable, effective and safe medicines, but also of delivering valuable, reliable and trustworthy information about appropriate doses and dosing intervals and about likely effects and side-effects of these treatments. Drug development is a process carried out by *sponsors* (mainly pharmaceutical companies) and its acceptability is ultimately judged by *regulators*. It is an extremely complex business and the risks are high, but the potential rewards are also considerable.

It takes many years for a project to reach development. First, basic research must be undertaken to validate concepts and mechanisms. Assessments of commercial potential for diseases and therapies are also needed and these will continue throughout the life of a project. Next, a lead compound must be identified for a particular indication. This will then be subjected to a battery of screening tests to assess its potential in terms of therapeutic activity. Back-up compounds will also be investigated. If a compound looks promising, it will also be evaluated from both safety and practical points of view. Will it be easy to formulate? How many steps are involved in the synthesis? How difficult will it be to manufacture in large-scale quantities? Before a treatment can go into development, not only must satisfactory answers have been obtained to all these questions but a viable pharmaceutical formulation permitting further study must be

Statistical Issues in Drug Development/2nd Edition   Stephen Senn
© 2007 John Wiley & Sons, Ltd

available. This can be an extremely delicate matter, involving work to develop suitable solutions, pills, patches or aerosols as the case may be.

If and when a molecule is accepted into development, animal studies will be undertaken in order to check safety and to establish a dose at which studies in humans may be undertaken. Once basic toxicological work has been undertaken, 'phase I' may begin and the first such studies may start. These will be single-dose studies in which lower doses are tried first and cautiously increased until a maximum tolerated dose may be established. In many indications such studies are carried out on healthy volunteers, but where the treatment is highly aggressive (and hence intended for serious diseases) patients will be used instead. In the meantime, longer-scale toxicological studies with animals will have been completed. Pharmacokinetic studies in humans will be undertaken in which the concentration–time profile of the drug in blood will be measured at frequent intervals in order to establish the rate at which the drug is absorbed and eliminated. These studies together, if successful, will permit multiple-dose studies to be undertaken.

Once maximum tolerated doses have been established, phase II begins and dose finding studies in patients are started. This is usually an extremely difficult phase of development but, if the drug proves acceptable, the object is that preliminary indications of efficacy should be available and that a firm recommendation for doses and dose schedules should emerge. Once these studies have been completed, the pivotal phase III studies can begin. These have the object of proving efficacy to a sceptical regulator and also of obtaining information on the safety and tolerability of the treatment.

A successfully completed development programme results in a dossier – an enormous collection of clinical trial and other reports, as well as expert summaries covering not only the clinical studies as regards efficacy and safety but also preclinical studies and other technical reports as well as details of the manufacturing process. If successful, the package leads to registration, but even during the review process, phase IV studies may have been initiated in order to discover more about the effect of the treatment in specialist subpopulations, or perhaps with the object of providing data to cover price negotiations with *reimbursers*.

> **Regulatory dossier**: A mountain of documents which takes a forest of trees to obscure the wood.

Once a drug has been launched on the market, the process of monitoring and 'pharmacovigilance' begins in earnest, since the drug will now be used by far more persons than was ever the case in the clinical trials in phases I to III, and rare side-effects, which could not be detected earlier, may now appear. Some further phase IV postmarketing studies may be initiated and further work extending indications or preparing new formulations may be undertaken.

1.2 THE ROLE OF STATISTICS IN DRUG DEVELOPMENT

There is no aspect of drug development in which statistics cannot intrude: from screening chemicals for activity to forecasting sales. Because the efficacy and safety of treatments has to be judged against a background of considerable biological variability, all of the judgements of efficacy boil down in the end to a numerical summary of evidence whose message can only be understood with the help of the science of statistics. It is the norm that clinical trials are planned jointly by a statistician and a physician. Statisticians are also becoming more active in the shaping of projects as a whole. Furthermore, whereas in the past in Europe, the expert reports for a dossier would largely be a subjective qualitative assessment of evidence from individual trials, regulators increasingly expect to see quantitative summaries, so called meta-analyses. Hence statistics is increasing its empire throughout the drug development process.

For many years now, the Food and Drugs Administration (FDA) in the United States has employed statisticians to assist in its review process, and this is now gradually being imitated in Europe by various national regulatory agencies, although the European Medicines Agency (EMEA) has yet (as far as I am aware) to follow suit. Statistical issues have long been covered by FDA general guidelines and there are now separate specific statistical guidelines produced by the Committee for Proprietary Medicinal Products (CPMP) in Europe, and by the Japanese Ministry of Health and Welfare. The International Conference on Harmonisation (ICH) is also addressing the subject. There are also many national and international societies specifically for statisticians in the pharmaceutical industry. The exact duties of the statistician working in drug development are covered in some detail in Chapter 5.

1.3   THE OBJECT OF THIS BOOK

As implied by our chapter quotations, this book is about figures, words and opinions; more precisely, it is an attempt to give a largely verbal account of the various opinions that are held by those who figure. The purpose is not to present an authoritative prescription as to how to deal with each particular application of statistics in drug development. I myself am far too cynical to believe that such statements are possible. Instead, the object is to make the reader think about genuine statistical controversies in drug development. In many cases the issues are deep, and thinking about them will increase understanding about scientific problems of evidence and inference as they relate to pharmaceuticals and their role in medicine and health, whether or not the reader's thinking about them concludes in resolution of the issues in question to his or her satisfaction. I hope the process is not only beneficial but enjoyable.

In complete contrast to my first book, *Cross-over Trials in Clinical Research* (Senn, 1993, 2002), this book includes very few concrete examples. There are a number of reasons, of which two are particularly important. First, it is not my object to teach the reader how to *calculate* anything. There is no need, therefore, of data to calculate upon. Second, the book is deliberately minimalist and I have eliminated anything that interferes with proceeding to discussing the issues.

The scope of the book is statistics in drug development in humans. I have taken this to include issues concerning the value of drugs that we may develop (Chapter 24) and also in monitoring drugs that we have developed (Chapter 23). With the exception of these two chapters, however, the book as a whole is concerned with matters affecting clinical trials in phases I to IV. There are many other areas in which statistics in the pharmaceutical industry are important thus I have not covered, including, for example, chemometrics and classification of molecules in research, screening for efficacy, toxicology, pharmaceutical development, stability testing, process optimization and quality control. If I have left these out it was partly because one has to drawn the line somewhere but mainly because what I know about them could be written on the back of an envelope. This does not mean I have left them out without regrets: I would have enjoyed learning about them, but it would have been unrealistic to have included them and, in any case, I wanted a book that reflected my actual experience of drug development. I hope that the book nonetheless serves to give an impression of how wide the subject is, but the reader should bear in mind that it is wider yet than covered in these pages.

1.4   THE AUTHOR'S KNOWLEDGE OF STATISTICS IN DRUG DEVELOPMENT

The fact that I have eliminated from this book the subjects about which I know nothing does not mean that I am equally knowledgeable about all those that remain. I think it is appropriate for me to warn the reader of strengths and weaknesses. If we exclude the chapters in Part 1, then chapters 6 through to 18 are strengths, as is chapter 22; chapters 19, 21 and 23 are weaknesses and chapters 20 and 24 fall somewhere between the two. Chapter 25 on pharmacogenetics, which is new, is a bit of an odd one out. My knowledge of genetics is poor. However, equally relevant to this chapter is an understanding of sources of variability and also of trial design, which are both areas in which I have researched extensively over the years. Extensive references, in many cases with recommendations for further reading, are given in each chapter.

1.5   THE READER AND HIS OR HER KNOWLEDGE OF STATISTICS

Ideally, nobody should study statistics who hasn't studied it already. The least stimulating aspect of the subject (I will not say the easiest since it has difficulties of its own), is the mechanics of calculation. Although many of the horrors of this topic have been eliminated by modern computing, it is inevitable that a first course in statistics will not avoid dealing with these algorithmic matters in some detail. (And those readers who find computing to be a horror in its own right have my sympathy.) Only in a second course, where many of the rudiments of 'how' have been answered, can the more interesting 'why', 'when' and 'whether to' questions be addressed.

> **Statistics**: A subject which most statisticians find difficult but in which nearly all physicians are expert.

Throughout this book it is assumed that the reader already has some basic familiarity with statistics, such as may be obtained, for example, by the excellent elementary text on medical statistics by Campbell, Machin and Walters (Campbell *et al.*, 2007). For a more detailed coverage I recommend Altman (1991) or van Belle *et al.* (2004), and for a more advanced level Armitage and Berry (2001). Some basic familiarity with statistics in clinical trials as covered, for example, in the classic text by Pocock (1983) is also assumed. Other treatments of statistics in clinical trials that I can recommend are the broad but elementary book by Wang and Bakhai (2006), the mathematically more advanced text by Matthews (2006), or the more comprehensive treatment by Piantadosi (2005). As regards the drug development process itself, I have found Hutchinson (1993) extremely useful to give to my own students wanting a quick introduction, and useful guides to the major classes of drug are Youngson (1994) and Henry (1994). Nevertheless, there is no heavy reliance on this assumed knowledge and the reader's memory will be jogged from time to time regarding relevant matters.

1.6 HOW TO USE THE BOOK

Part 1 consists of four chapters that give a crash course on statistics in drug development by presenting four different perspectives of the matter: historical, methodological, technical and professional. The least authoritative of these is the first, Chapter 2, which gives the historical view and where I have had to rely on secondary sources via the expert commentaries of others (with the exception of the history of the *t*-test, (Senn and Richardson, 1994) and Fisher's involvement in trials in humans (Senn, 2006), where I have undertaken some original researches myself). Nevertheless, if one does not consider the history of a subject, however crudely, one is all too vulnerable to the myth of 'present perfect' and I felt that it was important to cover history. Consideration of past imperfect helps to introduce a sense of proportion.

> **Analysis plan**: A detailed description of the intended analysis written before un-blinding data in the pharmaceutical industry and somewhat later, if at all, elsewhere.

The crucial chapters are Chapters 3 and 4, which give the 'iron rations' of the subject, covering basic statistical notions of causality and experimentation and introducing the two major schools of statistics: the frequentist and the Bayesian. (However, the general issue of Bayesian versus frequentist methods is too big for me to tackle seriously, preoccupying as it does many of the finest minds in the statistical profession. It cannot be entirely ignored, however, and it does break surface at various points throughout the rest of the book. Historical and philosophical accounts are given in my book *Dicing with Death* (Senn, 2003).) Chapter 5 explains something of the duties and concerns of the medical statistician working in drug development and may help to set the scene for the issues that follow. Chapters 2–5 together make a suitable one-day introductory course to clinical trials. Indeed, as mentioned in the preface to the first edition, they grew out of a course I gave while still working at CIBA-Geigy, which I left in 1995, and I have frequently given such courses both before and since the appearance of the first edition in 1997.

The issues themselves are covered in Part 2 and are grouped in chapters by broad theme which may be read in almost any order (or not at all) as the reader wishes. The chapters from Chapter 19 onwards are rather more technical and specialized than

Chapters 6–18, which are closely related to a postgraduate course I gave for many years at the University of Neuchatel, and it may help to have read some of these earlier chapters first. The grouping reflects drug development more than it reflects statistics. For example, if a purely statistical arrangement had been envisaged, there would have been a chapter on random-effect models, with entries on meta-analysis, multicentre trials and n-of-1 trials, rather than separate chapters on these topics with sections dealing with random-effect models. Certain such statistical topics are therefore more profitably hunted down via the index rather than the table of contents. The topics chosen are also those that are *particularly* relevant to drug development. Thus, topics that are relevant only because they affect the whole of statistics, such as, 'what should the role of robust statistics be?', are scarcely touched on. A few of the chapters in Part 2 have technical appendices, where I felt that the matters covered were not, or were not easily, available in the literature. These may be safely ignored by all but the more statistically minded.

In some of the chapters the reader will come across terms highlighted in bold type. This is an indication that these are important concepts and is usually a sign that there is an entry in the glossary. An exception is Chapter 2, where I have also highlighted the names of important historical figures.

The chapters can be used in a number of ways: by junior statisticians in order to get a quick overview of issues affecting a particular type of trial they are working on for the first time, by physicians and other life-scientists working in the pharmaceutical industry to help them discuss statistical issues with their statistical colleagues, and by university departments as the basis for student seminars and journal clubs.

Finally, for those who find controversy unsettling, I can do no better than quote the heroine of William Boyd's *Brazzaville Beach*: 'I have taken new comfort and refuge in the doctrine that advises one not to seek tranquility in certainty, but in permanently suspended judgement.' From *Brazzaville Beach* by William Boyd, published by Sinclair-Stevenson. Reprinted by permission of The Random House Group Ltd.

References

Altman DG (1991) *Practical Statistics for Medical Research.* Chapman and Hall, London.

Armitage P, Berry G, Matthews JNS (2001) *Statistical Methods in Medical Research* (4th edition). Blackwell Science, New York.

Campbell M, Machin D, Walters S (2007) *Medical Statistics: A Textbook for the Health Sciences,* (4th edition). John Wiley & Sons, Ltd, Chichester.

Henry J (ed.) (1994) *British Medical Association: New Guide to Medicines and Drugs.* Dorling Kindersley, London.

Hutchinson DR (1993) *How Drugs are Developed.* Brookwood Medical Publications, Richmond on Thames.

Matthews JNS (2006) *An Introduction to Randomized Clinical Trials.* Arnold, London.

Piantadosi S (2005) *Clinical Trials: A Methodologic Perspective.* John Wiley & Sons, Inc., New York.

Pocock SJ (1983) *Clinical Trials, A Practical Approach.* John Wiley & Sons, Ltd, Chichester.

Senn SJ (1993) *Cross-over Trials in Clinical Research.* John Wiley & Sons, Ltd, Chichester.

Senn SJ (2002) *Cross-over Trials in Clinical Research* (2nd edition). John Wiley & Sons, Ltd, Chichester.

Senn SJ (2003) *Dicing with Death.* Cambridge University Press, Cambridge.

Senn SJ (2006) An early 'Atkins' Diet': RA Fisher analyses a medical 'experiment'. *Biometrical J* **48**: 193–204.

Senn SJ, Richardson W (1994) The first t-test. *Statistics in Medicine* **13**: 785–803.

van Belle G, Fisher LD, Heagerty PJ, Lumley TS (2004) *Biostatistics: A Methodology for the Health Sciences* (2nd edition). John Wiley & Sons, Inc., Hoboken.

Wang D, Bakhai A (eds) (2006) *Clinical Trials: A Practical Guide to Design Analysis and Reporting.* Remedica, London.

Youngson RM (1994) *Prescription Drugs.* Harper-Collins, Glasgow.

Part 1

Four Views of Statistics in Drug Development: Historical, Methodological, Technical and Professional

... when the usual symptoms of health or sickness disappoint our expectation; when medicines operate not with their wonted powers; when irregular events follow from any particular cause; the philosopher and physician are not surprised at the matter, nor are ever tempted to deny, in general, the necessity and uniformity of those principles by which the animal economy is conducted. They know that a human body is a mighty complicated matter, that many secret powers lurk in it, which are to us altogether beyond our comprehension...

David Hume, *An Enquiry Concerning Human Understanding*

A Brief and Superficial History of Statistics for Drug Developers

O that this all important science might become part of University Education
                                        Florence Nightingale (writing about statistics)

2.1   INTRODUCTION

Statistics is the science of collecting, analysing and interpreting data. Statistical theory
has its origin in three branches of human activity: first, the study of mathematics as
applied to games of chance; second, the collection of data as part of the art of governing
a country, managing a business or, indeed, carrying out any other human enterprise;
and third, the study of errors in measurement, particularly in astronomy. At first, the
connection between these very different fields was not evident but gradually it came
to be appreciated that data, like dice, are also governed to a certain extent by chance
(consider, for example, mortality statistics), that decisions have to be made in the face of
uncertainty in the realms of politics and business no less than at the gaming tables, and
that errors in measurement have a random component. The infant statistics learned
to speak from its three parents (no wonder it is such an interesting child) so that, for
example, the word *statistics* itself is connected to the word *state* (as in *country*) whereas
the words *trial* and *odds* come from gambling and *error* (I mean the word!), has been
adopted from astronomy

   Because of its close relation to the mathematics of probability, it is worth, however,
drawing one distinction between the science of *probability* as understood by statisticians
and mathematicians and the science of *statistics* proper. The former starts with known or
presumed laws and uses the calculus of probability to say something about the chance
of given events occurring. (For example, given a fair die, what is the probability of a total
score of exactly 8 in two rolls?) The latter starts with data and (given some knowledge
of the circumstances under which they were obtained) tries to deduce something about
the state of nature. (For example, given the results of a number of rolls of a die, can
I say whether it is fair or not?) This latter problem is an example of what is known

Statistical Issues in Drug Development/2nd Edition   Stephen Senn
© 2007 John Wiley & Sons, Ltd

as *inverse probability* (Dale, 1991) which, either directly or indirectly, is the concern of statistics.

Statistics is thus also the science of inferring facts about nature given the evidence available. Therefore, it is closely related to the branch of philosophy known as epistemology. It may surprise those who are unfamiliar with statistics to learn that statisticians and philosophers have worked on the same problems. For example, the nature of probability itself (is it a subjective feeling, a relative frequency or a propensity of systems?) is a matter for philosophical speculation.

In this chapter we shall follow the development of probability and statistics more or less chronologically from the 17th century as it appears in a study of the mathematicians who contributed to these developments. When coming to medical statistics, we shall then return in time to pick up some of the developments made by biologists and physicians.

2.2 EARLY PROBABILISTS

A number of 17th-century mathematicians, notably **Pierre Fermat** (1601–1665), **Blaise Pascal** (1623–1662) and **Christian van Huygens** (1629–1695), made important contributions to the theory of probability. Hacking (1975) has made the claim that probability emerged as a concept around about the middle of the seventeenth century, and then developed rapidly but was scarcely known in modern form before this time. The contribution of Fermat and Pascal through their correspondence of 1654 discussing problems put to Pascal by the French gambler the Chevalier de Méré, is particularly important and often taken as being the start of the subject. Much of these early researches into probability problems consisted of deriving mathematical laws for enumerating ways in which particular types of events may occur. One well known illustration of such a law, the binomial law, is given by Pascal's triangle (Pascal is the author of an elegant treatise on this triangle proving many results which, although already known, had not been proved before. See Edwards (2002) for a scholarly examination of Pascal's work.)

The first few rows of Pascal's triangle (which carries on for ever) are given in Figure 2.1. (Armitage, a famous medical statistician, gives an amusing account of a

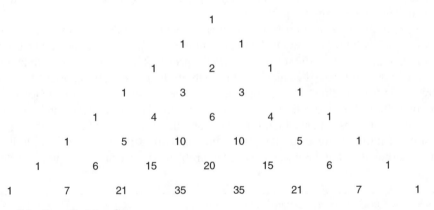

Figure 2.1   Pascal's triangle.

rather large Pascal triangle with 125 rows constructed by him, Godwin and Lindley, which was pasted to the wall of the office in which they worked during the Second World War. See Barnard and Plackett (1985).) Here, each number in a given row is the sum of the numbers nearest to it in the row above. For the first and last numbers in a row there is one such nearest number; for others there are two. For example, to use Pascal's triangle to enumerate the number of ways in which three heads may be obtained in five tosses of a coin we use the *fourth* entry in the *sixth* row (the first entry corresponds to 0 heads and the first row to 0 tosses) giving the answer 10. Since the total of all of the entries in the sixth row is 32 (corresponding to $2^{6-1} = 2^5$), then if on a single toss a head is just as likely as a tail, the probability of obtaining three heads in five tosses is 10/32. This general approach of calculating the ratio of favourable outcomes to total possible outcomes plays an important role in many probability calculations. Fermat's and Pascal's work can be regarded as a contribution to the theory of the binomial distribution, still applied today for studying binary outcomes. In the context of the clinical trial these might be dichotomies of the form survive/die, cured/not cured and satisfactory/unsatisfactory although, of course, unlike head/tail, such events would not be regarded as being equally likely. (The more general formula for the binomial distribution deals with such cases.)

2.3 JAMES BERNOULLI (1654–1705)

James (or Jakob, Jacques, etc) Bernoulli has been designated 'father of the quantification of uncertainty' (Stigler, 1986) and his *Ars Conjectandi*, published posthumously in 1713, is a landmark in the mathematics of probability. There are so many notable mathematicians among members of the well-known Bernoulli family of Basle (eight according to Bell (1953) but twelve according to Stephen Stigler and Boyer (1991)) that there is often confusion as to which is meant (uncertainty as to the father of the quantification of uncertainty?). Among statisticians, at least, *Bernoulli* without further qualification means, or ought to mean, *James* (the first James Bernoulli of note), who was Professor at the University of Basle from 1687 until his death in 1705. Figure 2.2, based on Bell (1953) and Boyer (1991) gives a pedigree. The Bernoullis with dashed boxes are those admitted to the pantheon by Boyer but not by Bell, although, rather confusingly, Bell charts Nicholas II but, perhaps showing a mathematician's prejudice against probabilists, does not count him among the great. However, not only is it thanks to Nicholas's actions in publishing his uncle James's work after his death, that *Ars Conjectandi* finally emerged to public scrutiny, but Nicholas himself made important contributions to the theory of probability as has now been made clear in Ander's Hald's masterly two-volume history of statistics (Hald, 1990, 1998). (Nicholas Senior's role in all this is merely to father a dynasty of mathematicians!)

James Bernoulli's skill in developing the methods of the calculus and his general familiarity with limits was put to a remarkable use in developing what we now call *Bernoulli's weak law of large numbers*. This sought to relate the observed relative frequency of successes in a large series of trials to the individual probability of success using a probabilistic law. It is an attempt to answer questions such as 'if the probability of obtaining a 5 in a single roll of a die is 1/6, in what sense may I expect that, given a large number of rolls, the proportion of 5s will be approximately 1/6?' Bernoulli's result is central to the science of statistics but its interpretation remains controversial.

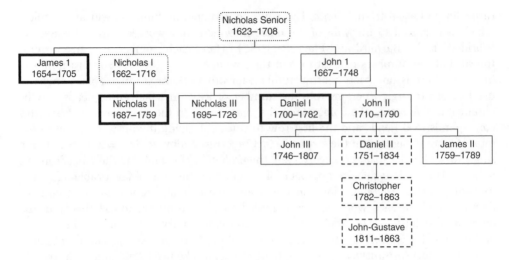

Figure 2.2 Family tree of the Bernoullis (based on Boyer, 1991). Nicholas Senior and Nicholas I were not mathematicians. James I, Nicholas II and Daniel I are particularly important in the history of statistics. Daniel II, Christopher and John-Gustave are not included by Bell (1953) but are included by Boyer (1991) and Stigler (1986).

2.4   JOHN ARBUTHNOTT (1667–1753)

A famous example of applied statistics in the 18th century is Arbuthnott's paper of 1710 *An argument for Divine Providence, taken from the constant regularity observ'd in the births of both sexes* (Arbuthnot, 1710), which used the fact that the probability was minute that the yearly observed excess of male compared female births (if christenings could be accepted as a measure) in London from 1629 to 1710 was due to chance (if it were assumed that male and female births were equally likely) as an argument that the Almighty must be intervening for good in the affairs of mankind by providing a greater number of the frailer sex. (Here frailer must be understand in its statistical sense! Women are the stronger sex.) Arbuthnott's analysis was improved upon by a **Bernoulli** (**Nicholas II**, 1687–1759, this time, nephew of James, and mentioned above) who, however, may have held rather different opinions regarding the value of this demonstration of Divine Providence.

John Arbuthnott earned his living as a teacher of mathematics and translated Huygens' (see above) treatise on probability into English. Unlike most mathematicians and statisticians, he evidently had a keen appreciation of practical economics as he then studied medicine and became a fashionable physician.

2.5   THE MATHEMATICS OF PROBABILITY IN THE LATE 17TH, THE 18TH AND EARLY 19TH CENTURIES

These developments are too numerous to cover in detail, but a few lines of work in particular are extremely important. The first is the development of the mathematics of insurance, associated in particular with the rise of commerce in Holland and in Britain. The Dutch politician **John** (Jan, Johan, etc) **de Witt** (1625–1672) and the English astronomer **Edmund Halley** (1656–1742) introduced methods for the calculation of annuities, the latter constructing a life table from records of vital statistics of the city of Breslau (Wroclaw). Halley's work was extended by the French-born English mathematician **Abraham de Moivre** (1667–1754), who also did important work on the binomial distribution, and by **John Simpson** (1710–1761), who was a weaver who supplemented his income by teaching mathematics. (Simpson is also honoured eponymously among mathematicians through *Simpson's rule*, a method for approximating the area under a curve. In drug development, areas under the curve are commonly calculated in bioequivalence and dose-proportionality studies, although the simpler trapezoidal rule is more usually employed.)

Modern survival analysis, an important tool of statistical analysis in drug development today, can be regarded as having its origins in the work of De Witt, Halley, de Moivre and Simpson and other mathematicians of the 17th and 18th centuries who worked on life tables and annuities.

A further important impetus for the development of probabilistic study came from the study of 'errors' in observation in astronomy and surveying, where scientists began to realize that, although individual errors were not predictable, their distribution *en masse* followed particular 'laws'. The study of this phenomenon and methods for dealing with it led to much important work by mathematicians, such as on the Normal distribution and on methods for combining observations, in particular the method of least squares. Among the many mathematicians who worked on these problems, particularly notable are the Swiss mathematician **Leonhard Euler** (1707–1783), the German astronomer and cartographer **Tobias Mayer** (1723–1762), and especially the French mathematicians **Pierre-Simon Laplace** (1749–1827) and **Adrien-Marie Legendre** (1752–1833) and the German mathematician **Carl Friedrich Gauss** (1777–1855). The Normal distribution has a central place in the subject of statistics today and the method of least squares is one of the most common methods of statistical estimation.

2.6 THOMAS BAYES (1701–1761)

A woman aged 40–44 at parturition is more likely to have a baby suffering from Down's syndrome than one aged 20–24, but to conclude, *therefore*, that any newborn baby suffering from Down's syndrome is more likely to have been born to a woman aged 40–44 than to one aged 20–24 is quite false. To solve this sort of problem we use one of the most important theorems in statistics namely *Bayes' theorem*.

Suppose we label the two classes of mother as 'young' and 'old' (ignoring all other age groups) and suppose that the probability of an old mother having a child with Down's syndrome is 1 in 40 (= 0.025) and for a young mother it is 1 in 200 (= 0.005). Suppose, furthermore, that the probability of any baby at all (irrespective of chromosomal status) having a young mother is 3 in 10 (0.3) and of having an old mother is 1 in 100 (0.01). Use of Bayes' theorem then shows that the relative probability of a Down's syndrome baby having a young mother is $(0.005 \times 0.3)/(0.025 \times 0.01) = 6$. Thus the Down's syndrome baby is six times as likely to have had a young mother as an old mother. (Of course the probabilities used in calculating this example are purely illustrative and should not be taken seriously.)

Until relatively recently, little was known about the Bayes of *Bayes' theorem*, but it is now known that he was a nonconformist minister in Tunbridge Wells who was elected a Fellow of the Royal Society in 1742. His *An essay toward solving a Problem in the Doctrine of Chances* (1764) was published after Bayes' death by his friend Richard Price in 1763 (see Barnard, 1958). There is a very vigorous modern school of statistics which is referred to as Bayesian because of the importance of Bayes' theorem in its approaches.

History, n. An account mostly false, of events mostly unimportant, which are brought about by rulers mostly knaves, and soldiers mostly fools.

Ambrose Bierce.

2.7 ADOLPHE QUETELET (1796–1874)

The Belgian Adolphe Quetelet is an important, if curious, figure in the history of statistics: mathematician, astronomer, man of letters and, ultimately, statistician. He was the first to attempt a systematic application of statistical methodology to what we should now call sociology and although, in Stigler's assessment, 'Quetelet did not accomplish a great deal towards this end – in some respects he failed totally' (Stigler, 1986, p. 161) he had an extremely profound effect on the generations after him. Our chapter quotation is taken from marginal notes by Florence Nightingale on a book of Quetelet's (Diamond and Stone, 1981) (she read and re-read Quetelet); he was an important influence on Galton (see below) and the claim has even been made that James Clerk Maxwell gained the confidence to develop statistical mechanics to explain the behaviour of gases from the example of Quetelet (Gigerenzer *et al.*, 1989), inspired by the ability in sociology to show order arising out of chaos through the aggregation of the random behaviour of numerous individuals.

2.8 FRANCIS GALTON (1822–1911)

Galton was an eccentric amateur scientist who studied both medicine and mathematics and made important contributions to a number of fields (Forrest, 1974). Among his many discoveries and inventions were a method for classifying fingerprints, a machine for extracting wave energy, barometric maps (he was the discoverer and namer of the meteorological phenomenon of the anticyclone) and a feminine beauty map of Britain (whenever he passed a woman in the street he would make a mark on a paper cross he carried in his pocket recording her attractiveness or otherwise). He also made extensive studies in genetic heritability and was able to discover empirically the phenomenon of *regression* (now easily demonstrated mathematically).

Galton discovered that tall parents tend to have children who, while taller than average, are nevertheless smaller than their parents. They thus *revert to mediocrity* or *regress to the mean*. This phenomenon of regression is widespread and general so that, for example, patients who have been selected for a clinical trial on grounds of high blood pressure may, *on purely statistical grounds*, be expected, other things being equal, to show an improvement in blood pressure when measured again. This omnipresent, but widely ignored, feature is an important reason for the unreliability of uncontrolled studies and it is a sad fact that medical researchers are still regular and gullible victims of this phenomenon.

Finally, as an example of Galton's approach to statistics one might cite his investigation of the efficacy of prayer. He concluded that it didn't work because prayers were said almost daily all over the country for the longevity of the monarch, yet, when British monarchs were compared to a control group of members of the aristocracy, it was found that their life span was shorter on average.

2.9   KARL PEARSON (1857–1936)

The man who brought Galton's work into the mathematical statistical mainstream was Karl Pearson, after whom the Pearson correlation coefficient and Pearson chi-squared tests are named (Porter, 2005). He made rapid progress in providing techniques for calculating the various coefficients that Galton's insight required and also, along with his colleagues **Walter Frank Raphael Weldon**, and later **George Udney Yule**, generalized the work to many dimensions (in this he was partly anticipated by **Francis Ysidro Edgeworth**). He also studied general families of distributions related to the Normal distribution. Much of modern statistical terminology originated with Pearson (*contingency table, goodness of fit, histogram,* to list a few). He was the founder of the discipline of *biometrics* (a word which used to be used and continues to be used to designate statistics when applied to the life sciences but is now increasingly misapplied to the unique identification of individuals using biological measurement) and also of the prestigious journal *Biometrika,* and his department at University College London may claim to be the first at which the subject could be studied.

2.10   'STUDENT' (1876–1937)

William Sealy Gosset studied mathematics and chemistry at Oxford and went to work for the brewers Arthur Guinness in Dublin, Ireland in 1899 (Pearson, 1990). The standard statistical techniques used at the time required large numbers of observations (perhaps as many as 200). Gosset's practical work, however, faced him with the problem of drawing inferences on the basis of small samples and he obtained leave to study with Karl Pearson at University College London from September 1906 to spring 1907. The results of his labours were the discovery of the *t*-distribution and its associated test. He published under the pseudonym 'Student', which is why his distribution is often referred to as *Student's t.* An early connection of the *t*-test to drug development is that the data Student used to illustrate his techniques were taken (incorrectly!) from a paper by Cushny and Peebles (Cushny and Peebles, 1905) describing an early cross-over trial of the effectiveness of optical isomers as hypnotics (Senn and Richardson, 1994).

2.11   R.A. FISHER (1890–1962)

Possibly the single most important figure in 20th-century statistics is R.A. Fisher. He made many original contributions to almost every branch of statistics including correlation, regression, significance tests, the theory of estimation, analysis of variance and multivariate analysis (Box, 1978). Indeed many of these and other fields in statistics were first developed by him. He also carried out a parallel career as a geneticist and has been described by Richard Dawkins as the greatest evolutionary biologist since Darwin (Dawkins, 1986). (In fact, although Fisher held chairs at University College London and Cambridge, he was never a professor of *statistics*.) Fisher worked for many years at the agricultural research station at Rothamsted and it was during his time there that he developed his influential ideas on experimental design. The use of blocks, factors, concomitant observations and, in particular, randomization have also been taken over in the design of clinical trials.

Although Fisher's legacy is of immense importance to medical statisticians, except indirectly through his work on genetics, he had little to do with medical statistics. One notorious exception is his criticism of Richard Doll and Bradford Hill's work on smoking and lung cancer.

2.12   MODERN MATHEMATICAL STATISTICS

Modern statistics is divided into two main camps. The larger frequentist (or classical) school, represents a synthesis and development of ideas originally proposed by Fisher and by his rivals, the Polish mathematician **Jerzy Neyman** (1894–1981) (Reid, 1982) and the English statistician **Egon Pearson** (1895–1980), the son of Karl. The smaller, but increasingly influential, Bayesian (or subjectivist) school has also adopted many ideas and techniques of Fisher, but its philosophy was developed by individuals such as the English philosopher **Frank Plumpton Ramsey**, the English geophysicist **Harold Jeffreys**, the Italian mathematician and actuary, **Bruno de Finetti** and the American mathematician and statistician **Jimmy Savage**. Although at the level of applied statistics there is considerable agreement in the results produced by the two schools, this is not always the case and interpretation is, in any case, always somewhat different. In particular, approaches to sequential analysis, a topic developed in the Second World War by the Romanian-Hungarian-American **Abraham Wald** (1902–1950), are quite different. (Wald is also the originator of modern decision theory, which has both frequentist and Bayesian variations.)

The general difference between the Bayesian and frequentist approaches can be summed up as follows. The frequentist starts with a model and sees whether it would reasonably be expected to produce the data observed. (In doing this he also has to take into account more 'extreme' data sets which the model *might* have produced.) This leads to an indirect judgement as to whether the model is reasonable. The Bayesian, on the other hand, calculates directly a probability that any particular model is true given the observed data only, but has to do this at the cost of giving probability a subjective interpretation and including as part of his specification of the problem, and before seeing the data, all other possible models that might have given rise to the data and a prior probability that each of these models is true.

Most statistical methods in current use in drug development today are frequentist, but Bayesian approaches are gaining in popularity, in particular in the field of pharmacokinetics but also in a regulatory context where medical devices are concerned. These matters are dealt with in more detail in Chapter 4.

2.13   MEDICAL STATISTICS

The story we have outlined so far has concentrated largely on the work of mathematicians. As Lancaster has pointed out, however, many of the significant mathematical advances in medicine, and more generally biology, were made by subject specialists rather than mathematicians (Lancaster, 1994). There are also a number of key figures who pursued both disciplines. We have already seen that Arbuthnott moved from mathematics to medicine and that Galton studied both. **Daniel Bernoulli** (1700–1782), nephew of James and cousin of Nicholas II) moved from medicine to mathematics and was responsible not only for an early development of the significance test (applied to a problem in astronomy) but also for an early attempt to model the benefits of vaccination against smallpox (Bailey, 1975).

Much important work, however, was not mathematical but directly statistical. For example, **Sir William Petty** (1623–1687) and **John Graunt** (1620–1674) were two amateurs with important statistical interests. Petty proposed that a central statistical office be established and suggested what uses might be made of the data collected. John Aubrey gives an interesting account of his statistical prowess. At the time of the war with the Dutch, he is supposed to have correctly predicted to one intending to recruit sailors in Ireland for the Navy that his target number of men would not be met. 'Sir William knew 'twas impossible, for he knew how many tons of shipping belonged to Ireland, and the rule is, to so many tons, so many men' (Aubrey, 1975). Graunt made detailed investigations of the bills of mortality in London. Petty's suggestions were not put into effect until the 19th century; the first census in Britain was in 1801 and it was not until **William Farr** (1807–1883) left his practice to take up an appointment to the General Registry Office in 1839 that Petty's ideas can really be considered to have come to fruition. Farr is one of a number of individuals in the 19th century connected with medicine (such as **Florence Nightingale**, 1820–1910 and her contemporary Galton) who came to appreciate the value of data in drawing conclusions. A notable instance is given by the French physician **Pierre Louis** (1787–1872). He collected data on blood-letting in phthisis (a term then used to cover various conditions now given a variety of names, one of which is pneumonia). The data might be presented thus:

	Bled for first time in first four days	Bled for first time in days five to nine
Number	23	27
Mean days pain	4	8
Mean days disease	17	20

His conclusion was that early blood-letting was effective. However, as was pointed out by the American physician **Elisha Bartlett** (1804–1855) in 1848, this does not constitute a proof of the efficacy of blood-letting, since no suitable control group to test *this* hypothesis is provided. A similar criticism still applies today for trials in which there is no placebo group, and this is an issue we shall consider in Chapter 15. Another important French physician is **Louis-Denis-Jules Gavarret** (1809–1890), an early proponent of applying the theory of probability to the estimation of rates. He showed how approximations to the binomial distribution based on the Normal distribution might be applied to assessing the reliability of rates and stressed the value of large numbers of cases in coming to reliable conclusions. (See the scholarly treatise by J Rosser Matthews (Matthews, 1995) for further discussion of these figures.)

In more modern times physicians have continued to be involved in medical statistics. There have been a number of notable cases of persons who have trained as physicians but decided ultimately to work as statisticians. Among many one might cite are the American physician Joseph Berkson, who did important work on survival analysis, the notable trialist David Byar, and Mitchell Gail, a former president of the American Statistical Association. Indeed, one of our (secondary) sources for this history of statistics, the Australian H.O Lancaster, was a pathologist and epidemiologist before taking up mathematical statistics (Fienberg, 1985; Senn, 2003). The rise of the modern medical discipline of epidemiology also means that there are now many scientists trained initially as physicians whose working tools are largely statistical and who have made and are making important contributions to the theory of medical statistics.

> The history of statistics is like a telephone directory: the plot is boring, full of numbers and the cast is endless.

2.14   STATISTICS IN CLINICAL TRIALS TODAY

The central idea in clinical trials today is that of concurrent control: comparing the effects of treatments at the same time in a single experiment. This idea did not really find widespread practice until after the Second World War but there were, of course, many earlier examples. Some are reviewed by Pocock (1983) in his book and also by Lancaster (1994) and Gehan and Lemak (1994), who suggest that the Islamic-Persian scholar **Avicenna** (980–1037) was an early proponent of the technique. **James Lind** (1716–1794) ran a clinical trial in 1747 to compare the effects of cider, oranges and lemons and four other treatments in 12 patients suffering from scurvy (two assigned to each treatment). The two given oranges and lemons recovered. There continued, of course, to be many clinical trials employing this general approach. We have, for example, already mentioned the cross-over trial (see also Chapter 17) reported by **Arthur Cushny** (1866–1926) and **Alvin Peebles** (1884–1917) in 1905 to test the effect of various optical isomers as hypnotics (Senn and Richardson, 1994).

The rational conduct of clinical trials is unthinkable today without statistical ideas. The first modern randomized clinical trials were carried out by the Medical Research Council in the United Kingdom and their prime mover was the statistician **Austin Bradford Hill** (1897–1991). The most important single application of medical statistics in drug development is to clinical trials. Although European regulatory agencies were slow to employ statisticians (in the United Kingdom, the first full time appointment was made in 1993), they have long been an important factor contributing to the strength of the US regulatory system and in Europe there are now also many working in regulation. The pharmaceutical industry itself, both in the United States and in Europe, has long employed statisticians and many have made important contributions to the theoretical and practical development of the subject. Statistical guidelines have now been agreed by The International Conference on Harmonization and published in *Statistics in Medicine*

(International Conference on Harmonization, 1999). A review of some current issues in statistics as applied to drug development at the turn of the millennium was given by Senn (2000).

History: The sum of the factual, less the forgotten, plus the fabricated.

2.15   THE CURRENT DEBATE

An extremely vigorous debate continues between Bayesian and frequentist statisticians. The frequentist is the majority school, at least as regards practice, but a survey of statistical methods actually applied will underestimate the inroads that Bayesian statistics has made. A survey of methodological papers published would show it to be important and growing in importance. **George Barnard** (1915–2002), an influential figure in the development of modern statistics and one who made contributions of relevance to both major traditions, made the claim that in fact there are four distinct systems with which all statisticians should be familiar: the Fisherian and Neyman–Pearson variants of the frequentist approach and the two major Bayesian variants, the semi-objective approach of Jeffreys and the currently dominant fully subjective De Finetti–Savage–Lindley approach. Barnard claimed (Barnard, 1996) that statisticians should settle for realizing that good work can be done in each tradition and that each is useful on occasion. He likened the controversies in statistics to those which arose in logic fifty years earlier and pointed out that logicians were now happy to state which particular set of foundational assumptions they were adopting when examining a given question.

Obviously, the choice between Bayesian and frequentist methods is *the* statistical issue, but if it deserves to be treated properly it needs a book devoted to it alone. In the first edition of this book I claimed that I was not the person to write it. Subsequently, I repented and in a fit of hubris attempted to treat it at some length in in my book *Dicing with Death* (Senn, 2003). The reader who is interested to know more may like to consult that work, which does, however, consider many other matters. The book by Howson and Urbach (1993) gives a partisan (Bayesian) though nonmathematical (but philosophically rigorous) evaluation and the more mathematical books by Barnett (1982), Lindsey (1996) and Royall (1999) are also useful.

This conflict will appear in various places, in particular in the chapter on sequential analysis, and the differences between the approaches are discussed in Chapter 4. However, it is not specifically covered here in the sense that this is not a book which tries to evaluate the general claims of either Bayesian or frequentist (classical) statistics to be *the* theory of statistical inference.

2.16   A LIVING SCIENCE

It is important to understand that statistics is a living science and that new techniques are constantly being developed. For example, three seminal papers on three statistical topics, generally important but specifically so for drug development, *generalized linear models* (Nelder and Wedderburn, 1972), *proportional hazards* (Cox, 1972) and the *log-rank test* (Peto and Peto, 1972) date from 1972; the key paper on *ordered categorical data* dates from 1980 (McCullagh, 1980), *Gibbs sampling* was introduced in 1990 (Gelfand and Smith, 1990), and the 1990s saw considerable methodological work on *meta-analysis, dose-finding, cross-over trials, equivalence studies, surrogate endpoints, repeated measures, survival analysis, multiple endpoints, sequential analysis, compliance* and *missing data* (to mention but a few areas of particular relevance to drug development). Since the turn of the millennium there has been further work on these topics and also considerable development of more complicated random-effect models, including hierarchical generalized linear models (Lee and Nelder, 2001), techniques for analysing micro-arrays (Landgrebe *et al.*, 2004), approaches to model selection and combination (Bretz *et al.*, 2004; Raab *et al.*, 2000), alternative approaches to dealing with multiplicity arising out of the work of Benjamini and Hochberg (1995), adaptive designs as introduced by Bauer and Kohne (1994) and work on analysis of trials with missing data (Molenberghs and Kenward, 2007).

There are now a number of journals devoted to medical statistics. *Statistics in Medicine* was founded in 1981 and has grown rapidly to have 24 issues and over 4000 pages a year. *Statistical Methods in Medical Research* is a general review journal founded in 1992; *The Journal of Biopharmaceutical Statistics* is specifically devoted to statistical issues in drug development and was started in 1991. New journals since the year 2000 include *Biostatistics* (2000), *Pharmaceutical Statistics* (2002) and *Statistics in Biopharmaceutical Research* (2007). Other journals of relevance that often have a strong statistical content are *Contemporary Clinical Trials, Clinical Trials, The Journal of Clinical Epidemiology* and the *Drug Information Journal* and, of course, many older statistical journals such as *Biometrics, Biometrika, The Journal of the Royal Statistical Society* and the *Journal of the American Statistical Association*, have papers on medical statistics.

The medical statistician also has the opportunity to join a number of specialist societies. The *International Society for Clinical Biostatistics* organizes an annual conference, as does the *Society for Clinical Trials*, and proceedings of these meetings are published in *Statistics in Medicine* and *Clinical Trials*, respectively. There are a number of organizations specifically for statisticians working in the pharmaceutical industry, such as the UK based PSI (Statisticians in the Pharmaceutical Industry) and there is a European Federation of Statisticians in the Pharmaceutical Industry (EFSPI), of similar national societies. Other national organizations such as the *American Statistical Association* and the French *Association pour la Statistique et ses Utilisations* have specialist sections.

The implication of these developments is that, inevitably, simpler techniques are replaced by more sophisticated ones. This trend can no more be resisted than can developments in chemistry and biology. Just as we cannot insist that the chemist must determine pH using titration and litmus paper because this is a simple method that we can understand and it was good enough in the 19th century, so we cannot insist that all comparisons be performed using the *t*-test because that is what we find discussed in our statistics primer and was 'state of the art' in 1908.

In short, in order to plan and analyse clinical trials effectively, cooperation between the statistician and the physician is essential. The earlier such cooperation begins (ideally when planning the drug development programme) the better the result for the company, for science and for future patients.

2.17 FURTHER READING

A famous, but rather dated, history of probability is given by Florence Nightingale David (David, 1962). For a necessary correction to her views on the Pascal and Fermat correspondence, see (Edwards, 2002). The general history of probability and statistics is very well served by Stigler (1986) and Hald (1990, 1998) and any serious researcher into the history of statistics will find the two articles by H.A. David (David, 1995, 1998) invaluable. An interesting essay on the language of statistics is Kruskal (1978). A concise review of the history of statistics is given by Fienberg (1992), who, however, badly underestimates the importance of Hald (1990). The development of Bayesian thinking is covered by Dale (1991). Other important works are those of Hacking (1975) and the two volumes of collected papers edited by Pearson and Kendall (1970) and Kendall and Plackett (1977). A number of Stephen Stigler's important original articles investigating the history of statistics have been collected in one volume (Stigler, 1999). Schwartz's charming book also includes much of historical interest (Schwartz, 1994) and a popular account of the history of statistics is given by Senn (2003). As regards medical statistics, the books by Gehan and Lemak (1994) and by Matthews (1995) are strongly recommended. For the interaction between William Farr and Florence Nightingale as regards medical statistics and the ultimately beneficial impact of this on the reform of the British Army, hygiene in hospitals and public health in Britain, the reader is referred to Hugh Small's enthusiastic biography of Florence Nightingale (Small, 1998).

For a brilliant and disturbing account of the rise of modern medicine and its generally harmful role in the treatment of disease until Lister's invention of antiseptic surgery in 1865, see *Bad Medicine* (Wootton, 2006).

References

Arbuthnot J (1710) An argument for Divine Providence taken from the constant regularity observ'd in the births of both sexes. *Philosophical Transactions of the Royal Society of London* **27**: 186–190.

Aubrey J (1975) *Brief Lives*. Folio Society, Bath Press, Bath.

Bailey NTJ (1975) *The Mathematical Theory of Infectious Diseases*. Griffin, London and High Wycombe.

Barnard GA (1958) Studies in the History of Probability and Statistics. 9. Bayes, Thomas, Essay toward solving a Problem in the Doctrine of Chances *Biometrika* **45**: 293–295.

Barnard GA (1996) Fragments of a statistical autobiography. *Student* **1**: 257–268.

Barnard GA, Plackett R (1985) Statistics in the United Kingdom 1939–1945. In: Atkinson AC, Fienberg SE (eds), *A Celebration of Statistics: The ISI Centenary Volume*. Springer, New York and Berlin, pp. 31–55.

Barnett V (1982) *Comparative Statistical Inference*. John Wiley & Sons, Ltd, Chichester.

Bauer P, Kohne K (1994) Evaluation of experiments with adaptive interim analyses. *Biometrics* **50**: 1029–1041.

Bayes T (1764) An essay towards solving a Problem in the Doctrine of Chances.

Bell ET (1953) *Men of Mathematics*. Penguin, Harmondsworth, Middlesex

Benjamini Y, Hochberg Y (1995) Controlling the false discovery rate – a practical and powerful approach to multiple testing. *Journal of the Royal Statistical Society Series B – Methodological* **57**: 289–300.

Box JF (1978) *R.A. Fisher, The Life of a Scientist*. John Wiley & Sons, Inc., New York.

Boyer CB (1991) *A History of Mathematics* (Revised by Uta C Merzbach). John Wiley & Sons, Inc., New York.

Bretz F, Pinheiro JC, Branson M (2004) On a hybrid method in dose finding studies. *Methods of Information in Medicine* **43**: 457–460.

Cox DR (1972) Regression models and life-tables (with discussion). *Journal of the Royal Statistical Society Series B* **34**: 187–220.

Cushny AR, Peebles AR (1905) The action of optimal isomers. II. Hyoscines. *Journal of Physiology* **32**: 501–510.

Dale AI (1991) *A History of Inverse Probability: from Thomas Bayes to Karl Pearson*. Springer, New York and Berlin.

David FN (1962) *Games, Gods and Gambling*. Griffin, London.

David HA (1995) First (questionable) occurrence of common terms in mathematical-statistics. *American Statistician* **49**: 121–133.

David HA (1998) First (?) occurrence of common terms in probability and statistics – A second list (vol. 49, pg 121, 1995). *American Statistician* **52**: 36–40.

Dawkins R (1986) *The Blind Watchmaker*. Longman, Harlow.

Diamond M, Stone M (1981) Nightingale on Quetelet. *Journal of the Royal Statistical Society Series A – Statistics in Society* **144**: 66–79.

Edwards AWF (2002) *Pascal's Arithmetical Triangle: The Story of a Mathematical Idea*. Johns Hopkins, Baltimore.

Fienberg SE (1985) Statistical developments in World War II: An international perspective. In: Atkinson AC, Fienberg SE (eds), *A Celebration of Statistics: The ISI Centenary Volume*. Springer, New York and Berlin, pp. 25–30.

Fienberg SE (1992) A brief history of statistics in three and one-half chapters: a review essay. *Statistical Science* **7**: 208–225.

Forrest DW (1974) *Francis Galton: the Life and Work of a Victorian Genius*. Paul Elek, London.

Gehan EA, Lemak NA (1994) *Statistics in Medical Research*. Plenum, New York.

Gelfand AE, Smith AFM (1990) Sampling-based approaches to calculating marginal densities. *Journal of the American Statistical Association* **85**: 398–409.

Gigerenzer G, Swijtinik Z, Porter T, Daston L, Beatty J, Krüger L (1989) *The Empire of Chance*. Cambridge University Press, Cambridge.

Hacking I (1975) *The Emergence of Probability*. Cambridge University Press, Cambridge.

Hald A (1990) *A History of Probability and Statistics and Their Applications before 1750*. John Wiley & Sons, Inc., New York.

Hald A (1998) *A History of Mathematical Statistics from 1750 to 1930*. John Wiley & Sons, Inc., New York.

Howson C, Urbach P (1993) *Scientific Reasoning: the Bayesian Approach*. Open Court, La Salle.

International Conference on Harmonisation (1999) Statistical principles for clinical trials (ICH E9). *Statistics in Medicine* **18**: 1905–1942.

Kendall MG, Plackett R (eds) (1977) *Studies in the History of Statistics and Probability*, vol 2. Griffin, London.

Kruskal W (1978) Formulas, numbers, words: statistics in prose. *The American Scholar* Spring: 223–229.

Lancaster HO (1994) *Quantitative Methods in Biological and Medical Sciences*. Springer, New York.

Landgrebe J, Bretz F, Brunner E (2004) Efficient two-sample designs for microarray experiments with biological replications. *In Silico Biology* **4**: 461–470.

Lee Y, Nelder JA (2001) Hierarchical generalised linear models: A synthesis of generalised linear models, random-effect models and structured dispersions. *Biometrika* **88**: 987–1006.

Lindsey JK (1996) *Parametric Statistical Inference*. Oxford Science Publications, Oxford.

Matthews JR (1995) *Quantification and the Quest for Medical Certainty*. Princeton University Press, Princeton.

McCullagh P (1980) Regression models for ordinal data. *Journal of the Royal Statistical Society B* **42**: 109–142.

Molenberghs G, Kenward MG (2007) *Missing Data in Clinical Studies*. John Wiley & Sons, Inc., Hoboken.

Nelder JA, Wedderburn RWM (1972) Generalized linear models. *Journal of the Royal Statistical Society A* **132**: 107–120.

Pearson ES (1990) *Student, A Statistical Biography of William Sealy Gosset* (Edited and augmented by RL Plackett with the assistance of GA Barnard). Clarendon Press, Oxford.

Pearson ES, Kendall MG (eds) (1970) *Studies in the History of Statistics and Probability. 1*. Griffin, London.

Peto R, Peto J (1972) Asymptotically efficient rank invariant test procedures (with discussion). *Journal of the Royal Statistical Society A* **135**: 185–207.

Pocock SJ (1983) *Clinical trials, A Practical Approach*. John Wiley & Sons, Ltd, Chichester.

Porter T (2005) *Karl Pearson: The Scientific Life in a Statistical Age*. Princeton University Press, Princeton.

Raab GM, Day S, Sales J (2000) How to select covariates to include in the analysis of a clinical trial. *Controlled Clinical Trials* **21**: 330–342.

Reid C (1982) *Neyman, from Life*. Springer, New York.

Royall R (1999) *Statistical Evidence: A likelihood paradigm*. Chapman & Hall/CRC, Boca Raton, FL.

Schwartz D (1994) *Le Jeu de la science et du hasard*. Flammarion, Paris.

Senn SJ (2000) Consensus and controversy in pharmaceutical statistics (with discussion). *The Statistician* **49**: 135–176.

Senn SJ (2003) *Dicing with Death*. Cambridge University Press, Cambridge.

Senn SJ, Richardson W (1994) The first t-test. *Statistics in Medicine* **13**: 785–803.

Small H (1998) *Florence Nightingale: Avenging Angel*. Constable, London.

Stigler SM (1986) *The History of Statistics: The Measurement of Uncertainty before 1900*. Belknap Press, Cambridge, MA.

Stigler SM (1999) *Statistics on the Table*. Harvard University Press, Cambridge, MA.

Wootton D (2006) *Bad Medicine: Doctors Doing Harm Since Hippocrates*. Oxford University Press, Oxford.

Design and Interpretation of Clinical Trials as Seen by a Statistician

. . . nor has rhubarb always proved a purge, or opium a soporific to everyone who has taken these medicines.

David Hume, *An Enquiry Concerning Human Understanding*

Two roads diverged in a yellow wood,
And sorry I could not travel both
And be one traveler, long I stood

Robert Frost, *The Road not Taken*

3.1 PREFATORY WARNING

The reader who has read Chapter 2 will realize that there is no such thing as a general consensus in statistics. Obviously there are many points on which most, if not all, statisticians agree but there are also many where there is no unanimity. (In this respect statistics is like physics where there is, for example, no general agreement over the interpretation of quantum mechanics.) What follows is my basic philosophy of statistics in clinical trials. Other statisticians may disagree. As with the rest of the book, however, the object is to raise issues, not to resolve them. As is the case for the following two chapters, many of the topic touched on here will be covered in greater death in individual chapters in Part 2.

3.2 INTRODUCTION

Clinical trials are experiments on human beings with the object of examining the effects of treatments. It is not always appreciated that there are two possible general aims for clinical trials. The first, is to assess the effects of treatment in the patients (or healthy volunteers) actually *studied*, and the second is to predict future effects of the treatments on patients **not** *studied* (Senn, 2004a). The first of these objectives is frequently overlooked because it is often falsely assumed to be a trivial matter of applying common sense. Hence, it is concluded that the only difficult part of analysing clinical trials consists in generalizing the results to future patients. It might be more accurate to say that the first objective is, in fact *very* difficult to achieve and the second is *extremely* difficult if not downright impossible.

In short, in a clinical trial the primary formal objective is to assess what effects the treatments *did* have on the patients studied in order to say what effects they *may* have. To say what effects the treatments *will* have or even *will probably* have, requires arguments that go well beyond any formal examination of the data.

3.3   DEFINING EFFECTS

It is best to start by defining effects of (or responses to) treatment and getting this fundamental notion clear first, because if this is not done much confusion follows. *The effect of any treatment for a given patient is the difference between what happened to the patient as a result of giving the treatment and what would have happened had treatment been denied.* (This is sometimes described as the **counterfactual** view of causality and has been extensively developed by Don Rubin and collaborators (Rubin, 1974).) The effect of a treatment is not, for example, the difference between the patient's state after treatment ('outcome') and his state before treatment ('baseline') although this *might* under certain circumstances be the way in which we should choose to *measure* such an effect. Actually, in general, this method of comparison with baseline is very poor. For example, we might have a number of patients present with multiple sclerosis. After ten years' treatment with a new drug, there is no difference between the current functional state of any of these patients and their state at presentation. If we make the mistake of defining the effect as being the difference between outcome and baseline then for each of these patients it would follow that there has been zero effect. Of course, since we know that patients with multiple sclerosis usually have a progressive worsening, the fact that these did not is a good indication that the drug is effective. In fact, in this case we should be very far from believing that the effect was zero.

Effect, *n*. The second of two phenomena which always occur together in the same order. The first called a Cause, is said to generate the other – which is no more sensible than it would be for one who has never seen a dog except in pursuit of a rabbit to declare the rabbit the cause of the dog.

Ambrose Bierce

3.4   PRACTICAL PROBLEMS IN USING THE COUNTERFACTUAL ARGUMENT

We have seen that causality has to be estimated by comparing the state of patients after treatment with the state they would have been in had treatment been denied. There are some practical difficulties in applying this concept.

The first is that effects have to be understood in terms of a choice. We may loosely refer to the effect of 'Treatment X' but what we really mean is the effect of giving 'Treatment X' *rather than* some alternative treatment – even if this 'treatment' is simply a placebo or even nothing at all.

The second problem is that although we can directly observe what happened after treatment, we cannot observe what *might* have happened. As a consequence, we are always forced not only to pay attention to the results observed but also to estimate what might have happened. In short, we need to construct a yardstick by which to judge the observed results.

The third problem concerns the construction of the yardstick itself. We need to know what would have happened to the patients had we treated them otherwise, but whatever approach we use will have its difficulties. For example, we may use the method of **historical controls** by which we compare our results to results obtained previously with different patients using the alternative treatment (which may be another treatment or no treatment at all), but the problem is that not only are the treatments different so are the patients and they may differ in important ways we cannot even measure. Another alternative that is possible with some diseases is the method of **baseline comparisons**, whereby patients are compared with their own baseline values. This method is subject to very many possible biases, among which **regression to the mean** (see below) and **time trends** (see discussion about multiple sclerosis above) are important.

These are the practical problems in using counterfactual. My former colleague Phil Dawid has also suggested that there are some more fundamental difficulties with the concept (Dawid, 2000a). However, I am not arguing here that the statistician should estimate counterfactuals for observations in order to estimate treatment effects, but merely that in considering the effects of treatments it is useful to have, at least at the back of one's mind, 'the road not taken'.

3.5 REGRESSION TO THE MEAN

This important phenomenon, encountered in Chapter 2, is difficult to grasp when first encountered and is therefore worth illustrating with an example. Figure 3.1 gives a plot of data obtained from sites on a road network in Lothian region over 4 years and reported by Senn and Collie (1988). A total of 3112 sites were cross-classified by the number of accidents reported in two two-year periods: 1 January 1979 to 31 December 1980 and 1 January 1981 to 31 December 1982. The figure gives a plot of the mean number of accidents that occurred in the second two-year period by sites that have been classified by the number of accidents that were observed to occur in the first two-year period. A line of exact equality is drawn on the graph and where a point falls below this, it indicates that the means of the number of accidents for those sites was less in the second period than the first. Since nearly all the points lie below the line, the plot seems to indicate an improvement in the accident rate. In general (there is one notably exception) this improvement is more marked for sites that had higher number of accidents in 1979–1980. The exception, corresponding to sites which had 12 accidents in the first year period, is probably a fluke, as means for very high values are based on very few sites.

Figure 3.2 is the corresponding plot seen from the other point of view. Here sites have been classified by the number of accidents they had in 1981–1982 and the mean

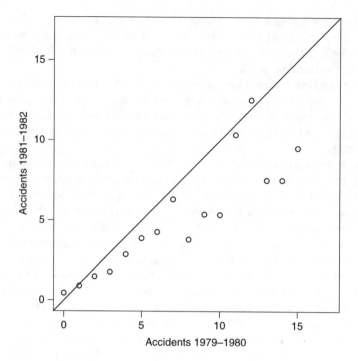

Figure 3.1 Mean accident rates in Lothian region in 1981–1982 classified by accident rate in 1979–1980.

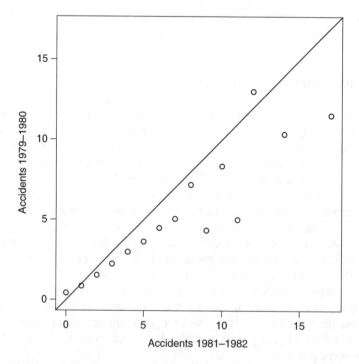

Figure 3.2 Mean accident rates in Lothian region in 1979–1980 classified by accident rate in 1981–1982.

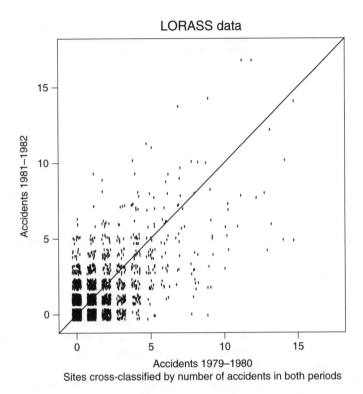

Figure 3.3　Bivariate distribution of accidents per site in Lothian region.

for 1979–1980 has been plotted. Since again the points appear to lie mainly below the line of equality, it now suggests that accidents were *less frequent* in the *earlier* period. We thus have an apparent contradiction.

In fact, both interpretations are wrong, as may be seen by considering Figure 3.3, which gives a bivariate representation of the number of sites cross-classified by the number of accidents which occurred in both periods. This distribution is, extremely stable, as may also be confirmed by studying Table 3.1. In fact, the mean number of accidents per site was 0.976 in the first period and 0.964 in the second. How has this paradox arisen? It has arisen through arbitrary classification. What the two diagrams hid was what was happening to the sites which had no accidents at all in one or other of the two periods. These sites, which are numerically by far the most important group in each marginal classification, actually showed a trend in the opposite direction to the other sites. On careful reflection it can be seen to be absolutely necessary that some such trend should occur somewhere. Unless *every single site* which had no accidents in the first period had no accidents in the second, the mean accident rate for such sites would have to be higher in the second period than in the first, since (by definition) the rate in the first is zero. If the overall mean number of accidents is to remain stable in the two periods, it thus follows that there must be some spontaneous improvement of the 'worst' sites to compensate. Thus, what we can expect for a stable distribution is that the 'worst' sites will improve and the 'best' sites will deteriorate, while the overall mean remains the same. This general phenomenon, which, as we explained in chapter 2, was discovered by Galton, is *regression to the mean*.

Table 3.1   Road sites in Lothian region cross-classified by number of accidents in two periods: frequencies and marginal means.

79/80	81/82 0	1	2	3 ...	Mean
0	1260	355	103	40	0.438
1	334	177	89	39	0.882
2	102	79	50	18	1.469
3	40	36	27	23	1.767
⋮					0.964
Mean	0.415	0.851	1.528	2.233	0.976

Now, of course, one may argue that the graphs are unfair, in that the scale of presentation obscured what was happening in the numerically extremely important sites with least accidents. This is a form of visual censorship which is, perhaps, unhelpful. In a clinical trial, however, an even more extreme form of censorship occurs: we omit to follow up altogether the less extreme cases we did not include. Furthermore, because we include patients on the basis of extreme values, we can expect regression to the mean and hence some spontaneous improvement unless this is overcome by some strong secular trend. In fact, the analogy with our road accident example would be to select for improvement sites which had a large number of accidents and only follow those up. Our road improvement schemes would then appear to have a dramatic effect.

The problem in clinical trials can be illustrated with Figures 3.4 and 3.5. Figure 3.4 shows simulated diastolic blood pressure in mmHg at 'baseline' and 'outcome' for a population of individuals. There is considerable variation in values and a strong but not perfect correlation, but the distribution of values at outcome is very similar to those at baseline. Also shown are cut-off boundaries for 'normotensive' and 'hypertensive' individuals at 90 mmHg.

Now look at Figure 3.5. This shows only the individuals who were 'hypertensive' at baseline. These are exactly the sort of individuals we would follow up in a clinical trial. Their values at outcome are on average lower than they were at baseline but it is clear that this is due to our method of sampling, which makes it impossible to include

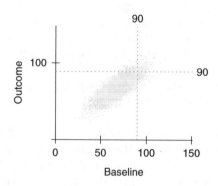

Figure 3.4   Simulated bivariate distribution of diastolic blood pressure in mmHg for a population.

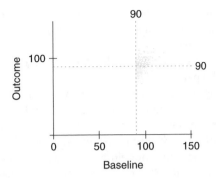

Figure 3.5   Bivariate values for the members of the population defined as 'hypertensive'.

compensating individuals whose values were below 90 mmHg at baseline but higher at outcome. Thus our method of sampling introduces a bias as regards using the before – after comparison to judge effects. This biasing effect is called regression to the mean.

3.6   CONTROL IN CLINICAL TRIALS

The way these difficulties are addressed in modern clinical trials is by using **concurrent controls**. An experimental treatment is studied at the same time as an alternative control treatment (which in some cases may be only a placebo). This eliminates any biases due to differences *between trials* since the data on both the experimental treatment and its control are obtained in the same experiment. (Obviously, within-trial differences are not eliminated so easily. The way in which they are dealt with should become clear in the sections on randomization and concomitant observations below.) For example, McQuay and Moore (1996) presented the results of 20 placebo-controlled trials of various treatments in painful diabetic neuropathy. The percentage of patients who had more than 50% relief varied from 50% to 90% in the active group and from 0% to 80% in the placebo group. Thus, for some trials the active 'response' was lower than was the placebo 'response' for some other trials. However, trial by trial, no response rate was lower for the active treatment group than for the accompanying placebo group and the response rate for the active group was, in fact, generally much higher.

The simplest trial using concurrent controls is the **parallel-group** design in two treatments, in which patients are allocated one of two treatments at random (see below). Other more complicated forms of design also serve the same general purpose, but for the moment it will be simplest if the reader has in mind a parallel-group study of this sort when considering the arguments which follow.

The idea behind the use of concurrent controls is so simple that it would scarcely seem to be worth discussing, yet, despite the essential simplicity of using concurrent controls, analyses of clinical trials commonly encountered in the medical literature betray the fact that *trialists often do not understand the implications of having adopted such a design*.

For example, it is quite common in placebo-controlled trials of hypertension to see separate estimates of the treatment effects, with associated standard errors. This practice is inconsistent with the aim of a controlled clinical trial for the following reasons.

First, such separate effects can only be calculated by using the baselines as the yardstick by which outcomes are judged. But if this process were adequate, there would be no need to use a control group.

Second, if such separate effects could be identified, then a far more efficient trial could be run by allocating all the patients to the experimental treatment. The placebo group is of no interest in its own right and hence, if it is believed that comparison with baseline is a meaningful option, either the trial could be run with half as many patients (dropping the placebo group) or for the same cost twice as many patients could be studied under the experimental group, thus providing more information.

Third, this sort of calculation does not eliminate the particular bias which concurrent controls are designed to eliminate. The results under placebo are only used indirectly to qualify the results for the experimental treatment. However, any chain is only as strong as its weakest link, and if this particular comparison is only performed informally, then it constitutes a weak link in the whole argument. To formalize the comparison requires us to complete the argument mathematically, say by subtracting the placebo result from the experimental one. Thus, the final figure upon which our interpretation came to rest would have to be a treatment **contrast** if we were to make the strongest use of the design of the trial.

Fourth, the calculation of standard errors in this way actually has no basis in statistical theory (Senn and Auclair, 1990). It usually proceeds by taking the standard deviation and dividing it by the square root of n, where n is the number of patients in the 'sample' (in this case the treatment group). What even experienced statisticians are sometimes inclined to overlook, however, is that this formula is the formula appropriate for a simple random sample from a specified population. But *the patients in a clinical trial cannot be regarded as a simple random sample (or even a representative sample) from any population of conceivable interest.*

Finally, it is appropriate to reinforce the general message. Controlled clinical trials demand controlled comparisons. These consist of direct comparisons between treatments, for example, in the form of differences.

3.7   RANDOMIZATION

Randomization is a word which is used to describe the allocation at random (using aleatory devices, such as, for example, dice, cards, lots or random number tables or generators) of treatments to the units in an experiment. In a clinical trial these units are most typically the patients, although occasionally a centre might be treated as a unit, and in **cross-over trials**, in which patients may receive two or more treatments, a treatment episode is the basic experimental unit.

It is pointless to beat about the bush and pretend that randomization is not controversial. It has remained controversial ever since it was introduced by R.A. Fisher into the design of agricultural studies in the 1920s and even statisticians disagree about its value. Many Bayesians (though there are some very prominent exceptions) regard it as irrelevant and most frequentists (again there are some exceptions) consider it important. Some possible justifications are considered below.

Even some harsh critics of randomization would concede that it has a role in blinded trials. This particular discussion will be deferred until later, when blinding itself will be discussed, and instead we shall consider the arguments for randomization, even where blinding is not intended.

Obviously, by virtue of having used concurrent controls, any observed difference between treatments in a clinical trial cannot be due to differences between trials. The patients being compared, irrespective of treatment, are in the same trial. This obvious point is worth labouring because it reinforces once again that *the basic logic of clinical trials is comparative and not representative*. If it were representative we should require patients who were 'typical'; the difference between patients from trial to trial would then not be an issue and we would not need concurrent controls. Nevertheless, even though the patients studied are studied in the same trial, there may be important differences between them. The purpose of randomization is to deal with this within-trial source of variation. It has nothing to do with differences between trials.

It is often said that the purpose of randomization is to ensure equality between the groups in a clinical trial as regards prognostic factors. This reason is, false or at the very least misleading. The two groups in a clinical trial will never be equal. What one can say is that on average, over all randomizations, the two groups will be equal. One can go even further and say that the probability of any particular degree of imbalance can be estimated if randomization has been used. A consequence of this is that this source of variability and uncertainty can be incorporated into the statistical and probabilistic calculations. There is thus an important point to be understood: namely, that the *inferential statistics calculated from a clinical trial make an allowance for differences between patients and that this allowance will be correct on average if randomization has been employed.* (This source of uncertainty is reflected in the standard errors, for example.) However, averages are not always appropriate. If I am cruising at 10 000 m above sea level in mid-Atlantic and the captain informs me that three engines are on fire, I can hardly console myself with the thought that, on average, air travel is very safe. On the other hand, if I am an aircraft insurer, it may be quite appropriate for me to use average probabilities of aircraft failure, if there is no way for me or my customers of identifying *at the time of insurance* which aircraft are more likely to fail. This is the basic point about randomization. It deals with the distribution of *unknown factors* since, for such factors, the average distribution is appropriate *faute de mieux*. It should not be used as an excuse for ignoring the effect of important and known factors, for here one can do better than simply using the average (Senn, 2005).

A related important reason is that it is a means of establishing **utmost good faith** between trialist and sponsor on the one hand and sponsor and regulator on the other. For example, even if a sponsor had balanced a clinical trial by known important prognostic factors (in practice this would be rather difficult, if not impossible) and these had been taken into account in the analysis, if he had allocated the patients according to a particular plan among many which might have satisfied the requirement for balance, the regulator might suspect his motives. He might suppose that some hidden characteristics of the patients were being used to give an advantage to the sponsor's drug. There is, in fact, evidence that there is a tendency for investigators to bias trials which are not randomized in favour of the experimental treatment. (See, for example, Chalmers *et al.*, 1983.)

Another reason is rather philosophical and has to do with replication of experiments. Suppose, for example, we insisted that in a clinical trial there was only one possible division of the patients into two groups that was acceptable. (Some division, perhaps, which made the two groups very evenly balanced in some way.) Having divided the patients in this way, we are indifferent as to which group received the experimental treatment and which received the control treatment. This final choice could be made on the toss of a coin. Now suppose we run the experiment and wish to assess how repeatable the result is. We do this by repeating the experiment as a whole. But if we repeat the experiment as a whole then we shall again find a group of patients, divide them in two again using the same rule, and again assign which group has the experimental treatment and which has control at the toss of a coin. Obviously we should have to repeat this procedure a number of times to assess the variability of our experiments. *The procedure we have described is a randomization procedure but one which takes place at the level of whole trials.* It is also one which would involve us in a great deal of work: drug development would take for ever. What we do instead is we look *within* the trial for replication. But to turn the argument inwards requires the same sort of repetition and arbitrary assignment within the trial. In short, it requires randomization at the level of patients.

To sum up. Randomization promotes confidence that we have acted in utmost good faith. It is not to be used as an excuse for ignoring the distribution of known prognostic factors. For a randomized trial, however, our probability calculations make an appropriate allowance for the distribution of unknown factors.

Randomization is also essential for effective blinding of a clinical trial.

3.8   BLINDING

It is obviously in the interest of a casino owner to have the fairest roulette wheel possible. If the wheel had any bias it might be detectable and a punter, by keeping records, could work out what it was. The wheel might then pay out at higher odds than those offered by the casino. Thus, to make the task of guessing which number will come up as hard as possible, the probability of any one number coming up should be the same as the probability of any other. We can take the argument one stage further and say that all sequences of numbers should be equally likely, for otherwise the punter could also improve his guess rate. Essentially, what we require is that the probability of all possible sequences should be identical. This is the property of random numbers.

Similarly, in a clinical trial the less pattern there is to our allocation, the more secure our blinding will be. This may be true even if the person being blinded is ignorant of the pattern employed. We can illustrate this with an example.

Suppose we run a placebo-controlled trial of an active treatment with 8 patients per centre in blocks of size 2 but do not inform the investigators. Suppose also that owing to an adverse experience the seventh patient treated in a centre has to have his emergency code opened and it is discovered that he received active treatment. Any investigator worth his salt will know that the block size used will either be 2, 4 or 8. His best guess of the treatment which the next patient will receive is 'placebo' irrespective of the block size. (For a block size of 8 this would have a 4/7 chance of success; for a block size of 4 the chance would be 2/3; and for a block size of 2 the guess is certainly right.) Now, as it turns out, the block size is 2 so that the guess is certainly right *irrespective of whether or not the investigator knows that the block size is 2.* The lesson to be learned is this: *the degree of blinding guaranteed cannot exceed the degree of randomization employed.* The important practical step to take is to increase the block size: whether the size of the block is known to the investigator is virtually irrelevant.

A further point to understand about blinding is that for the trial to be truly blind it is not sufficient for a patient or investigator to be in ignorance of the drug allocated. They must also, given knowledge of the treatments used in the trial, be in ignorance of the treatment *not* assigned (Senn, 1995). That is, although the ethical requirement that the patient should know which treatments are being compared in the trial should be fulfilled, for blinding to be complete a given patient should not be aware that one of these is being given to him or her. Suppose we designed a trial comparing two ACE (angiotensin-converting enzyme) inhibitors in hypertension. One (A) is to be given twice a day and the other (B) once a day. We do not wish to interfere with the natural schedule of administration by adding dummies and so forth, so that we run the trial using four groups of patients receiving either A or placebo to A twice daily or B or placebo to B once a day. Now, although the physician will not know whether any patient receiving a once-daily treatment will be receiving an active treatment or a placebo, she will know that such a patient cannot be receiving treatment A. Hence, not all contrasts are fully blinded. I have suggested that a trial which is partially blind in this way should be referred to as **veiled** (Senn, 1995). For example, suppose the doctor's prejudice led her to believe that patients might experience tolerability problems when treated once a day. This might cause her to exaggerate problems experienced by *all* patients on a once-a-day therapy. This causes no bias for the contrast comparing B with placebo to B, but if B is compared with A a bias is involved. (A strategy is available whereby A is compared with placebo to A and B with placebo to B and these comparisons are then compared to each other. But this double comparison carries a penalty in terms of variability.)

A further point about blinding of trials is that it gives no protection against the conclusion that the treatments are equivalent (Senn, 1994). Suppose I run a bioequivalence study as a two-period cross-over comparing a generic with a branded drug. I am in complete ignorance of the treatment code. However, I secretly take the blood samples from each healthy volunteer and mix those from period 1 with those from period 2, separating the resulting mixture into two phials. Obviously any reasonable analysis will conclude that there is no difference between treatments.

3.9   USING CONCOMITANT OBSERVATIONS

Contrary to what is commonly supposed, it is not necessary for clinical trials to be balanced in order to produce a valid comparison between treatments. Consider Table 3.2, which shows the cross-classification of numbers of patients by sex and treatment for a clinical trial. (Suppose, for argument's sake that the trial is in asthma and that we shall be measuring forced expiratory volume in one second, FEV_1.)

Table 3.2 Distribution of patients by sex and treatment in a clinical trial in asthma.

Sex	Treatment		Total
	Verum	**Placebo**	
Male	34	26	60
Female	15	25	40
Total	49	51	100

Table 3.3 Distribution of patients by sex and treatment in a second clinical trial in asthma.

Sex	Treatment		Total
	Verum	**Placebo**	
Male	26	26	52
Female	15	15	30
Total	41	41	82

Clearly this trial is badly unbalanced as regards the distribution of sex with respect to the two treatments. This does not mean, however, that it cannot be analysed in a way which deals with the unbalance of the sexes. Consider, for example, Table 3.3. Clearly, this table *is* balanced as regards the distribution of the two sexes within the two treatment groups. But this table was constructed simply by discarding 18 patients from the first table: 8 male patients receiving verum and 10 female patients receiving placebo. Now if a valid estimate can be obtained by a simple comparison of the mean results under each treatment from the second table, it would be ridiculous if, simply by virtue of having studied 18 further patients, we were *not* able to obtain a valid estimate from the first table. If the worst came to the worst, we could simply ignore the results from 18 patients.

In fact, things are not so bad. All we need to do is to reduce the results first of all to means within each of the four sex-by-treatment groups in Table 3.2. We then compare verum and placebo for each sex, obtaining two estimates of the treatment effect: one for each sex. These two estimates are then combined by averaging in some appropriate way.

Sex is an example of a dichotomous **covariate**. The technique above, sometimes referred to as **post-stratification** cannot be used for a continuous covariate such as height or baseline blood pressure. However, an analogous technique called **analysis of covariance** (see Chapter 7) can be used instead. This, for example, can deal quite successfully with observed imbalance in baseline blood pressure between the two groups in a clinical trial. Note that, contrary to what is commonly believed, converting the outcomes to differences from baseline does not deal with such imbalance. This is because the groups remain imbalanced whether the measures used are raw outcomes or differences from baseline. Only if differences from baseline were independent of the baseline values themselves would this imbalance be irrelevant. However, such independence does not apply. Other things being equal, the higher the baseline value the lower the difference (outcome – baseline) will be. (This statement requires careful thought and it must be understood in its strict mathematical sense so that -22 is lower than -13, which in turn is lower than 33 and so forth.) In fact, yet again we have an example of **regression to the mean**.

3.10 MEASURING TREATMENT EFFECTS

There is an inherent conflict in clinical trials in the aims of our measuring processes. Should we measure what the drug does or should we measure how well it does what we should like it to do? This is another controversial issue and (to add a personal note) I freely admit that, whereas I very strongly tended to the latter view at one time, I now tend to the former. The distinction can be made clear with reference to measuring FEV_1. It might be the case that, from the practical point of view of the patient's state of health, what is relevant is the absolute increase in FEV_1 brought about. It may be, however, that the drug acts in such a way that it increases FEV_1 in a percentage way, so that FEV_1 is X% higher than it *would have been*. (Don't forget to think counterfactually!) We therefore have a conflict here. Should we go for practical relevance and use absolute values, or measure most accurately what the drug actually does and use a logarithmic transformation? (A logarithmic transformation would convert constant multiplicative effects into constant additive ones.)

Most standard statistical models employ a notion of additivity (Senn, 2004a). That is to say, they presuppose a scale upon which the treatment effect acts additively. It is not often appreciated that they also presuppose *that the treatment effect is identical for every patient*. This may be taken as proof of the madness of statisticians, but it actually reflects something subtle. Suppose, for example, we ran a trial in 10 patients in which for the 5 patients given active treatment the values of the improvement in FEV_1 (outcome – baseline) at the end of the trial were −0.2, −0.1, 0.0, 0.2, 0.5 litres. Suppose that the corresponding figures for the 5 placebo patients were −0.5, −0.4, −0.3, −0.1, 0.2. One might be tempted to argue that the active treatment clearly does not work for every patient because two of the patients given active treatment have negative values, and in any case there is an overlap with the placebo group.

This argument is wrong, however. Again, *we must think counterfactually*. If we subtract 0.3 litres from the group given the active treatment, we obtain exactly the same values as for the placebo group. The results are thus entirely consistent with the position that every patient has received an improvement of 0.3 litres over what he would have received. (Here, of course, I have faked the results and they are too good to be true!) In fact, if the treatment worked in some patients and not in others we should expect an increase in the standard deviation in the treatment group. Even under such conditions, however, we should not be able to identify with absolute certainty *which* patients have benefited and which have not (Senn, 1998).

Thus, in assuming that the treatment effect acts identically for each patient, the statistician is simply adopting the simplest model consistent with the data: the statistical application of Occam's razor. There are two circumstances under which this model will be abandoned: (1) if genuine evidence arises that it is untrue, or (2) if continuing naively to assume that it is true will cause a problem in analysis. If neither of these conditions applies, then there is no point in not assuming such a simple model and the statistician may claim that those who don't adopt such an approach and produce more theories than are strictly required by the data should publish in *The Journal of Irreproducible Results*. As I have pointed out elsewhere, much of the hype regarding pharmacogenomics is posited on the false assumption that it has been demonstrated for most indications that patients respond differently to treatment (Senn, 2001, 2003, 2004b). In fact, for most indications this is not known to be true because the types of trial that would be capable of demonstrating it have not been run.

3.11 DATA GENERATION MODELS

In Chapter 4 we shall look at inferential statistics and try to explain the difference between two major approaches to statistics: the frequentist and the Bayesian. Before doing so, however, it is worth considering one matter which can affect approaches to inference even if one stays within, for example, the frequentist system and which has already been alluded to obliquely a number of times. This matter concerns what might be referred to as the *data generation model*.

In much of statistics, the notion of a population is stressed and the subject is sometimes even defined as the science of making statements about populations using samples. However, the notion of a population can be extremely elusive. In survey work, for example, we often have a definite population of units in mind and a sample is taken from this population, sometimes according to some well-specified probabilistic rule. If this rule is used as the basis for calculation of parameter estimates and their standard errors, then this is referred to as *design-based inference* (Lehtonen and Pahkinen, 2004). Because there is a form of design-based inference which applies to experiments also, we shall refer to it when used for samples as *sampling-based inference*.

In experiments, however, provided that we obtain suitable material, we rarely worry about its being representative. Inference is comparative and, as we have explained above, this is generally the appropriate attitude for clinical trials. If we randomize, then we can refer to the actual allocation as being a sample not from a population of *units* but from a population of *randomizations*. If we use the actual randomization rule as the basis for inference, then we may refer to this as *randomization based inference*.

In practice, we sometimes wish to include more factors in the analysis than dictated by the sampling strategy or the experimental strategy as the case may be. Furthermore, we accept that we can make inferences about observational studies which do not fall into either framework (Senn, 2004a). To do this we use *model-based inference*. In many ways this fits in best with either the propensity or subjective views of probability (see glossary entry under Probability) and less well with the frequency view, but as a statistical mode of inference this model-based approach is very common. Model-based inference is a technique of great flexibility because we are free to include as many factors as we wish in our model and we also give ourselves the freedom to remove any difficulties we wish by assumption. (This does not mean that we are always wise in exercising this freedom, but that is another matter.)

Now, it so happens that statisticians tend to learn the tools of the trade in courses of mathematical statistics which pay little attention to data generation models, although the *language* of such courses (which in fact are mainly about *symbols*) – to the extent that it makes contact with the real world – generally stresses *samples* from populations. What is covered, however, is inferential *models* and so, when statisticians first come to clinical trials from university, the techniques they use are often model based and the way they understand them is in terms of sampling. As regards calculation, often no harm is done, since the modelling approach is powerful, flexible and generally of great utility. As regards inference, no harm is generally done provided that comparisons between treatments are stressed. (But binary data can cause a problem. See, for example, Streitberg and Röhmel (1991) or Ludbrook and Dudley (1994a, b) for discussions.) However, as we have already discussed, there is a tendency to calculate standard errors for treatment means without thought about what these could mean.

This is not to say that I think that only randomization-based inference is valid for clinical trials: far from it. Model-based inference is extremely important. What is also important, however, is studying effects and estimating contrasts, whatever the statistical machinery used to do it. Thus my general advice for clinical trials is: (1) remember that they are experiments and (2) think comparatively.

An excellent and readable discussion of these matters will be found in Ludbrook and Dudley (1994a, b).

3.12   IN CONCLUSION

Your neighbourhood statistician may think in ways that you feel are downright peculiar. Have some sympathy with her. She is an irredeemable sceptic in a world full of random variation.

3.13   FURTHER READING

A concise introduction to clinical trials is given by Pocock (1996). For a perspective from a regulator see Temple (1982). A classic monograph on clinical trials is that of Pocock (1983). More modern and mathematical but highly recommended monographs are those of Matthews (2000) and Piantadosi (2005). For discussions of causality see Holland (1990), Cox (1992), Schwartz (1994) and Greenland (2000). Dawid (2000a, b) provides a criticism of counterfactuals. Discussions of blinding are given in Senn (1991, 1994, 1995) and general discussions of randomization in Cox (1958), Dudley *et al.* (1993), Kempthorne (1977) and Senn (2004a, 2005). Useful and interesting examples and discussion of regression to the mean will be found in Bland and Altman (1994a, b), Chuang-Stein (1993), Chuang-Stein and Tong (1997) and Stigler (1997).

References

Bland JM, Altman DG (1994a) Regression towards the mean. *British Medical Journal* **308**: 1499.
Bland JM, Altman DG (1994b) Some examples of regression towards the mean. *British Medical Journal* **309**: 780.
Chalmers TC, Celano P, Sacks HS, Smith H (1983) Bias in treatment assignment in controlled clinical-trials. *New England Journal of Medicine* **309**: 1358–1361.
Chuang-Stein C (1993) The regression fallacy. *Drug Information Journal* **27**: 1213–1220.
Chuang-Stein C, Tong DM (1997) The impact and implication of regression to the mean on the design and analysis of medical investigations. *Statistical Methods in Medical Research* **6**: 115–128.
Cox DR (1958) *Planning of Experiments.* John Wiley & Sons, Inc., New York.
Cox DR (1992) Causality – some statistical aspects. *Journal of the Royal Statistical Society Series A – Statistics in Society* **155**: 291–301.
Dawid AP (2000a) Causal inference without counterfactuals. *Journal of the American Statistical Association* **95**: 407–424.
Dawid AP (2000b) Causal inference without counterfactuals – rejoinder. *Journal of the American Statistical Association* **95**: 444–448.
Dudley RA, Harrell FE Jr, Smith LR, *et al.* (1993) Comparison of analytic models for estimating the effect of clinical factors on the cost of coronary artery bypass graft surgery. *Journal of Clinical Epidemiology* **46**: 261–271.
Greenland S (2000) Causal analysis in the health sciences. *Journal of the American Statistical Association* **95**: 286–289.
Holland PW (1990) Rubin model and its application to causal inference in experiments and observational studies. *American Journal of Epidemiology* **132**: 825–826.
Kempthorne O (1977) Why randomize. *Journal of Statistical Planning and Inference* **1**: 1–25.

Lehtonen R, Pahkinen EJ (2004) *Practical Methods for Design and Analysis of Complex Surveys.* John Wiley & Sons, Ltd, Chichester.

Ludbrook J, Dudley H (1994a) Issues in biomedical statistics – analyzing 2 × 2 tables of frequencies. *Australian and New Zealand Journal of Surgery* **64**: 780–787.

Ludbrook J, Dudley H (1994b) Issues in biomedical statistics – statistical inference. *Australian and New Zealand Journal of Surgery* **64**: 630–636.

Matthews JNS (2000) *An Introduction to Randomized Clinical Trials.* Arnold, London.

McQuay H, Moore A (1996) Placebo mania. Placebos are essential when extent and variability of placebo response are unknown. *British Medical Journal* **313**:1008.

Piantadosi S (2005) *Clinical Trials: A Methodologic Perspective.* John Wiley & Sons, Inc., New York.

Pocock S (1996) Clinical trials. In: Armitage P (ed.), *Advances in Biometry.* John Wiley & Sons, Ltd, Chichester and New York.

Pocock SJ (1983) *Clinical Trials, A Practical Approach.* John Wiley & Sons. Ltd, Chichester.

Rubin DB (1974) Estimating causal effects of treatment in randomized and nonrandomized studies. *Journal of Educational Psychology* **66**: 688–701.

Schwartz D (1994) *Le Jeu de la science et du hasard.* Flammarion, Paris.

Senn SJ (1991) Falsificationism and clinical trials. *Statistics in Medicine* **10**:1679–1692. [SeeComment in *Statistics in Medicine* **11**(9): 1263–1265 (1992)].

Senn SJ (1994) Fisher's game with the devil. *Statistics in Medicine* **13**: 217–230.

Senn SJ (1995) A personal view of some controversies in allocating treatment to patients in clinical trials. *Statistics in Medicine* **14**:2661–2674. [See Comment in *Statistics in Medicine* **15**(1): 113–116 (1996)].

Senn SJ (1998) Applying results of randomised trials to patients. N of 1 trials are needed [letter; comment]. *British Medical Journal* **317**(7157):537–538.

Senn SJ (2001) Individual therapy: new dawn or false dawn. *Drug Information Journal* **35**: 1479–1494.

Senn SJ (2003) Author's reply to Walter and Guyatt. *Drug Information Journal* **37**: 7–10.

Senn SJ (2004a) Added values: controversies concerning randomization and additivity in clinical trials. *Statistics in Medicine* **23**: 3729–3753.

Senn SJ (2004b) Individual response to treatment: is it a valid assumption? *British Medical Journal* **329**: 966–968.

Senn SJ (2005) Baseline balance and valid statistical analyses: common misunderstandings. *Applied Clinical Trials* **14**: 24–27.

Senn SJ, Auclair P (1990) The graphical representation of clinical trials with particular reference to measurements over time. *Statistics in Medicine* **9**: 1287–1302. [Published erratum appears in *Statistics in Medicine* 10(3): 487 (1991)].

Senn SJ, Collie G (1988) Accident blackspots and the bivariate negative binomial. *Road Traffic Engineering and Control* **29**: 168–169.

Stigler SM (1997) Regression towards the mean, historically considered. *Statistical Methods in Medical Research* **6**: 103–114.

Streitberg B, Röhmel J (1991) Alternatives to Fisher's exact test? *Biometrie und Informatik in Medizin und Biologie* **22**: 139–146.

Temple R (1982) Government view of clinical trials. *Drug Information Journal* **16**: 10–17.

4

Probability, Bayes, P-values, Tests of Hypotheses and Confidence Intervals

... what a long chapter of chances do the events of this world lay open to us!

Laurence Sterne, *Tristram Shandy*

My father, whose way was to force every event in nature into an hypothesis, by which rate never man crucified TRUTH at the rate he did

Ibid.

4.1 INTRODUCTION

The purpose of this chapter is to review some basic statistical concepts. Statistical calculation and algorithms are not covered since, as has already been explained, they do not form part of the subject matter of this book. I shall, however, attempt an illustration of the nature of an important divide in statistics: that between Bayesian or subjectivist statistics on the one hand and classical or frequentist on the other.

I shall motivate the discussion of the various statistical concepts which will be covered by considering a genuine and simple example of the application of statistical theories to everyday life. The example has nothing to do with medicine and is chosen because, although it is extremely trivial, it is easily comprehensible, concerns an occurrence which may be familiar to many readers and serves its didactic purpose well.

Statistical Issues in Drug Development/2nd Edition   Stephen Senn
© 2007 John Wiley & Sons, Ltd

4.2   AN EXAMPLE

When working on my word processor at home, as for example while working on this book, I frequently listen to music. My CD player permits me to play tracks in sequential or random order. When the *play* button is pressed, all tracks are played in sequential order. When the *shuffle* button is played, the tracks are played in random order, each track being played eventually and none being played twice. When I play a disc of popular music I often press the *shuffle* button. (I have a different policy for classical music!) However, the *play* button is next to the *shuffle* button. Occasionally, I press the *play* button by accident but, since I don't look at the buttons closely, I don't notice this at the time. On one occasion I had inserted the CD *Hysteria* by Def Leppard, which has 12 tracks, and pressed what I thought was the *shuffle* button. When the first track that played through my headphones was *Women* (henceforth referred to as W), which is the first track on the CD, I began to wonder if I had in fact, pressed the *play* button. We shall consider below approaches to answering this question.

4.3   ODDS AND SODS

Before confronting this problem, we consider a few basic rules about probability. The first is that, whatever interpretation we give to a probability, we shall represent probability as a number between 0 and 1, with 0 corresponding to impossibility and 1 to certainty. The second, the **addition rule**, is that, when considering two or more **mutually exclusive** events (by which is meant that both events cannot occur together), the probability that one or the other of them will occur is the sum of the individual probabilities. For example, suppose that the probability that an Austrian will win the gold medal in the next men's Olympic downhill skiing race is 0.3 and the probability that a Swiss will win is 0.25. Assuming that no skier has dual nationality, the probability that either a Swiss or an Austrian will win is $0.3 + 0.25 = 0.55$. The third rule, the **multiplication rule**, is an important definition. It says that if A and B are two events then the probability of A and B occurring equals the probability of A times the probability of B *given* A. Suppose, for example, that 1 in 12 persons working in the drug development department of a given pharmaceutical firm is medically qualified and that 1 in 4 such medically qualified persons is female. The probability of a person chosen at random being medically qualified is 1/12 and the probability of their being female given that they are medically qualified is 1/4. The probability of their being medically qualified *and* female is given by the multiplication rule and is $1/12 \times 1/4 = 1/48$. The probability of being female given being medically qualified is referred to as a **conditional probability**, the probability of being female and medically qualified as a **joint probability**, and the probability of being medically qualified as a **marginal probability**. If the probability of a person chosen at random within the same department being female is also 1/4 (irrespective of their qualification), then the marginal probability of being female is the same as the conditional probability and the two events are said to be **independent**. (Independence would, however, be most unlikely to apply in this case.)

Finally, we sometimes quote probabilities in odds form. If a horse has a chance of 1/7 of winning a race, it has a probability of 6/7 of not winning the race. The ratio of these two probabilities is referred to as the **odds** and (if quoted in the order not winning to winning) is clearly 6 to 1.

4.4   THE BAYESIAN SOLUTION TO THE EXAMPLE

We return to the problem with the CD player. The Bayesian solution to this problem proceeds as follows. First, I need to recognize that there are two basic competing possibilities. Either I pressed the *shuffle* button or I pressed the *play* button. We can refer to the first situation as hypothesis A (or simply A for short) and the second as hypothesis B (B for short). Second, I need to assign to each of these a **prior probability** (a probability *before* the evidence is obtained) that it is true. Let us suppose that the probability for A is 9/10 and for B 1/10. The next thing is to consider the probability of particular types of evidence given a hypothesis. This sort of conditional probability we shall refer to as the **likelihood**. Now suppose, for argument's sake, that B is true. Then the probability that the first track will be W is 1 and the probability that it will be something else (say X) is 0. Now suppose that A is true, then the probability that the first track is W is 1/12 and the probability of X is 11/12. The situation is summarized in Table 4.1.

Note that the prior probabilities total 1 when summed over the possible hypotheses $(9/10 + 1/10) = 1$. The likelihoods, on the other hand, sum to 1 for a given hypothesis $(1/12 + 11/12 = 1$ and $1 + 0 = 1)$ but do *not* sum to 1 over the hypotheses for a given event. For example, given that the first track observed is W, the likelihood under the *shuffle* hypothesis is 1/12 but under the *play* hypothesis is 1, so that the sum is 13/12.

Table 4.1 represents the position *before* obtaining the evidence. The final column lists four probabilities corresponding to four mutually exclusive situations: (1) I press *shuffle* and W is played; (2) I press *shuffle* and W is **not** played (X); (3) I press *play* and W is played; and (4) (a theoretical case only) I press *play* and W is **not** played. If the probabilities in the final column are added up, the total comes to 1. That is because these four cases cover all the probability between them and one and only one of them can apply. (The fourth case could have been ignored here, as it has probability zero, but this would not necessarily be so for all examples one might consider.)

After the CD has started playing, however, only two of these cases can still be deemed to apply. The second case clearly does not apply since evidence X does not obtain. (In fact, in the Bayesian solution to this problem, X has no direct role. In general, only the evidence observed is directly relevant.) However, the two probabilities of the two remaining cases must still add to 1, but as they stand the total comes to $9/(10 \times 12) + 1/(10) = 21/120$. If we scale both of the two remaining probabilities by dividing them by 21/120 then they will both total 1. Performing this calculation we obtain the results: probability A and $W = 9/21$ and probability B and $W = 12/21$. (The steps we have just completed correspond to applying **Bayes' theorem**.) These two probabilities are referred to as **posterior probabilities** (because they are probabilities after seeing the evidence, W) and are a form of conditional probability. Since W has

Table 4.1   Prior probabilities and likelihoods for the CD player example.

Hypothesis	Prior probability P	Evidence	Likelihood L	$P \times L$
A	9/10	W	1/12	$9/(10 \times 12)$
A	9/10	X	11/12	$9 \times 11/(10 \times 12)$
B	1/10	W	1	1/10
B	1/10	X	0	0

been observed, the only difference between the two cases is whether A or B applied. Hence the posterior probabilities are, effectively the posterior probabilities of the two theories: *shuffle* or *play*. Thus the probability that I pressed the play button is 12/21. This completes the solution.

> **Bayesian**: One who, vaguely expecting a horse and catching a glimpse of a donkey, strongly concludes he has seen a mule.

4.5 WHY DON'T WE REGULARLY USE THE BAYESIAN APPROACH IN CLINICAL TRIALS?

It is important to note straight away that some people think that we *should*. The following reasons are commonly given as grounds for not using the Bayesian solution.

(1) Two types of probability were required as input. One consisted of probabilities of evidence given theories. For example, the probability that the first track is W if I press *play* is 1, whereas if I press *shuffle* it is 1/12. These two probabilities are **likelihoods**, a term due to R.A. Fisher. This sort of probability arises from logical considerations of the situation and is largely uncontroversial. (Although it is true that, in treating this problem, I have assumed that which is not necessarily true, namely that the shuffle button chooses each track at random with equal probability. It might, for example, favour longer tracks.) The other probabilities were probabilities of theories *prior* to seeing the evidence and are thus called **prior probabilities**. Here, although some values of the probability would be ridiculous (for example if my intention is to press the *shuffle* button I can hardly accord it a probability of less than 1/2), there would not be any universal agreement over the value I should assign. Why not choose 99/100 or 8/10, for example, rather than 9/10 which I did choose? This sort of probability (the 'prior') is therefore subjective, but it is essential to the argument.

(2) Use of the Bayesian argument in its *full logical rigour* requires identification of *all* possible hypotheses. The likelihood given each of these hypotheses has to be established and each hypothesis has to be given a prior probability. This may be fair enough when considering a simple case such as my CD player, but it makes life very difficult in drug development. For example, if two drugs are different, there are infinitely many ways in which they can differ. Application of the Bayesian argument requires us to specify some sort of meta-theory which covers the way in which they differ. (If we are prepared to be slightly less rigorous as Bayesians we can avoid this problem, but then some of the philosophical advantages claimed for Bayesianism no longer apply.)

(3) In practice, despite the conceptual simplicity of the Bayes approach, it is computationally difficult to implement.

These, basically, are the major practical difficulties. There are a number of objections of a more philosophical nature, and it is only fair to add that the Bayesians, in their turn, have some pretty devastating philosophical objections to the alternative methods.

As regards the three practical criticisms, the Bayesians might reply as follows.

(1) Probability is subjective. Each of us will have different opinions as to the probabilities concerned and it is useless to pretend otherwise.

(2) You cannot come to a sensible conclusion about the truth of a hypothesis without considering all the alternatives.

(3) We are making great progress in the field of Bayesian computation. (In fact, since 1990 there has been such enormous progress in computation for Bayesian models, relying on simulation and hence, ironically, the long-run frequency properties of random numbers, that the third objection is hardly valid at all.)

4.6 A FREQUENTIST APPROACH

The frequentist approach to this sort of problem is closely related to the following philosophical position. If I have a theory which states 'all swans are white', then it doesn't matter how many white swans are observed, I cannot prove that it is true. However, a single swan of a different colour will succeed in proving that it is false. Now, if we return to the problem of the CD player, we can see that if the first track played is *not* W then the theory that I pressed *play* is wrong, whatever the prior probability of its being true. (It is worth pointing out that the Bayesian will also reach this conclusion.)

Unfortunately, however, in general our theories are not so simple and the evidence we obtain does not permit such clear-cut decisions. Even in our simple example, if the evidence W occurs, no such simple decision is possible.

The nature of statistical problems in general is such that usually all observable outcomes are possible under many theories, although they are not equally likely for every theory. (For example, in a randomized two-group parallel trial with many patients, a large difference in outcome between the two groups would seem to be most unlikely if the two treatments are in fact identical, but it is never *impossible*.) What the frequentist does is to replace the strictly logical argument,

(1) If A then *not* B,
(2) B
(3) therefore not A

with the argument

(1) If A then *probably not* B,
(2) B
(3) therefore not A.

Note that the third step is to be understood as being conventional. He decides to act as if A were a false hypothesis but accepts that it might conceivably be true.

There is, however, one formidable problem in applying this argument, and that is that there are all sorts of unlikely events which can occur which would not, in practice, lead us to reject a hypothesis. Consider, for example, a lottery with a million tickets, sold to a million persons (one each), and with a single prize and suppose that one of the tickets is owned by Mr Fred Bloggs. If the lottery is fair the probability that Fred Bloggs will win is one in a million. But the same is true for all of the 999 999 other persons who own a ticket. Therefore, if we reject the hypothesis that the lottery is fair because Fred

Bloggs wins, we should reject it whoever wins. This means that in practice two further conditions have to be satisfied to complete the frequentist's argument. First, we have to specify before the event which outcome(s) will lead to rejection of the hypothesis, and second, we have to have a good reason for specifying the particular outcomes we choose.

To return to the problem of the CD player, the frequentist might act like this. He might say, if the track W is played first (and only if this happens) I shall *assume* that I pressed *play*. Now if I did, in fact, press *shuffle*, then track W will be played first with probability 1 in 12. Therefore, under this circumstance the probability that I shall make an error is 1 in 12 and this is in fact the only observed outcome which will lead me to assume that I pressed play. On the other hand, if I pressed *play* then I shall never make a mistake using this rule. I thus have a perfectly objective description of the probabilities of the types of errors I can make using this approach.

To convert this approach to the language of **hypothesis testing**, we might (say) designate *shuffle* as the **null hypothesis** and *play* as the **alternative hypothesis**. We then recognize two types of error: a **type I error** is committed by rejecting the null hypothesis when it is true and a **type II error** is committed by rejecting the alternative hypothesis when it is true. The probability of making a type I error (given that the null hypothesis is true) is referred to as the **size** of the test (or sometimes as the **significance level**). The probability of *not* committing a type II error, given that the alternative hypothesis is true, is referred to as the **power** of the test. Here, the power of the test is 1 (or 100%). This is unusually high and is a consequence of the slightly unusual example.

However, at 1/12, the size of the test is rather larger than is usually considered conventionally acceptable: a 5% size is more usual. We now leave this specific example to discuss the frequentist approach to hypothesis testing in clinical trials.

4.7   HYPOTHESIS TESTING IN CONTROLLED CLINICAL TRIALS

Hypothesis testing is applied in controlled clinical trials as follows. We adopt a **null hypothesis** which represents a set of circumstances we are trying to *disprove*. A simple example of such a hypothesis in a placebo-controlled trial of a single active treatment in hypertension would be: *the effect of active treatment and placebo on blood pressure is identical.* (Obviously, in practice, such a hypothesis needs to be defined rather more precisely in terms of the measurements to which it refers: systolic or diastolic, particular time point or area under the curve, and so forth.) We next establish an alternative hypothesis, for example: the treatments and placebo have different effects on blood pressure. Note, that since the ways in which treatments can differ are essentially infinite (even as regards their effect on a single measure) such an alternative hypothesis is less well defined than the null hypothesis. In practice, for the purposes of specifying the statistical test to be used, we tend to use simpler versions of the alternative hypothesis. For example, we might suppose that the effect on blood pressure of active treatment compared to placebo is to change it by a value X for every patient, where X is unknown. For the purpose of planning the trial we might even have to posit a particular value for X (say a **clinically relevant difference**) in order to perform a **power calculation**. Note, however, that the role of these hypotheses is *not* to act as strict alternatives which *must* be accepted as being true if the **null hypothesis** is wrong, but rather to suggest what sort of test and what sort of trial might be successful in disproving the null hypothesis.

Once we have defined null and alternative hypothesis it is then often possible, using various theorems in mathematical statistics, to define a good statistical test. This test will use a **test statistic**. It will also be necessary to define a **critical region**. If the test statistic falls in the critical region, we reject the null hypothesis. For example, the test statistic might be **Student's *t* statistic** and we might decide to reject the null hypothesis if *t* is greater than 2 or less than −2. The critical region is then the values of *t* covered by 2 to infinity and −2 to −infinity. We shall have chosen the critical region in such a way that the probability of the test statistic falling in the critical region will be rather small (conventionally, 0.05 is the maximum value entertained) if the null hypothesis is true and higher if the alternative hypothesis is true. The test and the critical region together determine the probability of making a **type I error** given that the null hypothesis is true.

Of course, as was discussed above, there is another type of error, the so-called **type II error**, where we fail to reject the null hypothesis although it is in fact false. It is not, however, possible to simultaneously minimize both kinds of error. Therefore, what is conventionally done is to go for a test which will hold the type I error rate at some predetermined level and, subject to this constraint, make the type II error rate as low as possible. The **power** of the test is 1 minus the probability of making a type II error given that the alternative hypothesis is true. It is thus the probability of correctly concluding that the null hypothesis is false where the alternative hypothesis is true. For a given type I error rate the power can only be increased by reducing the variation, increasing the treatment effect or increasing the sample size. Since in practice there is little that can be done about the first two options, considerable weight is placed on the third, and power calculations have become an important aspect of clinical trials.

4.8   SIGNIFICANCE TESTS AND *P*-VALUES

The hypothesis testing framework described above is basically the system proposed by J. Neyman and E. Pearson (see Chapter 2). It can be regarded as the 'official' modern frequentist approach to clinical trials. In practice, an older approach due to R.A. Fisher (see Chapter 2) is often used.

There are two particular practical objections to the Neyman–Pearson approach which lead to Fisher's approach being used. (There are a number of philosophical ones which need not concern us here.) The first is that if I communicate the result of a test as 'null hypothesis rejected' this may be useless to a fellow scientist if he does not use the same type I error rate I do. Therefore, instead of determining a rule beforehand with an error rate which is acceptable to us and reporting the result as 'rejected' or 'not rejected', we report the results in a way that they can be used by anybody else to form their own test. So we can say 'significant at the 5% level but not significant at the 1% level'. This means that anybody using a Neyman – Pearson approach with a pre-determined 5% type I error rate would reject the hypothesis but someone with a 1% rate would not. We can go even further and give an exact **P-value**, say 0.032, which in this case would mean that anyone with a predetermined type I error rate of greater than or equal to 0.032 would reject the null hypothesis and anyone with a lower rate would not reject it.

This is one interpretation of the **P-value**. It is a way of communicating to individuals with different rules for rejecting or not rejecting null hypotheses whether they should reject this particular null hypothesis on the basis of the results of this test (Senn, 2002). In practice, the *P*-value is calculated as *the probability of observing a result as extreme or more extreme than the one observed given that the null hypothesis is true*. The way in which Fisher interpreted the significance test was that if the *P*-value was small you were left with the conclusion that *either the null hypothesis is not true or a very rare event has occurred*.

The second practical (and semi-philosophical) objection to the Neyman–Pearson approach is that it is often more natural to define the test statistic right away rather than the alternative hypothesis. In fact, most of the more common standard tests had already been derived by R.A. Fisher without reference to alternative hypotheses before the Neyman–Pearson theory was developed. Thus the posited alternative hypothesis in these formulations might unkindly be described as being an excuse for the test statistic adopted, rather than a reason.

Nevertheless, it is fair to say that there are some more complicated cases where it is perhaps easier to define the alternative hypothesis than the test and that the Neyman–Pearson theory then provides a way in which a test can be derived.

> **Statistician**: Someone who fondly imagines that the rest of the world is interested to know whether he or she bores as a Bayesian or a frequentist.

4.9   CONFIDENCE INTERVALS AND LIMITS AND CREDIBLE INTERVALS

One might conclude from reading the published account of a clinical trial that significance testing was the, 'be all and end all' of statistical analysis. In fact, a more useful application of statistics is in estimating the magnitude of effects. In providing an estimate it is also usual to include an estimate of its reliability. Two common approaches are to quote **standard errors** and **confidence limits**.

Confidence limits are an idea due to Neyman. (Fisher used a similar, but conceptually more difficult and controversial, idea of fiducial limits.) Neyman's idea can be explained like this. Conventionally, when testing the effects of treatment, we use the null hypothesis that they are equal and that the difference between them is zero. The framework of hypothesis testing, however, allows us to use any difference at all as a null hypothesis. Suppose in a given case we test a number of such null hypotheses at (say) the 5% level. For example, we might test the null hypothesis that the difference is 5 mm and then the null hypothesis that it is −7 mm and so forth. If we do this, we shall reject some of these 'null' hypotheses and not reject others. We can then collect all the null hypotheses that we would not reject in one set. Usually these will form one continuous interval and the limits of this interval can be established mathematically. The interval so derived then constitutes a **confidence interval** (in this case a 95% confidence interval) and the limits of the interval are **confidence limits** (in this case 95% limits). Values of the treatment effect lying outside the limits are then regarded as unreasonable values to entertain.

The Bayesian would stress, however, that the more practical concept is that of the **credible interval**. This would give an interval such that (say) the treatment effect lay between these limits with 95% probability. Of course, such an interval would have to be subjective and it would not be the same for me as for you. In many cases, however, if a so-called **uninformative prior** is used then for many applications the credible interval corresponds closely or even exactly to the confidence interval, so that two different interpretations of the same interval (or limits) can be given.

4.10 SOME BAYESIAN CRITICISM OF THE FREQUENTIST APPROACH

Some of the most common criticisms of frequentist approaches are the following.

1. They are conceptually complicated compared to the Bayesian approach, which uses the simple notion of the probability of a theory being true.
2. It is necessary, in order to apply them, to calculate the probability of events which did not occur.
3. They can be shown to be clearly irrational in given circumstances.

The frequentists might reply as follows.

1. The Bayesian simplicity is only apparent. The notion of a personal probability is actually extremely complicated and Bayesian calculations are usually more complicated than frequentist ones.
2. In order for the Bayesian to calculate a probability he has to consider all possible theories and, in order to assign probabilities coherently given these theories, he also has to consider all possible events.
3. The circumstances under which the results of frequentist calculations can be shown to be irrational are often those under which more knowledge is assumed to hold than is actually incorporated in the frequentist calculations. It should also be noted that in practice, although Bayesians will disagree with frequentists, they will not agree with each other.

> **Bayesian**: One who asks you what you think before a clinical trial in order to tell you what you think afterwards.

4.11 DECISION THEORY

The above discussion either has been in terms of *inferences*, or, where it has been about *decisions*, as when discussing hypothesis testing, has not addressed the consequences of making decisions. A theory developed by Wald in the 1940s, however, had the purpose of providing logical rules for making decisions using data given costs of various types of wrong decision. Depending upon whether prior probabilities were allowed to be used or not, the theory provided Bayesian and (sometimes) frequentist solutions.

Decision theory has since been extensively developed, especially in its Bayesian form. Sometimes, and in particular where eclectic borrowings from psychology and other disciplines have been made, for example for developing techniques for assessing personal probabilities, and where it has been used to solve genuine practical problems, the term **decision analysis** has been used instead. This requires that utilities be assessed for various outcomes. The most extreme of the Bayesian schools of statistics would insist that all statistical problems must be understood in terms of practical decisions and that for this purpose it is not enough to assess personal probabilities; it is necessary to assess personal utilities as well. Solutions to problems in which this is done are sometimes referred to as being *fully Bayesian* in order to distinguish from cases where prior probabilities are assessed but utilities are not.

4.12 CONCLUSION

Some of the concepts commonly used in reporting clinical trials are actually rather subtle and difficult. This is because cracking Nature's code in the presence of random variation and measurement error is itself difficult and subtlety is called for. The reader should be warned from this chapter that there is no general consensus among statisticians regarding statistical inference. It is small wonder, therefore, that many statistical issues in drug development are controversial. During my time in drug development I found it very useful to try and look at a number of problems both from a Bayesian and a frequentist perspective and this is the practice I recommend.

4.13 FURTHER READING

R.A. Fisher's own views on inference are outlined in Fisher (1956) For a modern text covering frequentist approaches see Cox (2006) and for a mathematically elementary but otherwise profound outline of the Bayesian approach see Lindley (2006). Likelihood approaches are covered in Lindsey (1996), Royall (1999), Pawitan (2001) and the classic by Edwards (1992). Classic expositions of the fully subjective Bayesian view of probability are give by Savage (1954) and de Finetti (1974, 1975) and the case for its use in science is made by the philosophers Howson and Urbach (1993). A comparative overview of the various statistical systems is given by Barnett (1999).

For criticisms of *P*-values see Freeman (1993), Goodman (1992) and Matthews (2001) and for a partial defence Senn (2001, 2002). For the case for frequentist approaches see Whitehead (1993). Enthusiastic advocacies of the application of Bayesian methods in medicine will be found in Berry (1993), Kadane (1995) and Lilford and Braunholtz (1996) and a more cautious assessment in Fisher (1996). For a regulatory endorsement of Bayesian methods see Campbell (2005). An elementary review of Bayesian, likelihood and frequentist approaches to statistics is given in my article in *Applied Clinical Trials* (Senn, 2003). Tutorials covering various applications of Bayesian methods are given by Fayers *et al.* (1997), Fryback *et al.* (2001) and Normand (1999) and monographs covering Bayesian applications to medical research or health care are Berry and Stangl (1996, 2000) and the books in this series by Parmigiani (2002) and Spiegelhalter *et al.* (2003).

References

Barnett V (1999) *Comparative Statistical Inference.* John Wiley & Sons, Ltd, Chichester.

Berry DA (1993) A case for Bayesianism in clinical trials. *Statistics in Medicine* **12**: 1377–1393.

Berry DA, Stangl D (eds) (1996) *Bayesian Biostatistics.* Marcel Dekker, New York.

Berry DA, Stangl D (eds) (2000) *Meta-analysis in Medicine and Health Policy (Biostatistics S.).* Marcel Dekker, New York.

Campbell G (2005) The experience in the FDA's center for devices and radiological health with Bayesian strategies. *Clinical Trials* **2**: 359–363.

Cox DR (2006) *Principles of Statistical Inference.* Cambridge University Press, Cambridge.

de Finetti BD (1974) *Theory of Probability,* volume 1. John Wiley & Sons, Ltd, Chichester.

de Finetti BD (1975) *Theory of Probability,* volume 2. John Wiley & Sons, Chichester.

Edwards AWF (1992) *Likelihood.* Johns Hopkins University Press, Baltimore.

Fayers PM, Ashby D, Parmar MK (1997) Tutorial in biostatistics Bayesian data monitoring in clinical trials. *Statistics in Medicine* **16**: 1413–1430.

Fisher LD (1996) Comments on Bayesian and frequentist analysis and interpretation of clinical trials – Comment. *Controlled Clinical Trials* **17**: 423–434.

Fisher RA (1956) Statistical methods and scientific inference. In: Bennet JH (ed.), *Statistical Methods, Experimental Design and Scientific Inference.* Oxford University Press, Oxford.

Freeman PR (1993) The role of *P*-values in analysing trial results. *Statistics in Medicine* **12**: 1443–1452; discussion 1453–1448.

Fryback DG, Stout NK, Rosenberg MA (2001) An elementary introduction to Bayesian computing using WinBUGS. *International Journal of Technology Assessment in Health Care* **17**: 98–113.

Goodman SN (1992) A comment on replication, *P*-values and evidence. *Statistics in Medicine* **11**: 875–879.

Howson C, Urbach P (1993) *Scientific Reasoning: the Bayesian Approach.* Open Court, La Salle.

Kadane JB (1995) Prime-time for Bayes. *Controlled Clinical Trials* **16**: 313–318.

Lilford RJ, Braunholtz D (1996) The statistical basis of public policy: a paradigm shift is overdue [see comments]. *British Medical Journal* **313**: 603–607.

Lindley DV (2006) *Understanding Uncertainty.* John Wiley & Sons, Inc., Hoboken.

Lindsey JK (1996) *Parametric Statistical Inference.* Oxford Science Publications, Oxford.

Matthews RAJ (2001) Why should clinicians care about Bayesian methods? *Journal of Statistical Planning and Inference* **94**: 43–58.

Normand SL (1999) Meta-analysis: formulating, evaluating, combining, and reporting. *Statistics in Medicine* **18**: 321–359.

Parmigiani G (2002) *Modeling in Medical Decision Making: A Bayesian Approach.* John Wiley & Sons, Ltd, Chichester.

Pawitan Y (2001) *In All Likelihood: Statistical Modelling and Inference Using Likelihood.* Clarendon Press, Oxford.

Royall R (1999) *Statistical Evidence: A Likelihood Paradigm.* Chapman & Hall/CRC, Boca Raton, FL.

Savage J (1954) *The Foundations of Statistics.* John Wiley & Sons, Inc., New York.

Senn SJ (2001) Two cheers for *P*-values. *Journal of Epidemiology and Biostatistics* **6**: 193–204.

Senn SJ (2002) A comment on replication, *P*-values and evidence S.N.Goodman, Statistics in Medicine 1992; 11: 875–879. *Statistics in Medicine* **21**: 2437–2444.

Senn SJ (2003) Bayesian, likelihood and frequentist approaches to statistics. *Applied Clinical Trials* **12**: 35–38.

Spiegelhalter DJ, Abrams KR, Myles JP (2003) *Bayesian Approaches to Clinical Trials and Health-Care Evaluation.* John Wiley & Sons, Ltd, Chichester.

Whitehead J (1993) The case for frequentism in clinical trials. *Statistics in Medicine* **12**: 1405–1413.

5

The Work of the Pharmaceutical Statistician

He unravels the web or argument and pieces it together again; folds it up and lays it aside, that he may examine it more and at his leisure. He hugs indecision to his breast and takes home a modest doubt or a nice point to solace himself with it in protracted, luxurious dalliance.

William Hazlitt, *The Spirit of the Age*

5.1 PREFATORY REMARKS

The medical statistician is someone who looks up the number of patients you need in a table and comes up with the answer 'too many'. Then, when the trial is over, he presses a button on his computer and produces a report that nobody can understand.

I hope that you don't believe this, but I fear you may. This chapter is an attempt to define the work of the medical statistician a little more accurately. On the whole it will cover the work of a medical statistician engaged in planning and analysing clinical trials in phase II and phase III as this is where the majority of statisticians working in drug development will be employed. There are, however, other areas where statisticians may work: phase I studies, portfolio management and drug monitoring, for example. These areas are covered in the chapters on specific issues in the second section of this book but are not otherwise dealt with here.

This chapter will consider various duties of the statistician. It may be that the details will be somewhat at variance with the practice in some drug companies. However, the broad outline ought to be similar. As is the case with the rest of this book, only drug development proper is covered. The emphasis is also on clinical trial design and analysis, although various authors have made the point that the role for statistical thinking in drug development is much wider (Grieve, 2002; Senn, 2003). The reader who is interested in the wider work of the pharmaceutical statistician may be interested to consult Porter (1993) as regards manufacturing support and Lendrem (2002) as regards nonclinical support more generally. Training issues are covered in Chuang-Stein (1996).

Statistical Issues in Drug Development/2nd Edition   Stephen Senn
© 2007 John Wiley & Sons, Ltd

5.2   INTRODUCTION

What makes a good experiment? Is it one which has been precisely controlled and for which the protocol is full of phrases like 'the volunteer will eat a standard breakfast consisting of two croissants, one cup of coffee, a pat of butter and 30 g of jam'? Is an even better experiment one which specifies the type of fruit to be used in making the jam, whether the croissants are to have been made with butter or not, and how many spoons of sugar (if any) are allowed in the coffee?

Obviously, attention to details of control can be important in an experiment, but this alone is not what makes a good experiment. The purpose of an experiment is to provide salient information: information which will enable one to distinguish between the plausibility of theories on the basis of the data obtained. The means by which one may make such distinctions are, in the broadest sense, *statistical*. They are made with the help of measurements or data and the statistics which summarize them. An important part of the statistician's work consists in performing the analysis of such data but, just as the chemist in performing a chemical analysis can hardly be expected to perform a decent job if you come to him or her saying 'I mixed this substance with the following reagent and these are the results,' so the statistician can hardly be expected to give effective advice if you say 'I carried out a trial according to the following protocol and would now like you to analyse the resulting data.'

One may put it more strongly than this. Just as with a chemical analysis, so with a clinical trial: you have to have established the way in which the results will be analysed in order to perform it properly. If you have designed a clinical trial effectively, then you must know what the analysis will be. If you know what the analysis will be, there can be no reason for you to consult the statistician for advice as to how to analyse it once the trial is run. Hence, the only sort of person who needs the statistician's help once the trial is run is the sort of person who needs his or her help when the trial is designed. Thus, the time to first consult the statistician is either before or when the trial is planned or not at all.

To return to our discussion of experiments, a good experiment is one which may reasonably be expected to be salient. Obviously, other things being equal, a large experiment is better than a small one, and one which is too small is unlikely to be salient. Hence the belief has arisen that the major function of the statistician in designing an experiment is to use his theories to determine the sample size. In fact, sample size is only one aspect of the problem and its importance has been overrated.

According to Neville Shute, anybody could build a bridge that didn't fall down but only an engineer could build one that *just* didn't fall down. Similarly, given enough time, enough money and enough patients and enough trial and error (in fact, far too many trials are an error), the effects of a drug will be determined. The task, though, is to do this at a reasonable cost in terms of money and human suffering and this is where the statistician can help.

> 'To call in the statistician after the experiment is done may be no more than asking him to perform a postmortem examination: he may be able to say what the experiment died of.'
>
>   R A Fisher

5.3   IN THE BEGINNING

From one point of view a drug development programme could be regarded as one long, complicated and evolving experiment. There is a strong interdependence between its various stages. Indeed, nowadays, regulatory agencies even expect to see formal overviews or meta-analyses of the results. These overviews are statistical in nature. It thus follows that the time to start consulting the statistician is not when the first trial plan is being drafted but even earlier and that he or she should be closely involved in designing the development programme as a whole.

5.4   THE TRIAL PROTOCOL

There are five major purposes to a clinical trial protocol, which can be summarized by a mnemonic which uses the five vowels. The purposes have to do with, **a**nticipation, **e**thics, **i**nference, **o**rganization and **u**tmost good faith. (For the purpose of discussion I shall assume that the trial protocol and case record form are used together as one single document.)

Anticipation is a necessary aspect of the protocol. It enables the persons involved to run a thought experiment from which, by recording in great detail which treatments will be given, which manouevres performed and which measurements taken, the likely course of the experiment can be anticipated. Thus, writing a detailed protocol is an important (if frequently tedious) discipline to be observed if problems in running the experiment are to be anticipated and hence allowed for and (if possible) avoided.

The *ethical* requirement is extremely important. A detailed protocol is essential in order to fulfill the ethical requirement for the following reasons. (1) The ethical committee (independent review board in the USA) must have a clear idea of what is intended if they are to make a reasoned judgement as to whether the trial is justified. (2) The patient cannot give informed consent unless the basis for that information is established. (3) If the protocol is not clearly defined, then the trial is in danger of being changed in midstream without returning to the ethical committee (or re-establishing informed consent), and as a consequence the ethical safeguards will be rendered ineffective. (4) It is unethical to waste patients' time to no good purpose and a poorly defined experiment is more likely to be a poorly executed one.

Both major schools of statistical *inference*, the Bayesian and the frequentist, require prior consideration of possible analyses at the time trials are run. The Bayesian school requires specification of prior probabilities. To make these genuine priors they have to be truly 'prior' and hence determined before the data are obtained. The frequentist school requires specification of the tests that will be performed and the decisions that will be made depending on various outcomes. For both schools, in order to design salient experiments, it is necessary to pay attention to very many aspects of design.

Medical statistician: One who will not accept that Columbus discovered America. . . because he said he was looking for India in the trial* plan.

*A cross-over trial.

The *organizational* purpose of a trial is also essential. The activities of a great many persons (trial physician, trial nurse, trial logistics, clinical research associates and monitors, database managers, regulatory personnel, statisticians and so on) have to be coordinated in order to bring the trial to a successful conclusion. The trial protocol is not the only document used in this, but it is the prime medium of communication.

As in insurance, so in drug regulation: standards of *utmost good faith* have to prevail if the process is to work, and the randomized clinical trial and the rules regarding its conduct provide the necessary 'fiduciary framework'. The sponsor is granted the privilege of performing an experiment and a subsequent analysis which the regulator will use. This privilege carries responsibilities with it. It is not enough for a regulatory agency to know that it is being presented with the truth and nothing but the truth. In order to come to a reasonable conclusion it has to have the whole truth also. The protocol is an important device for helping to ensure this. It fulfills this role as follows: (1) by stating clearly which data will be collected so that these can be accounted for once the trial is completed; (2) by formally declaring as irrelevant data not foreseen in the protocol; (3) by making it harder to hide the existence of unsuccessful trials.

As key co-authors of the trial protocol, the study physician and the statistician are involved with all of these aspects. Obviously the degree of their involvement in these various aspects is not identical and there are some aspects, for example the ethical (but see discussion of efficiency below), where the statistician's involvement is small. One aspect which is important to them both is the inferential one. We shall now proceed to look in more detail at this aspect of the protocol.

5.5   THE STATISTICIAN'S ROLE IN PLANNING THE PROTOCOL

A statistician in drug development is like a catalyst in a chemical reaction: neither necessary nor sufficient for the *process* but capable of improving yield considerably. Nevertheless, because efficiency is an ethical imperative in drug development, the statistician cannot be left out. The statistician's duty is to ensure, with the help of the physician or life-scientist with whom (s)he cooperates, that the trial is designed in such a way that a proposed analysis has a decent chance of reaching a useful conclusion. One factor, among many, affecting this probability is the number of patients recruited to the trial. The following two examples, based loosely on real life, illustrate, however, that frequently far more than sample size is involved.

Example 5.1
It is desired to investigate the therapeutic affect in asthma of a long-acting bronchodilator, to be given twice daily, by comparing it over three months to an established shorter-acting bronchodilator to be given four times a day. The statistician has been asked to determine the sample size. The physician informs him that the most important measurement is forced expiratory volume in one second (FEV_1) and that patients will be brought into the clinic on six separate occasion throughout the trial and have their FEV_1 measured. An immediate question for the statistician in determining the sample size is whether the mean of these measurements should form the basis for analysis or whether it should be based on individual measurements. In exploring the matter further, however, the statistician realizes that the measurements will be taken in the morning some two to three hours after the patient has taken medication and cannot,

therefore, form the basis of comparison of a long-acting and short-acting treatment. He suggests using peak expiratory flow (PEF), a measurement which the patients can take at home on waking, as a basis for comparison. This leads to a discussion of the relative merits of the two measures, it being recognized that, other things being equal, FEV_1 is more reliable but that here other things are not equal, since not only is the timing of the measurements not the same but the frequency is also different (PEF can be measured every day).

Example 5.2
It is desired to estimate the effect of a particular treatment on the rate of loss of bone mineral density in a prevention trial for osteoporosis. A dose-finding trial using several doses and a placebo is to be run in phase II, and there is extreme interest in an early conclusion in order that a definitive study using a suitable dose may be started. The physician has proposed a trial with a two-year treatment. The statistician obtains suitable estimates of the standard deviation of bone mineral density. In order to minimize the sample size she determines to use analysis of covariance. A clinically relevant difference is determined for the rate of change of bone mineral density and a sample size is calculated. Once recruitment time for the necessary number of patients is included, however, it is realized that the trial as a whole will take nearly three years and this is considered too long. The physician proposes to cut treatment time by one year. The statistician realises that this may imply a halving of the clinically relevant difference and hence lead to a considerable increase in recruitment time unless more centres are recruited. The cost of the trial will be increased and the total time saved will not be one year. Indeed, if care is not taken, the trial may actually take longer. This leads to an investigation by statistician and physician as to what is the best choice of a length of treatment for this trial.

In both of these examples, the task of the statistician has widened considerably beyond that of simply determining the sample size. Of course, some of the points the statistician made to the physician could have been appreciated without his help. No one profession has a monopoly of logic. The point is that these sorts of matters are more likely to be discovered and explored if statistician and physician work together on all aspects of trial design and the statistician's responsibility is not narrowly defined.

5.6   SAMPLE SIZE DETERMINATION

Notwithstanding the above, sample size determination *is* an important part of trial design. One of the simplest techniques is frequently overlooked. If many successful trials of a given type have been run in a given indication, then the typical size of such a trial gives a good indication of what is likely to be successful. More formal methods are available and a common approach is sketched below.

First, the statistician and physician together need to identify a particular outcome variable including the particular time-point (or combination) which will be used. Next the statistician must identify an appropriate statistical test. A size of this test, or nominal significance level, (see Chapter 4) must also be identified. It will also be important to have obtained from previous trials, or some appropriate source, an estimate (sometimes no more than a guesstimate) of the likely variability of the particular measure chosen. The statistician also needs to establish a working alternative hypothesis. This is *not* a hypothesis which he believes *must* be true if the null hypothesis is not true but rather a conceivable hypothesis of potential interest. This is the most difficult of all the steps in fixing a power calculation and it is precisely for this most difficult step that the physician is called upon to make her greatest contribution. She must commit herself to a magnitude of effect which she would like to investigate. Typically the concept of the **clinically relevant difference** is used: sometimes defined as 'the difference one would not like to miss'. Finally, the statistician and physician must agree on the power of the procedure. These pieces of information, taken together with the general background knowledge of the trial, then provide the statistician with the basis for calculating, using the tools of mathematical statistics, the sample size required. Tables and computer programs are available for various standard designs. These matters are taken up more fully in Chapter 13.

Bonus: A means of rewarding employees for that serendipity that outweighs incompetence.

5.7   OTHER IMPORTANT DESIGN ISSUES

Other important issues are to do with the basic structure of trials. For example, what are the appropriate comparator treatments? How many should be studied simultaneously? Will the object of the trial be to find differences or to demonstrate 'equivalence'? Should a parallel group study or a cross-over trial be used? How many centres should be used? What should the block size be? If a cross-over trial is employed will it be necessary to use incomplete blocks? (These are designs in which each patient receives only a subset of the treatments being studied.) How long should the treatments be applied? When should values be measured? How should they be combined? Should the results be analysed sequentially? If the trial is to be blinded, how should this be achieved? Is stratification desired? What factors should be included in the analysis? What is the general approach to be adopted? What is the strategy for dealing with multiplicity of outcomes?

It is also important to appreciate that a clinical trial protocol will have to include a detailed specification of the intended analysis as well, of course, as the attendant sample size justification. Indeed, these statements will be needed in order to get ethical approval and, since there is an intimate relationship between design and analysis, it is necessary to know the intended analysis to judge the suitability of the design (Bailey, 1981).

5.8   RANDOMIZATION

The statistician has to ensure that the randomization is prepared according to the study design. The key features of the schedule such as block size have to be approved by the statistician. Typically for a double blind trial, only those involved in the packing of the supplies are aware of the final treatment assignments.

Two approaches to randomization are common: *pre-allocation* and *post-allocation* (Senn, 2004). In pre-allocation, treatment packs that are identical in appearance are prepared in random sequences and delivered to the centres. As each patient is recruited, he or she is given the available pack with the lowest randomization number. In post-allocation, the patient is entered onto the trial and the trial physician is then informed which pack the patient should be given. This latter form of randomization is safer where there is a danger that treatment packs can be distinguished from each other and is also more easily modified to allocate based on covariates (ABC) (Senn, 2004). It requires telephone- or web-based systems for implementation.

5.9   DATA COLLECTION PREVIEW

In many drug companies, once the protocol and case record form have been finalized a meeting is held which may go by a number of different names but which I will refer to here as the *data collection preview*. An appropriate person to organize and chair this will be the statistician and it is designed to cover in more detail than was possible in the trial plan particular issues regarding the handling of data from the trial. It is an opportunity, in particular, for agreement to be reached regarding the monitoring of the trial and the checking of data collected.

5.10   PERFORMING THE TRIAL

This is an extremely important aspect of the trial with which the statistician has very little to do although he or she can occasionally be required to give advice regarding blinding and randomization issues. I mention it here to remind statistical readers of the arduous, essential and often complex, work carried out by others in performing experiments that statisticians have helped to design.

5.11   DATA ANALYSIS PREVIEW

In many drug companies, as the time for analysis approaches but prior to un-blinding the data, a meeting is held to specify the likely form of the report to be produced, in particular as regards statistical analyses, tabulation and graphical presentation. At this meeting, which I shall refer to as the *data analysis preview*, clinical and statistical colleagues should agree any final details not covered by the specification in the report as well as the impact of any particular issues (perhaps unforeseen at the time of planning) which have arisen in conducting the trial. Typical aspects which may have to be given further consideration to that already provided in the protocol may have to do with protocol violators, drop-outs, and centres which failed to recruit a reasonable number of patients as well as general problems arising from concerns about data quality or as a result of monitoring the trial.

   At the data analysis preview it is common to update the prespecified analysis and issue a formal statistical analysis plan. The plan gives more detail on the analysis to be conducted than can usefully be included in the protocol, e.g. precise descriptions of how variables derived from the source data are to be calculated, A key component is a full specification of the tables, listings and graphical presentations to be produced. The analysis plan is discussed and agreed by the study team.

Many drug companies produce mock-up tables using available data based on fake treatment codes in advance of database finalization. While the actual results shown in the tables have no meaning, they can help to identify data issues and clarify the proposed presentation of the results.

5.12 ANALYSIS AND REPORTING

Once clinical development have completed their task of running the trial, monitoring it and verifying the accuracy and adequacy of the data, a data-clean certificate will usually be issued and the trial database is locked. The clinical data analyst is then able to begin converting the data for analysis. (In some companies this person will not be the same as the data-manager or the statistician. In others one or other of these persons will fulfil this function.) This may involve converting data from a primary database system such as ORACLE into data sets within a statistical system such as SAS. Such conversions are not fully automatic and it requires skill and experience to ensure that the relevant primary databases (trial data, randomization data, laboratory ranges and relevant medical dictionaries) are linked, that the data are converted to an appropriate format and sub-setted in an appropriate manner. At one time, the programs to perform this step might have been written once the trial was completed. Nowadays they will have been written well in advance and tested on subsets of the accumulating trial data using dummy treatment codes.

The next step, which is to list the data, will also have been prepared well in advance. Again this is a skilled undertaking as these so-called lists are, in fact, complex tables. It is falsely assumed by many to be simply a matter of pushing a few buttons, but in practice it requires days of programming and a great deal of attention to detail if the result is to prove satisfactory. Randomization codes are only broken once the data have been finalized and the first genuine listings can then be produced.

It is sometimes found in tabulating the data that further problems emerge. This may require further source verification and correction, and consequently a reopening of the primary database and, inevitably, a second conversion and tabulation once the database has been locked. Some sorts of errors can only be detected with knowledge of the treatment code. For example, a suspiciously high lung function reading for an asthmatic patient might have been quite plausible had the patient been receiving active treatment but less plausible under placebo. Obviously there are possibilities for bias attendant on such unblinded cleaning and usually a data trail log will be kept to show which values have been corrected and when, so that if necessary an auditor could look at this. Once the process of tabulation and is complete the analysis may proceed. This will involve the statistician in writing the necessary programs and executing them. Nowadays, nearly all of this work will have been done in advance. It involves, of course, correct identification of the appropriate techniques to be used and is much less likely to be dependent on data diagnostics than in the past. It will be driven instead by prior knowledge of the area of application. If the groundwork has been properly prepared in planning, both at protocol and data analysis preview, then this step will have been made easier.

Again, although in the end it may be reduced to running a suite of pre-prepared programs, analysis is far from being a matter of pushing a few buttons. It would not be exceptional for an analysis library to contain 50 programs, many of them consisting of hundreds of lines. The amount of work in documenting, analysing and reporting a trial can be judged by the fact that currently (2007), in what is a competitive business, consultancy firms will charge several tens of thousands of dollars for analysing a trial.

Once the analyses are complete, the statistician then writes his or her contribution to the integrated report. The medical writer should already have prepared a skeleton report including the introductory background sections, and will draft a summary of the results. The study physician will provide clinical interpretation. Finally, the study team including the statistician will review the whole in order to harmonize the contributions, agree any necessary amendments and have the report released.

The purpose of the report is to present thoroughly and unambiguously the data, the analysis and the interpretation in a way that maintains quite clearly the link to the protocol, and enables the regulator to understand clearly not only what was concluded and how this conclusion was reached but what it was intended to investigate and how it was planned to do so. In this way the trial is brought to its proper close. It is my firm belief that on the whole this task has been well done in the industry (Senn, 2002). Various guidelines, as well as the vigilance of the FDA and other regulators, have helped ensure that statistician and trial physician carry out this task properly (International Conference on Harmonization, 1996, 1999).

5.13 OTHER ACTIVITIES

Of course, there are many other things the statistician is called upon to do. These range from the sort of day-to-day organizational matters with which all professionals in drug development are faced, to more directly statistical matters such as carrying out formal overviews (meta-analyses) of clinical trials. It is extremely important to mention that close collaboration with trial physicians is essential and that the medical statistician must be able to communicate (explain and understand) with his or her medical colleagues.

Statistician: One who is to figures what a librarian is to words.

5.14 STATISTICAL RESEARCH

Finally, I should like to say something about the importance of statistical research to the statistician in drug development: if not always in terms of his or her active contribution, at least in terms of active consumption. (The process of keeping up with the literature and making an active effort to understand the results of the research of others.)

As should be clear from previous chapters, statistics is a living and evolving science. New techniques are continually being developed and implemented. My definition of a real mathematician is someone who can solve mathematical problems he or she has never encountered before. (In some cases, however, the more original part of his or her work would be in defining such problems.) *Mutatis mutandis* this is also true of statisticians. Although many statistical techniques currently employed in the pharmaceutical industry have been developed by statisticians working from university addresses, many have also been developed by persons working within the industry. As with any scientist, what a statistician brings to a job from a university education is a certain amount of intellectual capital. There is then a choice between two courses of action: either to invest further in the subject and see the capital grow, or to sit tight and attempt to live off it. The science of statistics develops so rapidly that the latter choice will leave the statistician intellectually bankrupt and useless well before the end of his or her professional life.

5.15   FURTHER READING

The most important standard covering statistical matters in drug development and regulation is the International Conference on Harmonization (ICH) Tripartite Guideline 'Statistical Principles for Clinical Trials'. Although based largely on existing regulatory advice (Committee for Proprietary Medicinal Products, 1995), this appeared only in 1998 (in other words, since the first edition of this book) and was subsequently published in *Statistics in Medicine* (International Conference on Harmonisation, 1999). Also of interest is the less extensive CONSORT (Consolidated Standards of Reporting Clinical Trials) statement covering reporting of clinical trials in the medical literature (Altman, 1996; Moher *et al.*, 2001). Various matters to do with quality in analysing clinical trials are covered in Senn (2000b).

The statistician working in drug development is increasingly likely to become involved with data-monitoring committees. Although unlikely to be a member of such a committee, he or she may have to prepare statistical analysis plans for sequential trials or be involved in coordinating activities or data preparation. Useful references are Grant *et al.* (2005) and the comprehensive book in this series by Ellenberg *et al.* (2003). Statistical issues to do with sequential trials are covered in Chapter 19.

The so-called Pocock report (Pocock *et al.*, 1991) is now mainly of historical interest but was influential in promoting the role of the statistician in drug regulation in the UK and Germany. That role had already been well accepted in the USA for many years. See O'Neill (1991) for an account. More recent accounts of the situation in Europe are given in EFSPI Working Group (1999), Lewis (1996) and Morgan *et al.* (1999); however, even these are now mainly of historical interest. Sadly even in 2007 many European countries still do not employ permanent statisticians in their regulatory agencies. The Royal Statistical Society report on first-in-man studies contains much of relevance to statisticians working in phase I (Working Party on Statistical Issues in First-in-Man Studies, 2007).

The work of the medical statistician is described from an academic perspective by Pocock (1995) and that of the industry-based consulting statistician by Lendrem (2002) and Porter (1993). Time allocation and budgeting matters for collaborating statisticians are covered by Lesser (1996) and Lesser and Parker (1995). It is generally the case that even a postgraduate degree in medical statistics cannot prepare you completely for working in the pharmaceutical industry. On-the-job training of statisticians is covered by Chuang-Stein (1996). The vexed question of whether or not statistics is or should be a profession in the sense of accountancy or the law was considered by Andy Grieve in his presidential address for the Royal Statistical Society (Grieve, 2005).

At rather infrequent intervals, statistical issues in the pharmaceutical industry have been debated by the Royal Statistical Society. Three 'read papers' contain much of relevance to the work of the pharmaceutical statistician. Even though the first (Lewis, 1983), appeared nearly twenty-five years ago (at the time of writing), it is interesting to note that a number of the issues are still live. The second paper (Racine *et al.*, 1986) is an early exposition of the use of Bayesian methods within the pharmaceutical industry, which, despite the fact that it pre-dates the Markov chain Monte-Carlo revolution introduced by Gelfand and Smith (1990) is still ahead of current practice in many respects. The third (Senn, 2000a) was written by me and, as might be expected, touches on a number of issues covered in this book.

Finally, anybody working in the pharmaceutical industry must expect that his or her work will frequently be viewed with suspicion. In that connection, two of my articles (Senn, 2002; Senn, 2006) may be of interest.

References

Altman DG (1996) Better reporting of randomised controlled trials: the CONSORT statement [editorial] [see comments]. *British Medical Journal* **313**: 570–571.

Bailey RA (1981) A unified approach to design of experiments. *Journal of the Royal Statistical Society Series A – Statistics in Society* **144**: 214–223.

Chuang-Stein C (1996) On-the-job training of pharmaceutical statisticians. *Drug Information Journal* **30**: 351–357.

Committee for Proprietary Medicinal Products (1995) Biostatistical methodology in clinical trials in applications for marketing authorizations for medicinal products. CPMP Working Party on Efficacy of Medicinal Products Note for Guidance III/3630/92-EN. *Statistics in Medicine* **14**: 1659–1682.

EFSPI Working Group (1999) Qualified statisticians in the European pharmaceutical industry: report of a European Federation of Statisticians in the Pharmaceutical Industry (EFSPI) working group. *Drug Information Journal* **33**: 407–415.

Ellenberg S, Fleming T, DeMets D (2003) *Data Monitoring Committees in Clinical Trials: A Practical Perspective.* John Wiley & Sons, Ltd, Chichester.

Gelfand AE, Smith AFM (1990) Sampling-based approaches to calculating marginal densities. *Journal of the American Statistical Association* **85**: 398–409.

Grant AM, Altman DG, Babiker AB, *et al.* (2005) Issues in data monitoring and interim analysis of trials. *Health Technology Assessment* **9**: 1–238, iii–iv.

Grieve AP (2002) Do statisticians count? A personal view. *Pharmaceutical Statistics* **1**: 35–43.

Grieve AP (2005) The professionalization of the 'shoe clerk'. *Journal of the Royal Statistical Society Series A – Statistics in Society* **168**: 639–654.

International Conference on Harmonisation (1996) Guideline for good clinical practice. International Conference on Harmonisation. http://www.emea.europa.eu/pdfs/human/ich/013595en.pdf.

International Conference on Harmonisation (1999) Statistical principles for clinical trials (ICH E9). *Statistics in Medicine* **18**: 1905–1942.

Lendrem D (2002) Statistical support to non-clinical. *Pharmaceutical Statistics* **1**: 71–73.

Lesser ML (1996) Guidelines for budgeting biostatistics involvement in research projects. *Statistics in Medicine* **15**: 2127–2133.

Lesser ML, Parker RA (1995) The biostatistician in medical research – allocating time and effort. *Statistics in Medicine* **14**: 1683–1692.

Lewis JA (1983) Clinical trials – statistical developments of practical benefit to the pharmaceutical industry. *Journal of the Royal Statistical Society Series A – Statistics in Society* **146**: 362–393.

Lewis JA (1996) Statistics and statisticians in the regulation of medicines. *Journal of the Royal Statistical Society Series A – Statistics in Society* **159**: 359–362.

Moher D, Schulz KF, Altman DG (2001) The CONSORT statement: revised recommendations for improving the quality of reports of parallel-group randomised trials. *Lancet* **357**(9263): 1191–1194.

Morgan D, Bacchieri A, Bay C, *et al.* (1999) Qualified statisticians in the European pharmaceutical industry: Report of a European Federation of Statisticians in the Pharmaceutical Industry (EFSPI) Working Group. *Drug Information Journal* **33**: 407–415.

O'Neill RT (1991) The biometrical role in United States drug regulation. In: Vollmar J (ed.), *Biometri in der chemisch-pahramzuetischen Industrie.* Gustav Fischer, Stuttgart, pp. 31–42.

Pocock SJ (1995) Life as an academic medical statistician and how to survive it. *Statistics in Medicine* **14**: 209–222.

Pocock S, Altman D, Armitage P, *et al.* (1991) Statistics and statisticians in drug regulation in the United Kingdom. *Journal of the Royal Statistical Society Series A – Statistics in Society* **154**: 413–419.

Porter MA (1993) The role of the statistician in industry. *Statistician* **42**: 217–227.

Racine A, Grieve AP, Fluhler H, Smith AFM (1986) Bayesian methods in practice – experiences in the pharmaceutical industry. *Journal of the Royal Statistical Society Series C – Applied Statistics* **35**: 93–150.

Senn SJ (2000a) Consensus and controversy in pharmaceutical statistics (with discussion). *The Statistician* **49**: 135–176.

Senn SJ (2000b) Statistical quality in analysing clinical trials. *Good Clinical Practice Journal* **7**: 22–26.

Senn SJ (2002) Authorship of drug industry trials. *Pharmaceutical Statistics* **1**: 5–7.

Senn SJ (2003) Lost opportunities for statistics. *Pharmaceutical Statistics* **2**: 3–4.

Senn SJ (2004) Added values: controversies concerning randomization and additivity in clinical trials. *Statistics in Medicine* **23**: 3729–3753.

Senn SJ (2006) Sharp tongues and bitter pills. *Significance* **3**: 123–125.

Working Party on Statistical Issues in First-in-Man Studies (2007) Statistical issues in first-in-man studies. *Journal of the Royal Statistical Society, Series A* **170**: 517–579.

Part 2

Statistical Issues: Debatable and Controversial Topics in Drug Development

Information is something one goes out to seek and puts away when found as you might do a piece of lead: ponderous, useful, unvibrating, dull. Whereas knowledge comes to one, this sort of knowledge, a chance acquisition preserving in its repose a fine resonant quality.

Joseph Conrad, *Chance*

6

Allocating Treatments to Patients in Clinical Trials

Every medical man commits that act of treachery, Mr. Blake, in the course of his practice . . . Every doctor in large practice finds himself, every now and then, obliged to deceive his patients.

Wilkie Collins, *The Moonstone*

. . . every free man automatically participated in the sacred drawings, which took place in the labyrinths of the god every sixty nights and which determined his destiny until the next drawing.

Jorge Luis Borges, *The Lottery in Babylon*

6.1   BACKGROUND

The purpose of a clinical trial is to improve our knowledge of treatments in order that future patients may benefit. The patients actually recruited on a clinical trial have not presented for this reason, however. They expect their physician to treat them with the best treatment available, although they may, of course, be prepared to make some sacrifice in the interest of others. (In the case of chronic diseases there is also the possibility that they themselves may be numbered among the future beneficiaries.) On the other hand, to make wise choices as to treatment, one has to know something about the alternatives and this means that to get precise information about the value of a given treatment, one will also have to study other treatments which may turn out to be inferior. Furthermore, because patients vary over time and from centre to centre and because physicians and facilities vary also, in order to deal with these sorts of bias the ideal solution will be to study patients under various alternatives concurrently. There is thus a dilemma facing the physician in a clinical trial: how does the physician as scientist satisfy the physician as healer and vice versa?

An important element in such conflicts between healer and scientist is the degree of knowledge possessed by the physician. This will have increased by the end of the trial and, if the results are studied during the course of the trial, will increase to some degree before. It is thus possible that a choice which was not believed to be against patients' interests at the beginning of the trial will become unacceptable by or before the planned end. Patients are also far from homogenous and this creates further concerns both for healer and scientist. The healer may feel that there may be a greater justification for allocating more severely ill patients to an experimental treatment, especially where there is a moderately efficacious standard therapy. Those who are severely ill may be inadequately served by the standard and hence prepared to accept the risks of the experimental therapy. The scientist may be concerned that differences between patients allocated to different treatment groups may invalidate comparisons of the treatments.

The most common methods of allocation in clinical trials involve some form of randomization. Simple randomization, for example, would require that every possible split of a given set of patients into two groups was equally likely. Although for even a moderately sized trial, a great imbalance in numbers assigned to experimental and control group would be unlikely using this approach it is, nevertheless, more usual to randomize subject to the constraint that numbers shall be equal. In fact, trialists often go further than this and use the method of randomized blocks.

Randomized blocks are associated with R.A. Fisher and his work at the agricultural research station of Rothamsted in Harpenden. For the purpose of a carrying out a trial in agriculture, fields would be divided into plots. Sometimes the field would have a particular fertility gradient so that (say) the northwest end might be more fertile than the southeast end. A design which was sometimes used in such circumstances was to group the plots in blocks of roughly equal fertility. Treatments were then randomized to blocks so that they were equally well represented in each block. In a clinical trial, however, the patients cannot be gathered together before the trial and divided into similar groups by prognostic factors; instead they have to be treated as they present. Nevertheless, for reasons of balancing treatments over all patients, it is useful to regard a group of consecutively presenting patients as a block. Randomization can then be carried out in terms of these blocks. For example, if two treatments are to be given, verum (V) and placebo (P) and block sizes of 6 are chosen, then every 6 patients will be allocated 3 to V and 3 to P at random. This may be done by choosing, for any given block, one of 20 possible sequences of V and P (such as VVPPPV, VPVVPP and so forth) at random. If for any reason one then fails to recruit the planned numbers of patients at a given centre, it will then nevertheless be the case that the numbers of patients on the two treatments at that centre will be approximately equal. Table 6.1 gives an example of blocking a trial of two treatments, A and B, using a block size of 4.

Simple randomization is a method which by virtue of its very unpredictability affords the greatest degree of blinding. Some form of randomization is indispensable for any trial in which the issue of blinding is taken seriously, but it is, of course, also employed even where blinding is not possible (as in trials of surgical procedures) or is unnecessary. Randomization has its critics both from the ethical and the scientific points of view. On the one hand, there is concern that the method will be unfair to some patients in the trial by allocating them a treatment apparently without any consideration of their actual state of health. On the other hand, the scientific criticism argues that the method allows a degree of chance difference between treatment groups which may invalidate the analysis. (It is ironical that these two criticisms tend in different directions. As we shall see, the critics of randomization ethics would like the treatment groups to be more different than would be produced by randomization and the critics of randomization as a scientific device would like them to be more similar.)

In this chapter we consider various issues to do with allocating treatments to patients. These issues are not, of course, purely statistical: in many cases they are largely ethical. However, because, among other reasons, the number of patients it is necessary to recruit

Table 6.1 Randomized blocks for a trial with two treatments and block sizes of 4.

Patient	Block No.	Block sequence	Treatment
1	1	BAAB	B
2	1	BAAB	A
3	1	BAAB	A
4	1	BAAB	B
5	2	ABAB	A
6	2	ABAB	B
7	2	ABAB	A
8	2	ABAB	B
9	3	BAAB	B
10	3	BAAB	A
11	3	BAAB	A
12	3	BAAB	B

on a clinical trial is an important statistical issue and because this in its turn has ethical implications, the statistical dimension to these issues is also extremely important.

6.2 ISSUES

6.2.1 Placebo run-ins

Many trials are planned with a placebo run-in, that is to say a period before the trial proper starts and during which *all* patients receive placebo. There seem to be two common reasons. First, the run-in period may permit the trialist to operate some screening procedure, in particular as regards compliance with a treatment regime, which may help to decide which patients will enter the trial proper. Second, it is argued that a run-in period is necessary to permit a 'clean' comparison of the treatments in the trial.

The first claim has been the subject of some study and researchers have come to different conclusions. On the plus side is that the patients selected, and thus eventually randomized to treatment, will have a higher than average compliance. The negative aspect of such run-ins is that they are not very good predictors of the patient's compliance in the trial itself. Furthermore, although a lower number of patients may be randomized to treatment, the total time each randomized patient will be under study will be increased and, of course, a larger number of patients will have to be screened in the first place. In short, it is far from being necessarily the case that having a run-in period will increase the efficiency of a trial (Brittain and Wittes, 1990; Schechtman and Gordon, 1993). The second claim is rather more problematic but we defer considering it until an ethical difficulty with placebo run-ins has been addressed.

A placebo in a randomized clinical trial is no bar to operating informed consent. The physician can say to the patient: 'If you agree to enter this trial you will have half a chance of receiving the new treatment under study and half a chance of receiving an inactive treatment. You will not be told which you have received and I will not know either until the trial is over.' Furthermore, the patient could, in principle, read the whole protocol. (I would maintain that the patient ought to have this right in practice.) No such policy of honesty is possible for a placebo given in a run-in period, for the point is that all patients will receive it. However, the doctor is hardly likely to say 'You will be given an inert substance in the first two weeks to check your compliance,' and if she did, she would hardly have much faith in its utility for this purpose (Senn, 1997). Further still, quite apart from the ethical problems with the deception involved, a deception which has been cheerfully admitted in print by trialists, the efficacy of this stratagem must in any case rely on what I have called *the argument from the stupidity of others*: trialists are clever and know that a good trial has a placebo run-in, whereas patients are stupid and don't.

There are two simple alternative strategies to using a placebo in the run-in. The first is to give all the patients the active treatment and the second is to withhold treatment altogether for the period of the run-in. The usual objection to the first strategy brings us to the second of the reasons for a placebo run-in discussed above: the need for a clean comparison. It should be realized, however, that the usual purpose of a clinical trial is to study the steady-state effect of treatments and for this purpose it makes little difference what treatment was used in the run-in: by the time the drug comes to be studied it will have worn off. Of course, for certain rapidly progressing acute diseases (such as infections), to give all patients the experimental treatment would defeat the object of the exercise: they might all benefit in a nonreversible way. However, run-in periods are in any case unsuitable for such conditions. Of course, in some cases, we may wish to study the onset of action of a treatment and then an active run-in would not be suitable. Then the other alternative of having a wash-out without treatment must be considered. Lying to the patient is not an acceptable alternative (Senn, 2001, 2002).

A further problem with a run-in period is that it may compromise the generalizability of the results (Berger *et al.*, 2003). As I have already argued, patients in a clinical trial should not be regarded as a representative sample of some target population anyway, so this is a controversial issue. Nevertheless, a sponsor can hardly be surprised if, proof of efficacy only having been achieved as a consequence of some elaborate screening strategy, the regulator then demands that this be reflected in labelling and marketing of the drug.

6.2.2   Placebos as comparators

Clinical trials appear to be easiest to interpret if the comparator is a placebo. One justification is that this enables measurement of a pure effect of treatment (the difference with respect to treatment) which in any case permits a valid indirect comparison between different treatments of the specific pharmaceutical effect. This comparison is valid provided the effect is additive even if placebos have different effects in different circumstances.

Where there is an effective treatment already available, however, then there may be ethical objections to allocating patients to placebo. Hence this practice has received considerable criticism.

My view is that one must make a distinction between the sort of chronic disease in which patients may try a number of treatments during the course of therapy, including from time to time none, and serious life-threatening diseases in which this is not the case and the effect of a choice of treatment is not reversible to any appreciable degree.

For such diseases, where an effective treatment is available it must be offered. However, I would go further and say that for such diseases it will also usually be unacceptable to withhold the effective therapy from patients even if it is hoped that the new therapy may be better.

This means that all patients must receive the effective therapy as a background treatment. The experimental therapy can then only be used as an add-on, and for this purpose a placebo add-on may indeed be used as a comparator (Senn, 2001, 2002). Thus the placebo-controlled trial becomes acceptable after all. It may be argued that this sort of comparison is not pure, but such pure comparisons are a myth. Nourishing food, clean water and fresh air are all essential to the health of human beings and are the most effective of remedies. (The reader who doubts this should consider our general definition of effects and what would happen to patients who were denied these remedies.) We constantly run trials in which these background therapies are available to all patients and in my view there is no reason not to run trials where more obviously pharmaceutical remedies are used as background treatment for all patients. Once this is understood, the room for placebos is seen to be larger than supposed and the ethical objections to them not as serious as supposed.

However, there are cases where standard treatments make better comparators and there are also occasions when we might wish to have an open trial (perhaps with an 'untreated' group) and hence where placebos are not indicated.

6.2.3 Randomization and balance

A false claim that is sometimes made for randomization is that it will balance the characteristics of the patients in the two groups (Senn, 2005). Randomization will not even guarantee that the numbers in the treatment and control group are equal, although for a large trial the proportions will usually be similar. In fact, we commonly block randomization to ensure that numbers are closely balanced (see above.) Alternative approaches are sometimes considered for making sure that the numbers on each treatment are approximately equal while maintaining an element of unpredictability. For example, Efron (1971) suggested a biased coin approach to randomization which tends to produce stronger balance than randomization.

In general, randomization will not balance the groups by prognostic factors; it is rather that given any nominated prognostic factor it is impossible to predict whether, as a result of the randomization, the experimental or the control group will have the more favourable allocation. This is also true as regards any future patients to be recruited to the trial if the current allocation is studied. Randomization is an allocation mechanism which has no *tendency* to favour one group over another as regards *any* prognostic factor. There are certainly mechanisms which tend to produce greater imbalance. For example, allowing physicians to decide which patients should go in which group is a method which appears to favour the experimental treatment to a greater degree than does randomization. On the other hand, there are allocation mechanisms which force a greater degree of balance (at least as regards known prognostic factors). If, however, randomization does not produce balanced groups in a clinical trial, in what sense can it be acceptable? To understand this it is necessary to appreciate the role of balance in inference.

As we pointed out in Chapter 3, balance is not necessary in order to make *valid* inferences in a clinical trial. (This issue is also discussed further when we come to consider the role of baselines in the analysis of clinical trials in Chapter 7.) Baselines are factors which cannot be balanced perfectly between groups, so that if perfect balance were a requirement for validity of statistical inference this would be a fatal flaw for all clinical trials. The issue of covariates is not really an issue of *balance* but one of *conditioning*: that is to say, it is not necessary for factors to be balanced; it is necessary to account for them in analysis in some way. Furthermore, if the real issue of covariates is conditioning not balance, the real issue of balance is *efficiency* not *validity*.

This point was alluded to in Chapter 3 and can be shown very simply by considering a trial in blood pressure in which we compare two similar groups of patients (assume that as regards *relevant* factors they are identical) one of which has been given a verum and the other a placebo. Let us suppose that the total number of patients is 100 and the proportion in the verum group is p and that in the placebo group $(1 - p)$. Now, it is true that unless $p = 1 - p = 1/2$, and there are 50 patients per group, even in the case where the verum does not work, we do not expect the *total* blood pressure in the verum group to be the same as in the placebo group. Nobody, however, uses such a foolish statistic (although it would give a valid comparison for the case $p = 1/2$). Everybody recognizes, of course, that there is no such problem when comparing the *mean* blood pressures in the two groups. Such a comparison is valid, even when the groups are unequal. Let us call the observed difference of the means between the two groups t.

Although it is certainly true that a valid comparison can be made of the effect of verum compared to placebo using t whether there are 25 patients in the one group and 75 in the other or 40:60 or 50:50 or, indeed, any such split except 0:100 or 100:0 (for which no estimate would be possible), the information given by such comparisons is *not* identical in every case. This is recognized by the variance of t, which is in fact proportional to the sum of the reciprocals of the two sample sizes; thus, if the split is 25:75, the variance is proportional to $1/25 + 1/75 = 0.053$. On the other hand, if the split is 50:50, then the variance is proportional to $1/50 + 1/50 = 0.04$. This shows the value of balance. The variance is lower in the balanced case, but nobody denies that the comparison would be valid in either case.

Now suppose that we did not know what the split was for a given trial. It seems that we should be at a loss to know how to calculate the variance of t since, clearly, it is very different for different splits. Of course, such a case is quite unrealistic; in practice we should have to have observed the numbers in each sample in order to have calculated the mean, but let us suspend disbelief and suppose that the split of patients has been lost but we know the total number of patients overall and the mean results in each group and also have some suitable measure available of the variability of individual results. (Let us suppose, just for argument's sake and in order to permit us to simplify the discussion, that this individual variance is 1. Then the variance of the treatment estimate is $1/(np) + 1/\{n(1 - p)\}$ where n is the number of patients altogether.)

We shall still, however, be at a loss to know how to calculate the variance of t. Suppose, however, that we know we have randomized patients with equal probability to the two groups. We will then know with what probability any particular split arose. With each split we can associate two things: (i) the probability of its having occurred and (ii) the consequent variance if it did occur. In Table 6.2 these two things have been calculated, not for a trial with 100 patients as that would give a tediously long table, but for a trial with 10 patients.

In table 6.2, not only have the individual probabilities and associated variances been calculated but also the expected variance. Now, we may note the following about

Table 6.2 Completely randomized trial with two groups, 10 patients. Possible splits of numbers (given that there is at least one patient in each treatment group) together with associated probabilities, variances and calculation of expected variance.

Split of patients	Probability a	Variance b	Product $a \times b$
1:9	$10/1022 = 0.0098$	$1/1 + 1/9 = 1.111$	0.011
2:8	$45/1022 = 0.0440$	$1/2 + 1/8 = 0.625$	0.028
3:7	$120/1022 = 0.1174$	$1/3 + 1/7 = 0.476$	0.056
4:6	$210/1022 = 0.2055$	$1/4 + 1/6 = 0.417$	0.086
5:5	$252/1022 = 0.2466$	$1/5 + 1/5 = 0.4$	0.099
6:4	$210/1022 = 0.2055$	$1/6 + 1/4 = 0.417$	0.086
7:3	$120/1022 = 0.1174$	$1/7 + 1/3 = 0.476$	0.056
8:2	$45/1022 = 0.0440$	$1/8 + 1/2 = 0.625$	0.027
9:1	$10/1022 = 0.0098$	$1/9 + 1/1 = 1.111$	0.011
Total	1		**0.46**

the expected variance. (1) It is rather larger than the minimum value of 0.4. (2) It nevertheless provides a reasonable approximation to all the variances except for the most extreme splits (1:9, 2:8, 8:2 or 1:9). These cases together account for 11% of all randomizations. (3) Whatever the inadequacies of this individual measure, it is hard to think of any convincingly superior measure of the true actual variance which does not require knowledge of the actual split of numbers.

Given knowledge of the true split, nobody would propose using this average measure. For example, if the split actually were 5:5 we would consider it rather peculiar to use the average variance of 0.46, rather than the given value of 0.4. *However, trialists who insist on balancing their trials by some covariate factor, such as sex of patient, but who do not recognize the factor in the model they employ for analysis are doing something rather analogous to this* (Senn, 2004, 2005).

To see why this is so, consider now a more realistic example, in which the *n* patients are divided equally into the two groups and the true population variance is unknown but has to be estimated from the data. This is done by estimating the variance separately within each treatment group and averaging the result. This avoids the systematic effect of treatment itself inflating the estimate of the variance. Now suppose, however, that there is an important prognostic factor, so that the measured outcome will differ between patients given the same treatment according to the value of this prognostic factor. If we continue to use the same approach to calculating the variance of the trial, then in general the variance estimate will be inflated by this factor. Now, if we have randomized to treatment, but failed to measure this factor, this will be quite appropriate. The treatment estimate will vary according to the actual split of the prognostic factor and will thus have a higher variance, but it turns out that this higher variance is estimated correctly on average and *where we cannot do better we have to be satisfied with averages*.

Randomized clinical trial: A type of experiment that any damn fool can analyse and frequently does.

If we arrange matters so that the groups are perfectly balanced as regards this prognostic factor, then obviously the treatment estimate will not reflect any chance difference between the groups as regards *this* factor. However, the variability of results within the groups *will* be influenced by this factor. (In fact its influence *within* the group will be at its greatest.) Hence, the within-groups variance cannot be used as the valid basis for calculating the variance of the treatment estimate. If we also eliminate the effect of the prognostic factor from the variance estimate, then there is no contradiction.

R.A. Fisher, who introduced randomization into experimentation, has been misrepresented (or misunderstood) as regards the device. He did not oppose balancing experiments for given factors where this was feasible. He only insisted that since balancing removed the influence of these factors on the treatment estimate, their influence also had to be removed from the estimate of the variance of the treatment estimate. Furthermore, he pointed out that, although balancing automatically removed the effect of prognostic factors from estimates, this was not the only way to do it. He did, in fact, develop analysis of covariance to do just that. (The credit for developing this technique is shared with A.L. Bailey (Bailey, 1931; see David, 1995). The important point was to remove the effects of factors coherently throughout.

As I have explained, balance is essentially an issue of efficiency, not of validity (Senn, 1994, 1995a). Randomization is a way of choosing between equally (or approximately equally) efficient experiments. There can usually be no reason for refusing to make this choice at random. Where this is the case, the regulator has every reason to be suspicious if the sponsor refuses to randomize.

6.2.4   Stratification

Randomization does not guarantee perfect balance. In fact, for a very large trial where the probability of extreme imbalance is very low, the probability of *perfect* balance is also low. This means that if we regard a prognostic factor as being important, then since we have claimed that balance is a question of efficiency, a design which was perfectly balanced as regards this prognostic factor would *never* be less efficient than a randomized design and would nearly always be more efficient.

However, balancing patients in a clinical trial is not always an easy matter. For a given prognostic factor, one way of achieving balance is by stratification. For example, if we wish to balance numbers by sex we can maintain two randomization lists, one for females and one for males. Whether to stratify or not is a practical issue which many trialists have to face. From the inferential point of view there are few disadvantages. If a given factor is regarded as being prognostic and if therefore (as it probably ought to be) the factor is to be included in the model for analysis, that analysis will be more efficient if the levels of the factor are equally distributed between the treatments. (This does not require, for example, that there be equal numbers of males and females in the trial, simply that the males shall be divided equally between treatment and control and the females also.) Nevertheless, stratification does introduce a complication into running clinical trials and it is not possible to do it for all factors deemed prognostic. This has led some trialists to propose the technique of minimization as a means of allocating treatments.

6.2.5   Minimization

Some critics of randomization (those who have never actually planned any trials) appear to adhere to a 'freeze – thaw' theory of clinical trials: patients may be put into cold storage and warmed up when the trial is ready to start. If this were possible one could divide the patients into very well-matched groups for treatment. As it is, patients require treatment when they present. Therefore if one wishes to balance patients by some characteristic one has to do so on an ongoing basis as they are recruited consecutively. In principle, this can be done by stratification. In practice it becomes rather difficult to handle if there are more than one or two prognostic factors for which one wishes to balance. An alternative is to assign the next patient in a way which minimizes imbalance and according to some score which reflects the current distribution of factors. An informal approach to balancing for prognostic factors, known as minimization, was proposed by Taves (1974) and Pocock and Simon (1975) and an approach which combines the unpredictability of Efron's biased coins approach but which, by making explicit and formal use of the effect of balance in prognostic factors on the variance of the treatment estimate, is generally more efficient than minimization, has been proposed by Atkinson (1982). In what follows we illustrate Taves's minimization.

> **Minimization**: A curious form of arithmetic in which apples are added to pears to produce turkeys.

For example, consider a placebo-controlled trial of a long-acting beta-agonist in asthma where we wish to balance patients by sex and use of steroids as a concomitant medication. Suppose that we have been using minimization and that 60 patients have been recruited to date and that the position is as given in Table 6.3.

Now the 61st patient can be of one of four types: MS, MN, FS, FN. For the purpose of allocating him or her we ignore the cross-classification and take the relevant factors singly. Taking the single factors, we add up the numbers of the given type in each treatment group. The position is as given in Table 6.4. The 61st patient would now be allocated to the group with the lowest score. Thus, a male steroid user (MS) would be

Table 6.3   Example 6.1: Disposition of patients in a clinical trial of asthma by treatment and by sex and by concomitant steroid use.

Sex	Treatment		Total
	Beta-agonist (A)	Placebo (B)	
Male (M)	16	14	30
Female (F)	14	16	30
Total	30	30	60
Concomitant medication			
Steroid (S)	20	19	39
No steroid (N)	10	11	21
Total	30	30	60

Table 6.4 Minimization scores for four types of patient who might be recruited as the 61st patient for Example 6.1.

Treatment	MS	MN	FS	FN
Beta-agonist	36	26	34	24
Placebo	33	25	35	27

allocated placebo, as would a male non-steroid user (MN). Both types of female patient (FS and FN) would be allocated to the beta-agonist.

For handling continuous covariates (in this case, for example, one might be interested in baseline FEV_1) some prespecified dichotomization could be employed. Alternatively, one could use (say) the median value to date and note how many in each group were less than or greater than this. (It is also possible that some scheme could be developed which actually worked on the mean values in the groups but, if we wish to take the issue seriously then the approach of Atkinson (1982) is available.) The minimization procedure is usually started off by assigning the first patient at random. Where, during the subsequent course of minimization, the score is tied between groups, one has to have some alternative means of proceeding. One could, of course, use a rule such as, 'always divide arbitrarily in the opposite direction to the last arbitrary division', but it would probably be more usual to have prepared a randomization list in advance to deal with such cases. Useful accounts of minimization are given by Pocock (1983) and Matthews (2006).

In analysing such a trial one would then include steroid use and sex in the model for analysis. Of course, as already explained, one could include sex and steroid use in the model for analysis in the randomized trial in any case. The advantage of the minimized trial would be that the degree of balance would generally be greater and therefore analysis would be more efficient. In order to get some impression of the potential utility of this, one may compare the efficiency of a trial which is *perfectly* balanced with the *expected* efficiency under randomization. The efficiency of the minimized trial would then be expected to lie somewhere between the two. Thus the perfectly balanced trial gives the limit of what may be achieved by minimization. If we consider the case where a continuous covariate will be fitted, and take the perfectly balanced trial to have a variance of 1, then it may be shown that the randomized trial with equal numbers n in the two treatment groups has an expected variance of $1 + 1/(2n - 4)$. Figure 6.1 provides a plot of the variance against n. It can be seen that as the sample size grows, the advantage of the minimized trial in this respect diminishes rapidly.

As has been argued above, minimization should not be used as a justification for ignoring prognostic factors in analysis. The controversy with minimization is whether or not the fact that one has adjusted for the prognostic covariate adequately reflects the restriction on allocation it imposes. Consider the simple case where one simply wishes to balance the numbers in a trial. The trialist who sees no value whatsoever in randomization could agree to use some patterned scheme such as choosing between ABBAABBA etc. or BAABBAAB etc. at random to start off. (Let us call this *purposive* allocation.) The trialist who concedes some value to randomization could randomize every pair of patients, one to A and one to B (in fact, use the method of randomised blocks with a block size of 2.) In the first case there are only 2 allocations possible, in the second case there are 2^n. However, neither of these two numbers is as large as the total number of allocations, $(2n!)/(n!n!)$ which permits equal balance and both, for

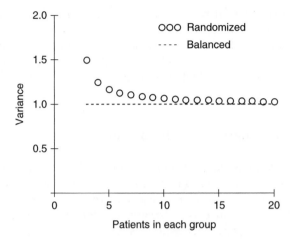

Figure 6.1   Efficiency of a randomized trial compared with a perfectly balanced one.

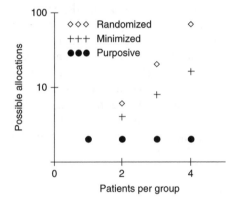

Figure 6.2   Possible allocations as a function of the number of patients in each treatment group for three approaches to balancing numbers. (Note that the vertical scale is a log-scale.)

example, would arbitrarily exclude schemes such as AAABBBBA which also satisfy the requirements for balanced numbers. Figure 6.2 shows a plot of the number of allocations possible as a function of the number of patients n in each group for randomization and the two other schemes discussed here.

Whether such arbitrary restrictions form a disadvantage for minimized designs is a hotly debated point. Some regulatory statisticians, for example, have expressed their reservations in print (Day *et al.*, 2005). Minimized designs are more open to manipulation. For example, in an open trial, by keeping track of the patients so far allocated, the trialist might be able to work out to which group a given patient would be assigned. Suppose that the experimental group is indicated. Then if the trialist considered that the patient had an unfavourable prognosis she might be tempted not to recruit the patient but wait for a further patient to present. Also, because the treatment allocation is less rich, the protection offered by blinding is not as great. The theoretical basis for randomization and certain nonparametric tests (that is to say, tests which use the actual randomization as a basis for inference) would also be lacking. It is a controversial point whether these constitute real or imagined disadvantages for the minimized design. It is also debated, however, whether minimization brings any real advantages compared to randomization (Senn, 2004), although some statisticians are enthusiastic about the possible advantages (Buyse and McEntegart, 2004). Thus we have an example of a genuine unresolved issue.

6.2.6   Superior alternatives to minimization

A further issue concerning classical minimization is that it is not actually based on sound design principles. The minimization score is an ad hoc sum of marginal totals. As already argued, the sole purpose of balance is to increase the efficiency of the treatment estimate. A standard result in classical regression theory states that the variance – covariance matrix of the parameter estimates is proportional to $(\mathbf{X}'\mathbf{X})^{-1}$, where $\mathbf{X}$ is the so-called design matrix, the matrix of covariates and treatment indicators. Now consider the case where a new patient arrives and is to be allocated a treatment. The covariates for this patient are what they are, but the final form of $\mathbf{X}$ once this patient has been allocated a treatment will be slightly different depending on whether the patient is given placebo (say) or verum. For each of these two cases the resulting $(\mathbf{X}'\mathbf{X})^{-1}$ matrix will be slightly different and if we are particularly interested, as we surely will be, with the diagonal element of this matrix that provides the multiplier for the variance of the treatment estimate, then all we need to do is calculate for which of the two cases this element will be smaller and allocated the patient accordingly.

This, essentially, is the proposal of Atkinson (1982). Unlike minimization it is not arbitrary but targets directly the criterion that is needed to ensure optimization. Given that it is trivial with modern computing power to implement this algorithm, there seems no point in using classical minimization.

6.2.7   Cut-off designs

It has been proposed that not all patients may be prepared to accept the risk of being allocated an experimental treatment, perhaps because of fear of side-effects, but that those who are more severely ill may be prepared to run this risk. It may be that the moderately ill patients have a treatment which, while far from perfect, is adequate, whereas those who are severely ill get inadequate relief. That being so, physicians may object to randomizing the moderately ill but be prepared to allocate the severely ill to treatment. A form of design which has been proposed under such circumstances is the cut-off design (Trochim and Cappelleri, 1992). Here moderately ill patients are assigned the standard treatment. The more severely ill may be randomized to experimental or standard treatment and the most severely ill will be given the experimental treatment. In the cut-off design, this allocation is done on the basis of an observed covariate. This might be the baseline measurement on the outcome variable of interest, but this is not essential. Figure 6.3 illustrates the position for a trial of hypertension in which baseline blood pressure is used to allocate patients to treatment.

In the cut-off trial there are then three 'regions' for allocation. If the middle randomized region is eliminated so that the two outer regions meet, we then have the extreme example of a cut-off design, the regression discontinuity design. In analysing the cut-off

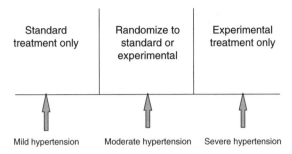

Figure 6.3   Schematic representation of a cut-off design.

design, since a covariate has been used as the basis of allocation, it follows, of course, that the covariate must be included in any model for analysis (see Chapter 7.) Various assumptions are necessary concerning the relationship between the outcome and the covariate. One that is **not** necessary is that the covariate used for assignment be measured without error: provided that one adjusts for the measured covariate there is no problem. It is also **not** necessary to adjust for further covariates which are correlated with the covariate, X, used for assignment (or at least, it is no more necessary than for any other design): this is because such further covariates are only confounded with the treatment allocation to the extent that they are correlated with the covariate used for allocation, so that adjusting for this covariate adjusts for the others to the extent that it is necessary to do so.

It is necessary, however, that the functional relationship between covariate, X, and outcome, Y, be correctly modelled. Consider, for example, allocating patients in an AIDS trial to treatment on the basis of a CD4 count being below some threshold k. This is equivalent to allocating them on the basis of $\log X$ being less than $\log k$, or X^3 being less than k^3 and so forth. (Any transformation which preserved the ranking of the X values would do.) Each of these rules would give the same allocation of patients. If we have to take account of each rule, however, we should have to model all these relationships, which would be impossible. In practice we use one only, the most common choice being the straightforward linear rule. Just how strong the necessary assumptions are may be seen by realizing that the allocation rule effectively uses the indicator function, $I(X)$ where, for the regression discontinuity design, $I(X)$ takes on just two values depending upon whether $X < k$ or $X \geq k$. But the indicator function itself is perfectly confounded with treatment, so that if we were to adjust for the indicator function it would be impossible to estimate the treatment effect. Therefore, contrary to what is sometimes supposed, adjusting for X is *not* equivalent to adjusting for the allocation mechanism. The equivalence instead is dependent on the assumption that the indicator variable's effect on outcome can be estimated from the effect of X on outcome within each group.

A further problem with cut-off designs is that they preclude any serious attempt at blinding treatment. Without the unpredictability of allocation which randomization provides, there can be no truly blinded trial. This in turn makes employment of a placebo also impossible, or at least futile. If anything, the ethical problems of using placebos would be even greater than for a run-in. One could hardly claim that it was

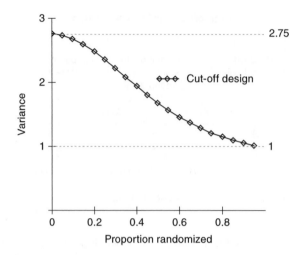

Figure 6.4   Variance of a symmetric cut-off design as a function of the randomized proportion of patients.

unethical to allocate an experimental treatment to patients unless they were severely ill but at the same time be prepared to withhold from moderately and severely ill patients alike whether they were receiving a placebo or an experimental drug! Hence any patients on placebo in such a trial would have to be informed that they were taking this.

None of this means that cut-off designs will never deliver a valid estimate of the treatment effect but, unfortunately, the difficulties above are not the only problems. There is also a cost in efficiency. Figure 6.4 gives the large-sample variance of the treatment estimate for a symmetric cut-off design compared to the corresponding randomized design with variance 1. The middle portion of patients is supposed randomized in equal numbers to experimental and control treatment, and the proportion of patients in the upper tail deliberately assigned to experimental treatment (say) is the same as the proportion in the lower tail deliberately assigned to the control treatment. The variance of the design is plotted as a function of the middle randomized proportion. As this proportion increases to 100%, the design becomes a completely randomized design. For a middle proportion of zero, the design is a regression discontinuity design and it can be seen from the figure that for such a design the variance is about 2.75 times as great as for a randomized design.

This considerable inefficiency also undermines the ethical argument in favour of a regression discontinuity design. Suppose a randomized design would require 200 patients but we accept that only the severely ill may be given the experimental treatment. We could then run a randomized trial in which 100 severely ill patients were given the experimental treatment and 100 such patients were given the control. This device would then meet head-on the criticism that the less severely ill may not be used to test a potentially dangerous experimental treatment. If, on the other hand, we run a regression discontinuity trial with equal power, we shall have to allocate 275 severely ill patients to the experimental treatment and 275 less ill patients to the control treatment. Thus, to give any ethical room whatsoever for the regression discontinuity would require the further moral constraint that severely ill patients must not be given the control treatment. This might apply if patients were so ill that they demanded the experimental treatment because it represented their only hope. In practice, however, the potential patients for a clinical trial form a very small subset (from a limited number of centres) from all patients of a similar condition. It then becomes rather strange to maintain that it is ethically unacceptable to offer a given patient half a chance of receiving an experimental therapy but perfectly acceptable to offer many more (those not in collaborating centres) no chance at all.

In fact, it is very difficult to find circumstances in which the regression discontinuity design can win the ethical argument against the randomized design. Suppose that $2n$ patients are to be recruited to a randomized design comparing an experimental treatment, E to a standard therapy, S. Suppose that all patients suffering from the disease are potential candidates for the trial and that half (by definition) are severely ill and half less so. Two possible randomized designs are considered, R1 and R2, and as a third alternative, a regression discontinuity design, D. For R1 $2n$ patients of both sorts will be randomized irrespective of severity, n to each of E and S. For R2 again $2n$ patients will be randomized but they will all be severely ill. (The patients not randomized will not be recruited to the trial but will, of course, be given the standard therapy, S.) For D, $2.75n$ severely ill patients will be given E and $2.75n$ fewer ill will be given S. Suppose, just for argument's sake, that as soon as the results are known the patients will be switched to the superior treatment, which may, of course, prove to be either E or S. Table 6.5 gives the total number of patients allocated to the inferior treatment for each of the three possible designs and each of the two eventualities.

It then follows that the only circumstance under which more patients are allocated to the inferior treatment under randomization than using a regression discontinuity design is if R2 rather than R1 is used and if the experimental treatment is eventually proved superior. Under those circumstances $0.25n$ more patients will have been allocated to the inferior treatment under randomization. If, on the other hand, the conventional treatment proves superior, then $1.75n$ patients will have been allocated to the inferior treatment by using the regression discontinuity design. The comparative advantage for the randomized design in the one case to the regression discontinuity design in the other is thus $1.75n:0.25n$ or 7 to 1. Now one might, of course, maintain that one carries out clinical trials expecting the experimental treatment to be superior (although I would maintain that it is really a hope rather than an expectation), in which case this apparent 7 to 1 disparity for the regression discontinuity design represents reasonable odds to accept. However, if one is so confident of success, it seems rather odd to maintain that it is unethical to randomize the less ill, and if it is not unethical to do so then we are able to use R1 rather than R2, in which case the regression discontinuity design is never superior.

Table 6.5 Number of patients allocated to the inferior treatment by trial design and eventual outcome.

	Trial design		
Eventual outcome	**R1**	**R2**	**D**
S superior	n	n	$2.75n$
E superior	n	$3n$	$2.75n$

6.2.8   Comprehensive cohort designs

There are occasions when patients will be offered the opportunity to enter a clinical trial and to be randomized to treatment and will refuse, but nevertheless then be faced themselves with deciding between the treatments to be compared. For example, the indication might be breast cancer and the choice might be between mastectomy and conservative treatment. Such a situation would be extremely rare in drug development but it might conceivably occur in a phase IV trial comparing two marketed products. If patients who refuse to be randomized are nevertheless followed up (this would also be unusual unless the condition were life-threatening) and will in any case choose one of the two treatments being compared, then data are available for two treatments for two types of patients: randomized and non-randomized. Olschewski *et al.* (1992) have named this type of trial a 'comprehensive cohort' design.

For such a design, provided each treatment is chosen by some patients who refuse randomization, it then becomes possible to obtain treatment estimates for the random-ized and non-randomized patients. If these are compared and found to be different, there are then two possible opposing interpretations. The first is that the randomized patients are an unrepresentative group of the whole as regards their response to treatment. (The treatment estimate from the randomized group lacks external validity.) The second is that the two non-randomized treatment groups are not comparable to each other from the outset and that this disparity cannot be corrected for by analysis. (The treatment estimate from the non-randomized group lacks internal validity.) To decide between these two interpretations would be very difficult in any given situation.

If one holds to the view that clinical trials are a means of determining what the treatment can do not what it will do, then the evidence from the non-randomized group will be regarded as largely irrelevant. If, on the other hand, one takes a more 'representative' view of clinical trials, then one might argue that the results from the non-randomized patients must also be considered. (Note, however, that these patients taken alone are also not representative so that some pooled compromise between the two estimates would be needed.)

Using estimates from non-randomized patients requires a strong assumption. It is tempting to analyse the problem in terms of an initial choice between randomization and no randomization and to allow for the effect of *this* choice, for the effect of treatment and for some interaction between the two. (It is the interpretation of this interaction which forms the controversy.) If instead we regard the patients as having chosen randomization, or treatment A or treatment B, then only for the randomized group is the effect of treatment capable of being separated from the effect of *choice* of treatment without making prior assumptions. (Of course, if the effect of a treatment cannot be separated from the effect of choosing it, this separation is in any case of no practical relevance. The point is, rather, that patients of a given type may have chosen a given treatment but they could in principle be persuaded to choose differently if provided with knowledge about the true effects of a treatment.)

Quite apart from any other obstacles which lie in the way of their being adopted, comprehensive cohort designs are unlikely to become important in drug development for the reasons that there are few circumstances in which a patient refusing randomization is likely to be faced with a choice between a drug in development and a standard therapy and, furthermore, could then be followed up. Nevertheless, such designs raise issues which are worth considering.

6.2.9   'Play the winner' and 'bandit' designs

As we have already seen, the ethical paradox of randomized clinical trials is that future patients may expect to benefit from the knowledge gained but that not all current patients (those allocated to the inferior treatment) will. Such designs also invite a rather strict operational separation between the patients currently being treated and those who will be treated at some future stage once the new drug has been registered (if it proves successful). An alternative approach would be to make no such distinction and run trials as if one wished to minimize the number of patients allocated to the inferior treatment (including those allocated to the trial) over some plausible future horizon.

Suitable trials are so-called 'bandit designs' (Berry and Eick, 1995), named after a problem in gambling which may be stated thus. *You are faced with a casino which contains a number of one-armed bandits. each has an unknown and possibly different pay out rate. Given a certain amount of time to play, what strategy should you adopt?* Three possible strategies would be: (1) Move around the casino playing one coin in each bandit until you find one which pays out, then stick with this forever afterwards no matter what happens. (2) Play each of the bandits a number of times no matter what the result (in other words also play losing bandits) in order to estimate accurately what the pay-out rate is for each bandit and then play the best. (3) Always move on to the next bandit when you have lost on the current one, but stick with any bandit for as long as you win on it. Obviously, the first strategy risks sticking with a bandit which, just by chance, happened to perform well once and is unlikely to do so again, whereas the second risks losing a great deal of money before choosing the best bandit, and the third is rather short sighted: previous wins are ignored and only the most recent counts.

A trial which is somewhat in the spirit of the third strategy above is the so-called 'play the winner' trial. Here one requires some definition of a successful treatment. The first patient to be treated can be allocated at random; thereafter, the same treatment will be used until a failure is encountered. Thus in a trial comparing two treatments (A and B) in which the first patient had received B, the following sequence of successes (S) and failures (F) would be matched by the accompanying sequence of treatments:

B	B	B	A	A	A	A	A	B	B	A	B	B
S	S	F	S	S	S	S	F	S	F	F	S	

Obviously, such a design will, in the long run, tend to allocate more patients to the successful treatment. In fact, if θ_A is the probability of success on treatment A and θ_B is the probability of success on treatment B, then, for a large trial, the expected proportion of patients allocated to A will be $P_A = (1 - \theta_B)/(2 - \theta_A - \theta_B)$. So, for example, if the probability of success with treatment A were 0.8 and that with treatment B were 0.4, so that $\theta_A = 0.8$ and $\theta_B = 0.4$, then the proportion of patients allocated to the superior treatment, A, would be 0.75 and the proportion allocated to the inferior treatment would be 0.25. The overall proportion of successes for such a trial would be $0.75 \times 0.8 + 0.25 \times 0.4 = 0.7$. This may be compared to the proportion of successes for a randomized group trial with equal numbers on each treatment, which is clearly $(0.8 + 0.4)/2 = 0.6$.

Note, that these proportions are true in the long run. If a clinical trial is stopped after a short while and all future patients are then allocated to the treatment which has proved best so far, with no option to reverse this policy, then the randomized trial may be expected to perform better, because it will estimate the true advantage more accurately by virtue of studying equal numbers under both treatments and will thus have a lower probability of making a mistake about the superior treatment.

If, however, some sort of adaptive design *is* wanted, then 'play the winner' is a poor choice. Nothing much is learned by this design, since, even where a treatment has notched up a string of successes, a single failure would lead to the alternative treatment being tried, even though this might previously have led to failure every time it was used. The allocation system has a very short memory and the expected future proportion of patients who will be allocated to the superior treatment is almost the same after a few patients as it is after many. A logical strategy would be expected to allocate more patients to the more successful treatment as knowledge of the treatments was gained. There is a theory of clinical trials which permits such a strategy and this is the theory of bandit designs.

Among the controversial issues which arise with bandit designs are the following. (1) A strategy which is optimal for treating a large number of future patients is not necessarily optimal for treating the next patient. For example, a Bayesian analysis of patients treated so far might lead us to conclude that our best estimate of which of A and B is superior is B. This suggests that if we are only interested in what is best for the next patient, that patient should be treated with B. It may be, however, that although we believe that B is better than A, we are not very confident that this is so, in particular because very few patients have been treated with A. In that case it might be of more interest for future patients if we study A in order to define its effects more precisely. To the extent that such policies are adopted, such designs do not entirely avoid the ethical difficulties associated with randomization. (2) Blinding becomes extremely difficult for such designs. (3) Effectively an absolute definition of success is needed. We have already discussed that the effect of treatment is to be judged counterfactually: we compare what happened to what would have happened. In a randomized trial the control group helps us to do this, but we have to accept that we cannot judge for a single patient whether the treatment was effective and can only judge whether it was so for at least some members of the group. For 'play the winner' and 'bandit' designs, however, we need to be able to judge the success of the treatment on a case-by-case basis. Suppose that there is a secular improvement over time. For a randomized design this will not cause a problem because we shall continue to study both treatments over time. For other sorts of design, however, we may be stuck with one treatment without realizing that the other treatment would also do well. A good investigation and discussion of various sorts of bias which may arise in operating adaptive designs is given by Bather (1992).

A further practical problem in running such designs is that the intervals at which patients arise may not permit one to determine the outcome of all previous treatments when deciding the current one. A suitable modification can deal with this. More serious is the fact that a binary outcome is required and this may force an arbitrary dichotomization. In principle this too could be overcome.

6.2.10   Problems with blinding

In Chapter 3, blinding was discussed briefly and it was explained that there are occasions where for practical reasons trials cannot be run in a completely blinded fashion. For example, if we wish to compare two different treatments as regards compliance then

Table 6.6 A possible schedule for a trial with double dummy loading.

Time	Treatment A	Treatment B
Morning	Verum A	Placebo to A
	Placebo to B	Verum B
Evening	Placebo to A	Placebo to A
	Placebo to B	Verum B

there are very many circumstances under which running the trial in a blinded fashion might eliminate the advantage one treatment might have compared to another. Suppose that we are comparing two treatments for hypertension, one to be given once daily (A) and the other twice daily (B). It is plausible, other things being equal, that the less onerous schedule of administration of A may lead to greater compliance. However, to fully blind the trial would require dummy loading so that patients being given A were treated twice daily also. In practice double dummy loading would be used so that the two schedules might be as in Table 6.6.

Clearly this arrangement eliminates any advantage in schedule of A. Similar problems arise when comparing treatments in which the route of administration is different: for example, oral forms with suppositories.

It may have to be accepted, therefore that there are certain purposes of clinical research for which blinding is inappropriate. The trial must either be run in an open fashion or 'veiled' (Senn, 1995b) as discussed in Chapter 3. In the example above we could create four treatment groups by adding two placebo regimes. The first would consist of placebo to A given once daily and the second of placebo to B given twice daily. Patients would then know which regime they were on but not whether they were receiving active treatment or placebo. To be fully blinded, the comparison of A and B would have to proceed via a double contrast of each active treatment with its own placebo and these differences would then be compared with each other. As discussed in Chapter 3, this procedure entails a considerable increase in variance. This double contrast might be appropriate if the trial were also being used for the purposes of making a classic therapeutic comparison between A and B. However, for the purpose of examining compliance itself, this would be inappropriate and a direct comparison of A and B would be needed.

The addition of extra placebo patients adversely affects efficiency and there are many circumstances under which it should be accepted that the most sensible course is to run the trial in an open fashion. It may be possible to include other safeguards such as blinded review of certain outcomes, but the fact that the most sensible design for some practical and economic 'phase IV' type questions is an open-label study is probably insufficiently appreciated.

References

Atkinson AC (1982) Optimum biased coin designs for sequential clinical trials with prognostic factors. *Biometrika* **69**: 61–67.

Bailey AL (1931) The analysis of covariance. *Journal of the American Statistical Association* **26**: 424–435.

Bather J (1992) Response adaptive allocation and selection bias. In: Flournoy N, Rosenberger WF (eds), *Adaptive Designs*. Institute of Mathematical Statistics, Hayward, CA.

Berger VW, Rezvani A, Makarewicz VA (2003) Direct effect on validity of response run-in selection in clinical trials. *Controlled Clinical Trials* **24**: 156–166.

Berry DA, Eick SG (1995) Adaptive assignment versus balanced randomization in clinical trials: a decision analysis. *Statistics in Medicine* **14**: 231–246.

Brittain E, Wittes J (1990) The run-in period in clinical trials. The effect of misclassification on efficiency. *Controlled Clinical Trials* **11**: 327–338.

Buyse M, McEntegart D (2004) Achieving balance in clinical trials. *Applied Clinical Trials* **13**: 36–40.

David HA (1995) First(questionable) occurrence of common terms in mathematical statistics. *American Statistician* **49**: 121–133.

Day S, Groulin J-M, Lewis JA (2005) Achieving balance in clinical trials. *Applied Clinical Trials* **14**: 24–26.

Efron B (1971) Forcing a sequential experiment to be balanced. *Biometrika* **58**: 403–417.

Matthews JNS (2006) *An Introduction to Randomized Clinical Trials*. Arnold, London.

Olschewski M, Schumacher M, Davis KB (1992) Analysis of randomized and nonrandomized patients in clinical trials using the comprehensive cohort follow-up-study design. *Controlled Clinical Trials* **13**: 226–239.

Pocock SJ (1983) *Clinical trials, A Practical Approach*. John Wiley & Sons, Ltd, Chichester.

Pocock SJ, Simon R (1975) Sequential treatment assignment with balancing for prognostic factors in controlled clinical trial. *Biometrics* **31**: 103–115.

Schechtman KB, Gordon ME (1993) A comprehensive algorithm for determining whether a run-in strategy will be a cost-effective design modification in a randomized clinical trial. *Statistics in Medicine* **12**: 111–128.

Senn SJ (1994) Testing for baseline balance in clinical trials. *Statistics in Medicine* **13**: 1715–1726.

Senn SJ (1995a) Base logic: baseline balance in randomized clinical trials. *Clinical Research and Regulatory Affairs* **12**: 171–182.

Senn SJ (1995b) A personal view of some controversies in allocating treatment to patients in clinical trials [see comments]. *Statistics in Medicine* **14**: 2661–2674. [Comment in *Statistics in Medicine* **15**(1): 113–116 (1996)].

Senn SJ (1997) Are placebo run ins justified? *British Medical Journal* **314**: 1191–1193.

Senn SJ (2001) The misunderstood placebo. *Applied Clinical Trials* **10**: 40–46.

Senn SJ (2002) Ethical considerations concerning treatment allocation in drug development trials. *Statistical Methods in Medical Research* **11**: 403–411.

Senn SJ (2004) Added values: controversies concerning randomization and additivity in clinical trials. *Statistics in Medicine* **23**: 3729–3753.

Senn SJ (2005) Baseline balance and valid statistical analyses: common misunderstandings. *Applied Clinical Trials* **14**: 24–27.

Taves DR (1974) Minimization: a new method of assigning patients to treatment and control groups. *Clinical Pharmacology and Therapeutics* **15**: 443–453.

Trochim WM, Cappelleri JC (1992) Cutoff assignment strategies for enhancing randomized clinical trials. *Controlled Clinical Trials* **13**: 190–212.

6.A TECHNICAL APPENDIX

6.A.1 The variance of a completely randomized design as a function of the proportion of patients in each treatment group

Consider a two parallel group randomized clinical trial. Let σ^2 be the variance of individual outcomes. Let n_1 be the number of patients in the first group and n_2 be the number in the second group. The mean in the first group has variance σ^2/n_1 and that in the second group has variance σ^2/n_2. Since these means are independent, the difference between the two means has variance

$$\sigma^2 \left(\frac{1}{n_1} + \frac{1}{n_2} \right). \tag{6.1}$$

If there are N patients in total and the proportion in group 1 is p, then $n_1 = Np$ and $n_2 = N(1-p)$. Substitution for n_1 and n_2 in (6.1) yields the variance

$$\sigma^2 \left(\frac{1}{Np} + \frac{1}{N(1-p)} \right). \tag{6.2}$$

6.A.2 The efficiency of randomized, minimized and cut-off designs

In order to compare the efficiency of the designs (as opposed to approaches to analysis) we assume that the same analysis, namely analysis of covariance, will be used in all three cases. For the cut-off designs we shall assume that we are allocating treatment on the basis of an observed baseline, and for the minimized design that we are using some allocation mechanism which reduces the disparity in this baseline. (See also Chapter 7 for discussion of efficiency and analysis of covariance.)

Assume that we have a trial comparing an experimental treatment with a control treatment with equal numbers, $n_1 = n_2 = n$, of patients in the two groups. Let X be a baseline with variance σ_X^2 and let Y be an outcome of interest. Let x be the difference between X and the mean of X over both treatments. Let σ^2 be the conditional variance of Y given X. Let t be an indicator variable with $t = 1/2$ in the experimental group and $t = -1/2$ in the control group.

We are interested in estimating the treatment effect, τ (which we assume is constant for all patients given treatment) using analysis of covariance. The variance of the treatment estimate is

$$\mathrm{var}\,(\hat{\tau}) = \frac{2\sigma^2}{n} \frac{\sum x^2}{\sum x^2 - 2 \left(\sum tx \right)^2 / n.} \tag{6.3}$$

The variance (6.3) may thus be factorized into two parts. The first, $A_1 = \left(2\sigma^2/n \right)$, is common for any distribution of covariates of baseline and, since it is a function of the conditional variance of Y given X, reflects the *general* consequence of including X in our model. The second factor, $A_2 = \left\{ \sum x^2 - 2 \left(\sum tx \right)^2 / n \right\}$, depends on the *actual observed* distribution of the covariate. A_2 may also be written as

$$A_2 = \left\{ \left(\sum x^2 \frac{-2 \left(\sum tx \right)^2}{n} \right) + \frac{2 \left(\sum tx \right)^2}{n} \right\} \Big/ \left(\sum x^2 \frac{-2 \left(\sum tx \right)^2}{n} \right)$$

$$= 1 + \left(\frac{2 \left(\sum tx \right)^2}{n} \right) \Big/ \left(\sum x^2 - 2 \frac{\left(\sum tx \right)^2}{n} \right). \tag{6.4}$$

Note that if $\sum tx = 0$, $A_2 = 1$. Otherwise $A_2 > 1$. Now

$$\sum tx = \frac{n\bar{x}_t}{2} + (-n\bar{x}_c/2) = \frac{n\bar{x}_t}{2} + \frac{n\bar{x}_t}{2} = n\bar{x}_t. \qquad (6.5)$$

Hence, the condition that $A_2 = 1$ reduces to the condition that the mean deviations in the two groups are identically zero, or equivalently, that the means in the two groups are identical. This is perfect balance. For anything less than perfect balance, a penalty in efficiency is paid. We are now in a position to discuss the relative efficiency of our three designs: the randomized clinical trial, the minimized clinical trial, and the cut-off trial.

Obviously, the degree of imbalance observed in a randomized clinical trial will vary randomly. On average the difference at baseline between groups will be zero. This does not imply, however, that the average value of A_2 will be 1. A_2 is, in fact related to familiar quantities from the analysis of variance: the numerator of the second term is simply the between sum of squares and the denominator is the within sum of squares for a one-way layout with n observations in each group. Since the sum of squares between has one degree of freedom, it is equal to the mean square between, MSB, whereas the within sums of squares has $2(n-1)$ degrees of freedom and hence is $2(n-1)$ MSW, where MSW is the mean square within. Hence,

$$A_2 = 1 + \frac{\text{MSB}/\text{MSW}}{2n - 2}. \qquad (6.6)$$

However, for a Normally distributed baseline, MSB/MSW is an F variable with 1 and $2n - 2$ degrees of freedom. Since the mean of an F variable with denominator degrees of freedom ω, is $\omega/(\omega - 2)$, in this case the mean is $2n - 2/(2n - 4)$. Hence, $E[A2] = 1 + 1/(2n - 4) = (2n - 3)/(2n - 4)$.

For a minimized trial $1 \le E[A_2] \le (2n - 3)/(2n - 4)$. Thus for reasonably large trials, the gain in efficiency compared with randomized trials is negligible and may not offset the other losses (loss in blinding, inferential problems and so forth).

Now suppose that a group of patients is included in a clinical trial because they have measured values in excess of some threshold k. We then have $X > k$. X now has a *truncated* Normal distribution. Let $\phi(u)$ be the probability density function of a standard Normal distribution and $\Phi(u)$ be the distribution function (cumulative density function). Let $a = (k - \mu)/\sigma_X$ and $Z = (X - \mu)/\sigma_X$, then $P(X > k) = P(Z > a) = 1 - \Phi(a)$. Now, if $x < k$ then $P(X = x \text{ and } X > k) = 0$; on the other hand, if $X > k$ then $P(X = x \text{ and } X > k) = f(x)$. Hence, if $F(X)$ is the distribution function of X it follows from the general definition of conditional probability whereby $P(B|A) = P(A\&B)/P(A)$ that the conditional distribution of X given $X > k$ is $f(X)/\{1 - F(k)\} = \phi(Z)/\{1 - \Phi(a)\}$. Hence

$$E[X/X > k] = \int_k^\infty Xf(X)\,dX/[1 - F(k)]$$

$$= \int_a^\infty (Z\sigma + \mu)\phi(Z)\,dZ \bigg/ [1 - \Phi(a)]$$

$$= \mu + \sigma\phi(a)/[1 - \Phi(a)]. \qquad (6.7)$$

Now, if we wish to study the efficiency of a symmetric randomized cut-off with patients allocated to control, randomization, or experimental treatments according to $Z < -a$, $-a \leq Z \leq a$ or $Z > a$, then we simply need to substitute $\mu = 0$ and $\sigma = 1$ in (6.6) to obtain the expected mean standardized baseline values in the extreme experimental groups. (The expected value in the middle group is, of course, 0 and the value in the lower group is simply the negative of that in the upper.)

However, if we look at *all* patients receiving experimental treatment, then we will expect to find that half of those in the randomized portion will receive it also. In fact, half of all patients will receive the experimental treatment and, since $1 - \Phi(a)$ will receive it because their baselines are extreme, the fraction of all patients receiving it who have extreme baseline values is $1 - \Phi(a)/(1/2) = 2\{1 - \Phi(a)\}$. The expected mean value for randomized patients is zero, hence, from (6.6), the expected mean value for patients receiving experimental treatment is simply

$$E(\bar{x}_t) = \frac{2\{1 - \Phi(a)\}\phi(a)}{1 - \Phi(a)} = 2\phi(a)\sigma_X. \tag{6.8}$$

Now from (6.5) and (6.8), $E[\sum tx] = 2n\phi(a)\sigma_X$, from which $E\left[2(\sum tx)^2 / n\right] = 8n\{\phi(a)\}^2\sigma_X^2$. However, the total sum of squares is not affected by having adopted a cut-off design. Therefore, if the sum of squares between are increased by a certain amount, the sum of squares within must be reduced by the corresponding amount. Hence, since

$$E\left[\left\{\sum x^2 - 2(\sum tx)^2 / n\right\}\right] + E\left[2(\sum tx)^2 / n\right] = \sigma_x^2(2n - 1),$$

$$E\left[\left\{\sum x^2 - 2(\sum tx)^2 / n\right\}\right] = \sigma_x^2\left[(2n - 1) - 8n\{\phi(a)\}^2\right].$$

Allowing that since the denominator is always positive, then for large n the expectation of the ratio of these quantities will be approximately equal to the ratio of the expectations and is thus

$$E[A_2] \approx 1 + \frac{8n\{\phi(a)\}^2}{2n - 1 - 8n\{\phi(a)\}^2}$$

which for large n further simplifies to

$$E[A_2] \approx 1 + \frac{8n\{\phi(a)\}^2}{2n - 8n\{\phi(a)\}^2},$$

$$\approx 1 + \frac{4\{\phi(a)\}^2}{1 - 4\{\phi(a)\}^2} \tag{6.9}$$

$$\approx \frac{1}{1 - 4\{\phi(a)\}^2}.$$

However,

$$\phi(a) = \frac{\exp(-a^2/2)}{\sqrt{2\pi}}. \tag{6.10}$$

Substituting (6.10) in (6.9) we obtain

$$E[A_2] \approx \frac{1}{1 - 2\exp(-a^2)/\pi}. \tag{6.11}$$

For $a = 0$, which corresponds to the extreme case of a cut-off design in which no patients are randomized (the regression discontinuity design), $E[A_2] \approx 2.75$. For $a = \infty$ we have a completely randomized design and $A_2 \approx 1$.

6.A.3   The proportion of patients allocated to the superior treatment in a 'play the winner' trial

We shall use a mixture of two slightly different approaches to find a solution. Consider two treatments A and B with probability of success θ_A and θ_B respectively, and let us suppose, for argument's sake, that $\theta_A > \theta_B$. If we let S stand for success and F stand for failure and regard each combination of treatment and outcome as a success, then we can represent the trial as a Markov chain with states AS, AF, BS and BF and transition matrix, **M**, as given in expression (6.12):

$$\begin{array}{c} & & \textbf{Initial State} \\ & & \begin{array}{cccc} \text{AS} & \text{AF} & \text{BS} & \text{BF} \end{array} \\ \textbf{Final State} & \begin{array}{c} \text{AS} \\ \text{AF} \\ \text{BS} \\ \text{BF} \end{array} & \begin{bmatrix} \theta_A & 0 & 0 & \theta_A \\ 1-\theta_A & 0 & 0 & 1-\theta_A \\ 0 & \theta_B & \theta_B & 0 \\ 0 & 1-\theta_B & 1-\theta_B & 0 \end{bmatrix} \end{array} \tag{6.12}$$

We wish to find the n-step transition matrix as n goes to infinity. Let us now introduce a second argument. Consider the expected run length, ERA, with treatment A, when we have just had a patient who has failed with treatment B. This is given by the sum of $1 \times (1-\theta_A) + 2 \times \theta_A(1-\theta_A) + \cdots + n \times \theta_A^{n-1}(1-\theta_A) \ldots$ and is $\text{ERA} = 1/(1-\theta_A)$. Similarly, the expected run length when we have just given a patient treatment B must be $\text{ERB} = 1/(1-\theta_B)$. From this, we deduce that the proportion of patients given A is

$$P_A = \text{ERA} \big/ (\text{ERA} + \text{ERB}) = \frac{1-\theta_B}{2 - \theta_A - \theta_B}. \tag{6.13}$$

The proportion of patients given B, P_B, is similarly deduced and is in any case $1 - P_A$.

This is our solution, which we may now check as follows. Since we know the conditional probabilities of success or failure given the treatment, we simply multiple these by P_A and P_B as appropriate to find the column vector, **D** of steady state probabilities for the four states:

$$\mathbf{D}' = \frac{1}{2 - \theta_A - \theta_B} [(1-\theta_B)\theta_A, \quad (1-\theta_B)(1-\theta_A), \quad (1-\theta_A)(\theta_B), \quad (1-\theta_A)(1-\theta_B)] \tag{6.14}$$

We may confirm this solution by checking that **MD** equals **D**, which it does. Hence **D** is the required steady-state solution we are seeking. It follows that (6.13), which is the sum of the first and second elements of **D**, is the solution we require for the proportion of patients allocated A.

The probability of success (unconditional as regards to treatment) for any patient, is given by the sum of the first and third probabilities and is

$$\frac{\theta_A + \theta_B - 2\theta_A\theta_B}{2 - \theta_A\theta_B}. \tag{6.15}$$

This may be compared with the corresponding figure for a standard randomized design, which is clearly $(\theta_A + \theta_B)/2$. The difference between (6.15) and this is

$$\frac{(\theta_A - \theta_B)^2}{2(2 - \theta_A - \theta_B)}, \tag{6.16}$$

which, clearly, is never negative.

Baselines and Covariate Information

There are others, again, who will draw a man's character from no other helps in the world, but merely from his evacuations; but this often gives a very incorrect outline, – unless, indeed, you take a sketch of his repletions too; and by correcting one drawing from the other, compound one good figure out of them both.

Laurence Sterne, *Tristram Shandy*

7.1 BACKGROUND

The 'bare bones' controlled clinical trial consists of two treatments, a set of patients, an allocation rule and some measured outcomes. This is all that is *necessary* to investigate the effect of a treatment. However, it is frequently the case that useful background information can be obtained by measuring various characteristics of the patients before the trial starts. These measurements may be of three sorts: (1) so-called demographic characteristics of the patient which are either unchanging (such as sex) or change only slowly (such as height) or at the same rate for all patients (such as age) during the course of the trial; (2) proper 'baselines': measurements before treatment of the outcome variable; (3) baseline correlates: measurements taken at outset which may be expected to vary during the course of the trial, but which are not on the same variable as that used to measure outcome. These distinctions are largely arbitrary, and indeed, from the statistical point of view all three can be regarded simply as covariates. However, physicians sometimes give the proper baseline a particular significance in defining effects. For a trial in which more than one outcome is being measured (which is the norm) a variable can be in category 2 for one analysis and in category 3 for another: for example, airways resistance (RAW) and peak expiratory flow (PEF) measured at baseline in a trial in which both are being used to determine efficacy. For some outcomes, in particular survival, no proper baseline can be defined, although I suppose one could regard age, which is otherwise a category 1 variable, as survival to date. (Alternatively, we could regard age at death as the outcome variable and survival from randomization to treatment as the outcome corrected by age at time of randomization.) I shall use the term 'covariates' to cover all three types of variable.

This particular heading is one under which many (but not all) of the issues are not controversial among statisticians. It is rather that statisticians have not always succeeded in persuading physicians of their point of view. Both statisticians and physicians are generally agreed on the value of such baseline information. The issues are to do with ways of using it.

A technique which statisticians favour for dealing with continuous covariates is analysis of covariance. This is a method of adjustment for variables analogous to stratification. Indeed, if a binary covariate is fitted using analysis of covariance it produces the same treatment estimate as stratifying on that covariate. Hence 'analysis of covariance' is a term which is used generally by statisticians to cover all forms of adjustment for covariates, even dichotomous ones. Of course, true stratification could also be adapted for continuous covariates. For example, in a placebo-controlled trial of a beta-agonist in 160 asthmatics (80 in each arm) we might calculate the median peak expiratory flow (PEF) at baseline for all patients (the median over both groups). We might then consider a cross-classification of patients as in Table 7.1.

Depending on the randomization, a would be some number between 0 and 80 but in practice generally close to 40. Where a is not equal to 40 the trial is not perfectly balanced as regards the constructed dichotomous variable, but this can easily be adjusted for by comparing like with like: constructing a treatment estimate for the high PEF stratum and one for the low PEF stratum and then combining the two. Of course, even within strata the mean values of PEF could differ between treatment groups and, indeed, even where the groups were balanced with respect to median PEF and a was equal to 40, mean PEF could be different at baseline from group to group. Analysis of covariance is an analogous way of controlling for such *means* rather than according to *numbers* in a given artificially constructed stratum.

A diagramatic representation of analysis of covariance is given in Figure 7.1. Outcomes are plotted against baselines for two treatment groups. The baselines are very different from one group to the other and would correspond to a regression discontinuity design (see Chapter 6) rather than a randomized trial. Nevertheless, in theory, even in a randomized trial this sort of difference could arise (with extremely small probability) and the diagram serves to make the point. The estimate of the treatment effect is given by the difference between the two lines at the mean value of the baseline and is thus an attempt to answer the question: 'if both groups had had average overall baseline values, what treatment difference would we have seen?'. Since the lines are presumed parallel, this difference at the overall mean is the same as the difference of the lines at any point, including the origin: It is thus equal to the difference in intercepts.

Table 7.1 Numbers of patients in a clinical trial of asthma cross-classified by baseline PEF and treatment given.

		Treatment		
		Placebo	**Beta-agonist**	**Total**
Baseline compared to median	**High PEF**	a	$80 - a$	80
	Low PEF	$80 - a$	a	80
	TOTAL	80	80	160

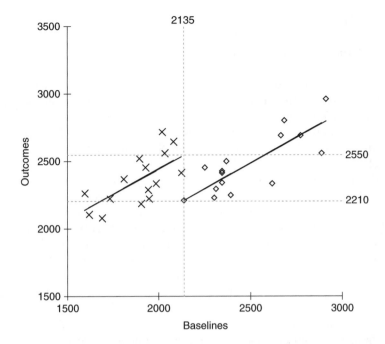

Figure 7.1 Baselines and outcomes for FEV_1 in ml for a two-parallel-group trial in asthma. The control group values are indicated by diamonds, the treatment values by crosses. The estimated treatment effect (about 340 ml) is given by the difference between the two fitted lines.

It is also possible in an analysis of covariance to adjust outcomes using individual slopes rather than a postulated common slope. This is not my usual habit in analysing trials and unless I state so specifically I shall not include this further refinement under the heading of analysis of covariance. This point is discussed in section 7.2.7 below. Stratification and analysis of covariance, when carried out on strongly prognostic factors, not only adjust for observed imbalances but even where (in fact especially where) such factors are balanced, bring with them a strong reduction in variance of the estimated treatment effect and a consequent increase in power.

Finally, it is perhaps worth mentioning one slight difference between analysis of covariance fitting a binary covariate and stratifying on the covariate. As mentioned above, the treatment estimates are identical. However, the variance estimates are not quite the same. Consider a simple example of a two-armed clinical trial with n patients in each of the four possible cross-classifications of binary covariate and treatment, so that there are $4n$ patients in total. Analysis of covariance will fit an overall intercept, a treatment effect and a covariate effect, leaving $4n - 3$ to estimate variability. Stratification will fit an intercept and treatment effect for each stratum, leaving $2n - 2$ degrees of freedom for error for each stratum and hence $4n - 4$ degrees of freedom in total, one fewer than for analysis of covariance. This missing degree of freedom corresponds to the treatment-by-stratum interaction and, indeed, if this interaction is fitted the residual variance will be identical to stratification. However, when an interaction is fitted the definition of a main effect is partly arbitary and one has to proceed with care. See Senn (2000) and also section 7.2.7 and Chapters 14 and 16 for further discussion.

7.2   ISSUES

7.2.1   'Testing' for baseline balance

Hardly a statistician of repute can be found to defend the practice common among physicians of comparing the treatment groups in a randomized clinical trial at baseline using hypothesis/significance tests on covariates. The reason for the statistician's dislike is that such a test appears to be used to say something about the adequacy of the *given allocation* whereas it could only be a test of the allocation *procedure*: the randomization process itself.

If the test of baseline balance *is* used to say something about the allocation procedure, then its use is unexceptionable. Berger has argued persuasively that statisticians have been too complacent about the possibility that the randomization procedure may be subverted by treating physicians or other parties (Berger, 2005a, b). In my view, it must then be accepted that the purpose of such a test is that of quality control: the trial either passes or it is rejected as being unusable (Senn, 2005b). It cannot, in that case, form part of the general strategy for *analysing* a trial. However, this is precisely what frequently happens: the baseline test of balance is used to decide whether and which covariates should be used to adjust the treatment effect. In the remainder of this section, this use will be discussed.

A hypothesis test is an attempt to say something about a 'deep structure': either a population from which a given sample has been drawn, or a set of outcomes associated with possible allocations of treatment to patients from which a given allocation has been chosen, or some general probabilistic process which is postulated to give rise to a given data set. When, for example, one compares two ACE inhibitors at outcome as regards diastolic blood pressure and one notes that the difference is 'significant', one is saying that the difference seems to be rather large if chance is the only explanation and that therefore one prefers to suppose that chance is *not* the whole explanation. In a carefully controlled experiment, the conclusion then goes beyond the observation that results are different from one treatment group to another, to the inference that the treatment must be having an effect on the outcomes.

However, randomization *is* a chance mechanism. Therefore, if at baseline we conclude that the observed difference is greater than we care to believe may be attributed to chance, we shall have to conclude that randomization has not taken place (or that the values have been disturbed since). In fact, trialists are most reluctant to agree this conclusion. Consequently, they accept that when a significant result occurs, it is a type I error. They then go further, however, and take the result as being some comment on the adequacy of the sample. This is an abuse of the procedure (Altman, 1985; Senn, 1994c, 1995a).

It should also be noted that if the object of a test of significance is to guard against the ill effects of chance imbalance, it cannot do this. A covariate could pass a test of baseline balance and yet the probability of declaring a significant result at outcome (using a nominal 5% level) for an ineffective treatment given the observed degree of imbalance could be nearly 50% (Senn, 1994c).

In short, the test of baseline balance is a misuse of the significance test. The fact that it is frequently performed does not constitute a defence any more than the fact that antibiotics are commonly employed to 'treat' viral infections proves that they are effective antivirals. And the fact that baseline tests are commonly performed without much apparent harm is no more of a defence than saying of the policy of treating colds with antibiotics that most patients recover. It should be noted, that testing for baseline balance is often *perceived* as being a regulatory requirement. However, the European statistical guidelines do not condone the practice.

7.2.2 Balance and randomization

This point was discussed in Chapter 3, where it was shown that balance is not necessary for correct inference. Stratification as illustrated in section 7.1 and/or analysis of covariance can be used to deal with the distribution of observed covariates. The point is rather that the standard methods of statistical analysis make an *average* allowance for covariate imbalance. This average allowance is not perfect but it is logically adequate where no further information is available (Senn, 2005a).

However, my view is that if and when further covariate information comes to light the average allowance is no longer adequate: for trials which are more balanced than the average, inferences are likely to be too conservative, whereas for those which are more unbalanced than average, they are likely to be too liberal (Senn, 2005a). Analysis of covariance is an appropriate way for the frequentist to deal with covariate information. Corresponding approaches may be used by Bayesians. However, as regards unobserved covariates, both Bayesians and frequentists are left with the average allowance. The question then arises whether this average allowance is appropriate. The answer is, in my view, that it *is* appropriate provided that randomization has been employed. This then is the value of randomization. It enables appropriate inferences to be made given that important *unmeasured* prognostic factors may exist.

7.2.3 Will simple analysis of change scores deal with imbalance?

A popular outcome measure with trialists is the difference from baseline, or the *change score* (outcome−baseline). It is sometimes supposed that using a score defined in this way without further adjustment ('simple analysis of change scores') will deal with imbalance in a proper baseline variable. This is incorrect. Consider the case of a trial in blood pressure. If patients in one group in a trial of hypertension have a higher baseline measurement for systolic blood pressure on average than patients in another, then we should expect, other things being equal (including treatment effects) that they would also have a higher systolic blood pressure at trial outcome. We should not, of course, expect the difference between groups to be exactly the same at outcome as at baseline: although the correlation between the two is positive it is not, in general, unity.

It turns out, however, that because the correlation between baseline and outcome is generally less than 1, the correlation between baseline and change score is generally negative. It thus follows that an observed difference between groups at baseline is predictive not only of a difference in raw outcomes but also of a difference in change scores (albeit in the other direction). Hence, if the treatment is at an unfair *disadvantage* compared to placebo when its effects are measured in raw outcomes (owing to an imbalance in baselines), it will have an unfair *advantage* if change scores are used. The solution is to use analysis of covariance. Analysis of covariance produces a measure which is adjusted by baseline in such a way that the result is uncorrelated with the baseline. Usually this corresponds to subtracting a fraction between 0 and 1 of

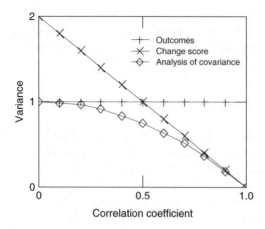

Figure 7.2 Variance of three estimators as a function of the correlation coefficient where the variances of baselines and outcomes are the same.

the baseline from the outcome measure, and under such circumstances the analysis of covariance estimator lies between the simple analysis of change score and raw outcomes estimators.

The analysis of covariance estimator also has the advantage that its variance is generally lower than that using raw outcomes or simple analysis of change scores. Figure 7.2 takes the case where the variances of baselines and outcomes are equal and plots the variance of the three estimators as a function of the correlation between baseline and outcome. It will be seen that the analysis of covariance estimator is everywhere superior to the other two and that the change-score estimator is actually inferior to raw outcomes (which is a constant whatever the correlation coefficient) unless the correlation is greater than 0.5.

7.2.4 Is clinical relevance a relevant consideration when choosing whether to use change scores or raw outcomes as the efficacy measure?

In this context, clinical relevance is a red herring as the following arguments show.

(1) If clinical relevance were to have something to do with the issue, then any difference in the results observed, according to whether change scores or raw outcomes were used, ought to have something to do either with some property of the treatment being studied, or with the disease, or with the patients recruited, or with all three. This is not the case. It is a property of chance only. If we define the treatment effect as being the difference treatment − placebo, then for any trial in which the baseline values are higher in the treatment group the measure based on raw outcomes will be higher than that based on change scores, whereas if baselines are higher in the placebo group the reverse will be the case, and for the ideal trial, in which baselines were perfectly balanced, *the answer would be the same.* If one used these measures in a long series of trials, in some trials one would be greater and in other trials the other and on average they would give very similar

results. In fact, using raw outcomes, change scores or analysis of covariance gives exactly the same answer in the long run. The *expected* values of these measures are identical for a randomized trial: the issue is really 'which measure is the most reliable?'.

(2)　The answer is 'analysis of covariance'. If we employ analysis of covariance using the baseline as a covariate, it makes absolutely no difference whether our measure is raw outcomes or change scores. Formally, as regards the estimate of the treatment effect and its standard error, exactly the same result is produced (Laird, 1983). Hence, provided analysis of covariance is employed, the whole debate is rendered irrelevant.

(3)　The treatment can only affect the outcomes. It cannot affect the baselines. If the treatment has had an effect, then it has affected the difference in outcomes between the two groups. The only function that the baselines could possibly fulfil would be to guide our inference as to what this difference would have been in the absence of any difference in the effects of the treatment. However, it remains true that it is the difference at outcome that has been affected by the treatment.

(4)　Suppose that a physician is unimpressed by these arguments and insists that he wishes to use change scores for measuring the treatment effect. Suppose that we are running two trials in order to satisfy the FDA requirement. I offer him the following bet. We are each to predict from the first trial on the basis of our preferred measures (change score in his case and analysis of covariance in mine) what the result (active − placebo) will be in the second trial, and, in order to make the bet especially interesting to him, I shall offer him a concession. The effect we shall try to predict in the second trial will be as defined using the change scores. I will use analysis of covariance to predict change score effects and he will use change scores to predict change score effects. Whoever gets the closer prediction wins, the stakes to be even. Should he accept? No. I have an odds-on chance of winning!

7.2.5　Can baselines be used to define effects?

We saw in Chapter 3 that they cannot. The effect of a treatment is the difference between what happens when treatment is given and what would have happened had treatment been denied. In controlled clinical trials we choose to measure differences between the effects of treatments: the effect of giving a verum rather than a placebo. Difference from baseline cannot be used to *define* an effect. This does not mean that it cannot be used to *measure* an effect. It can be so used if we strongly believe that the baseline value is the value we would have seen had treatment been denied. However, the very fact that we feel it is necessary to carry out a clinical trial means that we lack this confidence.

7.2.6　Should percentage change from baseline be used as a measure?

The popularity of this measure is difficulty to justify. It is unlikely to have very good distributional properties for the purpose of statistical analysis. If it is believed that the treatment effect is likely to be multiplicative, so that it will induce a percentage change in the counterfactual difference, for example by increasing FEV_1 by 15% above the level it would have had, then a log transformation is desirable. If baseline information is to be incorporated in the analysis, then a logarithmic transformation of the baselines should be employed and they should be fitted in an analysis of covariance.

7.2.7 Can analysis of covariance be used if the relationship between baseline and outcome is not constant from one treatment group to another?

It would certainly make analysis of covariance easier to interpret if the slopes of outcome on baseline were the same from treatment group to treatment group. If this is not the case it is evidence that the treatment effect is not simply additive on the chosen scale: that the treatment may have a different effect depending on the baseline value. Note, however, that this is just as much of a problem for other approaches. The change score approach also assumes that the relationship between outcome and baseline is identical from treatment group to treatment group. Therefore, if the treatment effect is different depending on the level of the baseline then the single answer which an analysis of outcomes only would produce is just as misleading and also less precise than a single answer based on analysis of covariance. To object to using analysis of covariance on these grounds and then resort instead to an analysis of raw outcomes or change scores is like saying 'crossing the English Channel in a rowing boat is dangerous, I prefer to swim'. In any case, the analysis of covariance estimator will nearly always lie between the estimator based on raw outcomes and that based on change scores. To be prepared to accept either of these two while criticizing analysis of covariance would be a most peculiar position to defend.

It should also be noted that under a null hypothesis of strict equality of the treatments there can be no treatment by baseline interaction, although it is conceivable that a chance imbalance could occur and that patients who react in one sort of way could have ended up in one group rather than another. This particular possibility does not strike me as worth worrying about.

However, care must be taken when using analysis of covariance and fitting a baseline-by-treatment interaction. It is dangerous to fit such a model unless you have first centred the baselines by subtracting the overall mean value. This is because otherwise the treatment effect is estimated at the covariate origin which, for uncentred values, is a baseline value of zero (in many cases this corresponds to a dead patient!). In fact it is probably safer always to centre the baselines anyway. This ensures that the origin is at the mean baseline value and hence that a treatment effect at the origin (the intercept) is the same as that for the average patient. A nice example of how including interactions in a model can easily lead to inferential confusion is given by Chuang-Stein and Tong (1996) and further discussed by Senn (2000). (This example is discussed more fully in Chapter 14.) It is probably prudent to follow the advice given in ICH9 (International Conference on Harmonisation, 1999) and fit a model without interactions as the primary analysis.

7.2.8 What should we do when we have more than one covariate?

Analysis of covariance can be used to adjust for a number of covariates. Since we are only really interested in the effect of treatment on outcome, it is not important to be able to identify the individual effects of various covariates (except perhaps to gain intelligence for the planning of future trials) and it is simply the joint effect of them all which is important. A useful feature of the randomized clinical trial is that, although covariates are often heavily confounded with each other, they are rarely strongly confounded with treatment. This means that a reduction in variance is usually to be gained by fitting covariates.

Nevertheless, the more covariates that are collected the greater the chance of accidental confounding. Strong confounding with the treatment effect will lead to an increase in the variance of the estimated treatment effect and, in the absence of any further wisdom to inform our analysis, it would be right and proper that it did so. If we had good reasons *a priori* for believing that a given factor, for example birth sign, had no effect on outcome, however, we would be foolish to run the risk of paying the penalty to which an unthinking algorithm for estimation must inevitably be subject when covariate and treatment group are confounded. In my opinion, the wisest course open to the frequentist is to make a list, prior to looking at the outcomes, of covariates suspected to be important and to fit these regardless.

A special case arises where we have repeated measures of a proper baseline. The mean of these is likely to be more strongly correlated with the outcome than any single measure and will also show a lower degree of confounding with treatment than the most confounded of the various measurements on which it is based. There will usually be little value in fitting these measurements separately and the mean may be used instead. Frison and Pocock have investigated this approach in detail and found it to be valuable (Frison and Pocock, 1992). An exception might be when the interval between baseline measurements is fairly long compared to the interval to outcome. It is possible that one could then correct not only for the observed baseline level of patients but also for a trend in baselines. For the case with two baselines, fitting the mean and the difference of the baselines would be formally equivalent to fitting them both separately. Another way of looking at this particular point is to say that if within-patient errors follow some sort of autoregressive process, then more recent baselines will be more highly predictive than earlier ones. It might then be inefficient to fit a mean of them all and wiser to fit them separately. It will usually be inappropriate to fit the last baseline only, however.

This issue is examined in more detail in the technical appendix (Section 7.A). See also Bristol (2007) for simulation results.

7.2.9 The fact that covariates can be correlated with each other causes a problem for analysis of covariance

This is sometimes maintained. In fact this is not really a problem as long as – which is likely to be the case in a clinical trial – the main focus of interest is the effect of treatment. Consider a trial consisting of old women and young men. Obviously we shall not separate the effect of sex and age very well and estimates of their effects will have very high variances. However, the joint effect of age and sex may be very successfully estimated and provided that the experimental treatment and control are both well represented in the two demographic groups, we shall estimate the effect of treatment well and if the response is different in the two demographic groups there will be value in having sex and age in the model.

7.2.10   Does the fact that baselines are measured with error invalidate analysis of covariance?

Some statisticians have maintained that it does (Chambless and Roeback, 1993), but this is wrong in the context of the randomized clinical trial (Senn, 1994a,b, 1995b). The randomized trial permits a valid analysis even where no baselines are measured. If we take the Bayesian view, however, that information cannot be ignored, then when we have measured some covariate we have obtained information we must act on. Instead of using an analysis which corresponds to a probability-weighted average over all possible distributions of the covariate, we must replace it with one which corresponds to the particular distribution observed. However, we are only required to condition on what is observed and what we have observed is the observed covariate!

The false argument which is often produced starts from the true observation that if a factor is measured with error, the relationship of an outcome with that factor will be attenuated. The simplest example is treatment itself. If some of the patients have been allocated to the wrong treatment it is clear that, unless we correct for this error, we shall underestimate the difference between groups. Similarly, if blood pressure at baseline is measured with error then we shall underestimate the influence of 'true' blood pressure on outcome. Therefore, it is argued, if we correct for an observed imbalance in blood pressure at baseline, we shall under-correct because the coefficient by which we shall correct will be too small. This conclusion is false because it implicitly assumes that the true mean difference in blood pressure at baseline must be the same as the observed difference or at the very least that it has the same expectation. In fact, if blood pressure is measured with error the variance of observed blood pressure must be higher than the variance of true blood pressure. Hence, since the mean of both over all randomizations is zero, it follows that on average, given an observed difference, the true difference must be smaller (that is to say, closer to zero). It turns out that this further attenuation compensates exactly for the attenuation in the relationship between outcomes and baselines and therefore that analysis of covariance using observed baselines is not only adequate but better than attempts to improve it.

> Measuring the effect of a drug as the difference between an outcome and a baseline established after the start of treatment is like measuring how high an athlete can jump from the top of his head. It gives midgets a sporting chance but it is no way to run the Olympics.

7.2.11   When is a baseline not a baseline?

A baseline is not a baseline when it is measured after the start of treatment and may itself reflect the effect of treatment. Where this is the case, adjusting for such baselines, whether by simple differencing to produce change scores, or by forming a ratio or by analysis of covariance can be extremely misleading. Unfortunately, there are areas

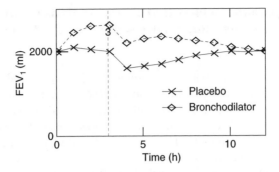

Figure 7.3 Time course of FEV$_1$ for a provocation test in asthma comparing a bronchodilator in which the challenge is given three hours after the start of treatment.

where this practice is common. For example, in trials of asthma to investigate the so-called late-phase or slow reaction patients are frequently given a provocation test after treatment has been initiated (Senn, 1989). Figure 7.3 illustrates a possible time course for such an experiment comparing a bronchodilator to a placebo. FEV$_1$ values are frequently expressed as a percentage drop from the control value taken just before the provocation test is administered. That this can be very misleading, however, is not hard to see and is illustrated in Figure 7.4. Where two treatments are being compared, given a large enough trial and given that the effects of treatments are reversible, the absolute values in FEV$_1$ must eventually come together. If, however, the percentage drop measure is studied, they will never come together, if there is an appreciable difference at the time that the control value is taken, because it simply reflects the treatment effect at that time in inverse form. (The higher the control value, the greater, other things being equal, the size of the drop.)

This illustrates the general problem with using late baselines. They remove part of the treatment effect and this can yield surprising results.

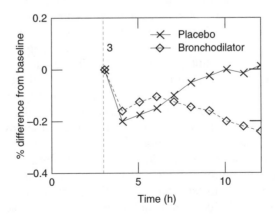

Figure 7.4 The results from the experiment shown in 7.3 expressed as percentage difference from a 'baseline' measured just before provocation but three hours after treatment.

7.2.12   Lord's paradox implies that where analysis of covariance and change from baseline analyses disagree the former cannot be trusted

Although most statisticians accept the arguments we have proposed here, that analysis of covariance will appropriately deal with an observed imbalance in true baselines but the simple analysis of change scores will not, some have advanced the contrary argument that unlike the simple analysis of change scores it will produce biased estimates (Liang and Zeger, 2000; Samuels, 1986). To understand the argument we make a slight diversion to consider Lord's paradox.

In a disturbing paper in the *Psychological Bulletin* in 1967, Lord considered a case where two statisticians analysing a data set come to radically different conclusions (Lord, 1967). We adapt the example here to the context of a clinical trial. Consider a two-armed trial in hypertension with diastolic blood pressure (DBP) as the outcome variable. Now suppose that in each arm the DBP at outcome is the same as it was at baseline but that the baseline values differ considerably from one arm to another. If a within-patient test of the difference between outcome and baseline is carried out for each arm, neither of these tests will be significant since each difference is zero. It also follows, of course, that since a two-sample t-test of the change scores will be comparing two mean differences of zero it will also be nonsignificant. Now suppose, however, that we carry out an analysis of covariance. The regression of outcome on baseline is likely to be less than 1. Thus the difference at outcome, which is the same as the difference at baseline, will only be corrected by a fraction of the difference. In consequence, the corrected difference will not be zero and may, indeed, be significant. This is Lord's paradox.

Some have taken this to mean that analysis of covariance is biased when the baseline difference is not zero (Liang and Zeger; 2000, Samuels, 1986). But it is trivial to construct counterexamples where this is not the case. Suppose that we design a bizarre clinical trial in which we only recruit patients in two strata: those with a DBP of 95 mmHg and those with a value of 100 mmHg, values between or outside these limits being excluded. Now suppose that in the first stratum we randomize patients 3:1 placebo to verum and that in the second stratum we randomize them 1:3 and that we have 400 patients in each stratum. An unbiased estimate can be produced by stratification, that is to say by comparing the 300 placebo patients in the first stratum to the 100 verum patients, the 100 placebo patients to the 300 verum patients in the second stratum, and averaging these two results. However, the treatment estimate will be exactly the same as that which would result by using the baseline value as a covariate. On the other hand, simply comparing all 400 patients under verum to all 400 under placebo in terms of change score will most definitely not produce an unbiased estimate.

Further useful discussion of Lord's paradox will be found in Holland and Rubin (1983) and Wainer and Brown (2004). Suffice it to say here that although there are certainly some epidemiological studies for which analysis of covariance will not deal appropriately with baseline imbalance, for controlled clinical trials, including nonrandomized designs such as the regression discontinuity design discussed in Chapter 6, analysis of covariance is an appropriate approach to adjustment. On the other hand, there are almost no circumstances under which this claim could be made for the simple analysis of change scores. The implicit assumption that is being made in assuming that the simple analysis of change scores will produce an unbiased estimate is that the difference that would be seen at outcome in the absence of any treatment effect is the difference that was observed at baseline. This ignores the regression effect. In a randomized clinical trial the regression is towards zero, the average difference over all randomizations, and it turns out that analysis of covariance estimates this regression effect appropriately. In other sorts of study the situation may be more complex and there will certainly be many data sets encountered in epidemiology for which neither analysis of covariance nor simple analysis of change scores would produce an unbiased estimate of the causal effect of treatment. However, for clinical trials, ANCOVA is appropriate.

Further discussion will be found in Senn (2006) and in Van Breukelen (2006).

7.2.13 The propensity score is a superior alternative to adjusting for confounders than analysis of covariance

In an influential paper in *Biometrika*, Rosenbaum and Rubin discussed the possibility of using what they called the propensity score for adjusting for confounders (Rosenbaum and Rubin, 1983). The idea is that a stratification be made on the probability of assignment to treatment or control as a function of covariates. In a classic randomized clinical trial, of course, the probability of assignment to either group is 1/2 irrespective of any covariate. The philosophy of the propensity score would then be that there is but a single stratum, that with score 1/2, and so no adjustment is necessary. This is, of course, equivalent to the familiar argument that for a classic randomized trial no adjustment is necessary.

In the bizarre example of the previous section, allocation to verum occurs with probability 1/4 if the baseline DBP is 95 mmHg and 3/4 if DBP is 100 mmHg and so the propensity score takes on these two values. Thus, the philosophy of stratifying by the propensity score agrees perfectly with the argument we propounded there: that adjustment using these strata (or equivalently using analysis of covariance) was indicated.

Nevertheless, it is my view that the propensity score is both superfluous and misleading. Essentially my position is that there is nothing more and beyond analysis of covariance, which dictates that we must adjust for covariates because they are predictive of outcome not because they are predictive of assignment. Consider, for instance, a clinical trial in asthma with two strata at randomization according to whether patients are currently on steroids or not, and suppose that the outcome variable was FEV_1, which one would usually analyse using a linear model. If the allocation ratio, which would most commonly be 1:1, were the same in the two strata then the treatment estimate would be the same whether or not one stratified the analysis. The propensity score would be the same for the two strata and this would suggest that according to that philosophy no adjustment was required. However, if as might plausibly be the case, FEV_1 were different between the two strata, the standard error of the overall treatment estimate would be quite different depending on whether or not steroid use was in the model. The philosophy of analysis of covariance, which chooses factors that are predictive of outcome, would have it in the model. The propensity score philosophy, which chooses factors that are predictive of assignment, would not. In my view this is a mistake.

Thus, I do not accept that the propensity score is a useful alternative to analysis of covariance. In my opinion it will produce either similar or inferior inferences.

7.2.14   The fact that the precise relationship between covariate and outcome is unlikely to be linear makes analysis of covariance unusable

One sometimes encounters this claim, but it is illogical. As John Tukey put it, 'Adjustments are not expected to be perfect – they are only supposed to help!' (Tukey, 1993, p. 273). Suppose that the true relationship between covariate and outcome is some nonlinear function. It is extremely likely that a linear approximation to this relationship will be better than nothing. One can always regret the fact that the adjustment that has been carried out is less than perfect, but as an approximation to the 'truth' a linear adjustment is likely to be better than nothing. Hence, imperfection in adjustment cannot be grounds for rejecting adjustment altogether.

Too little use is probably made in the analysis of clinical trials of various possible smooth adjustments. For example, as a superior alternative to forming different age groups of patients such as ≤ 45, 46–55, 56–65, 66–74, ≥ 75, and then stratifying the analysis, various smooth adjustment procedures could be considered. In making sure that regulatory confidence is maintained, an important consideration is that the adjustment procedure can be prespecified and, if necessary, repeated. Fitting *b*-splines of age would satisfy these requirements here. Some suitable modelling techniques are discussed by Harrell in his excellent book (Harrell, 2001). The point is that the relationship between covariate and outcome is not itself of direct interest. It just needs to be modelled in a way that increases understanding of the relationship between treatment and outcome and the precision with which this is estimated.

If, on the other hand, it is feared that the outcome itself will not be Normally distributed conditional on the fitted model and a suitable generalized linear model cannot be found, then various mixed strategies permit one to perform a partial adjustment and then proceed to a nonparametric analysis (Koch *et al.*, 1998; Lesaffre and Senn, 2003).

References

Altman DG (1985) Comparability of randomized groups. *Statistician* **34**: 125–136.

Berger VW (2005a) Quantifying the magnitude of baseline covariate imbalances resulting from selection bias in randomized clinical trials. *Biometrical Journal* **47**: 119–127.

Berger VW (2005b) *Selection Bias and Covariate Imbalances in Randomized Clinical Trials*. John Wiley & Sons, Ltd, Chichester.

Bristol DR (2007) The choice of two baselines. *Drug Information Journal* **41**: 57–61.

Chambless LE, Roeback JR (1993) Methods for assessing difference between groups in change when initial measurements is subject to intra-individual variation. *Statistics in Medicine* **12**: 1213–1237.

Chuang-Stein C, Tong DM (1996) The impact of parametrization on the interpretation of the main-effect terms in the presence of an interaction. *Drug Information Journal* **30**: 421–424.

Frison L, Pocock SJ (1992) Repeated measures in clinical trials: analysis using mean summary statistics and its implications for design [see comments]. *Statistics in Medicine* **11**: 1685–1704.

Harrell FE (2001) *Regression Modeling Strategies*. Springer, New York.

Holland PW, Rubin DB (1983) On Lord's Paradox. In: Wainer H, Messick S (eds), *Principles of Modern Psychological Measurement*. Lawrence Erlbaum Associates, Hillsdale, NJ.

International Conference on Harmonization (1999) Statistical principles for clinical trials (ICH E9). *Statistics in Medicine* **18**: 1905–1942.

Koch GG, Tangen CM, Jung JW, Amara IA (1998) Issues for covariance analysis of dichotomous and ordered categorical data from randomized clinical trials and non-parametric strategies for addressing them. *Statistics in Medicine* **17**: 1863–1892.

Laird N (1983) Further comparative analyses of pre-test post-test research designs. *The American Statistician* **37**: 329–330.

Lesaffre E, Senn S (2003) A note on non-parametric ANCOVA for covariate adjustment in randomized clinical trials. *Statistics in Medicine* **22**: 3583–3596.

Liang KY, Zeger SL (2000) Longitudinal data analysis of continuous and discrete responses for pre-post designs. *Sankhya – The Indian Journal of Statistics Series B* **62**: 134–148.

Lord FM (1967) A paradox in the interpretation of group comparisons. *Psychological Bulletin* **66**: 304–305.

Rosenbaum PR, Rubin DR (1983) The central role of the propensity score in observational studies for causal effect. *Biometrika* **70**: 41–55.

Samuels ML (1986) Use of analysis of covariance in clinical trials: a clarification. *Controlled Clinical Trials* **7**: 325–329.

Senn SJ (1989) The use of baselines in clinical trials of bronchodilators. *Statistics in Medicine* **8**: 1339–1350.

Senn SJ (1994a) Methods for assessing difference between groups in change when initial measurement is subject to intra-individual variation [letter; comment] [see comments]. *Statistics in Medicine* **13**: 2280–2285.

Senn SJ (1994b) Repeated measures in clinical trials: analysis using mean summary statistics and its implications for design [letter; comment]. *Statistics in Medicine* **13**: 197–198.

Senn SJ (1994c) Testing for baseline balance in clinical trials. *Statistics in Medicine* **13**: 1715–1726.

Senn SJ (1995a) Base logic: baseline balance in randomized clinical trials. *Clinical Research and Regulatory Affairs* **12**: 171–182.

Senn SJ (1995b) In defence of analysis of covariance: a reply to Chambless and Roeback [letter; comment]. *Statistics in Medicine* **14**: 2283–2285.

Senn SJ (2000) The many modes of meta. *Drug Information Journal* **34**: 535–549.

Senn SJ (2005a) Baseline balance and valid statistical analyses: common misunderstandings. *Applied Clinical Trials* **14**: 24–27.

Senn SJ (2005b) Quantifying the magnitude of baseline covariate imbalances resulting from selection bias in randomized clinical trials – Comment. *Biometrical Journal* **47**: 133–135.

Senn SJ (2006) Change from baseline and analysis of covariance revisited. *Statistics in Medicine* **25**: 4334–4344.

Tukey JW (1993) Tightening the clinical trial. *Controlled Clinical Trials* **14**: 266–285.

Van Breukelen GJ (2006) ANCOVA versus change from baseline had more power in randomized studies and more bias in nonrandomized studies. *Journal of Clinical Epidemiology* **59**: 920–925.

Wainer H, Brown LM (2004) Two statistical paradoxes in the interpretation of group differences: Illustrated with medical school admission and licensing data. *American Statistician* **58**: 117–123.

7.A   TECHNICAL APPENDIX

7.A.1   Concerning change scores, raw outcomes and analysis of covariance

Consider a two parallel group study comparing a verum to a placebo and employing simple randomization and suppose that the treatment effect, τ, is additive. Let $X_{i,t}$ and $Y_{i,t}$ be a baseline and an outcome respectively for the ith patient in treatment group t, where $t = \text{v}$ for verum and $t = \text{p}$ for placebo. Suppose that there are n_v patients in the verum group and n_p in the placebo group. Construct a score $D_i(b) = Y_{i,t} - b\, X_{i,t}$, where b is some constant. Any estimator of the treatment effect of the form

$$\hat{\tau}(b) = \bar{D}_{.v}(b) - \bar{D}_{.p}(b) = (\bar{Y}_{.v} - \bar{Y}_{.p}) - b(\bar{X}_{.v} - \bar{X}_{.p}) \qquad (7.1)$$

is unbiased over all randomizations. Some special cases of (7.1) include $\hat{\tau}(0)$, the treatment estimate based on outcomes alone and $\hat{\tau}(1)$, the simple analysis of change scores estimator. The covariance of (7.1) with the baseline difference is

$$\mathrm{cov}[\hat{\tau}(b), (\bar{X}_{.v} - \bar{X}_{.p})] = q(\sigma_{xy} - b\sigma_x^2) \qquad (7.2)$$

and the variance is

$$\mathrm{var}[\hat{\tau}(b)] = q(\sigma_Y^2 + b^2\sigma_X^2 - 2b\sigma_{xy}), \qquad (7.3)$$

where $q = (1/n_v + 1/n_p)$. A necessary condition for such a treatment estimate to be independent of the mean baseline difference is that (7.2) equals zero, from which $b = \sigma_{XY}/\sigma_X^2 = \rho\sigma_Y/\sigma_X = \beta$. This is also the value of b for which (7.3) is a minimum. Hence, an appropriate strategy (from two perspectives) to take account of the mean baseline difference is to adjust the treatment difference by β, the regression of Y on X. Note that if the variances of baseline and outcome are equal (which does not have to be the case but might sometimes be an appropriate assumption), then the regression of Y on X is the correlation coefficient, ρ. Note also that $\hat{\tau}(\beta) = (1-\beta)\hat{\tau}(0) + \beta\hat{\tau}(1)$ and that since in practice β will usually be less than 1, the covariance adjusted outcome will usually lie between the raw outcomes and change-score estimator.

If we consider the three special cases then from (7.3) we have formulae for the variances as

$$\mathrm{var}[\hat{\tau}(0)] = q\sigma_y^2, \qquad (7.4)$$

$$\mathrm{var}[\hat{\tau}(1)] = q(\sigma_Y^2 + \sigma_X^2 - 2\rho\sigma_X\sigma_Y) \qquad (7.5)$$

and

$$\mathrm{var}[\hat{\tau}(\beta)] = q(1-\rho^2)\sigma_Y^2. \qquad (7.6)$$

It this follows that $\mathrm{var}[\hat{\tau}(1)] < \mathrm{var}[\hat{\tau}(0)]$ iff $\beta = \rho\sigma_Y/\sigma_X > 1/2$ and of course that $\mathrm{var}[\hat{\tau}(\beta)]$ is less than the other two variances unless either $\rho = 0$ or $\rho\sigma_Y/\sigma_X = 1$.

In practice, however, the nuisance parameters σ_X, σ_Y and ρ are not known and have to be estimated if analysis of covariance is to be applied. In that case, the variance formula given by (7.6) is not quite right and must be multiplied by a further factor

$$F = \frac{\sum\limits_{p,v}(x - \bar{x}_{..})^2}{\sum\limits_{p,v}(x - \bar{x}_{..})^2 - (\bar{x}_{.v} - \bar{x}_{.p})^2}. \qquad (7.7)$$

This factor is never less than 1 and is only equal to 1 when the baselines are perfectly balanced. Hence, there is some penalty involved in analysis of covariance. Where proper baselines are concerned, however, it is rarely the case that the penalty imposed by (7.7) outweighs the advantage brought by (7.6).

7.A.2   Choice of baselines to fit

Let X_1 and X_2 be two baselines and Y an outcome measured on a given patient and suppose that these have all been standardized so that they have mean and variance 1. Suppose that the correlation matrix is

$$\Sigma = \begin{bmatrix} 1 & \rho_{12} & \rho_{13} \\ \rho_{12} & 1 & \rho_{23} \\ \rho_{13} & \rho_{23} & 1 \end{bmatrix} = \left[\begin{array}{c|c} A & B \\ \hline B' & 1 \end{array} \right],$$

where the rightmost side of this expression is a partitioned matrix. A is the correlation matrix for the baselines with each other, and B is the vector of correlations of baselines with outcomes. Let $X = [X_1 \quad X_2]$ and $x = [x_1 \quad x_2]$ be vectors of baselines as random variables and observed values respectively. Suppose that we are interested in adjusting for both baselines then

$$E[Y \,|X = x] = xA^{-1}B$$

and

$$\mathrm{var}[Y \,|X = x] = 1 - B'A^{-1}B \qquad (7.8)$$

where

$$A^{-1} = \begin{bmatrix} 1 & -\rho_{12} \\ -\rho_{12} & 1 \end{bmatrix} (1 - \rho_{12}^2)^{-1}.$$

If, on the other hand, we adjust only for the second baselines, we have

$$E[Y \,|X_2 = x_2] = \rho_{23} x_2 , \qquad (7.9)$$

$$\mathrm{var}\,[Y \,|X_2 = x_2] = 1 - \rho_{23}^2.$$

The condition that $(7.9) = (7.8)$ is that $\rho_{13} = \rho_{12}\rho_{23}$ or that the partial correlation of first baseline and outcome should be zero given the second baseline. This condition is extremely unlikely to be met in practice. Under other circumstances $(7.8) < (7.9)$.

Now suppose that we construct a new random vector $Z = (Z_1, Z_2) = (X_1 + X_2, X_1 - X_2)$. Then

$$E\,[Y \,|Z = z] = z \begin{bmatrix} (2 + 2\rho_{12})^{-1} & 0 \\ 0 & (2 - 2\rho_{12})^{-1} \end{bmatrix} \begin{bmatrix} \rho_{13} + \rho_{23} \\ -\rho_{13} + \rho_{23} \end{bmatrix}$$

and

$$\mathrm{var}\,[Y \,|Z = z] = 1 - [\rho_{13} + \rho_{23} \quad -\rho_{13} + \rho_{23}] \begin{bmatrix} (2 + 2\rho_{12})^{-1} & 0 \\ 0 & (2 - 2\rho_{12})^{-1} \end{bmatrix} \begin{bmatrix} \rho_{13} + \rho_{23} \\ -\rho_{13} + \rho_{23} \end{bmatrix}$$

$$(7.10)$$

On the other hand, if we only condition on the sum of the two baselines, we have

$$E(Y\,|Z_1=z_1) = \frac{z_1(\rho_{13}+\rho_{23})}{2+2\rho_{12}}$$

and

$$\mathrm{var}(Y\,|Z_1=z_1) = 1 - \frac{(\rho_{13}+\rho_{23})^2}{2+2\rho_{12}}. \qquad (7.11)$$

The condition that $(7.11)=(7.10)$ is that $\rho_{13}=\rho_{23}$. This condition may apply approximately in many cases, especially where the period of baseline observation is short compared to the period of treatment. Under other circumstances $(7.10) < (7.11)$.

8

The Measurement of Treatment Effects

But with proper medical treatment the rheumatism would soon have ceased; or even, without medical treatment, under the ordinary oscillations of natural causes.

Thomas De Quincey, *Confessions of an English Opium Eater*

A calculation of consequences is no more equivalent to a sentiment, than a seriatim enumeration of square yards or feet touches the fancy like the sight of the Alps or Andes.

William Hazlitt, *The Spirit of the Age*

8.1 BACKGROUND

A disease may have many symptoms and a treatment may have many effects. A particular disease may affect individuals differently and so may a given treatment. We do not study all individuals to whom we may eventually apply the treatment but a rather unrepresentative subset who form the patients in our clinical trial. We should like to be able to use the experience gained with these patients to say something about future patients. Measuring to the best extent that we are able what a particular treatment does is not the same as measuring how well it does what we should like it to do. Furthermore, certain standard statistical tools require measurements of a particular form. All of these are reasons why the measurement of effects in a clinical trial is not necessarily a simple matter. They are also reasons why measurement is not just the concern of the physician but also the concern of the statistician.

Some of the issues have already been touched on in Chapters 3 and 7; others will be dealt with when we come to consider multiplicity in Chapter 10, and also safety of treatments in Chapter 23. (In particular, some matters regarding survival analysis will be touched on in that chapter.) Other remarks and issues to do with measurement will be found in various chapters on more particular specialist matters: for example, Chapter 21 which deals with pharmacokinetics and Chapter 24 which deals with pharmaco-economics. In this chapter we shall cover those important issues which remain.

Statistical Issues in Drug Development/ 2nd Edition Stephen Senn
© 2007 John Wiley & Sons, Ltd

8.2   ISSUES

8.2.1   Additivity

If the effect of a given treatment for asthma is to increase forced expiratory volume in one second (FEV_1) 12 hours after treatment by 300 ml above what it would have been without treatment, (whatever it would have been), then the treatment is additive on the FEV_1 scale. If it increases FEV_1 by 15%, however, then while it increases a value which would have been 2000 ml by 300 ml, it only increases a value which would have been 1500 ml by 225 ml, and one which would have been 1000 ml is only increased by 150 ml. Thus, treatment is not additive on the FEV_1 scale. However, if we take logarithms of the data then we can restore additivity, as is illustrated in Table 8.1.

It can be seen from the table that, although the treatment is not additive on the original scale, it is additive on the log scale, the difference being $\log 1.15 \cong 0.14$. (Following the usual conventions in statistics, natural logarithms are taken. If logs to base 10 were taken, this would make no difference to the additivity phenomenon, although the differences observed would be $\cong (\log_{10} e) \times 0.14 \cong 0.434 \times 0.14 \cong 0.061$.) In fact, for most treatments and measurements, it is far more reasonable to suppose that the treatment is additive on the log scale rather than on the original scale, although, of course, there is no requirement for it to be additive on either. (The log scale is theoretically attractive for any measurement with an absolute zero, since it has the feature that when its inverse transformation, the antilogarithm, is applied to any predicted value, the value cannot be negative (Keene, 1995).) Some of these points are illustrated in more detail below.

Another transformation which is commonly employed by statisticians is the logit transformation. Suppose we are interested in looking at the effect of a treatment on the probability of survival of patients over a given time period. The probability of survival will lie between 0 and 1 for any patient. If we use the probability scale to make our analysis we may come to some conclusion such as (say) the effect of treatment is to increase the probability of survival by 0.23. Suppose, however, that we now wish to apply the treatment to a type of patient whose probability of survival without treatment we believe to be 0.86. Applying our treatment estimate would lead to the nonsensical conclusion that her chances of survival were now $0.86 + 0.23 = 1.09$! This can be avoided if, instead of using a scale like the probability scale, which is bounded by 0 and 1, we use a scale which, although related to it, is not so bounded. An example of such a scale is the logit scale and it is defined by

$$y = \text{logit}(p) = \log\left(\frac{p}{1-p}\right) = \log(p) - \log(1-p).$$

Table 8.1   Effect of a bronchodilator on absolute and log FEV_1.

FEV$_1$ (ml)			logê(FEV$_1$)		
Counterfactual	**Actual**	**Difference**	**Counterfactual**	**Actual**	**Difference**
1000	1150	150	6.91	7.05	0.14
1500	1725	225	7.31	7.45	0.14
2000	2300	300	7.60	7.74	0.14

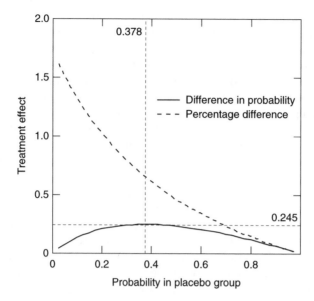

Figure 8.1   Difference and proportionate difference in probability of success, for a treatment group compared with a placebo group, as a function of probability of success in the placebo group, where the treatment effect, τ, is assumed additive on the logit scale and equal to 1.

Figure 8.1 shows the effect of a treatment which is additive (and equal to 1) on the logit scale, as a function of probability of success in the placebo group: both in terms of a difference in probability and also that difference expressed as a proportion of probability in the placebo group. The figure shows that the maximum effect in terms of difference occurs at a placebo probability of success of just under 0.4, for which value the effect is just under 0.25. The treatment effect in proportionate terms shows a steady decline with rising placebo probability of success. Of course, in logit terms the effect is constant and equal to 1.

A number of issues one associated with transformation. An important one, to do with the choice between clinical and statistical relevance, will be dealt with separately below. Another has to do with the reporting of results from trials and 'utmost good faith'. An unscrupulous trialist could try a number of transformations of the data, omit to mention that this has been done and selectively report only the most favourable. Clearly, this biases the results. Perhaps for this reason, regulators (and referees of papers) have sometimes looked unfavourably on transformations of data carried out by the sponsor (or author). This particular issue can be simply resolved, however, if the sponsor specifies the transformation to be undertaken in the protocol. Often there is no reason why this should not be done and there will also be background knowledge and arguments which indicate which transformation will be useful. Such prespecification ensures that the choice of analysis is not dictated by the result. A further issue which this raises, however, is that it is not always entirely reasonable to suppose that the choice of transformation ought *never* to be dictated by the result. Generally, a correct transformation will be more sensitive and hence more powerful. It might therefore be argued that the best transformation is the one which indicates the most significant result! (Note, also, that diagnostic examinations of data are more properly carried out on residuals rather than on raw data. Since residuals are the differences between observed data and those predicted by a model, this implies that an analysis of the effect of treatment has already taken place.)

I have rarely found this to be a particular difficulty in running clinical trials. I have frequently used transformations and have nearly always been able to prespecify them in the protocol, not least because by the time the issue becomes really serious, which is to say in phase III, a particular trial is one among many trials for a particular drug, which itself is usually one among many drugs which have been tried for a particular indication. To overturn a choice of transformation which has been based on such experience, as well as on prior considerations, on the basis of results from a given trial, requires very strong evidence indeed. I have generally found no problem in sticking to the intended analysis. If, occasionally, *force majeure* indicates that an alternative analysis should also be tried, then, of course, the fact that the intended transformation was specified in the protocol means that both analyses will be presented. If the results of the two analyses conflict, then the sponsor will have to accept that the regulator *may* find the results unconvincing. It is difficult to find any way around this. Indeed, it may well be that this is a right and proper difficulty. Where the class of possible models to be considered cannot be restricted *a priori*, then there is uncertainty as to which is correct. One may then expect that all analyses carried out under such circumstance, whether Bayesian or frequentist, *ought* to carry this uncertainty, at least to some degree, into the conclusions. (Note that attempting to establish by pretesting which model is correct and then, once a final choice of model has been made, behaving as if this model were the only possible one to entertain, gives a misleading impression of the uncertainties involved.)

It is perhaps also worth noting that economic pressures have increasingly driven statisticians into using prespecified analyses and transformations. It is now usually the case that programming for analysis is carried out prior to data unblinding, simply in order to speed up the development process. As a result, the time to look at data prior to determining the analysis has shrunk. (Nowadays the time from database lock to first draft of the statistical analysis might be a few days: a process which would have taken several weeks at one time. Of course, the total time for analysis is still weeks, it is just that it starts earlier.) This puts a considerable premium on predetermined analyses, since the time to modify, let alone write, new programs is just not there. The effect this has on analysis is, in many cases, beneficial but it is not without its drawbacks.

8.2.2   Individual response

As was pointed out in section 3.9, standard statistical models assume additivity on some appropriate scale (Senn, 2004a). There are a number of reasons why this is so. First, such models are simpler to apply and interpret. Second, other things being equal, simpler models should be preferred to more complex ones. Third, it turns out that in many types of clinical trial it is impossible to distinguish whether an effect is the same for every patient or not. There is thus no evidence for or against additivity. Fourth, in such trials it also follows that there is no harm in assuming additivity as regards formal analysis of the data. The exceptions to the above situation are certain types of repeated measure designs, most notably cross-over and n-of-1 designs.

This does not appear to prevent physicians and even some statisticians from over-interpreting data from standard clinical trials in terms of individual response. In fact, much of pharmacogenomics is carried out on the basis of the untested assumption that the variation in 'response' we see in clinical trials is largely due to genetic differences between patients. Suppose, however, that were we to treat a given patient again the patient would show a quite different response. This would imply that this source of variation could not possibly be genetic. But very few clinical trials have a structure that would make the investigation of this point possible (Senn, 2001, 2004c).

The reason we carry out clinical trials and feel it necessary to study many patients is that we do not find case studies convincing: a single patient may improve when treated but he might have improved anyway, therefore his improvement may have nothing to do with treatment. But to attempt to identify responders and nonresponders in a clinical trial is to abandon the logic of the trial and analyse the results as if they belonged to a series of independent case studies. The most that can be done for trials in which patients have not been repeatedly measured is to examine additivity at the group level: to check, for example, whether women react differently to treatment from men (see Chapter 9).

I will illustrate the difficulty of establishing individual response by considering what has been quoted as a particular requirement of the FDA, namely that a bronchodilator should have 15% bronchodilation in terms of FEV_1 to be assumed effective at a given time. At first sight, this sounds like a straightforward requirement, but it raises a number of issues. Suppose, for example, we wish to show bronchodilation at 12 hours. The following questions might be put.

1. Do we need to satisfy the requirement in a single-dose study or at steady state?
2. Do we need to *'prove'* it applies, for example by showing a lower confidence interval above 15%, or does it simply refer to an observed value?
3. Do we measure the effect compared with placebo or baseline?
4. Is the requirement a mean requirement over all patients or an individual requirement?
5. For individuals, should we use single measurements or means over many observation?

As soon as these questions are put, we begin to appreciate that the requirement is not straightforward and is in fact ambiguous as stated.

My opinion is that the answer to (1) probably ought to be 'at steady state' and that to (3) definitely ought to be 'compared with placebo' since asthmatics are well known to be both suggestible and subject to diurnal rhythms. In the case of question (2) it might seem logical to require a lower confidence interval above 15% but this may be too strong a requirement to be practical. (It will certainly have a considerable impact on the sample size required.) As regards questions (4) and (5), however, my opinion is that *if* the answer to question (4) is that an individual requirement is indicated, then this requirement is only logical if the answer to question (5) is that the long-term mean effect for a given patient is needed.

To see why, consider the following model. Assume for argument's sake that the treatment is truly additive on the log scale and that the effect is on average 18% in FEV_1 (treatment compared with placebo). Assume that the logarithms of FEV_1 are Normally distributed with mean $0.166 = \log(1.18)$. Now suppose that we compare the active treatment to placebo a number of times, n, for each patient (having taken suitable precautions regarding wash-out and so forth) and that we are therefore able to obtain n determinations of the treatment effect for each patient. (I ignore difficulties with period effects here, as they do not really affect the validity of the argument and can be dealt with at the expense of a slightly more complex formulation of the problem.) We suppose that as n increases, by averaging over n we obtain for each patient some estimate of the true average effect of the treatment for him or her. Suppose that the standard deviation of these long-term averages (again in terms of log FEV_1) is about 0.05. In that case we can calculate the proportion of patients for whom the *true* bronchodilating effect is in excess of 15%, and we shall find that this is the case for 70% of the patients. However, since we shall also have n estimates of the treatment effect for each patient, we can calculate a standard deviation of these treatment estimates for every patient. Suppose that the typical value of such a standard deviation is about 0.18. This implies that the standard deviation of treatment effects (if these are based on one comparison only per patient of placebo and active treatment) will be very much higher than that based on the mean of n determinations. In fact, the standard deviation of such a single determination will be the square root of the sum of the two variances involved (both between and within patients) or $\sqrt{(0.18^2 + 0.05^2)} \cong 0.19$. Now, calculating the proportion of patients on this basis who have at least 15% bronchodilation, we come up with the less impressive figure of 55%. Figure 8.2 shows the percentage of patients apparently satisfying the FDA's criterion as a function of the number of determinations of the treatment effect.

The moral here is not that we have to measure patients for ever, but that we have to be very careful when looking at individual response. My view is that the figure of 80%, corresponding to long-term or 'true' effects, would be the correct one to quote when attempting to answer the question 'what percentage of patients have a true benefit of 15% from the drug?' A careful statistical analysis based upon a random effects model, and using a design in which each patient is measured twice on placebo and twice on the active treatment, will suffice to answer this question, but a naive analysis will not. (See also Chapter 18, n-of-1 trials.) Furthermore, if the patients have only been measured once on each drug then it will be impossible to tell how much of the observed variability in the estimated treatment effect for each patient is pure 'noise' and how

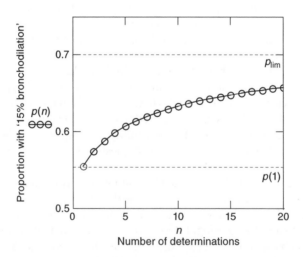

Figure 8.2 Proportion of patients showing an apparent mean bronchodilation of 15% as a function of the number of times, n, that the treatment effect (active compared with placebo) is measured for each patient. See text for further explanation.

much represents genuine individual response to treatment. Under these circumstances it would not be possible to distinguish between the claim that only 55% of patients have adequate bronchodilation and the claim that 100% do.

For an example of a careful analysis of an analogous situation with osteoporosis, see Hassager *et al.* (1994). These authors reviewed three published studies in which there were apparently considerable differences in response to hormone replacement therapy. By carefully modelling the effect of measurement error on bone mineral content they were able to show that it was plausible that patient-by-treatment interaction was much smaller than had been supposed and that nearly all patients benefitted from therapy.

8.2.3   Clinical versus statistical relevance

It is my opinion that this apparent conflict is not as great as is sometimes supposed. Consider the plot in Figure 8.1. It is clear that the treatment effect in *practical*, which is to say *clinical*, terms may be very different depending on the success rate which would be observed under placebo. For example, if the probability of success under placebo is 0.1, then a logit of 1 leads to a proportionate *improvement* of the chance of success of 1.32 times (the success rate is 2.32 times what it would be under placebo), whereas if the placebo probability is 0.9, the proportionate improvement is only 0.07. This sort of difference may have important policy implications.

This does not constitute a reason for abandoning the additive logit scale (if the treatment truly is additive on this scale) for any other clinically relevant scale. The truth is that it is impossible for us to run clinical trials in such a way that not only do all patients recruited in a given trial have the same background level of risk but also so that we can study every possible level of background risk. We are therefore forced to find a way of translating effect from one level of risk to another both within and beyond trials. The best way to do this is undoubtedly using an additive scale if one can be found. Provided the use of such scales is understood, an estimated treatment effect can then be used in conjunction with a given background level of risk to provide a prediction of the effect of the treatment. An example of using this approach to decide whether a particular treatment will be of value to a given patient given some knowledge of the background risk is provided by Glasziou and Irwig (1995)

Another way of looking at this, admirably expounded by Lane and Nelder (1982), is to maintain a distinction between estimation and prediction and to recognize that though the former may lead fairly directly to the latter in simple cases, more generally it may require some further modelling effort to predict once an analysis of a data set is complete (Senn, 2004b).

Nevertheless, this issue can cause some problems, especially where a clinical trial permits one to measure many things and it is not clear which is the most important. There is a certain conflict between trying to find out exactly what a treatment does and trying to discover how well it does what we should ideally like it to do. It seems to me that the latter is a proper object where we consider that the trial will be used to inform a global decision: we shall either treat all patients of a given broad type in the future with the given treatment or none. If however, we consider that the object of a trial is to permit a patient (with her physician) to come to a personal decision as to which treatment is best, and if we accept that patients may have different priorities, then there is no single clinically relevant measure anyway, even if constructed as a combination of others. Under such circumstances, it seems to me that the statistical approach of seeking an additive scale (or scales for many measures) is the most appropriate. This issue receives a further airing in Chapter 10.

8.2.4 Dichotomizing continuous measurements

This is a very bad and all too widespread habit. Between statisticians there is not really much of an issue here, yet it is still a common wish of physicians to be able to divide patients into sheep and goats on the basis of a continuous outcome measure. Quite apart from the fact that it is both conceptually false and entirely arbitrary to divide patients into responders on the basis of whether they achieved a given target fall in blood pressure or cholesterol, or a given rise in FEV_1, or exercise time, or CD4 count, or whatever the case may be, such a procedure simply throws away information. It is ironic that when faced with a dichotomous outcome, standard statistical procedures, such as logistic regression or probit analysis, attempt to reconstruct a continuous 'proto-measurement' which is presumed to give rise to the dichotomous values.

To return to FEV_1 as an example, the dichotomizer might compare outcome with baseline (ignoring possibly important trend effects and measurement error) and then label a patient as responder (1) or nonresponder (0) on the basis of bronchodilation being above or below 15%. The results are then handed over to the statistician, who will have to find some way of modelling the binary outcome. This requires modelling probability of success as a function of the covariates and treatment given. To ensure that this is constrained to lie in the limits 0 to 1, a tolerance function in terms of a continuous unmeasured variable will be invoked, the choice of which (for example, Normal, logistic, extreme value) determines which link (inverse cumulative Normal, logit, complementary log-log) will be used. This can then be fitted using generalized linear models. How much better to use the actual and genuine values!

> **Dichotomy**: A means by which regulators, destroy information, increase the size of clinical trials, delay treatment for patients and cost the economy millions. See *Responder analysis*.

In fact, as is well known, the sign test has a Pitman asymptotic efficiency (Garthwaite *et al.*, 2002) of $2/\pi \approx 64\%$, which is to say that, other things being equal, a trial would appear to need to have $\pi/2 \approx 1.57$ as many patients to have the same power if analysed in terms of a dichotomy rather than a continuous measure. However, this underestimates the losses considerably. This efficiency figure applies when the optimal cutpoint, which will divide patients into two equal classes, has been chosen to define the dichotomy. The more general situation is given by Figure 8.3. Furthermore, if the dichotomy is itself based on change scores then the change scores themselves will be an inefficient use of the baseline information (Senn, 2005) as discussed in Chapter 7. This loss could be partially recovered by including the baseline as a covariate in an analysis of the dichotomy using logistic regression. However, some irreparable damage

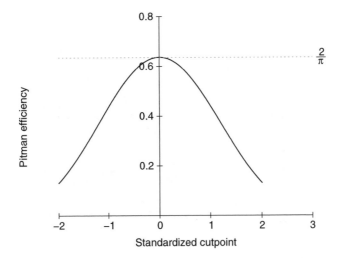

Figure 8.3 Pitman efficiency of a dichotomy compared to the original measure as a function of the cutpoint.

will have been done by the transformation and the recovery will not be complete. In short, the losses of precision in dichotomizing are considerable (Senn, 2003).

Some dichotomies are particularly objectionable. For example, a definition of response in hypertension that is sometimes encountered (see Goetghebeur *et al.* (1998) for an example) is that this is achieved if diastolic blood pressure (DBP) has reduced *either* by 10% *or* from ≥ 95 mmHg to ≤ 90 mmHg. However, this implies that a reduction of 10 mmHg and 9.9% from 101 mmHg to 91 mmHg does not constitute a response, whereas a reduction of 5 mmHg and 5.3% does. This is clearly absurd. The response region defined by this measure is given by Figure 8.4. This sort of dichotomy is likely not only to lead to a loss in efficiency but to produce inappropriate divisions of patients in terms of response. It goes beyond a mere loss of precision to achieve a genuine distortion.

8.2.5   Measuring trend effects

In Chapter 7 we saw that, in a controlled clinical trial, difference from baseline and absolute outcomes are actually two ways of measuring the same thing and, indeed, if a baseline is fitted as a covariate the result of using these measures is formally equivalent. When we have a number of measures taken during the course of a trial, then rather more options are available to us and which we choose depends largely on the way we expect the treatment to work.

We can, of course, analyse the individual measurements, either independently at each time point (that is to say, repeating the same form of analysis using the different time points) or globally using a so-called repeated measures analysis. (Some issues to do with this will be treated in Chapter 10 and need not concern us here.) An alternative is to use the so-called *summary measures* approach, whereby, in an initial stage, we combine the multiple measures on individual patients into statistics which are then, in a second stage, analysed further. A very simple and obvious summary measure is the

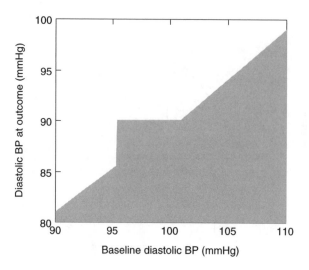

Figure 8.4 Response region (solid) for a common definition of response in hypertension.

arithmetic mean. This would usually be a suitable measure for any chronic disease in which the treatment is expected to provide a degree of relief which sets in rapidly and is then fairly steadily maintained. Bronchodilators used to treat asthma might be a good example.

If the treatment has an effect which is slowly accumulating, however, then it may be argued that the average effect over the course of the trial is not of interest. An example of such a disease might be osteoporosis in postmenopausal women where, in the absence of treatment, one may expect a gradual but fairly steady loss of bone mineral density. Hormone replacement therapy might have the effect of reducing the rate of loss. In a 12-month trial, in which measurements are made at 3-month intervals, to take the average of the responses at 3, 6, 9, 12, months is (effectively) to estimate the treatment effect at $7^1/_2$ months, whereas it may be greatest at 12 months. Only to use the readings at 12 months, however, seems unduly wasteful. An alternative is then to estimate the trend effect over the 12 months. This can be done, for example, using ordinary least squares (the standard regression option in most statistical packages). When this is done, the standard approach is to include the baselines in the measurement of the trend effect. It is important to note, however, that although regression may appear to be a complicated statistical procedure, all that the estimate of the slope amounts to is a weighted sum of the observed outcomes. For example, in the 12-month trial considered above, if we choose to estimate the treatment effect as a rate of change per three months, and we code the outcomes at baseline, 3, 6, 9 and 12 months as Y_0, Y_1, Y_2, Y_3 and Y_4, then the estimate is simply $b_1 = (2Y_4 + Y_3 - Y_1 - 2Y_0)/10$. Actually, for this sort of measure, exactly the same arguments apply as for difference from baseline. As always, we are interested in estimating a causal effect and a similar argument can be adduced to show that if the baseline is to be used at all, it should be fitted in an analysis of covariance. It turns out that this is formally equivalent to doing an analysis of covariance on the measure $b_2 = (2Y_4 + Y_3 - Y_1)/10$. Furthermore, in terms of statistical significance, for a rate assumed constant, there is effectively no difference between a rate per year and a rate per three months: only a fourfold scaling factor. Therefore, as regards significance, $b_3 = 4b_2 = (4Y_4 + 2Y_3 - 2Y_1)/5$ will give the same result. And, if a truly linear relationship holds, then the effect rate per one year is the same as the effect at one year. It can thus be seen that just using the final value alone, Y_4, can also be regarded as estimating the same thing as using b_3. Using b_3 in preference to using Y_4 can then be justified by saying that an estimate of the effect of treatment after one year superior to simply using the one-year measurement alone can be obtained by adjusting it using information obtained from previous measures. Effectively, a sort of smoothing takes place in which to 4/5 of the final measurement 2/5 of the penultimate is added and 2/5 of the first post treatment is subtracted.

Of course, this would not be a good thing to do if the treatment effect were not growing with time. If the treatment effect at the end of the trial is very similar to the treatment effect at the beginning, then it is clear that we may expect that Y_1 will be approximately equal to Y_4 and that b_3 will estimate only 4/5 of the treatment effect at the expense of having added a lot of irrelevant noise. A very plausible alternative estimate of the effect at the end would simply be the average throughout. Under those circumstances, we might be interested in using as our estimate $b_4 = (Y_1 + Y_2 + Y_3 + Y_4)/4$.

Thus, although final values, means and trends appear to be estimates of very different things, there are circumstances under which they can be regarded as estimates of the same thing. It would be very nice to know, when planning a given trial with repeated measures, which form of summary measure (assuming that general approach has been chosen) would be the most sensitive. Obviously, background knowledge will be of help here. Where this is not sufficient to resolve the issue, then the temptation will be to decide on the basis of an inspection of the data. This is not necessarily inappropriate but there are two points to watch out for. First, as we have already discussed, regulatory authorities prefer prespecified analyses. Second, contrary to what is sometimes maintained (Matthews *et al.*, 1990), an inspection of individual time plots for given patients is not necessarily an appropriate way to determine which form of summary measure should be used (Senn, 1990; Senn *et al.*, 2000). There are two reasons. The first is that noise (random variation) may obscure the nature of the signal (systematic effects) which should be extracted. The second reason is that the signal to be extracted is only that which relates to the effect of treatment itself. This may be overlaid by other signals, for example the secular trend (which may be quite complex) to which all patients are subject independently of the treatment they are assigned. This secular trend is irrelevant to the choice of summary measure. The summary measure only needs to reflect the treatment effect, which is (essentially) the difference between groups. Defining the difference between groups may itself be difficult (for example, should one transform to logs first or not), but often a standard linear model fitted independently at each time point will enable an identification of an appropriate summary measure to be made.

As an alternative, a compromise between either fitting a mean or fitting a trend using ordinary least squares is to fit a regression through the origin. Where this is adjusted for baselines it corresponds (for our example) to using the combination $Y_1 + 2Y_2 + 3Y_3 + 4Y_4$. Unlike, the conventional estimates of slope, this statistic has the interesting property that none of the values affected by the treatment enters negatively (Senn *et al.*, 2000). As a consequence, it can be regarded not only as a slope estimate but also as a (weighted) mean estimate or, indeed, as some sort of compromise between the two.

Obviously, very many other choices of summary measure are possible.

8.2.6   A potential issue with mixed models applied to repeated measures

This issue is related to the one described in the preceding section. Mixed-model approaches have grown dramatically since the first edition of this book, largely owing to advances in computing. For example, an excellent book in the same series as this one, which has appeared since the first edition, is entitled *Mixed Models in Medicine* and gives detailed advice on applying `proc mixed` of SAS to the analysis of repeated-measures design (Brown and Prescott, 1999, 2006). A simple alternative to the repeated measures approach is the summary measures approach. In some circumstances the two will lead to similar inferences. However, the summary measures approach, by combining the measures according to some weighting scheme prior to analysis, will not necessarily combine these in the most efficient way (Senn *et al.*, 2000).

As an example, consider a trial with three equally spaced measurements and no missing values and suppose that we believe that the treatment effect is constant during the period of observation. A simple summary-measures approach will use the unweighted mean of these three observations for each patient and then proceed to analyse these statistics. This corresponds to a linear combination with weights 1/3, 1/3, 1/3. We can call this the naive combination. If, however, a mixed modeling approach is used, the observed correlation structure will be exploited to find an efficient combination of the observations. Suppose, to take an example, that the variances are all the same and that the correlation is 0.8 between neighbouring observations but is 0.4 between the first and last observations. The optimal linear combination now has weights of the form 1, −1, 1. Just like the naive combination, the sum of the weights is 1. However, the variance of the naive combination will be approximately 30% higher.

From one point of view this illustrates the superiority of the mixed-models approach. However, in this particular instance the result is somewhat disturbing. It seems rather unnatural to add the value for the first and last visit together and subtract the value for the visit in the middle as a way of judging the efficacy of the treatment. It requires a lot of faith in the model being used.

To take a concrete example which highlights this point, consider a famous data example due to Thall and Vail (1990) and adapted from a trial reported by Leppik *et al.* (1987) which has been widely used to provide a test data set for illustrating the performance of repeated-measures analyses. (It has been cited over 80 times.) In the example as adapted, a number of patients have been allocated to one of two anti-epileptics and the number of seizures in each of four periods has been recorded. A summary measures approach would quite naturally use the totals from the four periods (Senn, 2006a). Thus, the success of the drugs will be judged by the total number of seizures. However, if we used some mixed nonlinear model (perhaps some combination of Poisson regression with some correlation structure), it is likely that such simple totals would not be used but that some more complicated combination of the four values would appear. It cannot even be excluded (although it may be unlikely) that one of the period totals might appear with contrary sign, which might be disturbing.

The issue here is not just one of simplicity versus complexity. My personal view is that in the use of covariates and measurements generally there is much to be gained by using more complex models. This was the view as regards use of baselines and other covariates expounded in Chapter 7. The issue here, however, is to do with modelling of the relationship between outcome measures themselves rather than between outcome measures and baselines. This raises the problem of 'correction' for post-baseline covariates, which was covered in the last chapter. The moral is that one may need to be cautious in using certain types of mixed model and reflect carefully on what is happening. A summary-measures approach may be a useful back-up analysis.

8.2.7 Using surrogate endpoints

A surrogate endpoint is one which is chosen as an indicator of efficacy in lieu of the one of substantive interest. For example, in a trial of a treatment for osteoporosis we might be interested in reducing the fracture rate but measure bone mineral density (BMD) instead, or in a trial in AIDS we might ultimately be interested in mortality but analyse CD4 counts instead. The idea behind using a surrogate endpoint is that an impression of efficacy may be obtained sooner or more cheaply. There are some indications where such endpoints are commonly used. For example, high blood pressure is not in itself a problem, although it can be the cause of many problems. In a sense, therefore, if we measure blood pressure rather than the problems it causes, we have used a surrogate endpoint.

> The difference between a surrogate and a true endpoint is like the difference between a cheque and cash. You can often get the cheque earlier but then, of course, it might bounce.

The advantage of using such endpoints is clear. We may reasonably hope to obtain an indication of efficacy for less trouble than by using the true endpoint. The disadvantage is that we may deceive ourselves as to the efficacy of a treatment. Consider, for example, the case of osteoporosis above. Loss of bone mineral density leads to a weakening of bones and an increased risk of fracture. However, if a treatment increases density at the expense of adversely affecting the construction of the bones, it may actually have a harmful affect on the fracture rate. This sort of example implies that the adequacy of a surrogate measure may depend on the treatment. For example, both hormone replacement therapy and bisphosphonates may reduce bone mineral loss, but since they act in different ways it is conceivable that one might have a beneficial effect on fracture rate and the other a harmful one. FDA draft guidelines for osteoporosis issued in 1994 reflected this, requiring fracture studies for bisphosphonates but accepting BMD for hormone replacement (Division of Metabolism and Endocrine Drug Products, 1994).

As Prentice pointed out in an important paper (Prentice, 1989), this sort of consideration implies that the fact that one endpoint is highly correlated with another does not prove that it is an adequate surrogate. The key question one must ask about a surrogate endpoint is this: 'Does knowledge of the surrogate value make knowledge of the treatment given irrelevant for the purpose of predicting the true outcome?'. If the answer is 'no', it implies that the treatment has an effect on the outcome which is not captured by the surrogate endpoint. This makes it a potentially dangerous choice for analysis.

This in turn raises a further dilemma. The only way in which the 'Prentice criterion' can be proved to apply is to run a trial with a given treatment and analyse both true and surrogate endpoints. But if an adequate analysis of true endpoints is possible, then the surrogate endpoints are superfluous. The solution would then seem to be rather like the story of the mice who decided that the cat could be rendered harmless if a bell could be tied around its neck: the problem of the nasty cat which would creep up unawares on the mice was merely replaced by the equally difficult one of finding a mouse who could creep up safely on the cat. The problem of surrogate endpoints is a problem of 'belling the cat': to prove that the endpoints are adequate you have to run the sort of trial the endpoints were supposed to enable you to avoid. One might argue that this just shows how unsound the whole business of using surrogate endpoints is and that they should therefore not be employed at all, but this in itself raises problems. In some indications it would dramatically increase the number of patients we had to study and this might be regarded by some as being unethical. We may not be able to prove that a beneficial effect on a surrogate endpoint will eventually be translated into true benefit, but suppose that we strongly believe it. Are we then justified in continuing to randomize patients to a treatment we now believe is inferior? On the other hand, if belief alone justifies the choice of treatment, who needs evidence and whose belief is acceptable?

A concrete example may be helpful in highlighting the dangers. In discussing surrogate endpoints, Fleming (1996) draws attention to the case of the Cardiac Arrhythmia Suppression Trial (CAST) comparing encainide and flecainide to placebo. That these drugs were extremely beneficial in suppressing arrhythmia had been established beyond doubt. Much to the surprise of many cardiologists, however, CAST showed that the drugs tripled the death rate. Since 200 000 Americans were being treated annually with these drugs for what is a serious condition, thousands of deaths must have resulted annually from their use in the USA alone.

The example supports the case which some would make: in the ethics of choice, belief alone is not enough; what is needed is knowledge.

8.2.8   Titrations

For certain types of trial measurement is by titration. For example, in angina a patient may be asked to perform an exercise until a given degree of pain is experienced. In asthma it may be established at what dose of a metacholine challenge a 20% drop in FEV_1 is induced. There are many other examples of such measures.

What is often overlooked, however, is that the process of titration destroys the meaning of other measurements. Just as it is meaningless to measure the pH of an acid once it has been neutralized by a base, it is extremely misleading to take other measurements in a clinical trial once a titration has been performed (Senn, 1989, 1993). For example, there is not much point in using pain or FEV_1 as outcome measures in angina or asthma once exercise test titrations or methacholine challenge titrations have been carried out.

Furthermore, where such repeated titrations are being carried out over time, very strong assumptions are required. Consider a case in which repeated titrated histamine challenges are used in a single-dose trial of a beta-agonist in asthma to examine the time course. Suppose, say, that three challenges are carried out at 4-hourly intervals. After the first challenge, if the treatment is successful, patients on active treatment will have received more histamine than those on placebo. From this point on the groups are unbalanced. Either the results of the second and third challenges must then be given a conditional interpretation, or we must assume that all effects of the histamine are completely reversible. But if, for example, histamine can interfere in some way with binding of the beta-agonist to the effect-site, then it is conceivable that the duration of action of the drug will be affected by the titration. Hence extreme caution in interpretation is needed.

One difficulty which this problem raises is that patients may be self-titrating. Suppose, for example, that patients suffering from hay-fever are more likely to go out on sunny days in the country during the pollen season if given a partially effective treatment than are those who are untreated. (Let us call this *rural mobility*.) They may then titrate to a certain degree. Since rural mobility is enjoyable, we will then fail to capture the full benefit of the drug by measuring hay-fever symptoms alone. We would have to measure rural mobility as well. (If they were fully titrated by symptoms, then only rural mobility would capture the effect of treatment.) The possibility of this sort of thing is a potential worry for the interpretation of all clinical trials and raises two particular issues. First, that we may have to measure many different outcomes even where we think we are only interested in measuring one. Second, that where we simply wish to interpret one measure, it will be difficult to escape from the concept of intention to treat. We can only compare the policy of allocating one treatment to patients rather than another. What the patients then do with that allocation is beyond our control.

8.2.9   Number needed to treat (NNT)

These particular summaries of efficacy have attracted considerable controversy. For example, Altman *et al.* were so much in favour of these measures that they proposed as a reason for not using odds ratios that is was difficult to calculate NNTs from them (Altman *et al.*, 1996). Others have defended odds ratios and criticized NNTs for a number of reasons including the fact that they are extremely unlikely to be additive (Grieve, 2003; Hutton, 2000; Senn, 1998). NNTs have become so popular with the evidence-based medicine (EBM) movement that much effort is directed (I would say misdirected) to considering how NNTs may be calculated for continuous data. Thus the desire to produce NNTs has become a reason for dichotomizing measures, with all the disadvantages discussed in section 8.2.4 above.

NNTs are a measure of the number of patients that would have to be treated to gain one extra 'cure'. Now consider that for the control treatment the probability of an unsuccessful outcome is π_1 and the corresponding probability for the intervention group is π_2. The risk reduction is $\pi_1 - \pi_2$. For example, if 8 out of 10 control group patients have an unsuccessful outcome, and 7 out of 10 intervention group patients, we have $\pi_1 = 0.8$, $\pi_2 = 0.7$, $\pi_1 - \pi_2 = 0.1$. This implies that out of 10 patients who would have been treated with the control treatment, one fewer will have an unsuccessful outcome if treated by the intervention. The number of patients one needs to treat to gain one improvement is thus 10 and this is what is meant by the NNT. In general we calculate $NNT = 1/(\pi_1 - \pi_2)$.

Number needed to treat. The only way, we are told, that physicians can understand probabilities: odds being a difficult concept only comprehensible to statisticians, bookies, punters and readers of the sports pages of popular newspapers.

My own view is that these measures are an extremely misleading way to summarize the results of individual trials. The patients in a clinical trial are heterogeneous. It is highly unlikely that a single NNT applies to them. One could always expect to find subgroups for which the NNT was different. In other words, the measure is extremely unlikely to be additive. By the same token, since the patients in a clinical trial are unlikely to be exactly like the target population, the NNT for the trial may be misleading as regards the NNT in the population (Senn, 2004a).

Another argument that is sometimes advanced in favour of NNTs is that they are simple to interpret. The counterargument would be that a simple lie is being preferred to a complex truth. As Hutton has pointed out, differential equations are a difficult topic to understand but nobody suggests that their use should be removed from pharmacokinetics (Hutton, 2000). Similarly, log-odds-ratios are important and fundamental concepts in handling binary data. The fact that they bring with them some complexity cannot be grounds for eliminating them.

In short, although NNTs may have some utility at the point of prescription, where they would have to be individualized, they are extremely misleading at the point of analysis and should not be used to summarize individual trials, still less as the basis for a meta-analysis (Smeeth *et al.*, 1999).

8.2.10   Problems in using and interpreting sigma divided measures

A sigma divided measure is a measure of the treatment effect that relates the magnitude of the difference between groups to the variation within groups. For example, for a trial in blood pressure one could consider expressing the mean difference between treatment groups as a ratio of the pooled within-groups standard deviation. This is sometimes referred to as the *effect size*. One might consider relating the difference to the control group standard deviation only. Yet another possibility is to look at the difference between the two standardized means.

Assuming that the variance is the same in the two groups and that the data are Normally distributed, certain probabilities of apparent interest can be calculated from such quantities. For example, one may calculate the probability that a randomly chosen individual from one group has a higher value than a randomly chosen individual from another. This particular probability is made use of in approaches to determining the sample size for a Mann–Whitney–Wilcoxon test and also forms the basis of some modern approaches to nonparametric analysis. Another alternative is to calculate the area under both Normal distributions as a sort of measure of overlap (Rom and Hwang, 1996). Yet a third possibility is to calculate the probability that a randomly chosen individual under treatment will have a value higher than the control group mean (Acion *et al.*, 2006).

Because such measures are particularly popular in meta-analysis, where in particular the effect size was used by Glass (1976) in his pioneering work, they will be dealt with in some detail in Chapter 16. Here, it will simply be mentioned that such measures are problematic when randomization, rather than random sampling, is the basis for inference. The patients in a clinical trial are not representative of some target population. In particular, depending on circumstances that vary from trial to trial – such as entry criteria, the centres in which the trial is conducted, the precision with which measurements are taken and a host of other factors – the standard deviation may be expected to vary from trial to trial and there is no reason why it should be the same as in the target population (Senn, 1997). This is, of course, a matter that causes some problems for sample size determination, for which some past guess of the standard deviation is often used. However, for usual approaches to analysis, this causes no problems for interpretation. If the treatment effect is additive on the scale chosen then the effect is the same whatever the baseline risk and it will not vary in expectation from trial to trial. (Of course it will vary randomly.) By the same token, however, trials with different standard deviations will produce different effect sizes.

There is also a danger that the overlap in distributions will be determined in terms of causal probabilities. However, this is a straightforward mistake. For example, if every single patient in a clinical trial given active treatment has his or her FEV_1 increased by 200 ml compared with the value he or she would have had under placebo, there will still be an overlap between distributions and it will still be the case that some patients under placebo will have higher FEV_1 than some under active treatment. The probability of a response is 100%, but the probability that a randomly chosen patient under active treatment will have a higher value than a randomly chosen patient under placebo is far from this and says nothing directly about it.

Sigma divided measures should be avoided except where the problems with the data are so extreme (as for example in a meta-analysis combining different outcomes) that there is little alternative (Senn, 2006b).

References

Acion L, Peterson JJ, Temple S, Arndt S (2006) Probabilistic index: an intuitive non-parametric approach to measuring the size of treatment effects. *Statistics in Medicine* **25**: 591–602.

Altman DL, Deeks JJ, Sackett DL (1996) Down with odds ratios. *Evidence-Based Medicine* **1**: 164–166.

Brown H, Prescott R (1999) *Applied Mixed Models in Medicine*. John Wiley & Sons, Ltd, Chichester.

Brown H, Prescott R (2006) *Applied Mixed Models in Medicine* (2nd edition). John Wiley & Sons, Ltd, Chichester.

Division of Metabolism and Endocrine Drug Products (1994) *Guidelines for pre-clinical and clinical evaluation of agents used in the prevention and treatment of post-menopausal osteoporosis*. Food and Drug Administration, Rockville, MD.

Fleming TR (1996) Surrogate endpoints in clinical trials. *Drug Information Journal* **30**: 545–551.

Garthwaite PH, Joliffe IT, Jones B (2002) *Statistical Inference*. Oxford University Press, Oxford.

Glass GE (1976) Primary, secondary and meta-analysis of research. *Educational Research* **5**: 3–8.

Glasziou PP, Irwig LM (1995) An evidence based approach to individualising treatment. *British Medical Journal* **311**: 1356–1359.

Goetghebeur E, Molenberghs G, Katz J (1998) Estimating the causal effect of compliance on binary outcome in randomized controlled trials. *Statistics in Medicine* **17**: 341–355.

Grieve AP (2003) The number needed to treat: a useful clinical measure or a case of the Emperor's new clothes? *Pharmaceutical Statistics* **2**: 87–102.

Hassager C, Jensen SB, Christiansen C (1994) Nonresponders to hormone replacement therapy for the prevention of postmenopausal bone loss – do they exist. *Osteoporosis International* **4**: 36–41.

Hutton JL (2000) Numbers needed to treat: properties and problems (with comments). *Journal of the Royal Statistical Society A* **163**: 403–419.

Keene ON (1995) The log transformation is special. *Statistics in Medicine* **14**: 811–819.

Lane PW, Nelder JA (1982) Analysis of covariance and standardization as instances of prediction. *Biometrics* **38**: 613–621.

Leppik IE, Dreifuss FE, Porter R, *et al.* (1987) A controlled study of progabide in partial seizures: methodology and results. *Neurology* **37**: 963–968.

Matthews JNS, Altman DG, Campbell MJ, Royston P (1990) Analysis of serial measurements in medical research. *British Medical Journal* **300**: 230–235.

Prentice RL (1989) Surrogate endpoints in clinical trials: definition and operational criteria. *Statistics in Medicine* **8**: 431–440.

Rom DM, Hwang E (1996) Testing for individual and population equivalence based on the proportion of similar responses [see comments]. *Statistics in Medicine* **15**: 1489–1505. [Comment in *Statistics in Medicine* **16**(11): 1303–1306 (1997)].

Senn SJ (1989) The use of baselines in clinical trials of bronchodilators. *Statistics in Medicine* **8**: 1339–1350.

Senn SJ (1990) Analysis of serial measurements in medical research [letter; comment]. *British Medical Journal* **300**: 680.

Senn SJ (1993) Statistical issues in short term trials in asthma. *Drug Information Journal* **27**: 779–791.

Senn SJ (1997) Testing for individual and population equivalence based on the proportion of similar responses [letter; comment]. *Statistics in Medicine* **16**: 1303–1306.

Senn SJ (1998) Odds ratios revisited. *Evidence-Based Medicine* **3**: 71.

Senn SJ (2001) Individual therapy: new dawn or false dawn. *Drug Information Journal* **35**: 1479–1494.

Senn SJ (2003) Disappointing dichotomies. *Pharmaceutical Statistics* **2**: 239–240.

Senn SJ (2004a) Added values: controversies concerning randomization and additivity in clinical trials. *Statistics in Medicine* **23**: 3729–3753.

Senn SJ (2004b) Conditional and marginal models: another view – comments and rejoinders. *Statistical Science* **19**: 228–238.

Senn SJ (2004c) Individual response to treatment: is it a valid assumption? *British Medical Journal* **329**: 966–968.

Senn SJ (2005) An unreasonable prejudice against modelling? *Pharmaceutical Statistics* **4**: 87–89.

Senn SJ (2006a) Discussion on the paper by Lee and Nelder. *Journal of the Royal Statistical Society Series C – Applied Statistics* **55**: 173.

Senn SJ (2006b) Letter to the Editor: Probabilistic index: an intuitive non-parametric approach to measuring the size of the treatment effects by L. Acion, J.J. Peterson, S. Temple and S. Arndt. *Statistics in Medicine* **25**: 3944–3948.

Senn SJ, Stevens L, Chaturvedi N (2000) Repeated measures in clinical trials: simple strategies for analysis using summary measures. *Statistics in Medicine* **19**: 861–877.

Smeeth L, Haines A, Ebrahim S (1999) Numbers needed to treat derived from meta-analyses – sometimes informative, usually misleading [see comments]. *British Medical Journal* **318**: 1548–1551.

Thall PF, Vail SC (1990) Some covariance models for longitudinal count data with overdispersion. *Biometrics* **46**: 657–671.

8.A   TECHNICAL APPENDIX

8.A.1   Fifteen per cent bronchodilation

If the treatment estimate for a given patient is a mean of n comparisons of active treatment to placebo, then the variance of this measure over all patients is

$$\text{var}\,(\hat{\tau}_n) = \sigma_\tau^2 + \sigma_w^2/n, \tag{8.1}$$

where σ_τ^2 is the variance of the true treatment effect over all patients and σ_w^2 is the variance of a single contrast within a given patient. We then have

$$\text{prob}\,(\hat{\tau}_n > k) = 1 - \Phi\left(\frac{k - \mu_\tau}{\sqrt{\sigma_\tau^2 + \sigma_w^2/n}}\right) \tag{8.2}$$

and

$$\text{prob}\,(\hat{\tau}_\infty > k) = 1 - \Phi\left(\frac{k - \mu_\tau}{\sigma_\tau}\right), \tag{8.3}$$

where μ_τ is the expected value of the treatment effects and $\Phi(.)$ is the Normal distribution function.

In the example in section 8.2.2, we had $k = \log(1.15) = 0.140$, $\mu_\tau = 0.166$, $\sigma_\tau = 0.05$ and $\sigma_w = 0.18$. Substitution in (8.2) with $n = 1$ and in (8.3) gives probabilities of 55% and 70%, respectively.

9

Demographic Subgroups: Representation and Analysis

The play, I remember pleased not the million; 'twas caviare to the general.
William Shakespeare, Hamlet

But what's true of the general must be truish of the particular.
Howard Jacobson, Roots Schmoots

9.1 BACKGROUND

Our chapter quotations are a little confusing, since the messages are not in full agreement. Shakespeare is pointing out that tastes are not universal, whereas, if what Jacobson maintains is true, they should be universalish. Nevertheless, the quotations serve to introduce a difficulty: the statistician's art is practised in the hope that the properties of aggregates have some relevance to the individual but with the fear that they may not.

As we saw in the last chapter, an important goal of statistical analysis is to find an additive scale: a system of measurement which has the property that treatment effects so defined are constant from patient to patient. Note that this does not require that patients be homogenous with respect to demographic characteristics, but merely that they *react* to treatment in the same way given some suitable scale of measurement. We cannot, however, expect that our efforts will always be successful in this respect and therefore a particular worry in drug development is that there may be subgroups of patients for whom the treatment will have quite different effects.

It has also been the case that clinical trials have not been particularly representative as regards the patients studied. For example, it has been claimed that women have often been under-represented for various reasons, not least because fear of damaging the unborn has led sponsors to exclude many women of child-bearing age from their trials. A particular trial in which this certainly was the case was the Physician's Health Study (Hennekens and Eberlein, 1985) in which 22 071 male US physicians were the subjects in a factorial study designed to look at the possible prophylactic effects of aspirin and beta-carotene in heart-disease and cancer. In 1990 a political lobby in the USA, the Women's Congressional Caucus, disturbed by the example of the Physician's Health Study, lobbied to get women also represented in such trials.

In fact, subsequent research by Meinert *et al.* (2000), showed that the concerns of the Women's Congressional Caucus were unfounded. In 100 455 trials published in US journals between 1966 and 1998, 55% involved men and women, 12% involved men only and 11% involved women only (for 21% the policy could not be determined). For 724 trials in five leading journals, female subjects totaled 550 374 and male subjects only 355 614.

Neverthless, in order to remedy this presumed deficiency, in 1993 the Congress of the USA passed the National Institutes of Health (NIH) Revitalization Act, which specifically addressed the point and required the NIH to ensure that women and other demographic subgroups were adequately represented in clinical trials. In response, the NIH published guidelines to cover this issue for clinical trials which it sponsored (NIH, 1994). The FDA independently issued guidelines of its own. This legislation, and its associated guidelines, have brought to prominence many controversies regarding the treatment of demographic subgroups in clinical trials, but they were in any case already important. Indeed, the issue is an old one. In his masterly study, the *History of Statistics*, Stephen Stigler (Stigler, 1986) draws attention to a nineteenth-century debate regarding the quantification of social analysis. Keverburg, writing in 1827, pointed to the importance of representativeness and also its impossibility, arguing that there were so many reasons why groups could differ that none was like any other: detail was of the essence. Cournot (1801–1877), in 1838, made a criticism which tended to the opposite view: the greater the detail, the greater the scope for meaningless chance patterns. As Stigler puts it, 'How could a social scientist determine that he had sufficiently subdivided his data to permit a useful analysis? And, how could he guard against a selection effect that could come with too fine a categorization? The solutions did not come early. Indeed, they cannot be said to have been completely solved today' (p. 200).

We consider some of the issues below. In the discussion we shall refer to trials in which some attempt is made to fulfil specific demographic quotas as *discriminatory* (in the sense of positive discrimination). Other trials will be referred to as *conventional* trials. We shall also assume that whether or not it were considered to be of interest to make separate statements about the treatment effect for each sex, an important covariate such as sex would be fitted in any model used for analysis: in other words, that we would always stratify by sex. (See Chapter 7.) Since genotyping is an increasingly popular way of determining subgroups, some of the considerations in this chapter are also relevant to Chapter 25 on pharmacogenetics and vice versa. A recommended paper on equivalence and subgroups is that of Garrett (2003).

9.2   ISSUES

9.2.1   The adequate representation of women and other demographic subgroups

The issues here have to do with the way in which *adequate* is to be defined. Obviously no trialist is going to claim to have conducted a trial in which groups were *in*adequately represented, although she might, of course, claim that demographic subdivisions were unimportant. As soon as one attempts to define *adequate*, however, the real problems of demographic representation emerge. Below are listed some possible types of trial representing approaches to adequate representation (considering sex only and ignoring age, race, religion, social class and so forth).

Type I: Representation in the trial is to be proportionate to the representation in the target population. For example, if 9 out of 10 of all osteoporosis patients are women, then 90% of the patients in the trial must be women, and so forth.

Type II: Representation in the trial is to be such that equally precise statements may be made for women as for men.

Type III: Representation in the trial is to be such that there is adequate power to test treatment effects separately for men and women.

Type IV: Representation in the trial should be adequate to detect differences in the treatment effect in women and in men.

Exploratory analysis: The art of finding a Rembrandt in a Jackson Pollock

These are, in fact, quite different requirements and they have been arranged in order of difficulty for the trialist to achieve. The first, for example, *may* only have a marginal effect on total recruitment time (but see the discussion in Chapter 14) since, provided that centres are fairly representative of the general patient population and willingness to enter clinical trials is not different from sex to sex, this requirement would be almost naturally satisfied by any conventional trial. (In practice, however, things will not usually work out quite like this and there *will* be a delay in recruitment for such a discriminatory trial compared to a conventional trial.) Note, however, that the type I approach does not guarantee the representativeness of the sample. It is a form of *quota* sampling. It does not correspond to *stratified* sampling. For the latter, patients would have to be sampled *at random* from the strata defined by the sexes, whereas the type I approach merely assures that a convenience sample is obtained from each sex. This convenience sample may well be unrepresentative of the given sex.

If the concern in specifying adequate representation is one of equality of opportunity or sacrifice in clinical trials for or by the two sexes, such a trial will answer the objective. (But it does, not of course, guarantee such equality within the sexes: women of different social classes, for example, might have different opportunities.) If, however, it is desired to be able to make equally precise statements for men and for women, it will not. For that purpose, the second sort of trial above will be required and it will be necessary to recruit equal absolute numbers of men and women. This means that the sampling fractions for the two sexes will not be equal. Hence, since the rate limiting factor is usually the rate at which patients present, rather than the rate at which physicians can deal with them, then although the total number of patients required will not be increased compared to a conventional trial, there will be a considerable increase in recruitment time for all cases except that where the sexes can be recruited at an equal rate to the trial. An even greater delay will be experienced for any discriminatory trial in which it is deemed necessary to make statements which are as precise for each sex as is normally required for patients as a whole in a conventional trial, since this will also require a doubling

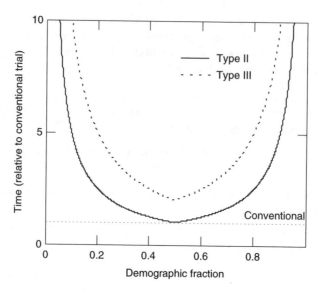

Figure 9.1 Recruitment times of type II and type III discriminatory trials relative to a conventional trial as a function of the demographic fraction.

of the number of patients studied. Figure 9.1 represents the recruitment time required for trials of types II and III compared to that for a conventional trial as a function of the *population* demographic fraction, where this is defined to be the proportion which women form of all eligible patients presenting and prepared to enter the trial. As can be seen, the effect on recruitment time can be considerable.

Even a type III trial, however, will not provide adequate power to test differences in response to treatment of men and women. There are two reasons. First, we may expect that the difference in the treatment effect between one sex and another will be smaller than the larger of the two effects. (If this were not the case it would imply that the treatment was harmful for one sex and beneficial for another: a so-called *qualitative interaction*.) Second, such interactive contrasts, have, in any case (other things being equal) higher variances. Thus a type IV trial will require even greater numbers of patients and recruitment times.

One might argue, of course, that these increases in recruitment times are acceptable if scientific truth is our object: it may be an unpleasant consequence of adequately representing demographic subgroups, but there can be no guarantees that drug development will be easy and if that *is* the consequence, we must accept it. There are, however, several difficulties with this argument. The first is that it is unclear where it should stop. Should we require this of all subgroups? Persons of East Asian origin, for example, form an important minority in many Western countries, yet their numbers are nevertheless not considerable when one comes to conducting clinical trials. It would obviously be impractical to have them represented in the same number as persons of European origin. Of course, we may wish to sell a drug in East Asian countries, in particular Japan. It may be, therefore, that the solution would be to conduct trials in the Far East to answer this question and certainly, to look at the problem from the opposite perspective, Japanese pharmaceutical companies carry out trials in Europe and America. A point must come, however, where this approach would have to stop. What about cross-classifications such as Japanese female children aged 10–15, for example? Absolute numbers will be even smaller in such groups. And what about other characteristics? It was claimed at one time (Coren and Halpern, 1991) that left-handed persons had an appreciably lower life expectancy than right-handed persons. (This claim is probably incorrect; Harris, 1993.) Should we not also recognize handedness as a subgroup? And what about blood groups, the human leucocyte antigen (HLA) system, eye colour and so forth. The list could be endless.

The second problem is an ethical one. As we have seen, the randomized clinical trial has been criticized because it requires physicians to allocate patients to treatments they believe (but are not sure) may be inferior. Appeal is often made to the concept of equipoise, but it is difficult to see how physicians can be in equipoise at the beginning of a trial, pretty certain as to which of two treatments is superior at the end, and not have moved some way from equipoise during the trial, except by willingly forgoing the ability to look at results as they accrue. Such a self-denying ordinance, while it could be defended as being in the interests of future patients, could not be presented as being for the benefit of those about to be treated. This is one reason why sequential analysis was introduced for trials in serious diseases (see Chapter 19). This problem arises in an acute form with any discriminatory trial of type III in a serious disease in which the demographic fraction is not close to 1/2. In that case, the trial will have recruited adequate numbers of one sex long before recruitment is finished for the other. Suppose, for argument's sake, that women are the faster recruiting sex. The very requirement for adequate numbers in each group means that an independent analysis could be carried out for women before results are available for men. Must results for future female patients be withheld until results are available for men? If, however, the results are analysed for women and found to be highly favourable, will physicians be justified in withholding from men the treatment proved better for women on the grounds that it hasn't yet been adequately studied for men?

Even a type II trial cannot escape these difficulties if the disease is serious. Consider an indication where potential female subjects for a trial present more frequently than males. Here, recruitment will stop for females at the point at which half as many female patients have been recruited as would be indicated for an independent analysis and at a point when males are still being recruited. It might be argued, therefore, that there is no problem since an independent analysis is inappropriate for females. But what about future recruitment of females? Will women from this point on be allocated to the standard therapy only? If one were to continue to recruit female patients to the trial, one could reach a conclusion much earlier than by insisting that from this time onwards only males should be recruited. Is one justified in instituting a policy which will withhold such a potentially early conclusion for female patients, especially since such a conclusion might in any case be of benefit to male patients also?

This last point is important. In practice we do not consider that *only* results studied for a given subgroup are relevant to that subgroup; we accept that results carry over to some degree. This is, in fact, a necessary condition for any science of statistics. At the very least we have to be prepared to act as if results from one individual had some relevance to another. In fact, both frequentist and Bayesian approaches to statistics allow ways in which this can be done. The Bayesian, for example, can place an *informative* prior on possible differences in treatment effects between subgroups. Such a prior would state that she believes with high probability that any possible difference between sexes as regards treatment effects will be fairly small. If the treatment effect itself has an *uninformative* prior (she has little prior notion what it will be), until a great number of patients have been studied, the more important uncertainty will be what the treatment effect might be for any sex, rather than how much it might differ between sexes. Under such circumstances, for example, even studying further female patients can be extremely valuable in providing more information about the effect of treatment in males. (The similar problem of interpreting factorial designs, in which combinations of two drugs are compared with the monotherapies and with placebo, has been considered in a Bayesian framework by Simon and Freedman (1997).)

The frequentist equivalent would be to posit some maximum possible difference between the sexes in the effect of treatment. In a common, but extreme, approach, this difference would simply be assumed to be zero until there was convincing evidence to the contrary. Where, some difference were allowed, it could then be decided that the object of any treatment estimate would be to minimize the maximum mean square error: the sum of the variance and square of the maximum bias. If this maximum bias were not considered to be too large, then for the usual number of patients, the variance would dominate. Hence, reducing this would be a more important object than eliminating bias. Thus, as in the Bayesian case, it would be valuable to study further female patients even where the object was to say something about the treatment of males.

We return to this discussion below when considering what effect subgroup differences should have on the analysis of results. For further discussion see Freedman *et al.* (1995), Garrett (2006), LaRosa *et al.* (1994), Merkatz *et al.* (1993), and Piantadosi and Wittes (1993).

9.2.2   Should we carry out separate analyses for subgroups?

The problem with carrying out such analyses include: (i) that individual subgroups will have inadequate numbers to provide suitably precise statements and (ii) that the more subgroups one studies the greater the chance of a fluke unusual result. These do not constitute grounds for not studying subgroups, but they do give grounds for caution. A better approach would be to carry out some sort of analysis whereby the effect for a subgroup is estimated as a weighted average of the overall treatment effect and the stand-alone estimate from that group. A similar approach has been used in random effects meta-analyses of clinical trials (with a given trial taking the role of the subgroup), but its implementation for subgroup analysis raises some difficulties and I am not aware that it has been used. Nevertheless, it bears investigation.

> **Statistician**: A harmless drudge, as opposed to *subgroup analysis*, an aimless dredge.

In figure 9.2, the mean square error of two estimates of the treatment effect for females is given as a function of the *trial* demographic fraction (females as a proportion of all patients in the trial). It is assumed that it had been suspected that the treatment effect might be less for women than for men and that, to err on the side of caution, the trial has been designed with total numbers equal to the numbers which would be required to achieve 80% power for a 5% significance level (two-sided) for a trial

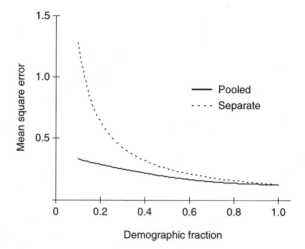

Figure 9.2   Mean square error for two estimates of the treatment effect for women, as a function of the demographic fraction.

in women only. Suppose that the treatment effect for women is, in fact, equal to that posited, but that the effect for men is half as great again. The figure shows the mean square error for the estimate of the effect for women (a) based on women only and (b) based on all patients. It will be seen that where the demographic fraction is high, the mean square errors are very similar. This is as it should be, since the trial will consist almost entirely of women and under such circumstances the pooled estimate will be almost identical to that based on women alone. For the case where the demographic fraction is small, however, it will be seen that by far the better policy is to pool. Of course, the problem in practice is that one does not know what the degree of bias is. My belief is that in many cases it will be considerably less than that considered here and so it appears that only for very large trials will it be worth producing separate estimates for the sexes. It may be, however, that at the end of a drug development programme there may be some value in producing separate estimates for each sex pooled across trials in a meta-analysis, since the superior numbers available may make bias, rather than random variation, the more important component of mean square error.

Of course, a straight choice between a separate estimate for each sex and a pooled estimate is the not the only one which may be made. For example, for a given degree of bias the optimal estimator would actually be some compromise between the two. Figure 9.3 illustrates the mean square error of the two estimators already considered and the optimal compromise for the case where the bias is assumed to be half of the treatment effect for women and the standard deviation is equal to the treatment effect as a function of the number of patients recruited to each of the two treatment groups for the case where the demographic fraction is 0.3. It can be seen that for lower sample sizes the pooled estimate is superior to the one using females only. (The point at which the two lines cross corresponds to a power of about 99% for a significance level of 5% two-sided.) However, the weighted optimal compromise is always superior to both.

In practice, the problem in using any weighted compromise is the impossibility of knowing what sort of degree of bias should be allowed for. (This is a crude version of the Bayesian problem of specifying a prior.) Indeed, a known bias is no problem at all since

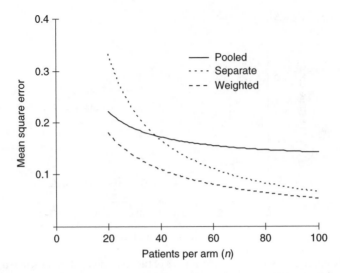

Figure 9.3 Mean square error for three estimators of the true treatment effect for women, as a function of the sample size n, in each treatment group, in a trial in which women form 30% of all patients, the individual standard deviation is equal to the treatment effect for women, and the treatment effect for men is 50% greater (or smaller) than that for women.

it can be adjusted for, enabling one to produce a mean square error which is simply equal to the variance. It may, however, be possible to place a plausible upper bound on the absolute value of the bias. In that case the optimal estimator lies between the weighted estimator corresponding to this bound and the pooled estimator. It may be that these limits are enough to enable a satisfactory inference to be made. Alternatively, the theoretical possibility of a fully Bayesian approach remains, although it would not be easy to implement. For an example of attempts to apply Bayesian thinking to this problem, see White *et al.* (2005).

One further point is worth making: looking for effects in subgroups is not a good way to rescue a disappointing trial. If the treatment effect in a given subgroup is larger than the trial average, it will be smaller than average in another subgroup. The trial as originally planned, however, recruited patients from both subgroups; it therefore remains a failure and regulatory authorities may properly take this point of view. It may be, of course, that such analysis can suggest in what sort of patients future trials might be run. This has two consequences. First, the potential market is less than supposed originally. Second, convincing proof of the efficacy of the drug, even in this subgroup, lies with future trials. It might be argued that even if a treatment is efficacious as a whole there is no proof of its efficacy in subgroups. This is, of course, true. However, believing *a priori* that subgroup differences will be relatively unimportant and continuing to concentrate on the results of a trial as a whole constitutes a consistent position. Looking for subgroup differences represents a retreat from this position and is potentially dangerous. It ought to be taken as an admission of a lack of confidence in the pooled estimate. For example, the Bayesian who embarks on this course will do well to have carefully specified the relevant prior probability distributions before examining the data. If he does not do this, he too is in danger of being over-influenced by chance variation.

9.2.3 The approach to be used in detecting differences

Suppose that one is not convinced by the arguments above which tend to show that, for the sorts of sample size usually entertained for clinical trials, given a straight choice between pooling and not pooling, the former is preferable, but wishes to explore, as fully as possible, the extent to which treatment effects differ between the sexes. Another controversy is then raised, namely whether one should test for treatment-by-sex inter-action or simply study the treatment effects separately for each sex.

If the object is truly that of studying differences between the treatment effects in the sexes, then I feel that the merits lie with a formal study of treatment-by-sex interaction. My arguments would be as follows. If it is purely an issue of estimating treatment effects for a given sex then either we are prepared to accept (until further evidence is provided) that treatment effects are similar enough for the two sexes for there to be no disadvantage in pooling, or we already fear that they may be considerably different, in which case pooling can only be justified where it is irrelevant (does not change the treatment effect) or we had some prior belief that effects may differ to some degree, in which case some sorted of weighted compromise is called for. In none of these cases does it seem to me that the actual evidence of the difference contributes much to the strategy. However, if the way in which the treatment effect may differ from sex to sex is of substantive interest, then producing two treatment estimates does not really answer the question. It is the difference between the two which is important, but this is nothing less than the interactive effect and to examine formally the difference between the two estimates corresponds to an examination (in terms of hypothesis testing or confidence intervals) of the interactive effect. This point is well made in three expository short pieces by Matthews and Altman in the *British Medical Journal* (Altman and Matthews, 1996; Matthews and Altman, 1996a,b).

9.2.4 Simpson's paradox; subgroup effects and interactions

Simpson's paradox is a phenomenon whereby an overall treatment effect in one direction is reversed in every stratum. It is named after a paper of 1951 in which it was extensively examined by E.H. Simpson (Simpson, 1951), although a related phenomenon had been discussed at least as early as 1899 by Karl Pearson (Pearson *et al.*, 1899). (See Aldrich (1995) for discussion.) A hypothetical example is given in Table 9.1, in which a trial has been run comparing two treatments in two strata of patients: moderately ill and

Table 9.1 Numbers surviving and dying by treatment and disease severity together with percentage surviving.

Treatment	Outcome	Stratum		
		Moderate	Severe	Both
A	Survived	30 (50%)	180 (30%)	210 (32%)
A	Died	30	420	450
	Total	60	600	660
B	Survived	240 (40%)	12 (20%)	252 (38%)
B	Died	360	48	408
	Total	600	60	660

severely ill. Overall the survival rate is 6% lower under A (32%) than under B (38%). In each of the two strata, however, the picture is reversed and the survival rate under A is 10% higher than under B (30% versus 20% and 50% versus 40%). If a generalized linear model is fitted with an identity link, then the result is significantly in favour of A if severity is used as a covariate and significantly in favour of B if it is not used ($P \cong 0.02$ in both cases).

Certainly the result is curious, but why is it a paradox? After, all we surely accept it as possible that more evidence can change our opinion about the truth of a situation, otherwise evidence would be superfluous (Senn, 2003). As Pearl points out, however, the paradox arises if we give a causal interpretation to what is observed (Pearl, 2000). A drug that increased survival for both the severely and moderately ill but reduced their survival chance overall would be truly paradoxical and of course we don't believe that this is possible. Furthermore, because we believe in the importance of temporal order when judging causality and because disease severity was determined prior to treatment, we would prefer the interpretation given by the analysis that conditions on strata and regards A as superior to B.

Of course, in a clinical trial we would never see imbalances like this at baseline and would therefore very rarely expect to be faced with Simpson's paradox. Its importance is far greater in an epidemiological context. For example, we might suspect when a new drug is launched on the market that patients with the most refractory disease might be more likely to take it. In the example there were 600 severe patients who took A and only 60 who took B, the numbers being reversed for moderate disease, so this might be a possible pattern if A were a newer treatment. Disease severity would then be a confounder for which it was appropriate to adjust.

In an epidemiological context we can always fear that there may be further confounders that we should have adjusted for. However, even in a clinical trial context we can always worry that, because of accidental bias, if only we look at enough strata we might eventually find a reversal. This stresses the importance of having thought carefully prior to analysis (and hence in practice prior to design) about what factors are likely to be of prognostic importance in analysing a trial (Senn, 1989, 1994, 2000).

Note that Simpson's paradox does *not* imply that an interaction is present (Senn, 2004). Indeed, the pure paradox occurs when the subgroup effect is the same but the average effect is different. There is some confusion over this point, however. The confusion arises, I think, because of log-linear models used in analysing contingency tables. Consider the case in Table 9.1. We can analyse this table using logistic regression and treating survived/died as an outcome and stratum and treatment as factors. Fitting treatment alone gives the following results for the effect of treatment B:

$$\text{Estimate} = -0.280, \quad \text{standard error} = 0.116, \quad \text{Wald statistic} = -2.42,$$

$$P\text{-value} = 0.015.$$

If stratum is added as a main effect, then the results for the effect of treatment B are:

$$\text{Estimate} = 0.459, \quad \text{standard error} = 0.209, \quad \text{Wald statistic} = 2.20, \quad P\text{-value} = 0.028.$$

(The Wald statistic is the ratio of estimate to standard error.) This demonstrates the effect reversal. However, an equivalent analysis is possible using log-linear models. This requires that survived/died, or outcome, is also treated as a factor and that the numbers of patients in the eightfold classification formed by the three factors, the frequencies, are modelled as a function of the three factors. The model that is equivalent to (and produces identical effects to) the logistic regression model ignoring stratum requires that the main effects of treatment, outcome are fitted and their interaction, and it is this interaction that gives what was the effect of treatment B in the logistic regression model. On the other hand, the model that is equivalent to fitting the main effects of stratum and treatment in logistic regression requires main effects of stratum, treatment, outcome and all two-way interactions, and it is again the interaction of treatment and outcome that is equivalent to the logistic regression main effect of treatment.

In other words, what is a main effect in logistic regression terms becomes an interaction in log-linear model terms. However, it is really the log-linear model that is the odd one out among generalized linear models as regards use of 'interactions' and, in more conventional terms, Simpson's paradox does not involve interactions.

See Garrett (2006) for further discussion of Simpson's paradox and Aldrich (1995) for a historical account.

9.2.5 Subgroups and nonlinear models

An advantage of a randomized clinical trial is that on average over all randomizations any covariates are balanced at baseline. This implies that a phenomenon such as Simpson's paradox is rather unlikely to arise in practice. For certain types of model it also implies that the expected value over all randomizations of a treatment effect that does not include a given covariate in the model is the same as the expected value that does include the covariate. For example, this applies to Normal linear models.

However, in general it is not true that means over models are the same as models over means and there are, in fact, many types of model commonly applied for which it will make a systematic difference to a treatment estimate, even in a randomized clinical trial, whether a prognostic covariate is included in the model or not (Gail *et al.*, 1984). For example, if logistic regression is used, the average log-odds will be different depending whether a balanced prognostic covariate is included in the model or not (Robinson and Jewell, 1991). A similar point applies as regards the log hazard ratio for a proportional hazards model (Ford *et al.*, 1995).

To illustrate this point, consider Table 9.2, which gives frequencies of patients in a clinical trial cross-classified according to treatment (A or B), strata of a factor with two levels and outcome (success or failure). The trial is perfectly balanced at baseline in that there are 100 patients within each stratum for each treatment. The odds ratios in stratum 1 and stratum 2 are

$$OR_1 = \frac{80/20}{60/40} = \frac{80 \times 40}{60 \times 20} = \frac{8}{3},$$

$$OR_2 = \frac{60/40}{36/64} = \frac{60 \times 64}{36 \times 40} = \frac{8}{3}$$

and so are identically equal to $8/3 = 2.67$.

Table 9.2 Numbers of patients in a clinical trial cross-classified by treatment, stratum and outcome.

Treatment	Outcome	Stratum 1	2	Both
A	Success	80	60	140
A	Failure	20	40	60
B	Success	60	36	96
B	Failure	40	64	104

However, if we ignore the strata, the odds ratio is

$$OR = \frac{140/60}{96/104} = \frac{140 \times 104}{96 \times 60} = 2.53.$$

This is not, in my view, a reason for preferring simpler models. On the contrary, it suggests that it may be naive to hope that the treatment estimate (for these types of models) can be simply transferred from trial to target population, since it would imply that differing background risk would produce different results for analyses that ignored the covariate. It also shows that one should be careful about drawing conclusions by comparing different models in terms of parameter estimates. As Lee and Nelder (2004) point out, it will usually be better to compare them in terms of predictions.

References

Aldrich J (1995) Correlations genuine and spurious in Pearson and Yule. *Statistical Science* **10**: 364–376.

Altman DG, Matthews JN (1996) Statistics notes. Interaction 1: Heterogeneity of effects. *British Medical Journal* **313**: 486.

Coren S, Halpern DF (1991) Left-handedness – a marker for decreased survival fitness. *Psychological Bulletin* **109**: 90–106.

Ford I, Norrie J, Ahmadi S (1995) Model inconsistency, illustrated by the Cox proportional hazards model. *Statistics in Medicine* **14**: 735–746.

Freedman LS, Simon R, Foulkes MA, *et al.* (1995) Inclusion of women and minorities in clinical trials and the NIH Revitalization Act of 1993 – the perspective of NIH clinical trialists. *Controlled Clinical Trials* **16**: 277–285.

Gail MH, Wiand S, Piantadosi S (1984) Biased estimates of treatment effects in randomized experiments with nonlinear regressions and omitted covariates. *Biometrika* **71**: 431–444.

Garrett AD (2003) Therapeutic equivalence: fallacies and falsification. *Statistics in Medicine* **22**: 741–762.

Garrett AD (2006) *The Role of Subgroups and Sub-Populations in Drug Development and Drug Regulation.* PhD, Open University, Milton Keynes.

Harris LJ (1993) Do left-handers die sooner than right-handers – Commentary. *Psychological Bulletin* **114**: 203–234.

Hennekens CH, Eberlein K (1985) A randomized trial of aspirin and beta-carotene among U.S. physicians. *Preventive Medicine* **14**: 165–168.

LaRosa JH, Seto B, Caban CE, Hayunga EG (1994) Including women and minorities in clinical research. *Applied Clinical Trials* **4**: 31–38.

Lee Y, Nelder JA (2004) Conditional and marginal models: Another view. *Statistical Science* **19**: 219–228.

Matthews JN, Altman DG (1996a) Interaction 3: How to examine heterogeneity. *British Medical Journal* **313**: 862.

Matthews JN, Altman DG (1996b) Statistics notes. Interaction 2: Compare effect sizes not P values. *British Medical Journal* **313**: 808.

Meinert CL, Gilpin AK, Unalp A, Dawson C (2000) Gender representation in trials. *Controlled Clinical Trials* **21**: 462–475.

Merkatz RB, Temple R, Sobel S, Feiden K, Kessler DA (1993) Women in clinical trials of new drugs – a change in Food and Drug Administration policy. *New England Journal of Medicine* **329**: 292–296.

NIH (1994) Guidelines for the inclusion of women and minorities as subjects in clinical research. *NIH Guide for Grants and Contracts* **23**.

Pearl J (2000) *Causality: Models, Reasoning and Inference*. Cambridge University Press, Cambridge.

Pearson K, Lee A, Bramley-Moore L (1899) Mathematical contributions to the theory of evolution. VI. Genetic (reproductive) selection: inheritance of fertility in man, and of fecundity in thoroughbred racehorses. *Philosophical Transactions of the Royal Society A* **192**: 257–330.

Piantadosi S, Wittes J (1993) Politically correct clinical trials. *Controlled Clinical Trials* **14**: 562–567.

Robinson LD, Jewell NP (1991) Some surprising results about covariate adjustment in logistic regression models. *International Statistical Review* **58**: 227–240.

Senn SJ (1989) Covariate imbalance and random allocation in clinical trials [see comments]. *Statistics in Medicine* **8**: 467–475. [Comment in *Statistics in Medicine* **10**(5): 797–799 (1991)].

Senn SJ (1994) Testing for baseline balance in clinical trials. *Statistics in Medicine* **13**: 1715–1726.

Senn SJ (2000) Consensus and controversy in pharmaceutical statistics (with discussion). *The Statistician* **49**: 135–176.

Senn SJ (2003) *Dicing with Death*. Cambridge University Press, Cambridge.

Senn SJ (2004) Conditional and marginal models: another view – Comments and rejoinders. *Statistical Science* **19**: 228–238.

Simon R, Freedman LS (1997) Bayesian design and analysis of two × two factorial clinical trials. *Biometrics* **53**: 456–464.

Simpson EH (1951) The interpretation of interaction in contingency tables. *Journal of the Royal Statistical Society, Series B* **13**: 238–241.

Stigler SM (1986) *The History of Statistics: The Measurement of Uncertainty before 1900*. Belknap Press, Cambridge, MA.

White IR, Pocock SJ, Wang D (2005) Eliciting and using expert opinions about influence of patient characteristics on treatment effects: a Bayesian analysis of the CHARM trials. *Statistics in Medicine* **24**: 3805–3821.

9.A TECHNICAL APPENDIX

9.A.1 Recruitment times

Consider a two-group parallel trial which is to be stratified by sex (that is to say, sex will be fitted as a main effect but not necessarily as an interaction). Let N be the target number of individuals to be studied in a conventional trial. Let the overall arrival rate for patients be r and let the population demographic fraction be f, and suppose that the arrival rate for women is fr and for men is $(1 - f)r$. Let tn be the time to recruit if there is no discrimination (tn stand for 'time no'), as in a conventional trial. Let tt (f) be the time to recruit if equal numbers of males and females are required for the same total power (*tt* stands for 'time total') as the conventional trial. Let $ti(f)$ be time to recruit if equal numbers of males and females are required for the same *individual* (*ti* stands for 'time individual') power for each sex as the conventional trial. Let

$$a(f) = \max\left[1/f,\ 1/(1-f)\right] \tag{9.1}$$

Then $tn = N/r$, $tt(f) = a(f)(N/2)/r$ and $ti(f) = a(f)N/r$. If we standardize these times with respect to the conventional trial, then we need to divide them by $tn = N/r$ to obtain

$$tn = 1,$$
$$tt(f) = a(f)/2, \tag{9.2}$$
$$ti(f) = a(f).$$

So, for example, for a trial in which 75% of the patients presenting are women we have $f = 3/4$, $a(f) = \max[4/3,\ 4] = 4$ and $tt(f) = 2$, $ti(f) = 4$.

9.A.2 The maximum possible difference in the treatment effects in the absence of qualitative interactions

Let the treatment effect for females be τ_f and that for males be τ_m. The difference is $\delta = |\tau_f - \tau_m|$. Suppose that there are no qualitative interactions and (without loss of generality) that $\tau_f \geq 0$ and $\tau_m \geq 0$. Suppose now that $\tau_f \geq \tau_m$. Then, for given τ_f the maximum value of δ is attained when $\tau_m = 0$, at which point it equals τ_f. Suppose now that $\tau_m \geq \tau_f$, then similarly we may show that the maximum possible value of δ is τ_m. Thus, in the absence of qualitative interactions, the difference in effects cannot be greater than the greater of the two effects.

9.A.3 Mean square error of pooled (over both sexes) and separate estimates of the effect for females as a function of the trial demographic fraction

Let f now stand for the *trial* demographic fraction with τ_f, τ_m and δ defined as above and t_f and t_m as the unbiased estimates of τ_f and τ_m. The absolute bias in estimating τ_f using the pooled estimate $t_p = f t_f + (1-f)t_m$ is $\beta = f\tau_f + (1-f)\tau_m - \tau_f = (1-f)(\tau_m - \tau_f)$, so that

$$\beta = (1-f)\delta. \tag{9.3}$$

Let γ^2 be the variance of the pooled treatment estimate, t_1. The variance of the unbiased (separate) treatment estimate, t_f, of τ_f, being based on the fraction f of the total patients, is γ^2/f. Hence the mean square errors are

$$\mathrm{MSE}\,(t_p) = \beta^2 + \gamma^2 = (1-f)^2\,\delta^2 + \gamma^2 \tag{9.4}$$

and
$$\mathrm{MSE}\,(t_f) = \gamma^2/f. \tag{9.5}$$

If the trial is planned on the assumption that $\tau_f = \tau_m = \tau$ and it turns out that $\tau_f = \tau$, then for 80% power and a 5% size of test (two-sided) $\gamma \cong \tau_f/2.8$. Suppose, however, $\delta = \tau_f/2$. Then

$$\text{MSE}\left(t_p\right) = (1-f)^2\,\tau_f^2\Big/4 + \left(\tau_f/2.8\right)^2 \tag{9.6}$$

and

$$\text{MSE}\left(t_f\right) = \left(\tau_f/2.8\right)^2\Big/f. \tag{9.7}$$

To obtain these factors as proportions of the square of the treatment effect we simply substitute $\tau_f = 1$ in (9.6) and (9.7). If we do this, taking, for example, a demographic fraction of $f = 1/4$, then we obtain $\text{MSE}(t_p) = 0.27$ and $\text{MSE}(t_f) = 0.51$.

9.A.4   The mean square error of pooled separate and optimally weighted treatment estimates as a function of the sample size

Now consider the optimal estimator, which consists of a pooled weighted sum of the two separate treatment estimates for each sex. The weight is w for the female group and $(1-w)$ for the male group. This will now be considered as a function of the total number of patients n of either sex in each treatment group for a fixed demographic fraction. The variances of t_p and t_f will also be considered as a function of n. This can be done very simply by noting that if σ^2 is the variance of the individual observations within strata and treatment groups then $\gamma^2 = 2\sigma^2/n$. Hence we may write

$$\text{MSE}\left(t_p\right) = \beta^2 + \gamma^2 = (1-f)^2\,\delta^2 + \frac{2\sigma^2}{n} \tag{9.8}$$

and

$$\text{MSE}\left(t_f\right) = \frac{2\sigma^2}{nf.} \tag{9.9}$$

Now define $t_w = wt_f + (1-w)t_m$ where w is to be determined so as to make the mean square error of t_w a minimum. We then have

$$E\left(t_w\right) = w\tau_f + (1-w)\left(\tau_f + \delta\right) \tag{9.10}$$

and

$$\text{var}\left(t_w\right) = \left(\frac{w^2}{f} + \frac{(1-w)^2}{1-f}\right)\frac{2\sigma^2}{n}, \tag{9.11}$$

from which we have

$$\text{bias}\left(t_w\right) = (1-w)\,\delta \tag{9.12}$$

and

$$\text{MSE}\left(t_w\right) = \{(1-w)\,\delta\}^2 + \left(\frac{w^2}{f} + \frac{(1-w)^2}{1-f}\right)\frac{2\sigma^2}{n.} \tag{9.13}$$

If (9.13) is minimized with respect to w, we obtain as a solution

$$w = \frac{2f + nf\,(1-f)\,\theta^2}{2 + nf\,(1-f)\,\theta^2}, \tag{9.14}$$

where $\theta = \delta/\sigma$ and is a measure of the importance of the true difference in the subgroups compared to variability. If we study (9.14), we see that where $\delta = 0$, and there is no bias, the optimal weighting is f. Hence the optimal estimator is the pooled estimator. As n goes to infinity, bias dominates variance, w approaches 1, and the optimal estimator is simply the separate estimate. In general some compromise is superior. Let $d = \delta/\tau_f$ and $\psi = \tau_f/\sigma$ so that $\theta = d\psi$. If ψ is very small, implying that precision is low, then again $w \cong f$, as is also the case for small n. Suppose that $f = 0.3$, and $\psi = 1$ with $d = 0.5$. Then from (9.14) for $n = 38$ we have $w = 0.65$. ($d = 0$ and the pooled estimate would give a ratio of parameter to standard error of about 4.4, which implies extremely high precision.) Since the pooled estimate will use a weight of 0.3 and the separate estimate will use a weight of 1, then for this particular parameter combination the optimal estimator represents approximately a compromise between the two. Substituting in (9.8), (9.9) and (9.13), we have $\text{MSE}(t_p) = 0.175$, $\text{MSE}(t_f) = 0.175$ and $\text{MSE}(t_w) = 0.114$.

10

Multiplicity

Pour bien savoir les choses, il en faut savoir le détail; et comme il est presque infini, nos connaissances sont toujours superficielles et imparfaites.
François, duc de La Rochefoucauld, *Réflexions ou Sentences et Maximes Morales*

*The fox knows many things – the hedgehog one **big** one.*
Archilocus

10.1   BACKGROUND

In its simplest form a clinical trial consists of a head-to-head comparison of a single treatment and a control in order to answer a single well-defined question. In practice, however, matters tend to be more complex. Suppose, for example, we wish to know whether a particular drug improves lung function in asthmatics. We have a number of possible continuous outcome measures: forced expiratory volume in one second (FEV_1), forced vital capacity (FVC), peak expiratory flow (PEF), airways resistance (RAW) and so forth. These are measures we can take many times in the course of a day. We might also be interested in the effectiveness of the drug from the point of view of the patient as regards severity and frequency of asthma attacks, breathing difficulties in general, quality of sleep and so forth. We may also wish to monitor the tolerability of the drug – its effect on tremor, heart rate, blood pressure (systolic and diastolic), QT interval, potassium levels – as well as to make a record of any side-effects.

There may also be occasions when we wish to compare more than two treatments. We may want a placebo and a standard therapy as a comparator, or we may wish to carry out a dose-finding study. We have also seen, in the previous chapter, that we may have legitimate reasons to study the effect of treatment in subgroups and that there may be many of these. These are all reasons why, in practice, a clinical trial may provide the possibility of making dozens, if not hundreds, of comparisons.

We touched on this problem in Chapter 9, where we drew attention to Cournot's criticism of multiple comparisons. To use the language of hypothesis testing, the problem is that as we carry out more and more tests, the probability of making at least one type I error increases. This probability of at least one type I error is sometimes referred to as the family-wise error rate (FWER) (Benjamini and Hochberg, 1995). Thus, controlling the type I error rates of individual tests does not guarantee control of the FWER. To put

Statistical Issues in Drug Development/2nd Edition   Stephen Senn
© 2007 John Wiley & Sons, Ltd

it another way, if, for a trial in which all treatments are identical, we carry out very many tests of significance (comparing different outcomes, in different subgroups and perhaps more than two treatments), it becomes highly likely that one of these tests will be significant. Therefore, it seems that simply obtaining such a result hardly provides grounds for concluding that there is a difference.

Some of the issues which arise in connection with this general problem are discussed below. Unless explicitly stated otherwise, it will be assumed that the general set-up is that of a clinical trial comparing two treatments only, but for which a large number of measures may be taken. Occasionally the case of more than two treatments is discussed.

Multiplicity continues to be a field of much research and controversy. Good reviews are given by Cook and Farewell (1996), Koch and Gansky (1996), and Wassmer *et al.* (1999) and a regulatory view by the Committee for Proprietary Medicinal Products (2002).

10.2   ISSUES

10.2.1   There should be only one significance test per trial

One way of dealing with the issue of multiplicity would appear to be to avoid multiple testing. If our object is to ensure that the probability of making at least one type I error per trial should be no more than α (usually the value chosen for α is 0.05), then a simple way of dealing with the issue is obviously to ensure that only one test of size α is carried out. (A possible strategy is to nominate a main outcome variable and test only this. This variable must be declared before data are obtained.) A practical argument which is put in favour of this approach is that the planning of a clinical trial is a complex issue which can only be successfully concluded if one has a very precise objective in mind. Where we wish to answer two or more questions with a single clinical trial, it will be impossible to do this optimally for each question. There is a danger that in trying to answer more than one question we shall produce a design which answers none effectively. Hence, in any case, quite apart from inferential and philosophical difficulties in carrying out more than one significance test, we ought to be designing trials to answer a single question.

The counterargument, however, is that we usually have many questions which we wish to answer in drug development. There is a practical (economic) and ethical imperative to answer these questions as efficiently as possible. It is ludicrous to refuse to look at other questions which could be answered to some degree in the same trial either because they cannot be answered perfectly (we would have designed a slightly different trial if this had been the main question) or because we fear that the probability of making at least one type I error will be increased (Lindsey, 1999).

10.2.2   Controlling the probability of making at least one type I error rate per trial is irrelevant

However many tests one carries out, the probability of making at least one type I error per test is not increased. Therefore, it can be claimed that, if all tests conducted are reported and the trialist takes the rough with the smooth, considering not only significant but nonsignificant results, then there should be no problem. (Note that even with this viewpoint, selectively reporting those tests which are significant, while ignoring the others, *does* cause a bias. However, if all tests which are to be performed are stated in the trial protocol, it may then be checked by the regulator that these and only these tests have been carried out.)

A counterargument is that some sort of mental selection process will inevitably take place between tests. If a number of tests are presented, then this selection will be influenced by the significance or otherwise of the test. Hence we shall over-stress the significant results. Only if this selection process takes place before the result will this danger be avoided, but this, effectively, leads back towards position 10.2.1.

10.2.3   The problem can be dealt with by constructing a global measure

One way of avoiding multiplicity in *testing* while allowing it in *measuring* is to combine the measures in some way prior to performing a test. This is a general approach often applied in quality-of-life assessments, for example. A great many questions (say n) are put with the object of measuring many aspects of the patient's life. These are than combined into a single score or index. A similar approach can be applied to deal with repeated measures over time. For example, we may obtain a great number (say n) of individual pain scores for every patient in a clinical trial. These may be reduced to a single score in some way. (A popular index is the SPID, the sum of the pain intensity differences from baseline.) In either of the above examples, therefore we shall have replaced n measurements by a single measurement. This single measurement can then be tested, thus, apparently, avoiding the problem of multiplicity. (Of course, the regulator must be convinced that the sponsor has not made the decision on how to combine the data after the trial results are in: this would give the sponsor sufficient leeway to influence the probability of success. This difficulty can be dealt with by specifying exactly the form of any summary measure or index to be used in the protocol.)

There are at least two objections to this approach. First, it makes most sense if what we are trying to do is to make some global decision for all patients. If we consider that individual patients may have different priorities, then we are simply destroying information by combining individual measures into a single global statistic. Second, even if we accept that such a global decision is important, there may be much disagreement among decision makers as to how individual measures should be combined. Indeed, Hilden (1987) has argued that permitting patients to come to rational decisions requires us not to combine measures globally on behalf of all patients but that if we insist on using significance tests to make such decisions we should allow each patient to specify the way such measures should be combined.

10.2.4   Where many outcomes are being compared, Bonferroni corrections should be performed

Suppose that n hypothesis tests are being performed comparing an active treatment with placebo on n outcomes, each test being carried out at level of significance α. (For the most popular level of significance we should have $\alpha = 0.05$.) In general, the probability of making at least one type I error depends upon correlations between the outcomes. For example, in the unlikely case of all tests being independent, the probability of making at least one type I error is 1 minus the probability that no test is significant, or

$$1 - (1 - \alpha)^n. \tag{10.1}$$

In general, tests will tend to be positively correlated and the probability of making at least one type I error may be expected to be less than (10.1). It is conceivable, though, that tests could be negatively correlated, in which case the probability of making at least one type I error would be greater than given by (10.1). It has been shown, however, that whatever the correlation structure, if each test is carried out at a nominal level of significance of α/n, then the probability of making at least one type I error cannot exceed α. This correction, dividing the level of significance by n (or alternatively multiplying the P-value by n) is referred to as the Bonferroni correction (Carlo Emilio Bonferroni, 1892–1960, was the Italian mathematician who first established the inequality which provides the correction. An excellent summary in English of his paper is given by Dewey who also includes a biographical note (Dewey, 1996).)

A number of criticisms may be made of this approach. First, that the power of individual tests carried out will be reduced (see Figure 10.1). For example, for a power of 80% for 5% size (two-sided), applying a Bonferroni correction to six outcomes reduces the power for a single test to 57%. (However, the power that at least one will be significant, what one might refer to as **disjunctive power** (Senn and Bretz, 2007) is not affected to this degree. In fact, the power that *at least one* endpoint will be significant can easily increase despite correction as the number of endpoints tested increases. This is illustrated by Figure 10.2, which shows the power of at least one result being significant for different numbers of tests, where the Bonferroni correction is applied. It is assumed that the trial is of sufficient size to give 80% power for a one-sided test at the 2.5% level if only a single outcome measure is taken. (Both Figures 10.1 and 10.2 are justified in the appendices.)

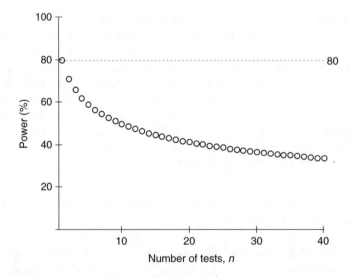

Figure 10.1 Power of individual tests given the Bonferroni correction, as a function of n, the number of tests. The power for a single unadjusted two-sided test is assumed to be 80% for 5% size.

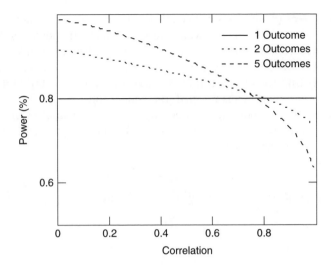

Figure 10.2 Disjunctive power (probability of at least one significant result) as a function of the common correlation coefficient for 1, 2 or 5 outcomes for a power of 80% for a single outcome.

Second, the situation may nevertheless arise where rather many tests will be significant at level α but none will be significant at level α/n. We may then formally be unable to declare the treatment as significant while strongly believing that this is so. (This suggests that in practice we do not necessarily come to conclusions about the efficacy of treatments by looking at results individually.) Third, the Bonferroni correction is rather pessimistic and will be conservative where, as may usually be expected to be the case, clinical outcomes are positively correlated.

Some improvements on the Bonferroni approach, for example Holm's procedure (Holm, 1979), are available as alternatives but they do not entirely escape the criticisms above.

10.2.5   The problem can be solved by using global multivariate tests

It is possible to construct procedures which simultaneously test the null hypotheses that a number of outcomes are identical for the two treatments. Such tests can use the empirical correlation structure of the observations and thus deal with the third of the criticisms of the Bonferroni approach. An example of such a test is Hotelling's T^2 test.

There are, however two important difficulties. First, although such tests make good use of the empirical correlation structure, they make no use of any knowledge about the likely effect of treatment. For example, in a trial comparing an experimental to a standard bronchodilator in asthma and for which FEV_1, FVC, RAW, and PEF were measured, the test would admit as alternative hypotheses not only the two 'consistent' hypotheses that all four measures might be better or that all four might be worse for the experimental treatment compared with the standard, but also the six hypotheses that any two measures might be better and any two might be worse as well as the four hypotheses that any three might be better and one could be worse and the four that any three could be worse and one might be better. In total, therefore, there are 14 mixed alternative hypotheses (if we take strict equality of treatments as being the limiting case of the experimental treatment being worse) among which the power of the procedure would be dissipated. These hypotheses are, however, extremely unlikely *a priori* and the procedure as a whole has low power for testing the hypotheses of interest. The second difficulty is that the question that is posed is itself of very little interest, so that even where the null-hypothesis is rejected, the conclusion reached is uninformative. It is analogous to an opinion-poll interviewer stopping an individual in the street, giving a list of several government policies and asking 'Do you disagree with *any* of these?'. The answer 'yes' is not very informative.

Multivariate analysis: A means of finding the answer when you don't know the question.

10.2.6   The problem can be managed by global univariate tests

The strategy discussed under Section 10.2.3 was to reduce the outcomes to a single measure by combining them. The disadvantage is that this combination involves a certain degree of arbitrary choice: different trialists would come up with different indices or summary measures. An approach which appears less arbitrary is to try to produce a single univariate test. For example, one procedure, due to O'Brien (1984), is to rank every patient on every outcome, sum the ranks, and compare the sums between treatment groups. (There are various ways this can be done.) Consider, however, the case where we have just two outcome measures. It is clear that this approach weights them equally. Equal weights are also, in a sense, arbitrary. It might be the case that most physicians would agree that one of the two measures was much more important than the other. Furthermore, the weights which fundamental factors receive are not invariant to choice of measures. In asthma, peak expiratory flow (PEF) and forced expiratory volume in one second (FEV_1) measure rather different things, the former is a flow measure and the latter a capacity measure. But forced vital capacity (FVC) is very similar to FEV_1. Therefore, if FEV_1, FVC and PEF are included in the same analysis using this approach, although each of the *measures* receives equal weight, capacity receives twice the weight of flow. This issue of partial redundancy of measures can be dealt with by taking explicit account of the correlation between them, and a number of schemes have been proposed by various authors (Cornelli and Klersy, 1996; O'Brien, 1984; Pocock, *et al.* 1987; Senn, 1989).

10.2.7   Where there are repeated measurements over time, the problem can be dealt with by modelling

The sort of modelling that is popular here, for example, is the random slopes model of Laird and Ware (1982). Some aspects of repeated measures modelling were discussed in Chapter 8, where, among other things, it was pointed out that this approach is not always robust and can lead to (implicit) curious measures of the treatment effect.

Nevertheless, the approach can be very efficient and yield useful inferences where the model is correct and will no doubt continue to be popular. It is dealt with in some detail in the book in this series on mixed models (Brown and Prescott, 2006).

10.2.8   A significant result for a prespecified outcome permits further valid analysis of secondary endpoints

This claim is sometimes made. Provided that a single prespecified analysis is significant, whether a global analysis as in Section 10.2.5 or Section 10.2.6 or of some single endpoint or of a set of endpoints with a level protected by adjustment as in Section 10.2.4, then the probability of making at least one type I error per trial is controlled. If one regards this error as being important, then one may consider that, an important guarantee having been provided, further analysis of an exploratory nature is permitted. Thus the primary analysis fulfills a sort of 'gate-keeper' function, whereby only trials that satisfy this entry requirement are then permitted to proceeed to secondary analysis. Certainly, the regulator is unlikely to allow secondary claims unless this minimal condition has been satisfied and, indeed, Robert O'Neill of the FDA has a paper with the suggestive title 'Secondary endpoints cannot be validly analyzed if the primary endpoint does not demonstrate clear statistical significance' (O'Neill, 1997). However, the title is not 'Secondary endpoints *can* be validly analyzed if the primary endpoint *does* demonstrate clear statistical significance,' and O'Neill does not suggest that this will always be acceptable.

In fact, this point of view – that provided some gate-keeper analysis is positive, secondary analyses may then be carried out safely – is open to criticism from both ends of the statistical spectrum. Those who are unconvinced of the necessity for adjustment at all will point out that the expected proportion of significant results for true null hypotheses is not increased however many tests you carry out. The only problem is in failing to accept the rough with the smooth and simply concentrating on that which is significant.

Those who believe in strong control of error rates will point out that one could nominate a 'man of straw' endpoint that was almost certain to yield significance and then regard oneself as entitled to look at anything one liked. For example, in a trial of osteoporosis in which it was important to show an improvement in fracture rates one could nominate the much weaker endpoint of bone mineral density as the primary one and then have a host of different fracture measures (overall, vertebral, wrist, hip and so forth) as secondary endpoints, claiming a therapeutically demonstrated success if at least one of these was significant. This type of criticism is discussed further in connection with the problem of comparing many treatments in section 10.2.9.

10.2.9   Where many treatments are being compared, a global test comparing all treatments should be carried out first

Such a test, for example, is an F-test associated with an analysis of variance. It is the practice of some statisticians to use this prior to carrying out individual pairwise comparisons. The idea is that we first attempt to answer the question 'Is at least one of the treatments different from the others?'. If we decide 'yes', we are then justified in examining further to try to pin down exactly what the differences are. Actually, to strike a technical note, although this controls what has been referred to as the global level α (Bauer, 1991), it does not control the multiple level α if there are more than three treatments. For example, if we were comparing three doses of a new formulation with a standard and a placebo, we might already know that the standard was superior to placebo. That being the case, we should expect that for a reasonably sensitive trial the global test of significance of equality of all five treatments would be rejected. However, if we hadn't included the placebo we should have had to carry out a global test comparing three doses to each other and to a comparator before proceeding to pairwise comparisons. Including a 'man of straw' treatment like a placebo, therefore, does not justify missing out this further step. Hence a cascade of tests, starting with the global test, might be called for.

To add a personal note, I never found in many years' experience of drug development that such global tests of significance were of any interest and soon stopped looking at them. (However, some statisticians would disagree with this attitude.)

10.2.10   Even where the probabilities of making at least one type I error are controlled, conditional error rates may not be

Consider a placebo (P)-controlled trial of n doses (D_1, D_2, ..., D_n) of a drug. Suppose that we compare each dose to placebo, do not compare the doses with each other and apply the Bonferroni correction by dividing the target significance level, α, by n, thus performing each test at level α/n. As a means of controlling the probability of making at least one type I error, this procedure is conservative. Now suppose that one is told that the contrast of the lowest dose against placebo ($D_1 - P$) is significant. Naturally, one might expect that the other contrast will also be significant because it seems reasonable that if the lowest dose is effective, the highest dose will also be effective. If all dose contrasts do, indeed, turn out to be significant, then this will increase one's confidence in the overall efficacy of the result.

There is, however, another subtle and not so pleasant reason why one might expect the other contrasts to be significant. Suppose that the lowest dose is in fact useless, but that the reason the first contrast is significant is that, just by chance, the placebo results are low. These results will be involved in calculating all the other contrasts. Hence, even if all doses are useless, the chance that any given further contrasts will be significant will exceed α/n and even α. In fact, the more doses are significantly different from placebo the more likely it is that the placebo result is unusual. Figure 10.3 illustrates the case where five doses are being compared with placebo and a Bonferroni correction has been applied to the conventional significance level of 0.05. In fact, each individual contrast of dose against placebo is tested at the 0.01 level. The figure gives the conditional probability that the nth contrast tested is significant given that all previous contrasts are significant. It will be seen that this probability rises to nearly 50% by the fifth contrast.

A similar position applies when one has correlated outcomes. For example, if I observe in a trial comparing an active treatment with a placebo that there is a significant difference in FEV_1 at the 5% level, then it is reasonable to expect that the probability of a significant difference in PEF at the 5% level will be much higher than 5%: not only because the observed difference may indicate that the treatment is efficacious but

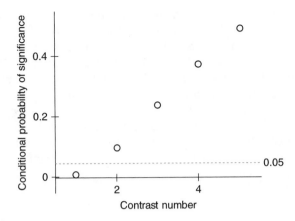

Figure 10.3   Conditional size of significance tests comparing five doses of a drug with placebo and carried out independently at the 0.01 level. The figure shows the probability under the null hypothesis of concluding that a given dose is significant given that all other doses tested to date are significantly different from placebo. Note that although the probability of the first result being significant is held at 0.01, the conditional probability of the second already exceeds 0.05.

because, even if the difference is spurious, the fact that measures tend to be correlated indicates that a further spurious difference is more likely.

10.2.11   A structured approach to testing can deal with the problem

A device which can be used to control the probability of making at least one type I error is to use a structured approach to testing. Return to the case where we are comparing n doses with placebo and let D_1 be the lowest dose, D_2 be the next lowest, and so forth through to the highest dose D_n. Now it may be that I would be reluctant to accept that any dose could be better than placebo unless all higher doses were all better. In that case, I might be prepared to operate a scheme whereby I first test the highest dose, D_n against placebo. Only if this contrast were significant would I proceed to test D_{n-1} against placebo. Using this procedure I could test each contrast at level α while holding the probability of making at least one type I error at α, whatever the situation regarding the truth or falsity of the various hypotheses. The above is a very crude scheme. There are many specialist multiple comparison tests which have been proposed for particular circumstances. For example, Dunnett's (for comparing a number of treatments to a control), the Newman – Keuls test, Duncan's test and so forth.

   The difficulty in implementing such procedures is in deciding on an appropriate structure for the alternative hypotheses and an associated strategy. The difficulty in interpreting such procedures is the general one which effects all hypothesis testing. Strictly speaking, such procedures correspond to a rule for action: the question, however, is whether scientists who operate such rules *actually* believe (or act according to) the rules and, in particular, whether they can persuade others to do so. This is especially problematic when one has a complex web of tests. Note that it is a weakness of both frequentist and Bayesian theories (but see below) that they implicitly deal with single decision (or at the very least inference) makers.

Marcus *et al.* developed a theory which can be used to construct general strategies and which has been very popular with theoretical statisticians of the Neyman – Pearson school. In the strategy of Marcus *et al.* (1976), the **closed test procedure**, we consider a set of hypotheses which are closed under intersection. (This is sometimes referred to as the *close* test procedure rather than the *closed* test procedure, a phrase which will be rejected here on linguistic grounds.) That is to say that if H_{0a} and H_{0b} are two null hypotheses we must also admit $H_{0a} \cap H_{0b}$ (that is to say H_{0a} 'and' H_{0b}) as a hypothesis and so forth. A hypothesis may then be rejected if it and all higher-level hypotheses formed through intersection with it would also be rejected. Consider the case where, following Bauer (1991), we are testing that three means are equal to zero. The closed set of all hypotheses is then:

Global null hypothesis

$$H_{111}: \mu_1 = 0, \mu_2 = 0, \mu_3 = 0.$$

Intersection null hypotheses

$$H_{110}: \mu_1 = 0, \mu_2 = 0, \quad H_{101}: \mu_1 = 0, \mu_3 = 0, \quad H_{011}: \mu_2 = 0, \mu_3 = 0$$

Individual null hypotheses

$$H_{100}: \mu_1 = 0, \quad H_{010}: \mu_2 = 0, \quad H_{001}: \mu_3 = 0.$$

Here, in operating the closed test procedure, if we wish to conclude that H_{100} is false, then we must reject not only the individual hypothesis H_{100} at the α level but also the two intersection hypotheses $H_{110} = H_{100} \cap H_{010}$ and $H_{101} = H_{100} \cap H_{001}$ at the α level as well as the global hypothesis $H_{111} = H_{110} \cap H_{101}$ also at the α level. This procedure is usually carried out in step-down mode. The global test is carried out first. If it is rejected then all the intersection tests at the next level down are carried out. The tests which are then rejected at this level dictate which further tests may be carried on down the cascade and so forth. Finally, if the procedure proceeds that far, the individual hypotheses are tested in order to see which are rejected. As Bauer points out, the procedure is *coherent* by definition, in that we are not allowed to conclude that a single hypothesis is rejected unless the higher-level hypotheses of which it is a part are also rejected. On the other hand, *consonance* is not guaranteed. We could, for example, reject the global hypothesis and no other, thus ending up with the conclusion that some hypotheses are false without knowing which.

The closed test procedure is attractive in that it provides an automatic and coherent approach to controlling the type I error rate. For any given case, however, the problem still remains of defining suitable test statistics with which to examine the null hypotheses. For the multiple treatment groups problem a cascade of F-tests is common. For multiple outcomes, because of the unknown correlation structure, it may be more difficult to identify valid but useful tests. The problem with the automatic application of the procedure is that by failing to order the hypotheses according to interest we may lose power to address the most important questions. However, this is only a problem with the automatic application. Orderings suggested by the alternative hypotheses can be taken into account, although, of course, the procedure then loses some generality. (Suppose, for example, that the regulator does not approve of the sponsor's ordering.)

The procedure presupposes, of course, what may seem intuitively reasonable but which is difficult to justify logically – that we wish to control the probability of making at least one type I error.

10.2.12 Bayesian statistics has the answer

Bayesian statistics has an answer for everything. In this case a multivariate prior for all the variables of interest would have to be specified and then updated using the multivariate likelihood to form a multivariate posterior distribution. (For methods of elicitating multivariate priors from experts, see chapter 5 of O'Hagan *et al.* (2006)). Ideally this would all have been embedded in a random-effects model which enabled one to predict for any new patient, using also multivariate data on him or her, the probability of any given multivariate prognosis. If one wished to recognize the fact that decisions are personal, this would then be combined with the patient's personal utility function (of multivariate outcomes) to produce an optimal strategy.

The only drawback to this solution is that it cannot be implemented.

The somewhat flippant preceding sentence was where this chapter ended in the first edition of this book. I still believe it is true that a fully Bayesian solution to this problem is impossible to implement. However, that is not a reason for not considering what might be done in practice. In that connection, an issue regarding choice of prior distribution is worth discussing and this is considered in the next section.

> **Bayesian statistics**: A means of finding the answer to *how* to find the answer but rarely, unfortunately, the answer.

10.2.13 Bayesian selection paradoxes

An interesting paradox has been raised by Phil Dawid (Dawid, 1994), which we will now attempt to discuss. In order to make this as simple as possible we will do this in terms of a rather unrealistic example. Imagine that we have selected one of a number of treatments from a trial of many treatments in which for each of the k treatments we have studied n patients and we wish to make a Bayesian statement about the 'true' population average outcome using the observed mean. The question is: does it make any difference to our inference if the treatment selected has been selected because it has the highest observed mean?

This example is actually unrealistic in two ways. First, we don't run trials with two experimental treatments unless they are different doses of the same treatment, which is not the case here; and second, for reasons discussed in Chapter 3, we are generally interested in controlled comparisons and not population averages. However, to avoid some complications we shall accept the example as described here with the further simplification that we will assume that the variance of individual responses is known and the same for each treatment.) We suppose that the sample mean for a given treatment i is $\bar{X}_i$ and is Normally distributed with variance σ_i^2/n.

It turns out that if we use a conjugate Normal prior for a treatment mean, with prior mean μ and prior variance γ^2, it makes no difference whatsoever whether the particular treatment about which we are making the inference is selected at random or as being the one which has the largest observed mean. Under the circumstances, Bayesian inference only needs the data for that treatment and the prior. It is irrelevant that the treatment was selected as being the largest among a group of treatments.

It is instructive to think about the meaning of the prior distribution in order to understand why this happens. Having a Normal prior distribution for a true population mean and then observing a sample from that population is formally analogous to the following. One has observed an infinity of population means (these are what make the prior); one has drawn a population at random from this infinity (but one does not know which one), observed a sample from it and now proceeds to make inferences about the mean. Thus implicitly, one is comparing the sample mean with an infinity of known *population* means. Thus the comparison with some locally observed sample means adds no further useful information and it is therefore also irrelevant whether the sample mean is the largest or not in this sample.

10.2.14 Controlling the false discovery rate

This particular topic is of greater significance to drug discovery than to development. Nevertheless, it has become so important in recent years that it is included here as it is beginning to have some influence on development also.

In an influential paper of 1995 that by the end of 2005 had attracted more than 1000 citations, Benjamini and Hochberg (Benjamini and Hochberg, 1995) drew attention to an alternative sort of error rate that it might be of interest to control. Consider the situation in Table 10.1, which is based on table 1 of their paper.

Here all entries in the table are frequencies. We suppose that m null hypotheses are being tested. U, V, T and S are unobservable random variables, whereas R is an observable random variable. That is to say, we can see how many hypotheses we reject, and this is R but we don't know how many are false, which is S. If V true hypotheses are rejected then what Benjamin and Hochberg refer to as the *per comparison error rate* (PCER) is $E[V/m]$, which is to say that it is the expected proportion of all hypotheses tested that are falsely rejected.

Now, suppose all null hypotheses are true, so that $m_0 = m$, then $m - m_0 = 0$ and therefore $S = 0$ and testing each hypothesis at level α will give $E[V/m] = \alpha$. In general, if there are some false null hypotheses, then the expected value of V will be less but the value of m will be unchanged so that the $E[V/m] < \alpha$. Thus the PCER is controlled at or below α by this strategy. On the other hand, the family-wise error rate (FWER) is simply the probability that at least one hypothesis is falsely rejected, and this is $P(V \geq 1)$. This

Table 10.1 Null hypothesis cross-classified by status (true or false) and decision taken (accept or reject).

	Accepted	Rejected	Total
True null hypotheses	U	V	m_0
False null hypotheses	T	S	$m - m_0$
	$m - R$	R	m

can be controlled at being less than or equal to α by testing each hypothesis at level α/m, as in the standard Bonferroni strategy.

Now consider, not the ratio of falsely rejected hypotheses to all hypotheses tested, but the ratio of false rejection to all rejections, $Q = V/(V+S)$. The expected value of this, Q_c, given by

$$Q_c = E[Q] = E[V/(V+S)] = E[V/R],$$

is what Benjamini and Hochberg call the *false discovery rate* (FDR).

As they point out, there are many circumstances under which it is more reasonable to control the FDR than to control the probability of making at least one type I error per experiment. For instance, if we are testing multiple endpoints for a given treatment compared with a control, it is some overall profile that we may be interested in. Another case they suggest is when investigating multiple subgroups. We might be prepared to accept some false positives in order to allow ourselves the ability to find some true positives. The third case they mention is that of screening various chemicals for potential drug development. This, in my view, is the most important. Use of the FDR gets around a particular difficulty to do with the number of treatments in an experiment. Consider two scientists working in a laboratory. Each is comparing members of a (different) class of compounds with a control in an in-vitro experiment. One is comparing three compounds and one is comparing six. Why should the one who is comparing six make a bigger adjustment for significance than the one who is comparing three? If the experiment involving six had been run as two experiments with three, a comparable adjustment would have been made. It seems more natural for each scientist simply to control the false discovery rate.

Of course, there are various technical issues in controlling the FDR and this fact is witnessed by the huge and growing literature in this field. These issues, however, are beyond the scope of this book.

References

Bauer P (1991) Multiple testing in clinical trials. *Statistics in Medicine* **10**: 871–890.

Benjamini Y, Hochberg Y (1995) Controlling the false discovery rate – a practical and powerful approach to multiple testing. *Journal of the Royal Statistical Society Series B – Methodological* **57**: 289–300.

Brown H, Prescott R (2006) *Applied Mixed Models in Medicine*. John Wiley & Sons, Ltd, Chichester.

Committee for Proprietary Medicinal Products (2002) *Points to consider on multiplicity issues in clinical trials*. European Medicines Evaluation Agency, London, http://www.emea.europa.eu/pdfs/human/ewp/090899en.pdf.

Cook RJ, Farewell VT (1996) Multiplicity considerations in the design and analysis of clinical trials. *Journal of the Royal Statistical Society Series A – Statistics in Society* **159**: 93–110.

Cornelli M, Klersy C (1996) Different methods to analyze clinical experiments with multiple endpoints: a comparison on real data. *Journal of Biopharmaceutical Statistics* **6**: 115–125.

Dawid AP (1994) Selection paradoxes of Bayesian inference. In: Anderson TW, Fang Ka-ta, Olkin I (eds), *Multivariate Analysis and its Applications*, vol. 24. Institute of Mathematical Statistics, Hayward, CA.

Dewey ME (1998) Bonferroni. In: Armitage P, Colton T (eds.) *Encyclopedia of Biostatistics*. John Wiley & Sons, Ltd, Chichester, pp. 420–421.

Hilden J (1987) Reporting clinical trials from the viewpoint of a patient's choice of treatment. *Statistics in Medicine* **6**: 745–752.

Holm S (1979) A simple sequentially rejective multiple test procedure. *Scandinavian Journal of Statistics* **6**: 65–70.

Koch GG, Gansky SA (1996) Statistical considerations for multiplicity in confirmatory studies. *Drug Information Journal* **30**: 523–534.

Laird NM, Ware JH (1982) Random-effects models for longitudinal data. *Biometrics* **38**: 963–974.

Lindsey JK (1999) Some statistical heresies. *Journal of the Royal Statistical Society Series D – The Statistician* **48**: 1–26

Marcus R, Peritz E, Gabriel KR (1976) On closed testing procedures with special reference to ordered analysis of variance. *Biometrika* **63**: 655–660.

O'Brien PC (1984) Procedures for comparing samples with multiple endpoints. *Biometrics* **40**: 1079–1087.

O'Hagan A, Buck CE, Daneshkah A, *et al.* (2006) *Uncertain Judgements.* John Wiley & Sons, Inc., Hoboken.

O'Neill RT (1997) Secondary endpoints cannot be validly analyzed if the primary endpoint does not demonstrate clear statistical significance. *Controlled Clinical Trials* **18**: 550–556.

Pocock SJ, Geller NL, Tsiatis AA (1987) The analysis of multiple endpoints in clinical trials [see comments]. *Biometrics* **43**: 487–498. [Comment in *Biometrics* **45**(3): 1027–1028 (1989)].

Senn SJ (1989) Combining outcome measures: statistical power is irrelevant [comment]. *Biometrics* **45**: 1027–1028.

Senn SJ, Bretz F (2007) Power and sample size when multiple endpoints are considered. *Pharmaceutical Statistics* **6**: 161–170.

Wassmer G, Reitmeir P, Kieser M, Lehmacher W (1999) Procedures for testing multiple endpoints in clinical trials: an overview. *Journal of Statistical Planning and Inference* **82**: 69–81.

10.A TECHNICAL APPENDIX

10.A.1 The power of individual tests when a Bonferroni correction has been performed

Let the sample size be such that an uncorrected test would have power $1 - \beta$ for a size $\alpha/2$. Let $k = \Phi^{-1}(1 - \alpha/2) + \Phi^{-1}(1 - \beta)$ where $\Phi(.)$ is the distribution (cumulative probability density function) of the standard Normal. Let the clinical relevant difference be Δ, the standard error be γ, the test statistic be t and z be a standard random variable. Then $\Delta/\gamma = k$. Check:

$$P[|t/\gamma| > \Phi^{-1}(1 - \alpha/2)] \cong P[t > \Phi^{-1}(1 - \alpha/2)\gamma] = P[z > \Phi^{-1}(1 - \alpha/2) - \Delta/\gamma]$$
$$= P[z > \Phi^{-1}(1 - \alpha/2) - k] = P[z > -\Phi^{-1}(1 - \beta)] = 1 - \beta.$$

Now, if we apply the Bonferroni correction, the power is approximately given by

$$P[t > \Phi^{-1}\{1 - \alpha/(2n)\}\gamma] = P[z > \Phi^{-1}\{1 - \alpha/(2n)\} - k].$$

Example: suppose $\alpha = 0.05$, $1 - \beta = 0.2$, then $\Phi^{-1}(1 - \alpha/2) = 1.96$ and $\Phi^{-1}(1 - \beta) = 0.84$ and $k = 2.8$. If $n = 6$, then $\Phi^{-1}[1 - \alpha/(2n)] = 2.638$, and we require $P(z > 2.638 - 2.8) = P(z > -0.162) = 0.57$.

10.A.2   The power of at least one test being significant when Bonferroni corrections are employed

This issue is difficult to address in generality because the answer is dependent on correlation between measures and also on clinically relevant differences for different measures and all sorts of correlation structures and patterns for differences can be envisaged. However, some qualitative feel for the effect can be gained by making two radically simplifying assumptions: first that the values are conditionally independent given some latent variable, and second that some common effect size (ratio of clinically relevant difference to standard deviation) is targeted. (It will also, of course, be assumed that the outcomes are Normally distributed.)

Let the latent variable be Λ, let the conditionally independent measures be correlated with Λ with correlation ρ, and suppose that the type I error rate to be tolerated is α, so that, if a Bonferonni correction is applied it will be α/n for each of n tests. Assume, without further loss of generality that the variance of a test statistic is 1 and that positive values of a test statistic will lead to rejection of the null hypothesis. In that case, the measures have conditional variance $(1 - \rho)$, whereas Λ has variance ρ and, for given $\Lambda = \Lambda$, $\Lambda > 0$, the probability of not rejecting the null hypothesis with a given test is

$$\Phi\left(\frac{z_{\alpha/n} - \Lambda}{\sqrt{1 - \rho}}\right),$$

where $\Phi(.)$ is the cumulative density of a Normal distribution and $z_{\alpha/n}$ is the critical (positive) value of the test. Hence, conditional on Λ the probability of at least one significant result among n is

$$1 - \left[\Phi\left(\frac{z_{\alpha/n} - \Lambda}{\sqrt{1 - \rho}}\right)\right]^{n}.$$

On the other hand, the probability density that $\Lambda = \Lambda$ is

$$\phi\left(\frac{\Lambda - \Delta}{\sqrt{\rho}}\right),$$

where $\phi(.)$ is the probability density of the standard Normal. Hence the power of rejecting at least one null hypothesis is

$$\int_{-\infty}^{\infty} \phi\left(\frac{\Lambda - \Delta}{\sqrt{\rho}}\right) \left\{1 - \left[\Phi\left(\frac{z_{\alpha/n} - \Lambda}{\sqrt{1 - \rho}}\right)\right]^{n}\right\} d\Lambda$$

$$= 1 - \int_{-\infty}^{\infty} \left[\Phi\left(\frac{z_{\alpha/n} - \Lambda}{\sqrt{1 - \rho}}\right)\right]^{n} d\Lambda.$$

(10.2)

10.A.3   Conditional type I errors for a number of treatments compared with a placebo

Consider a case with equal numbers of patients per group and where the common variance is known. Suppose that the means from the treatment groups have been divided by their standard errors so that each has variance 1. Under the null hypothesis these means have identical expectation. Suppose that this expected value is 0. The difference between any two standardized means has standard error $\sqrt{2}$. Let the treatment mean for placebo be m_0 and for the other treatments be $m_1, m_2, \cdots, m_n$. Let z_c be some critical value of the standard Normal to be determined by the target type I error rate and whether or not a Bonferroni correction is applied. For example, we might have $z_c = \Phi^{-1}\{1 - \alpha/(2n)\}$. Now suppose that we condition on a given value x of m_0, the mean for placebo. The difference from the ith treatment will be significant if $m_i - x > z_c\sqrt{2}$ or $m_i - x < -z_c\sqrt{2}$. This is equivalent to requiring that $m_i > x + z_c\sqrt{2}$ or $m_i < x - z_c\sqrt{2}$. However, since m_i has a standard Normal distribution the probability that this will occur is easily calculated as

$$\psi(x, z_c) = \Phi\left(x - z_c\sqrt{2}\right) + 1 - \Phi\left(x + z_c\sqrt{2}\right) \tag{10.3}$$

Since the means for the n treatments are independent, then the conditional probability that all n contrasts to placebo will be significant is given by

$$\{\psi(x, z_c)\}^n. \tag{10.4}$$

Now, if we take (10.4) multiply it by the marginal probability density function of the mean in the placebo group and integrate we shall obtain the probability that all n contrasts will be significant. This is given by

$$\varphi(n, z_c) = \int_{-\infty}^{\infty} \frac{1}{\sqrt{2\pi}} e^{-x^2/2} \{\psi(x, z_c)\}^n dx \tag{10.5}$$

Now, by the definition of conditional probability, the probability that contrast n is significant, given that the previous $n - 1$ contrasts are, is the joint probability that contrast n is significant and the previous $n - 1$ contrasts are significant, divided by the probability that the previous $n - 1$ contrasts are significant. But the joint probability in question is nothing less than the probability that all n contrasts are significant. Hence the conditional probability we require is

$$\xi(n, z_c) = \frac{\varphi(n, z_c)}{\varphi(n - 1, z_c)}. \tag{10.6}$$

Expression (10.6) can then be evaluated numerically for any given critical value.

Intention to Treat, Missing Data and Related Matters

In proving foresight may be vain
The best laid schemes of mice and men gang aft a-gley.

Robert Burns, *To A Mouse*

11.1 BACKGROUND

The essence of an experiment is that a scientist manipulates a condition to see what effect ensues. Interpretation is easiest if conditions that are not of primary interest are controlled. However, experiments go wrong. Although this can itself be extremely fruitful on occasion (consider, for example, the legend of Alexander Fleming and the accidental contamination of a culture plate by penicillin or Becquerel's discovery of radiation through unintentionally exposed photographic plates), it generally leads to difficulties in interpretation. In a clinical trial, the condition which is manipulated is that of the treatment of the patient. Except for single-dose pharmacodynamic studies and studies where the patient is treated in hospital, it is nearly always the case that some patients do not take their medicine as planned by the trialist. This lack of compliance can take a number of forms. The patient can drop out of the trial, take none of the medicine while pretending to do so, forget to take the treatment from time to time, or take it at the wrong time or in the wrong way. These would be examples where the patient did not follow the protocol and such deviations can make interpretation difficult. However, even where the protocol expressly mentions circumstances under which a patient may withdraw from treatment, such withdrawals may make the task of evaluating the results hard. A further problem for the trialist is that the participating physician may also not comply with the protocol. For example, she may include patients on the trial for which the inclusion criteria are not satisfied.

These sorts of occurrences are common and have to be faced in analysis. In particular, a decision has to be made as to which patients are to be included in the analysis of the trial results. Two phrases commonly used in this connection are 'per-protocol' and 'intention to treat' (or sometimes, 'intent to treat'). A 'per-protocol' analysis excludes all patients who are known not to have completed the trial as planned. It would thus exclude drop-outs, noncompliers and poor compliers, as well as the falsely included. An 'intention to treat' analysis actually analyses patients according to the treatment the trialist intended for them. Thus, a patient assigned to the active treatment, but who confessed to not taking it, would nevertheless be analysed as if she had received the active treatment. (Sometimes this is described as, 'if randomized then analysed', but see Section 11.2.8 below.) The regulator usually requires that an intention to treat analysis be carried out and it is often supposed that the sponsor would prefer a per-protocol analysis. Thus we have an issue which is presumed to divide the two sides of drug licensing.

One technical point that is perhaps worth mentioning is that the degree of compliance of a patient cannot be established perfectly. In the past, reliance was made on statements obtained from the patients themselves and also on 'pill counts': returned medication. At the time of the first edition I mentioned two recent technical developments that had opened up new possibilities (see Urquhart (1994) for a discussion). One was electronic monitoring: pill dispensers with an in-built microchip which will log when the dispenser was opened. The other was low-dose, slow-turnover chemical markers, which can be added to a treatment and then detected via blood sampling. (Obviously there are considerable practical problems with the latter.) These techniques made it a practical possibility to take degree of compliance into account in statistical analyses. However, my impression is that, despite the initial enthusiasm for these technological advances, they have been little employed in the ten years since the first edition. However, what have developed apace are statistical approaches to dealing with missing data and, indeed, there is now an excellent book in the same series as this one entitled *Missing Data in Clinical Studies* (Molenberghs and Kenward, 2007) with not only an extensive coverage of the theory but also much practical advice on implementation. Other books include Dodge (1985) and Little and Rubin (2002).

Although the issues of missing data and intention to treat are closely related, they are not identical. Intention to treat analysis is possible provided outcome and randomization data are not missing and (in its strict sense) impossible if they are. If data are not missing, then even if patients are noncompliant it is possible to analyse them as randomized provided only that their original treatment allocation is known. A per-protocol analysis requires knowledge of compliance. Also, depending on what one means by per protocol, it may or may not require complete outcome data. For example, one could simply say for a per-protocol analysis that one is only interested in patients who not only took the medicine as instructed but also recorded their outcomes.

However, there are clearly many circumstances under which it is highly misleading just to deal with the data one has as if they were a random sample of all the data one intended to have or would like to have. A famous nonclinical example is that which faced Abraham Wald (who was mentioned briefly in Chapter 2) in the work he did on aircraft survivability during the Second World War. Mangel and Samaniego (1984) describe it like this:

> Aircraft returning from missions have hits by enemy weapons distributed over various parts of the plane (e.g. wings, tail, fuselage etc.). The operational commander must decide... how to reinforce various parts of the aircraft to improve survivability... The operational commander does not know the distribution of hits on an aircraft that did not return. This is the basic difficulty of making a decision.
>
> (p. 259)

The problem has two traps for the unwary that Wald, of course, avoided. If one is not careful one assumes first that one should reinforce where the planes are most likely to be hit and second that the distribution of hits in returned planes provides a straightforward estimate of the overall distribution of hits. In fact, some places are more vulnerable than others and it is the distribution of hits in planes that did *not* return that is important, since this is indicative of vulnerability. If one could assume that hits were distributed at random over all planes (returning and nonreturning) then it would make sense to reinforce the places in the returning planes that had had the fewest hits.

11.2   ISSUES

11.2.1   The theoretical justification for intention to treat

A common justification for 'intention to treat' is in terms of the randomization theory of clinical trials as used in connection with frequentist hypothesis testing. In the simplest experimental situation, patients are randomized to two groups which are given different treatments. If a large difference is observed in outcome, then either this is due to chance assignment alone, or there must be an effect due to treatment. The probabilities associated with random assignment can be calculated and hence there is a basis for a test of significance. If, however, we only analyse a subset of patients, say ignoring drop-outs (that is to say, analysing 'completers' only), then there are now three possible explanations for the difference between groups: (1) chance assignment', (2) treatment', (3) the effect of noncompliance. It is then sometimes claimed that there is now no basis for a test of significance since where explanation (1) is rejected there is no means of deciding between (2) or (3).

Actually, for a test of strict equality between treatments, the argument is not quite correct. For example, suppose that noncompliance differs considerably between the two groups. In a double-blind trial there would seem to be only two possible reasonable explanations: either the difference is due to chance or it is due to treatment. Thus, the third explanation above can be reduced to the other two. It therefore seems unreasonable to suppose that the risk of showing a difference between treatments where the treatments are identical is increased by using an analysis of completers only. A further difficulty with the argument is that clinical trials are almost never analysed as randomized. Usually subcentre blocks are used but they are not used as strata in the analysis (see Chapter 14.) This undermines the practical importance of the pure randomization argument.

A further justification for intention to treat can be given in practical terms. If the main medical decision-maker is the physician, then what is relevant are his or her decisions. He or she decides whether to give a patient a particular treatment or not. In assessing the consequence of such a decision it is the total effect of the treatment which is relevant and this includes compliance. A better estimate of the practical consequence of allocating a treatment will be given by the intention to treat analysis. From the patient's point of view, things are perhaps a little more complicated. Here it may be more relevant to know the effect of the treatment *given* full compliance, although it might also be relevant to know the probability of complying.

For general discussion of intention to treat see Ellenberg (1996), Lewis (1988) and Lewis and Machin (1993). A very useful, and much-cited, survey of trials claiming to use intention to treat was carried out by Hollis and Campbell (1999), who concluded 'The intention to treat approach is often inadequately described and inadequately applied. Authors should explicitly describe the handling of deviations from randomized allocation and missing responses and discuss the potential effect of any missing response.' See also White and Pocock (1996). Intention to treat was something of a bête-noire of the late and great pharmacokineticist Lewis Sheiner, to the extent that he sometimes claimed that statisticians had ruined clinical research with their obsession with it. For an out-and-out attack on the concept (and some other attitudes) see Sheiner (1991).

11.2.2   The theoretical justification for per-protocol analysis

The justification of this is usually that it will lead to better estimates of the pure pharmaceutical effect of treatment where the treatment is effective. It is obvious that a treatment which is not taken cannot affect outcome. Therefore, including noncompliers in the analysis of an effective treatment will lead to a dilution of the treatment effect and, hence, a better estimate of this will be given by analysing the compliers only.

This argument is also not without its difficulties. It presupposes either that noncompliers do not differ in their state of health (apart from any benefit they would have received from the treatment not taken) from those who comply, or that the decision to comply is not itself influenced by treatment. But if patients who are dissatisfied with the effect of their treatment fail to comply, then excluding them from analysis will over-estimate the effect of the treatment.

Nevertheless, where we are interested in the pharmacological consequence of treatments it seems intuitively reasonable that some sort of adjustment for compliance is relevant. In this connection, an interesting distinction between explanatory (or scientific) trials and pragmatic trials was introduced by Schwartz, and colleagues (Schwartz *et al.*, 1980; Schwartz and Lellouch, 1967). For the former, a per-protocol analysis would be more relevant, whereas the latter might require intention to treat.

11.2.3   Beyond intention to treat and per-protocol

The two extreme positions amount to this. A per-protocol analysis assumes that information from noncompliers is irrelevant to judging the effect of a treatment. An intention to treat analysis assumes that it is only safe if all information regarding outcomes is analysed, treating noncompliers as if they were compliers. I have drawn attention to two scientific views of causality in drug development: the 'voluntary' (which I associated more with statisticians) and the 'mechanistic' (associated more with pharmacokineticists) (Senn, 1997). As regards the first I wrote:

> The voluntary view of causality is one which denies that causal statements can be given any meaning except in connection with actions which an agent can voluntarily alter. In most clinical trials this agent is implicitly taken to be a prescribing doctor because her cooperation with both trial and real world prescribing protocols can be assumed to a much higher degree than that of the patient. Thus the caricature pharmaceutical statistician

might remark sarcastically that a treatment which patients refuse to take but which a 'per protocol' analysis shows would be highly effective, if only patients *would* take it, is really no better than a treatment which all patients are prepared to take and which would be highly effective if only it weren't useless.

Regarding the second, I wrote:

> It is mechanistic in its view of causality: causes and effects are links between molecules and molecules and molecules and receptors and receptors and cells and so forth and ultimately these may be expressed in terms of differential equations governing the interaction of pharmaceuticals and body-systems. The caricature pharmacokineticist might remark sarcastically that the pharmaceutical statistician, with his intention to treat analyses, is embarked on medical sociology not biology.

These two extreme attitudes might be regarded as leading naturally to intention to treat in the first case and per-protocol in the second. These analyses are not, however, the only ones possible and there has been a great deal of attention to alternative approaches whereby the complex interactions between outcomes on the one hand and discontinuation and degree of compliance on the other, as well as the effect of treatment on both, are all modelled. The idea behind this is to recover, to an appropriate degree, the information on the effect of treatment given by noncompliers.

An early simple proposal as to how to do this was made by Gould (Gould, 1980). He suggested that patients could be divided into three groups: (1) those who discontinued for reasons which had nothing to do with the efficacy (or lack of it) of the treatment assigned to them; (2) those who discontinued for lack of efficacy; (3) those who completed. In analysis, group 1 could be ignored and patients from groups 2 and 3 could be given ranks as follows. All those who discontinued would be ranked according to the length of time they 'survived' on the trial. All completers would be given higher ranks than this, but they themselves would be ranked according to the outcome measure originally envisaged. Thus the first patient to drop out would be given the lowest rank and the completer with the best outcome the highest rank.

Since Gould's paper, numerous alternative approaches to the problems of compliance and missing data have been put forward. As regards compliance, two rather controversial papers from 1991 have been cited at least 100 times each (Efron and Feldman, 1991; Sommer and Zeger, 1991). As regards missing data, much-cited examples include Diggle and Kenward (1994), Greenland and Robins (1985), Laird (1988) and Smith and Roberts (1993), and the review papers by Rubin (1996) and Schafer and Graham (2002). Anther important paper is Robins and Gill (1997).

A key paper in the development of the subject pre-dates that of Gould (1980) and that is Rubin (1976). In it Rubin introduced the now-famous distinction between *missing completely at random, missing at random* and *missing not at random*. The first of these implies that although missingness may depend on observed covariates, it does not depend on outcomes observed or unobserved. The second allows that missingness may depend on observed outcomes (and covariates) but not on unobserved outcomes. The third applies where the missingness depends on unobserved values.

Some other relevant terminology is covered by Molenberghs and Kenward (2007) and concerns ways of handling measurements and missingness mechanism. *Selection models* consider marginal models for outcome measurements and model missingness conditional on outcomes. *Pattern-mixture models* consider missingness as a marginal process and measurement as a conditional process (a different response model for each pattern of missingness). Finally, we have shared-parameter models involving latent variables providing a connection between missingness and measurement.

Whatever framework is used, analysis is not a simple matter. In general, results are found to be rather strongly dependent on assumptions, but it would be wrong to suppose that this in itself is an argument against employing the methods. Simpler approaches may just produce consistent but wrong answers. The issue remains controversial and vexed. Where the regulator fears the influence of assumptions on the result, *some* of these fears at least can be allayed if the sponsor has specified in detail the approach to be used in the protocol. Of course, it can be reassuring to the regulator if the results are consistent whatever the assumptions, but the requirement that multiple analyses under different models should be significant can be expensive to the sponsor in terms of power or sample size (see Chapter 13) and, of course, there may be some indications for which the results of such analyses will never agree, whatever the sample size. (The fact that they may give quite different results is the reason why the field is so controversial in the first place.)

In addition to the issue of models of missingness, a further issue is to do with what one wishes to estimate. This is well covered by Molenberghs and Kenward (2007). They take the case of a trial with repeated measurements over time and consider three views, designated view 1, view 2a and view 2b. View 1 means that one is interested in the whole longitudinal sequence. This requires formulation of a longitudinal model. For view 2, of particular interest is the value at the end of the trial and this has two variants. For view 2a the end of the trial is the last planned occasion. For any patients who dropped out, data are missing. For view 2b the end of the trial is the end for that patient, that is to say (approximately) the last time the patient was observed.

11.2.4   Last observation (carried forward) analysis

This is a much-used and much-despised form of analysis. See, for example Mallinckrodt (2006) for a particularly withering attack. If we take view 2a from section 11.2.3, then last observation carried forward (LOCF) consists of replacing the missing value at the planned end of the trial by the last value that was observed. This is a form of what is called single imputation. However, there is another interpretation of last observation carried forward and that is the one expressed by view 2b in section 11.2.3 above. For view 2b, LOCF has the advantage that it is actually based on observed data. From this point of view, and particularly as a test of the null hypothesis that the treatments are identical, the properties of LOCF have been claimed to be not too bad (Shao and Zhong, 2003, 2006), although this claim has been disputed (Carpenter *et al.*, 2004) and more generally LOCF has come in for a great deal of criticism (Mallinckrodt *et al.*, 2004a, 2004d).

For view 2a, however, LOCF has two severe disadvantages. First, as a single imputation method it makes the very strong and unlikely to be realistic observation that patients could have been expected to continue to have the same general level had they stayed in the trial. The second is that it *is* a single imputation method and hence does not express the uncertainty inherent in imputation itself. See Section 11.2.8 for a discussion.

Both of these objections are serious; in particular, the second means that standard errors will be too small. Unfortunately, the first applies in part in general to nearly all approaches to missing data: they involve assumptions that are neither entirely realistic nor completely testable. The main objection in my view to LOCF, if one takes view 2a, is that it is too often used as a quick-fix lazy solution (I plead guilty on occasion) leading automatic acceptance where in fact careful thought and criticism are what is needed.

However, some of the alternatives do have a strong hypothetical or counterfactual flavour and it seems to me that their proponents have sometimes swept the problems under the carpet. As Shih and Quan (1997) have put it, 'We argue that the hypothetical complete-data marginal mean averaged over the dropout patterns is not as relevant clinically as the conditional mean of the completers together with the probability of completion or dropping out of the trial.' (p. 1225). They have suggested an analysis that consists of two stages. In the first one models the drop-out process itself and in the second the completers only. They then suggest ways in which the two pieces of information can be combined. Although this is not quite the whole truth (for example, there may be some further information on those who dropped out early), it is at least nothing but the truth in comparison with many alternative methods that have been proposed.

11.2.5   Missing completely at random

This is the simplest case of missingness and implies that conventional analysis methods can be used. Indeed, complete case analysis is possible. The main disadvantage is that this will involve a loss of information if some subjects provide incomplete information.

Another possibility may be to reduce the profiles to a suitable summary. Suppose, for example, that we were absolutely confident that the effect of treatment would be to improve reported values by a constant amount compared with placebo over the period of observation and that the reasons that some patients dropped out was completely unconnected with treatment. Under some circumstances a suitable measurement of the treatment effect would be the mean of all the visit measurements over the period of observation. Whether this was an efficient measure would depend on the correlation structure. However, in the unrealistic case of a trial with no baseline measurements and only two post-randomization values, this would be a completely efficient measure. Let us assume for argument's sake that the mean of all the post-treatment measures is an efficient measurement of the effect on that patient.

Now, if some patients have missing values, then a complete case analysis will discard them completely, leading to a loss of information. On the other hand, if we include all patients and perform a two-stage summary measures analysis by first calculating a mean of all values and then in a second stage use these as a raw input, we lose sight of the fact that the patients have been measured with varying precision. We shall combine the patient means with equal weight and lose efficiency (Senn *et al.*, 2000). (This issue was discussed in Chapter 8 and is analogous to that to do with weighting effects from different centres which is discussed in Chapter 14.)

In fact, suppose we are producing a treatment group mean using n patients and that for patient $i, i = 1, \ldots, n$ the variance of the treatment estimate will be V_i, where this reflects both the random variation in the true effect from patient to patient given the same treatment and also the number of times the values have been measured for a given patient. If we calculate the arithmetic mean of these estimates we have

$$V_a = \frac{1}{n^2} \sum_{i=1}^n V_i = \frac{1}{n} \bar{V}, \tag{11.1}$$

where $\bar{V}$ is the arithmetic mean of the various variances. However, the optimal estimator would weight with weights proportional to $w_i = 1/V_i$, so that the resulting estimator would have variance

$$V_{opt} = \frac{\sum_{i=1}^n w_i^2 V_i}{\left(\sum_{i=1}^n w_i \right)^2} = \frac{\sum_{i=1}^n w_i}{\left(\sum_{i=1}^n w_i \right)^2} = \frac{1}{\sum_{i=1}^n w_i} = \frac{1}{n} \bar{V}_h, \tag{11.2}$$

where $\bar{V}_h$ is the harmonic mean. However, unless all variances are identical, which implies that no patients have missing data, then the harmonic mean is less than the arithmetic mean, which implies a loss of efficiency by using the summary measures approach (Senn *et al.*, 2000). To recover the information correctly requires a move to a mixed-models approach and, indeed, ability to handle missing data is a key advantage of such methods.

The main problem with missing completely at random approaches is that it is hard to justify the key assumption.

11.2.6 Missing at random

From the practical point of view, this is the most important of the three cases of missingness. This is because missing completely at random is unlikely to apply and missing not at random is extremely difficult to deal with. I will not attempt here to summarize the huge literature on this subject but will refer the reader instead to the companion book in this series (Molenberghs and Kenward, 2007). There is no doubt that extremely important work has been and is being done in this area and that this is even beginning to feed into regulatory submissions. However, I will sound one note of caution about the supposed superiority of these approaches.

First, a number of simulations have shown how miserably last observation (carried forward) approaches perform compare with mixed-model approaches. However, in general one has to be very careful about assuming that simulations tell one what one thinks they do. For examples in other contexts where I have shown that they do not, the reader might be interested to consult Senn (1993, 1994, 1995, 1996, 2007). A key issue in comparing a simpler with a more sophisticated method is whether one has not implicitly assumed information that in practice one would not have.

Second, in my opinion, is that in some of their attacks on last observation approaches, some of its critics have rather over-egged the pudding. A typically misleading analysis looks at the result for each treatment arm separately and finds differences from method to method that are important when in fact the difference between methods when treatment effects (difference active versus placebo) are studied is less impressive. Note, by the way, that contrary to what is sometimes claimed, choice of response profile approach (slope, mean and so forth) does *not* depend on the shape of individual profiles.

It is governed by the way that the treatment *effect*, that is to say the difference between groups, changes over time (Senn *et al.*, 2000). Thus, for example, flattening of treatment curves over time which might occur with last observation carried forward is only an indication of a problem to the extent that it leads to a bias in the contrast.

Also, it seems to me that critics are expecting degrees of agreement that are just not reasonable in practice. To take an analogy, it is inevitable, for example, that parametric and nonparametric procedures will not always agree as regards significance of treatment effects, but this fact cannot on its own be taken to prove that either one or the other is unsatisfactory. Consider, for example, the generally excellent paper by Mallinckrodt *et al.* (2004d). I would not disagree with a major recommendation of this paper: 'Practice should shift away from using LOCF ANOVA as the primary analysis and focus on likelihood-based, mixed-effects model approaches develop under the MAR framework . . . ' (p. 161). However, in their paper the authors refer to an extensive study of 20 outcome variable in eight trials of duloxetine in depression (Mallinckrodt *et al.*, 2004b), which, because some trials had more than one dose of duloxetine, yielded a total of 202 comparisons with the placebo. This study seems also to be the one reported in more detail in Mallinckrodt *et al.* (2004c). Note that the first author is the same in these three papers. This cited study showed agreement and disagreement as regards statistical significance (which the authors accept is a rather poor measure). The results are as given in Table 11.1.

Of course, these 202 measures are based on only eight trials, and furthermore in some cases the placebo arm is used more than once for the same outcome. Nevertheless, as a purely descriptive summary, the result is not particularly alarming. For example, the tetrachoric correlation coefficient, which is based on assuming that the data are a discrete realization of a bivariate Normal (which at least approximately they are) is 0.85. Also note that although, as has quite correctly been pointed out, last observation analysis is not in general conservative, it *does* seem to be so on average in this case. Furthermore, the title of the paper by Mallinckrodt *et al.* (2004b) is, 'Interpretations of the efficacy of duloxetine are invariant to the choice of analytical technique – MMRM vs. LOCF', which hardly lends support to the notion that last observation analysis is problematic. Finally, many enthusiasts for mixed effect models have implicitly assumed that these provide impeccable yardsticks for judging other methods. This is far from being the case, *since they can give misleading inferences even when full data are present*. For example, the extremely popular random slope methods commonly employed corrects

Table 11.1   Cross-classification of two methods of analysis of 202 contrasts from 8 trials of duloxetine in depression. Based on Mallinckrodt *et al.* (2004b) and Mallinckrodt *et al.* (2004c).

		Last observation carried forward		
		Not significant	**Significant**	**Total**
Mixed model repeated measures	Not Significant	107	11	108
	Significant	25	59	84
	Total	132	70	202

differences at the end of the trial using differences at the beginning. That is to say, early measurements enter with opposite sign. (See the section on measuring trend effects in Chapter 8.) Thus a form of post-baseline correction is used. This technique can be extremely powerful provided that the assumptions underlying it are satisfied, but it is far from safe when they are not (Senn *et al.*, 2000). For an example where I consider that application of generalized mixed models has led dozens of researchers to the wrong conclusion see Senn (2006).

11.2.7   Missing not at random

The most difficult case for missing data is when they are not at random. I will not pretend to be able to contribute any penetrating insights to this problem except to mention the obvious point that, since missing not at random is a case where missingness depends on unobserved values, it depends on what you have observed whether you can claim something is missing at random or forced to concede that it may be missing not at random. The problem is always to know whether you have observed enough. This is very like the central problem of epidemiology, which is that successful adjustment for confounding depends on knowing what is relevant, how it is relevant and measuring it.

Chapter 4 of Molenberghs and Kenward (2007), which greatly extends the framework of Diggle and Kenward (1994), is recommended reading.

11.2.8   Concerning multiple imputation

Last observation carried forward analysis is a form of what is called single imputation: a missing value is replaced by a single imputed value. Quite apart from whatever other objections one may have about this procedure, depending on how the further analysis is carried out, a further problem can arise. Even if the resulting estimate is unbiased, the resulting variances of the estimate *may* be biased. The reason is not hard to see: the information is not genuine but the statistical algorithm may assume that the data are complete. Thus the amount of information is overestimated and hence declared standard errors are too small.

One approach is to generate an imputed value with a certain amount of random variation and then repeat this procedure many times. A series of treatment estimates ensues, each of which will differ slightly due to the differently imputed value. The declared variances for each imputation should be fairly similar and can be averaged and then a variance reflecting the extent to which results have differed from simulation to simulation can be added to reflect the true uncertainty. This procedure is called multiple imputation and is particularly associated with the work of Don Rubin (see Rubin (1996) and Schafer (1999) for reviews).

Since simulation is involved, multiple imputation shares with other simulation-based estimation procedures, such as the bootstrap and Markov chain Monte Carlo Bayesian approaches, the problem that it could conceivably produce different answers on different occasions even though the same data are involved. This might lead to some regulatory reluctance, although regulators have accepted the result of multiple imputations on occasion.

Multiple imputation is not, in fact, always necessary to produce correct variance estimates. It depends on the analysis strategy following single imputation. A simple example is given in the technical appendix.

11.2.9   Should false inclusions be analysed?

Perhaps because protocols are often complex, it is a common experience that some patients get included in trials who shouldn't be. For example, in a trial in asthma, patients might be required to be aged 18 to 65, with an FEV_1 which is 50–80% of that predicted by the patient's height age and sex, to be capable of showing a 15% improvement above baseline FEV_1 when given a bronchodilator, to be taking no concomitant medication, to have a normal ECG and no history of heart disease and not to have had any incident of respiratory infection within the last month and so forth. It may well be, however, that when the statistician comes to look at the results, one or other of these criteria will have been violated for some patients.

The argument against including such patients in analysis would be: (1) it was not the original intention to treat these patients; (2) since the inclusion criteria are not affected by treatment, excluding such patients cannot bias the results; (3) a better estimate will therefore be produced by excluding them. There are, however, a number of counterarguments. (1) More information is better than less. If the physician includes the patients in the trial, his or her subjective impression is no doubt that the patients are suitable. The objective criteria are, in any case, not perfect. Why, in that case, throw away the information provided by such patients? (2) Rectification schemes are known to be a poor approach to quality control. In the long run, allowing the statistician to exclude patients in analysis will encourage the physician to be less than vigilant in deciding who is included. The quality of trials will suffer. In fact, one of Deming's famous 14 maxims of quality was 'Cease dependence on inspection to achieve quality' (Deming, 2000). (3) As soon as such late exclusions are permitted, an arbitrary element is allowed in to trials, since not everyone will agree who should be excluded. For example, we may have mistakenly included a 17-year-old patient in the trial. The reason for excluding him was not scientific but ethical: not to expose a minor to an experimental treatment. But the fact of that exposure cannot be changed by excluding him from analysis. Therefore, it could be argued (and *was* argued on a trial with which I was involved) that the patient should be included for analysis. The regulator may, therefore, not wish to give the sponsor the leeway of excluding any randomized patients from the trial, fearing that this may be abused.

Lewis (1988) suggests that patients should usually be excluded from the efficacy analysis if they violate entry criteria and that this issue can be handled before unblinding the trial. My personal experience, however, has been that the more precise analysis has been that which does *not* exclude falsely included patients in the analysis and it has always been my practice to analyse the trial according to the motto: 'Inclusion criteria are to help the physician decide who should enter the trial, not to tell the statistician who should enter the analysis'. A compromise position is, in fact possible; an analysis could be performed which was stratified by inclusion status. This would probably produce an even more precise analysis, although, of course, it might allow the sponsor a certain degree of leeway (in defining strata) the regulator might not wish to see. Lewis and Machin (1993), in an excellent discussion of many of the issues affecting intention to treat policies, make the important point that there are occasions, where false inclusions should not be analysed. Suppose it were the case that the treatment had already proved itself generally and its efficacy was not in dispute but that there was some doubt whether in a particular more narrowly defined population it would be effective. If some patients from the wider population were mistakenly entered into this more precisely focused trial, an intention to treat analysis might give irrelevant answers.

Unfortunately, false inclusions are not uncommon. Much of the blame lies with trialists at sponsor headquarters who tend to pack protocols with inclusion criteria, wrongly, in my view, regarding this as the sign of a good trial. On the other hand, if a simple ethical step were introduced to good clinical practice, much could be done to eliminate the problem. The trial physician should be required to tell all patients at the end of the trial exactly what use, or not, has been made of their data. The prospect of having to tell a patient that the diary he or she has filled in every week for three months, as well as the four visits made to the clinic, not to mention all that work on the exercise treadmill and the three months making do with placebo, were all for nothing because the patient 's data will be thrown away, since the patient should never have been in the trial in the first place, should concentrate the physician's mind considerably.

11.2.10   Practical difficulties in applying intention to treat

The intention to treat philosophy works best in trials of serious diseases where survival is the outcome. Here it is usually possible to follow up most patients, whether or not they remain on the treatment originally allocated to them. The difficulty with trials in asthma, say, or hypertension, where regular measurements are made on patients, are that as soon as the patient drops out, measurements are no longer available. The trialist may thus be perfectly willing to apply the intention to treat philosophy but unable to carry it out.

Various devices are employed to deal with this. For example, the last available observation on the patient may be carried forward. This approach was discussed in sections 11.2.4 and 11.2.6. This is very common technique is often justified in the following terms. (1) It is a crude and simple attempt at imputation. It is an attempt to predict the value that would have been seen if the patient were available to be measured. (2) Even if this is criticized as being naive, it leads to an analysis which can be given an interpretation which does not depend on the reasonableness of the imputation. For example, in a three-month trial in asthma comparing a beta-agonist with placebo we should be able to answer the question: 'What will be the effect of treating patients with the beta-agonist at the moment when they stop treatment, whether because the three months are complete or because they withdraw from the trial?' (3) If the treatment has no effect, it is hard to see how this form of analysis could increase the probability of concluding that it is effective (Shao and Zhong, 2003).

Nevertheless, it remains a fact that intention to treat is easier said than done. In practice it is difficult to include all patients in an analysis, even if one wants to, and even where one does succeed it is not clear that such inclusion deals with all difficulties intention to treat is presumed to overcome.

There are two sorts of analyses of clinical trials: Intention to treat and intention to cheat.

11.2.11   Practical difficulties in applying per-protocol analyses

On the whole, these are less than that of applying intention to treat. One difficulty is in determining compliance. Relying on the patient is not always adequate. As mentioned in Section 11.1 above, it is possible to incorporate microchips into patient packs and measure, for example, the precise times at which containers were opened. This does not prove that the patient did not then flush the medication down the lavatory, but it goes some way to resolving the uncertainty as to whether and when treatment was taken.

A more important practical difficulty has to do with degree of compliance. It would usually be considered extreme to remove any patient from analysis who failed to comply on a single occasion. A worse record of compliance would usually be required. Of course, if the degree of compliance is included as a variable in the analysis, then some compromise between the extremes of intention to treat and per-protocol becomes possible as mentioned above. For example, the famous paper by Efron and Feldman cited previously considers just this possibility (Efron and Feldman, 1991).

11.2.12   The use of rescue medication

In some medical specialties it is usual for patients to have rescue medication. For example, in asthma, many asthmatics will carry a beta-agonist in an inhaler to deal with asthma attacks. This form of emergency treatment cannot reasonably be denied them in a clinical trial. A number of analysis strategies are possible for dealing with resort to rescue medication.

For example, the time until first use of rescue medication can be made the outcome of the trial, treating those who never use rescue medication as censored observations, rather as in survival analysis. The disadvantage of this is that it ignores second and third resort to rescue medication and makes rather poor use of the information available on those who never use it. To deal with this latter problem, Gould's method (see section 11.2.3) could be applied (Gould, 1980). A common approach is to ignore the problem altogether and analyse outcomes in the ordinary way making no use of the fact that the patient has taken rescue medication. This has evident disadvantages but in my opinion is definitely preferable to that of rescheduling visits and so forth because rescue medication has been taken. This is an even worse biasing manoeuvre as I shall now attempt to explain.

The reason we are reluctant to use a value measured after rescue medication has been taken is that we fear that it will have been affected by the extra medication. Ideally we should like to have available to us the reading the patient would have given had he or she not taken rescue medication. We feel that it is inappropriate to substitute for this 'counterfactual' measurement the value after rescue medication. However, if we reschedule the visit we shall be substituting another measurement for this counterfactual value. The question then is which of the two substituted measurements – 'post-rescue' or 'rescheduled' – will most closely resemble the counterfactual value we should like to use? It is by no means clear that the absolute difference between 'post-rescue' and 'counterfactual' will be greater than the difference between 'rescheduled' and 'counterfactual'. Consider the concrete case of rheumatism. The patient takes paracetamol when her rheumatism is very bad. But on a good day she takes none. If we are only prepared to measure her on good days, is this not more biasing than measuring her after she has taken paracetamol?

A further common strategy is to analyse the standard outcome and resort to rescue medication independently. In some cases each gives clear proof of the benefit of the treatment, but in general an appropriate combined analysis ought to improve matters. It may be that O'Brien's approach would be suitable (O'Brien, 1984) (see chapter 10) or that of Shih and Quan (1997).

References

Carpenter J, Kenward M, Evans S, White I (2004) Last observation carry-forward and last observation analysis. *Statistics in Medicine* **23**: 3241–3242; author reply 3242–3244.

Deming WE (2000) *Out of the Crisis*. MIT Press, Cambridge, MA.

Diggle P, Kenward MG (1994) Informative drop-out in longitudinal data analysis. *Journal of the Royal Statistical Society Series C – Applied Statistics* **43**: 49–93.

Dodge Y (1985) *Analysis of Experiments with Missing Data*. John Wiley & Sons, Inc., New York.

Efron B, Feldman D (1991) Compliance as an explanatory variable in clinical trials. *Journal of the American Statistical Association* **86**: 9–17.

Ellenberg JH (1996) Intention to treat versus as-treated analysis. *Drug Information journal* **30**: 535–544.

Gould L (1980) A new approach to the analysis of clinical drug trials with withdrawals. *Biometrics* **36**: 721–727.

Greenland S, Robins JM (1985) Estimation of a common effect parameter from sparse follow-up data. *Biometrics* **41**: 55–68.

Hollis S, Campbell F (1999) What is meant by intention to treat analysis? Survey of published randomised controlled trials. *British Medical Journal* **319**: 670–674.

Laird NM (1988) Missing data in longitudinal studies. *Statistics in Medicine* **7**: 305–315.

Lewis JA (1988) Statistical standards for protocols and protocol deviations. *Recent Results in Cancer Research* **111**: 27–33.

Lewis JA, Machin D (1993) Intention to treat – who should use ITT? [editorial]. *Br J Cancer* **68**: 647–650.

Little R, Rubin DB (2002) *Statistical Analysis with Missing Data*, 2nd edition. John Wiley & Sons, Inc., New York.

Mallinckrodt CH (2006) The test of public scrutiny. *Pharmaceutical Statistics* **5**: 249–252.

Mallinckrodt CH, Kaiser CJ, Watkin JG, Detke MJ, Molenberghs G, Carroll RJ (2004a) Type I error rates from likelihood-based repeated measures analyses of incomplete longitudinal data. *Pharmaceutical Statistics* **3**: 171–186.

Mallinckrodt CH, Raskin J, Wohlreich M, Watkin J, Detke MJ (2004b) Interpretations of the efficacy of duloxetine are invariant to the choice of analytical technique – MMRM vs. LOCF. *International Journal of Neuropsychopharmacology* **7**: S175–S175.

Mallinckrodt CH, Raskin J, Wohlreich MM, Watkin JG, Detke MJ (2004c) The efficacy of dulox-etine: a comprehensive summary of results from MMRM and LOCF_ANCOVA in eight clinical trials. *BMC Psychiatry* **4**: 26.

Mallinckrodt CH, Watkin JG, Molenberghs G, Carroll RJ (2004d) Choice of the primary analysis in longitudinal clinical trials. *Pharmaceutical Statistics* **3**: 161–169.

Mangel M, Samaniego FJ (1984) Wald, Abraham Work on aircraft survivability. *Journal of the American Statistical Association* **79**: 259–267.

Molenberghs G, Kenward MG (2007) *Missing Data in Clinical Studies*. John Wiley & Sons, Inc., Hoboken.

O'Brien PC (1984) Procedures for comparing samples with multiple endpoints. *Biometrics* **40**: 1079–1087.

Robins JM, Gill RD (1997) Non-response models for the analysis of non-monotone ignorable missing data. *Statistics in Medicine* **16**: 39–56.

Rubin DB (1976) Inference and missing data. *Biometrika* **63**: 581–590.

Rubin DB (1996) Multiple imputation after 18+ years. *Journal of the American Statistical Association* **91**: 473–489.

Schafer JL (1999) Multiple imputation: a primer. *Statistical Methods in Medical Research* **8**: 3–15.

Schafer JL, Graham JW (2002) Missing data: our view of the state of the art. *Psychological Methods* **7**: 147–177.

Schwartz D, Flamant R, Lellouch J (1980) *Clinical Trials*. Academic Press, London.

Schwartz D, Lellouch J (1967) Explanatory and pragmatic attitudes in therapeutic trials. *Journal of Chronic Diseases* **20**: 637–648.

Senn SJ (1993) Baseline distribution and conditional size [letter; comment]. *Journal of Biopharmaceutical Statistics* **3**: 265–276. [Published erratum appears in *Journal of Biopharmaceutical Statistics* **4**(3): 449 (1994)].

Senn SJ (1994) Methods for assessing difference between groups in change when initial measurement is subject to intra-individual variation [letter; comment]. *Statistics in Medicine* **13**: 2280–2285. [Comment in *Statistics in Medicine* **14**(20): 2283–2285 (1995)].

Senn SJ (1995) In defence of analysis of covariance: a reply to Chambless and Roeback [letter; comment]. *Statistics in Medicine* **14**: 2283–2285.

Senn SJ (1996) Baseline balance and conditional size: a reply to Overall et al. *Journal of Biopharmaceutical Statistics* **6**: 201–210.

Senn SJ (1997) Statisticians and pharmacokineticists: what can they learn from each other? In: Aarons L, Balant LP, Danhof M, *et al.* (eds), COST B1 medicine. The population approach: measuring and managing variability in response, concentration and dose. European Commission Directorate-General Science, Research and Development, Geneva, pp. 139–146.

Senn S (2006) Double hierarchical generalized linear models – Discussion. *Journal of the Royal Statistical Society Series C – Applied Statistics* **55**: 173.

Senn SJ (2007) Trying to be precise about vagueness. *Statistics in Medicine* **26**: 1417–1430.

Senn SJ, Stevens L, Chaturvedi N (2000) Repeated measures in clinical trials: simple strategies for analysis using summary measures. *Statistics in Medicine* **19**: 861–877.

Shao J, Zhong B (2003) Last observation carry-forward and last observation analysis. *Statistics in Medicine* **22**: 2429–2441.

Shao J, Zhong B (2006) On the treatment effect in clinical trials with dropout. *Journal of Biopharmaceutical Statistics* **16**: 25–33.

Sheiner LB (1991) The intellectual health of clinical drug evaluation [see comments]. *Clinical Pharmacology and Therapeutics* **50**: 4–9. [Comment in *Clinical Pharmacology and Therapeutics* **52**(1): 104–106 (1992)].

Shih WJ, Quan H (1997) Testing for treatment differences with dropouts present in clinical trials – a composite approach. *Statistics in Medicine* **16**: 1225–1239.

Smith AFM, Roberts GO (1993) Bayesian computation via the Gibbs sampler and related Markov-Chain Monte-Carlo methods. *Journal of the Royal Statistical Society Series B – Methodological* **55**: 3–23.

Sommer A, Zeger SL (1991) On estimating efficacy from clinical trials. *Statistics in Medicine* **10**: 45–52.

Urquhart J (1994) Why has patient compliance become important? *Clinical Research and Regulatory Affairs* **11**: 81–106.

White IR, Pocock SJ (1996) Statistical reporting of clinical trials with individual changes from allocated treatment. *Statistics in Medicine* **15**: 249–262.

11.A   TECHNICAL APPENDIX

11.A.1   Example to show that single imputation does not necessarily lead to incorrect variance estimation

Suppose that patients are due to be measured on two occasions post randomization, yielding values Y_1, Y_2, but that some are missing at random before the second occasion. A last observation carried forward approach is used and the second value is imputed using the first for such patients. We assume that there is no bias in this, so that we have the sort of condition where the effect of treatment is constant over a period of observation. (This might apply approximately, for example, for beta-agonists in asthma.)

We now proceed to calculate the mean of the two observations for every patient. (Actually, for this example this renders the imputation procedure pointless since the mean of the two observations will be the same as the mean of the first for those patients with imputed values but it will suffice to make the point.) Suppose that on a given treatment arm we have subjects $i = 1, \ldots, m_1$ with one measurement and subjects $j = 1, \ldots, m_2$ with two measurements and that $m_1 + m_2 = n$. We suppose that the summary measures (means in this case) from the first set of subjects are statistics S_i with sample mean $\bar{S}_1$, expectation μ and variance σ_1^2 and from the second set are statistics S_j with sample mean $\bar{S}_2$, expectation μ and variance σ_2^2, with $\sigma_1^2 > \sigma_2^2$. (The relative size of these two variances will depend on within- and between-subject variances but it is not necessary to know these in order to complete the argument.) Now suppose that we calculate the group mean as

$$\bar{S} = \frac{\sum\limits_{i=1}^{m_1} S_i + \sum\limits_{j=1}^{m_2} S_j}{n} = \frac{m_1 \bar{S}_1 + m_2 \bar{S}_2}{n}. \tag{11.3}$$

Expression (11.3) will have mean

$$E[\bar{S}] = \mu \tag{11.4}$$

and variance

$$V = \frac{m_1 \sigma_1^2 + m_2 \sigma_2^2}{n^2} = \frac{1}{n} \left(\frac{m_1}{n} \sigma_1^2 + \frac{m_2}{n} \sigma_2^2 \right) = \frac{1}{n} \sigma^2, \tag{11.5}$$

where $\sigma^2 = \theta \sigma_1^2 + (1 - \theta) \sigma_2^2$ and $\theta = m_1/n$.

We will estimate σ^2 using

$$\hat{\sigma}^2 = \frac{\sum\limits_{i=1}^{m_1} (S_i - \bar{S})^2 + \sum\limits_{j=1}^{m_2} (S_j - \bar{S})^2}{n-1}$$

$$= \frac{\sum\limits_{i=1}^{m_1} (S_i - \bar{S}_1)^2 + \sum\limits_{j=1}^{m_2} (S_j - \bar{S}_2)^2 + m_1 (\bar{S}_1 - \bar{S})^2 + m_2 (\bar{S}_2 - \bar{S})^2}{n-1}. \tag{11.6}$$

However,

$$m_1 \left(\bar{S}_1 - \bar{S} \right)^2 = m_1 \left(\frac{(n - m_1)}{n} \bar{S}_1 - \frac{m_2}{n} \bar{S}_2 \right)^2 = \frac{m_1 m_2^2}{n^2} \left(\bar{S}_1 - \bar{S}_2 \right)^2$$

$$m_2 \left(\bar{S}_2 - \bar{S} \right)^2 = m_2 \left(\frac{(n - m_2)}{n} \bar{S}_2 - \frac{m_1}{n} \bar{S}_1 \right)^2 = \frac{m_2 m_1^2}{n^2} \left(\bar{S}_2 - \bar{S}_1 \right)^2$$

$$(11.7)$$

Now since $\bar{S}_1, \bar{S}_2$ are independent with identical expectations from (11.7), we have that

$$E \left[m_1 \left(\bar{S}_1 - \bar{S} \right)^2 + m_2 \left(\bar{S}_2 - \bar{S} \right)^2 \right] = \left(\frac{m_1 m_2}{n} \right) \left(\frac{\sigma_1^2}{m_1} + \frac{\sigma_2^2}{m_2} \right) \qquad (11.8)$$

Hence, from (11.6) and (11.8) we have that the expected value of $\hat{\sigma}^2$ is

$$E \left[\hat{\sigma}^2 \right] = \frac{1}{n-1} \left[(m_1 - 1) \sigma_1^2 + (m_2 - 1) \sigma_2^2 + \left(\frac{m_1 m_2}{n} \right) \left(\frac{\sigma_1^2}{m_1} + \frac{\sigma_2^2}{m_2} \right) \right], \qquad (11.9)$$

which, with much tedious but elementary algebra, may be shown to be σ^2.

The demonstration is, in a sense, unnecessary since it is obvious that the distribution formed by the mixture of S_1, S_2 itself defines a new random variable S for which standard theorems of expectations of means ands sums of squares apply. How S arose is irrelevant.

12

One-sided and Two-sided Tests and other Issues to Do with Significance and P-values

The product of this carelessness thus far differs; always it is coarse and inelegant, but sometimes (say in 1–20th of the cases) it becomes specially legible
Thomas De Quincey, *Confessions of an English Opium Eater*

It is always good when a man has two irons in the fire.
Francis Beaumont and John Fletcher, *The Faithful Friends*

But yet I'll make assurance double sure
And take a bond of fate

William Shakespeare, *Macbeth*

12.1 BACKGROUND

A *P*-value is the probability of observing a value as extreme or more extreme than the value observed given that the null hypothesis is true. A problem is in deciding what constitutes a more extreme value. Consider a two-group clinical trial comparing an ACE inhibitor with placebo in hypertension and suppose that systolic blood pressure measured at some suitable time point is the outcome variable. Suppose that the difference, (placebo−active) is 12 mmHg. It seems clear that values of 13 mm, 14 mm and so forth are more extreme values but what about values of −13 mm and −14 mm: are these also more extreme? Deciding on this makes an important difference to the calculation of the *P*-value. Let t stand for any difference which might be observed. Then in the one case we need to calculate $P(t \geq 12\,\text{mm})$ and in the other case $P(t \leq -12\,\text{mm}$ or $t \geq 12\,\text{mm}) = P(t \leq -12\,\text{mm}) + P(t \geq 12\,\text{mm}) = 2P(t \geq 12\,\text{mm})$. It thus follows that, taking one view, the *P*-value (corresponding to the 'two-tailed' test) will be twice that obtained using the other (corresponding to the 'one-tailed test').

Now, it is a fact that in drug development two-tailed tests are commonly performed, whatever the comparator. (An exception is tests of equivalence where two one-sided tests are commonly performed. This confusing state of affairs will be covered in Chapters 15 and 22.) In this chapter we consider arguments in favour of and against two-sided and one-sided tests. We also consider some further matters, of the number of significant trials needed to support a claim, replication probabilities and P-values and supposed improvements to Fisher's exact test, because, although they are not directly related to the choice between one-sided and two-sided tests, they are related to wider issue of standards of evidence.

In discussing the various issues below we shall take the example of a trial comparing an active treatment with a placebo. Many of the issues raised in this chapter are treated in more depth by various papers of my own and the interested reader might like to consult Senn (2001, 2002, 2003, 2007).

12.2 ISSUES

12.2.1 Because we cannot exclude the superiority of placebo we must use two-sided tests

In the Neyman–Pearson theory of hypothesis testing, the nature of the alternative hypothesis helps to define the test. Let τ be the true difference between active and placebo. According to this theory, if we can write the following as our null and alternative hypotheses,

$$H_0 : \tau = 0, \quad H_1 : \tau > 0 \tag{12.1}$$

(which is to say that our null hypothesis is that there is no difference between treatments and that our alternative is that the treatment effect is positive), then we have a one-sided test. If, on the other hand, we write

$$H_0 : \tau = 0, \quad H_1 : \tau \neq 0 \tag{12.2}$$

(which is to say that our null hypothesis is as before but our alternative is simply that the treatment has some effect either positive or negative), then we have a two-sided test.

According to this view, the argument in favour of two-sided tests is simply that however implausible we may feel it might be, we cannot rule out the possibility that the active treatment is inferior to placebo. We are thus incapable of asserting the form of the alternative hypothesis associated with (12.1) and must use (12.2). This leads to two-sided tests.

12.2.2 Because we would never register a drug which was inferior to placebo we may use one-sided tests

According to this argument, the real purpose of drug development is to decide between null and alternative hypotheses as follows:

$$H_0 : \tau < 0, \quad H_1 : \tau > 0, \tag{12.3}$$

This is related to the famous distinction between explanatory and pragmatic trials made by Schwartz and Lellouch (1967). Here we are faced with the pragmatic task of choosing between the hypothesis that the drug is useless or worse than useless and the hypothesis that the drug brings some benefit. The argument in favour of this division of hypotheses is that the only relevance of the decision to be made is whether to register the drug or not, and for this purpose we make no distinction between a drug being useless and harmful: either will lead to failure to register. Suppose, now, that we use a one-sided test at the 5% level; then (assuming that there is only one trial and that this is in principle enough to support registration) we can construct the following table of **regulator's risk**.

Practical situation	Probability of registering the drug
The drug is harmful	< 0.05
The drug is useless	0.05
The drug brings some benefit	> 0.05

Thus, according to this argument, there is no need to use a two-sided test, since in the unlikely event of the drug's having a harmful effect the regulator's risk will be less than 0.05 anyway.

An argument against this view is that it sacrifices the scientific (explanatory) purpose to the practical (pragmatic) one. The significance test is a device which scientists universally use to decide which hypotheses to accept and which to reject. For this general inferential purpose the practical context is irrelevant. It may well be that a drug which is significantly worse than placebo will not be registered. However, a trialist who discovers that there is an otherwise significant difference in favour of placebo will in practice believe that active treatment is harmful. Thus, unless he carries out two-sided tests he will end up believing that there is some sort of difference between treatments in more than 1 in 20 of those cases where there is none. His significance tests will therefore be invalid. To guard against this he must use two-sided tests.

12.2.3   Label invariance requires us to use two-sided tests

This argument is related to Section 12.2.1. The two-sided test is **label invariant**. That is to say, we can reverse the labels on the treatments and still come to the same conclusion. (Note that in a sense this is true of the estimate of the treatment difference also. It only requires a change of sign when the labels are changed.) On the other hand, the one-sided test of significant is not label invariant unless, say, we regard $P = 0.95$ as giving the same information as $P = 0.05$, which would seem to bring us back to the two-sided test. The advantage of label-invariant procedures is that they reflect no differential assumptions regarding the treatments being compared. Of course, this may also be viewed as a weakness.

12.2.4   Unless we use one-sided tests when comparing a treatment with a placebo, we shall not be entitled to claim superiority of the treatment under any circumstances

The argument goes that unless we test an alternative hypothesis of the form $H_1 : \tau > 0$ rather than of the form $H_0 : \tau = 0$ we shall not, in rejecting H_0, be entitled to accept that the treatment is superior to placebo. Therefore we must use one-sided tests. This argument is not reasonable on two counts (Hauschke and Steinijans, 1996). First, the need to be able to assert a particular form of the alternative hypothesis does not justify our declaring by fiat that other forms may be discounted. Therefore, if there is no reason why the hypothesis $H_1 : \tau < 0$ may not be discounted as impossible, the hypothesis $H_1 : \tau > 0$ cannot be regarded as the only alternative to $H_0 : \tau = 0$ for the purpose of testing. Second, it is obvious that if we test $H_{1\,A} : \tau > 0$ against $H_0 : \tau = 0$ at size $\alpha/2$ and also $H_{1\,B} : \tau < 0$ against $H_0 : \tau = 0$ at size $\alpha/2$, then since it is impossible for both hypotheses to be rejected, the probability of rejecting one or the other given that H_0 is true is $\alpha/2 + \alpha/2 = \alpha$. So, by carrying out this procedure we shall maintain the type I error rate at α. Furthermore, we shall always reject the null hypothesis where the conventional two-sided test does so, and only reject the hypothesis when this does so. Hence these two one-sided tests are equivalent to the two-sided test. Therefore, carrying out a two-sided test and using the results to determine whether superiority, equivalence or failure to prove a difference applies is a perfectly acceptable procedure.

12.2.5   Because we have used two-sided tests in the past we must continue to do so

According to this argument it does not really matter whether the tests should be one- or two-sided. All those who take the view that the real set-up is that given by expression (12.3) will consider that we have really been carrying out one-sided tests in drug development for years but that the nominal level we have been using is not 1 in 20 but 1 in 40. It thus follows that if we were (a) to adopt the practice of always using one-sided tests but (b) retain practical consistency with what we have done in the past, we should start using one-sided tests at the 1 in 40 level. Operationally these would be indistinguishable from two-sided tests at the 1 in 20 level. After all, 5% and 2.5% are equally arbitrary standards. What is important is what the standard has become and this is either (depending on one's view) 5% two-sided or 2.5% one-sided.

12.2.6   The whole debate is irrelevant

This would certainly be the Bayesian point of view. It would suggest that three things are relevant to a correct decision: (a) prior belief in the relevant hypotheses, (b) data and (c) consequences of decisions. What the proponents of the various points of view are attempting to do is come to a decision without this complete specification. For example, the proponents of the view given in section 12.2.1 are ignoring consequences but giving some partial recognition to prior belief. (This is because they recognize that under any reasonable belief we cannot rule out entirely the possibility that the treatment may be worse than useless.) In practice, however the choice is not a stark one between believing that the treatment effect might be anything or that it can only be positive. Maybe negative values are less likely than positive ones but not impossible. On the other hand, the proponents of the view expounded in section 12.2.2 are giving some consideration of consequences but have not included prior belief in the specification. A fully Bayesian analysis would included both prior beliefs and consequences, would be different from case to case and would not be restricted to such extreme alternative strategies.

12.2.7   Should the two-sided *P*-value always be twice the one-sided value?

This controversy is a long-running one among theoretical statisticians. For example, it was debated extensively in Yates's famous read paper to the Royal Statistical Society (Yates, 1984) on the analysis of 2×2 tables. Table 12.1, which is based on Yates, illustrates the problem. The upper left-hand cell has a frequency of a. For a given value of a we can calculate the *P*-value using Fisher's exact test by conditioning on the row and column totals and calculating the probability of a split as extreme or more extreme than that observed. But how should we calculate what is a more extreme split? If performing a one-sided test, this is obvious. For example, suppose that the value of a is 1. Clearly a more extreme value is 0. Using $\cup$ to stand for 'or', the one-sided *P*-value is thus

$$P(a=0 \cup 1) = P(a=0) + P(a=1) = 0.00624 + 0.0553 = 0.0615.$$

If this is doubled, the *P*-value is 0.0123. However, an alternative argument notes that the expected frequency under independence for the cell in question is $7 \times 19/40 = 3.325$. Hence an observed value of 1 is a departure in absolute terms of 2.325. Values of 6 or 7 would yield deviations of 2.675 and 3.675. Thus an alternative definition of the two-sided *P*-value is to calculate

$$P(a=0 \cup 1 \cup 6 \cup 7)$$
$$= P(a=0) + P(a=1) + P(a=6) + P(a=7)$$
$$= 0.00624 + 0.0553 + 0.03056 + 0.0027 = 0.0948.$$

Personally, I prefer the doubling approached, which seems to have been R.A. Fisher's preferred method although, according to Yates (1984), this is only revealed in a letter to Finney. This letter was subsequently (to Yates's paper) reproduced on p. 89 of Henry Bennett's edition of Fisher's letters (Bennett, 1990). Fisher writes, 'I believe I can defend the simple solution of doubling the total probability... because it corresponds with halving the probability, supposedly chosen in advance, with which the one observed is to be compared.' This is consistent with regarding the usual type I error rate required by drug regulators to register a drug using placebo-controlled trials to be 1 in 40 as argued in section 12.2.5. However, for a contrary view see Cox and Hinkley (1974). For further discussion see Pawitan (2001).

Table 12.1   Hypothetical 2×2 contingency table based on Yates (1984).

			Totals
	a	$19-a$	19
	$7-a$	$14+a$	21
Totals	7	33	40

12.2.8   The two-trials rule

The requirement in the USA that results should be both demonstrable and repeatable has led the FDA to demand that two well-controlled trials should demonstrate efficacy. Although the FDA *may* permit exceptions where the disease is life-threatening or there is a long duration of treatment or either the disease or the outcome is rare (Ruberg and Cairns, 1998), such cases are the exception. This has a number of consequences, one of which, that the power of individual trials may need to be higher, is discussed in Chapter 13 and another of which, affecting the conduct of sequential trials, is discussed in Chapter 19. The relationship to meta-analysis is discussed in Chapter 16. Here we discuss, briefly, the influence of this rule on type I error rates. First, however, we should note that it is a mistake to suppose that the FDA applies this rule in an automatic and absolute way in the sense of requiring that each of two trials should be significant two-sided at the 5% level. For example, one significant result together with another suggestive result and overall significance in a meta-analysis might be acceptable. Nevertheless, it is perhaps worth discussing the effect of this most extreme version of the requirement for three reasons. First, it is adequate as a first approximation to the way in which the requirement is made; second, it may be useful to consider the implications of making the requirement in its most extreme form; and third, it is difficult to discuss the performance of more informal approaches.

Suppose that exactly two trials are run in phase III and that each must be significant two-sided at the 5% level. The operational type I error, that of registering a useless drug, then becomes $1/40 \times 1/40 = 1/1600$. This is because, taking the operational view, we simply regard a two-sided test at the 5% level as being a one-sided test at the 2.5% level as discussed above. Since each of the trials will be required to show a positive result in favour of the candidate for registration, this yields the type I error rate. Suppose that our test statistic is Normally distributed and that we have a reasonably large sample. We can then look at this in terms of the two standardized treatment scores, or 'z-statistics'. Each of these will be required to be greater than 1.96, the value of the standard Normal distribution corresponding to a 2.5% tail probability. Let us call this the *two-trials rule*.

Now, if the reason for this rule is simply that we want a type I error rate of $1/1600$, we can, in fact, replace it by a more efficient one. This is (assuming the trials are of equal precision) to require that the mean of the two z-statistics is greater than 2.28 (or, equivalently to require that their sum is greater than 4.56). This mean will have a variance of $1/2$ and hence a standard error of $1/\sqrt{2}$, and hence the standardized value of the Normal distribution corresponding to the critical value of 2.28 for the mean is $2.28/(1/\sqrt{2}) = 2.28 \times \sqrt{2} = 3.23$ which corresponds to a tail area of the Normal distribution of $1/1600$. Thus, this test also has the required type I error rate. Let us call a requirement that this test be significant the *pooled- trials rule*.

Both rules are illustrated in Figure 12.1, which shows the portion of the 'space' for the z-statistics from the two trials which leads to overall significance. For the two-trials rule, it is the area of the graph to the right of the vertical dashed line and also above the horizontal dashed line. For the pooled-trials rule it is the area to 'north-east' of the solid diagonal line. It can be seen that for this rule, large values of the z-statistic for one trial can compensate for values in the other.

The question then arises. Why should we prefer the two-trial rule to the pooled-trial rule, especially since, as can be demonstrated, the latter is more powerful or, for a given

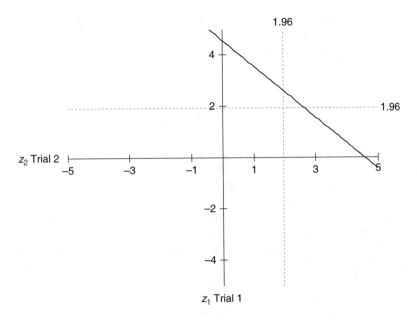

Figure 12.1 Illustration of the two-trials rule and the pooled-trials rule.

power, can be made more efficient in requiring fewer patients per trial? It would seem to me that there are only two possible answers (which are in fact related). The first is that we consider that the results are 'unpoolable': different things are being answered by the two trials, and there is no common question which can be answered by both, at least not in the crude sense proposed. Success is being demanded in two different tests, rather in the way that for some combined honours degrees it is required that the student passes in each subject and compensation from one subject to the other is not allowed, so that to be a graduate in economics and statistics, for example, you have to have proved yourself as an economist *and* a statistician.

The second is that we fear some sort of 'random gremlin' which affects trials and occasionally leads to spectacularly low but unrepeatable *P*-values which reflect not so much the effect of treatment but that the trial has 'gone wrong'. If this occurrence is fairly rare, a good level of protection will be afforded provided only that there is no tendency for the random gremlin to strike in one trial when it has struck in the other. Such common mode failure would vitiate the value of this protection. So once again its seems that the rule makes sense if the trials are rather different: if the protocols are different, different sorts of centres are used, the trial is run with different monitors and so forth.

However, it seems to be often the case that sponsors do the reverse. They produce two trials which are so similar that the protocols, monitoring procedures and so forth are effectively identical, and a centre in the one trial could equally well have been chosen as a centre in the other. That being the case it would seem to me that there is no argument against using the pooled-trials rule and, indeed, there is no argument against simply running a larger trial and requiring that the results be significant at the 1/1600 level one-sided (if this is the standard evidence required). What the purpose is behind the two-trials rule under such circumstances is anybody's guess.

This issue was discussed in the first edition of this book but since then has been discussed by a number of authors. Readers who would like to know more might wish to consult the following papers: Darken and Ho (2004), Fisher (1999), Rosenkranz (2002) and Shun *et al.* (2005).

12.2.9   Replication probabilities and *P*-values

Some further issues regarding interpretation of significance results and *P*-values are covered in the next chapter on determining the sample size. Here a specific issue regarding replication probabilities is discussed.

Suppose that we have observed a given (one-sided) *P*-value in a clinical trial say $P = \alpha_1$, what is the probability that in a second trial of similar precision for which we will also calculate a *P*-value, say, $P = \alpha_2$, that we will find that the *P*-value is now lower than the first. In other words, what is the probability that $\alpha_2 < \alpha_1$. In an interesting paper in *Statistics in Medicine*, Goodman (1992) showed that the answer would be $1/2$ under either of the following two circumstances: (a) one had an uninformative prior distribution for the treatment effect before running the first trial or (b) the true treatment effect was equal to the observed treatment effect from the first trial.

A heuristic justification of this result as regards the first case is as follows. If the two trials are identical then $P(\alpha_1 < \alpha_2) = P(\alpha_2 < \alpha_1)$. If, *P*-values being continuous, we can ignore $P(\alpha_1 = \alpha_2)$ as being negligible, then this implies that on average $P(\alpha_2 < \alpha_1) = 1/2$. This is not quite the same as saying that for a given value of α_1 one is justified in saying that $P(\alpha_2 < \alpha_1) = 1/2$ because one might, say, be able to recognize that α_1 was unusually low in which case one might rationally suppose that $P(\alpha_2 < \alpha_1) < 1/2$. However, one could only recognize such a case as having arisen using prior knowledge, which is excluded in the formulations here.

As regards the second case, then on average one expects any future test statistic to have the same value it had for trial 1. However, if the test statistic is symmetric and continuous, then this implies that on the original scale of measurement in 50% of the cases it will be less than in the first trial and in 50% of the cases more, but since the precision is the same as in the first trial this is true for the standardized test statistic also. But a value exactly equal to that in the first trial would give $\alpha_2 = \alpha_1$, so that half the time we shall see $\alpha_2 < \alpha_1$ and half the time $\alpha_1 < \alpha_2$ (if we ignore the case of exact equality).

Goodman's paper is valuable in informing trialists not to 'count chickens before they are hatched'. This is particularly important if one trial has been completed in a programme and is marginally significant. It should then be appreciated that (in the absence of any other information) it is not improbable that the next trial will be not significant.

However, it would be quite wrong to conclude that this is a reason for mistrusting *P*-values (Senn, 2002). There are many criticisms that can be made of *P*-values (some are considered in the next chapter) but this is not one of them. Bayesian probabilistic statements have to obey a very similar 'Martingale' property whereby what we see now is what we expect in the future. If it were the case that we knew with high probability that a significant *P*-value would be followed by an even more significant one then we would believe with high probability that further experimentation would on average leave us more certain than we now were regarding the falsity of the null hypothesis.

This would be a disastrous property of any system of inference since it would undermine the value of future evidence by confusing actual with anticipated evidence. Thus this particular property of *P*-values is highly desirable and in fact does not distinguish them from Bayesian statements.

12.2.10   Improving Fisher's exact test

An issue that surfaces from time to time is the alleged conservatism of Fisher's exact test, whether in its classic 2×2 form or used as a trend test. Indeed, Yates' paper, cited above, was written partly to defend the test (Yates, 1984). There are at least two issues. The first is that the test conditions on the margins of the table and thus assumes that there is no information to be extracted from them. I am not entirely persuaded that there is no information in the margins while not going as far as the position of Richardson, who suggests that the actual randomization process itself should govern the approach to analysing such tables (Richardson, 1994). In fact, I think that under most circumstances the information is so small as to be of little consequence. The exception is when all results are on the diagonal of the table. Consider, as a case in point, the disastrous outcome of the trial in TGN1412 when on 13 March 2006 out of 8 healthy volunteers treated the 6 who were given active treatment suffered severe side-effects in the form of cytokine storms. Fisher's exact test gives a one-tailed *P*-value of 0.036, which is thus not significant at the standard 2.5% level one-sided (Senn, 2006). However, the fact that the split of severe reactions is 6 to 2, which is exactly the same as the split of treatments, is itself suggestive. For a similar suggestive split see Senn (1988).

A test that does not condition on the margins is Barnard's test, which uses the maximum *P*-value obtained as a function of the unknown probability of an adverse reaction (Barnard, 1945). The value of this test for the TGN1412 example is 0.011 (one-sided). Of course, the TGN1412 example shows how irrelevant *P*-values can be on occasion. Neither Fisher's exact nor Barnard's test begins to do justice to how striking these results are. The reason is that they ignore further highly relevant information, namely that cytokine storms are extremely rare and that the onset of symptoms followed very closely on treatment administration (Senn, 2006, Working Party on Statistical Issues in First-in-Man Studies, 2007).

The second issue with Fisher's exact test is that it tends to be more discrete than some alternatives, that is to say involves fewer points in the sample space leading to distinct *P*-values. This means that greater power can be achieved by some alternatives. For example, Ivanova and Berger (2001) have taken the example of a 2×3 trend test and suggested that conventional trend scorings of 0, 1, 2 (or equivalently 0, 1/2, 1) might be replaced by scores such as 0, 0.49, 1 or 0, 0.51, 1. Since the average of 0 and 1 is 0.5 and not 0.49 or 0.51, this has the consequence that the test statistic takes on more values. For similar proposals see Cohen *et al.* (2000), Corcoran *et al.* (2000), Kim and Agresti (1995) and Korn (1987). However, as was shown by Tocher (1950) many years ago, use of an auxiliary randomization device restores the power disadvantage of Fisher's exact test. Of course many find the use of a randomization device repugnant, and so do I, but my repugnance extends to using the sample space itself as an auxiliary randomization device, which is essentially what such improvements suggest. For this reason I do not consider that Fisher's exact test should be replace by such approaches (Senn, 2007). For other reasons to use the exact test in clinical trials, based on the fact that patients are not sampled at random, see Streitberg and Röhmel(1991).

References

Barnard GA (1945) A new test for 2×2 tables. *Nature* **156**: 177.

Bennett JH (1990) *Statistical Inference and Analysis. Selected Correspondence of R.A. Fisher.* Oxford University Press, Oxford.

Cohen A, Sackrowitz HB, Sackrowitz M (2000) Testing whether treatment is 'better' than control with ordered categorical data: an evaluation of new methodology. *Statistics in Medicine* **19**: 2699–2712.

Corcoran C, Mehta C, Senchaudhuri P (2000) Power comparisons for tests of trend in dose-response studies. *Statistics in Medicine* **19**: 3037–3050.

Cox DR, Hinkley DV (1974) *Theoretical Statistics.* Chapman and Hall, London.

Darken PF, Ho S-Y (2004) A note on sample size savings with the use of a single well-controlled clinical trial to support the efficacy of a new drug. *Pharmaceutical Statistics* **3**: 61–63.

Fisher LD (1999) One large, well-designed, multicenter study as an alternative to the usual FDA paradigm. *Drug Information Journal* **33**: 265–271.

Goodman SN (1992) A comment on replication, p-values and evidence. *Statistics in Medicine* **11**: 875–879.

Hauschke D, Steinijans VW (1996) Directional decision for a two-tailed alternative [letter; comment]. *Journal of Biopharmaceutical Statistics* **6**: 211–218.

Ivanova A, Berger VW (2001) Drawbacks to integer scoring for ordered categorical data. *Biometrics* **57**: 567–570.

Kim D, Agresti A (1995) Improved exact inference about conditional association in 3-way contingency tables. *Journal of the American Statistical Association* **90**: 632–639.

Korn EL (1987) Data-randomized confidence intervals for discrete distributions. *Communications in Statistics – Theory and Methods* **16**: 705–715.

Pawitan Y (2001) *In All Likelihood: Statistical Modelling and Inference Using Likelihood.* Clarendon Press, Oxford.

Richardson JT (1994) The analysis of 2×1 and 2×2 contingency tables: an historical review. *Statistical Methods in Medical Research* **3**: 107–133.

Rosenkranz G (2002) Is it possible to claim efficacy if one of two trials is significant while the other just shows a trend? *Drug Information Journal* **36**: 875–879.

Ruberg S, Cairns V (1998) Providing evidence of efficacy for a new drug. *Statistics in Medicine* **17**: 1813–1823.

Schwartz D, Lellouch J (1967) Explanatory and pragmatic attitudes in therapeutic trials. *Journal of Chronic Diseases* **20**: 637–648.

Senn SJ (1988) A note concerning the analysis of an epidemic of Q fever. *International Journal of Epidemiology* **17**: 891–893.

Senn SJ (2001) Two cheers for p-values. *Journal of Epidemiology and Biostatistics* **6**: 193–204.

Senn SJ (2002) A comment on replication, p-values and evidence, S.N.Goodman, Statistics in Medicine 1992; 11: 875–879. *Statistics in Medicine* **21**: 2437–2444.

Senn SJ (2003) p-values. In: Chow SC (ed.), *Encylopedia of Biopharmaceutical Statistics.* Marcel Dekker, New York, pp. 685–695.

Senn SJ (2006) Comment on Farrington and Whitaker: Semiparametric analysis of case series data. *Journal of the Royal Statistical Society Series C – Applied Statistics* **55**: 581–583.

Senn SJ (2007) Drawbacks to noninteger scoring for ordered categorical data. *Biometrics* **63**: 296–299.

Shun Z, Chi E, Durrleman S, Fisher L (2005) Statistical consideration of the strategy for demonstrating clinical evidence of effectiveness – one larger vs two smaller pivotal studies. *Statistics in Medicine* **24**: 1619–1637; discussion 1639–1656.

Streitberg B, Röhmel J (1991) Alternatives to Fisher's exact test? *Biometrie und Informatik in Medizin und Biologie* **22**: 139–146

Tocher KD (1950) Extension of the Neyman–Pearson theory of tests to discontinuous variates. *Biometrika* **37**: 130–144.

Working Party on Statistical Issues in First-in-Man Studies (2007) Statistical issues in first-in-man studies. *Journal of the Royal Statistical Society, Series A* **170**: 517–579.

Yates F (1984) Tests of significance for 2×2 contingency tables. *Journal of the Royal Statistical Society A* **147**: 426–463.

13

Determining the Sample Size

Hain't we got all the fools in town on our side? and aint that a big enough majority in any town?
Mark Twain, *Huckleberry Finn*

Nothing comes of nothing.

William Shakespeare, *King Lear*

13.1 BACKGROUND

Clinical trials are expensive, whether the cost is counted in money or in human suffering, but they are capable of providing results which are extremely valuable, whether the value is measured in drug company profits or successful treatment of future patients. Balancing potential value against actual cost is thus an extremely important and delicate matter and since, other things being equal, both cost and value increase the more patients are recruited, determining the number needed is an important aspect of planning any trial. It is hardly surprising, therefore, that calculating the sample size is regarded as being an important duty of the medical statistician working in drug development. This was touched on in Chapter 5 and some related matters were also considered in Chapter 6. My opinion is that sample size issues are sometimes over-stressed at the expense of others in clinical trials. Nevertheless, they are important and this chapter will contain a longer than usual, and also rather more technical, background discussion in order to be able to introduce them properly.

All scientists have to pay some attention to the precision of the instruments with which they work: is the assay sensitive enough? is the telescope powerful enough? and so on are questions which have to be addressed. In a clinical trial many factors affect precision of the final conclusion: the variability of the basic measurements, the sensitivity of the statistical technique, the size of the effect one is trying to detect, the probability with which one wishes to detect it if present (power), the risk one is prepared to take in declaring it is present when it is not (the so-called 'size' of the test, significance level or type I error rate) and the number of patients recruited. If it be admitted that the variability of the basic measurements has been controlled as far as is practically possible, that the statistical technique chosen is appropriately sensitive, that the magnitude of the effect one is trying to detect is an external 'given' and that a conventional type I error rate and power are to be used, then the only factor which is left for the trialist to

Statistical Issues in Drug Development/2nd Edition Stephen Senn
© 2007 John Wiley & Sons, Ltd

manipulate is the sample size. Hence, the usual point of view is that the sample size is the determined function of variability, statistical method, power and difference sought. In practice, however, there is a (usually undesirable) tendency to 'adjust' other factors, in particular the difference sought and sometimes the power, in the light of 'practical' requirements for sample size.

In what follows we shall assume that the sample size is going to be determined as a function of the other factors. We shall take the example of a two-arm parallel-group trial comparing an active treatment with a placebo for which the outcome measure of interest is continuous and will be assumed to be Normally distributed. It is assumed that analysis will take place using a frequentist approach and via the two independent-samples *t*-test. A formula for sample size determination will be presented. No attempt will be made to derive it. Instead we shall show that it behaves in an intuitively reasonable manner.

We shall present an approximate formula for sample size determination. An exact formula introduces complications which need not concern us. In discussing the sample size requirements we shall use the following conventions:

α: the probability of a type I error, given that the null hypothesis is true.

β: the probability of a type II error, given that the alternative hypothesis is true.

Δ: the difference sought. (In most cases one speaks of the 'clinically relevant difference' and this in turn is defined 'as the difference one would not like to miss'. The idea behind it is as follows. If a trial ends without concluding that the treatment is effective, there is a possibility that that treatment will *never* be investigated again and will be lost both to the sponsor and to mankind. If the treatment effect is indeed zero, or very small, this scarcely matters. At some magnitude or other of the true treatment effect, we should, however, be disturbed to lose the treatment. This magnitude is the difference we should not care to miss.)

σ: the presumed standard deviation of the outcome. (The anticipated value of the measure of the variability of the outcomes from the trial.)

n: the number of patients in each arm of the trial. (Thus the total number is $2n$.)

The first four basic factors above constitute the *primitive* inputs required to determine the fifth. In the formula for sample size, n is a function of α, β, Δ and σ, that is to say, given the values of these four factors, the value of n is determined. The function is, however, rather complicated if expressed in terms of these four primitive inputs and involves the solution of two integral equations. These equations may be solved using statistical tables (or computer programs) and the formula may be expressed in terms of these two solutions. This makes it much more manageable. In order to do this we need to define two further terms as follows.

$Z_{\alpha/2}$:   this is the value of the Normal distribution which cuts off an upper tail probability of $\alpha/2$. (For example if $\alpha = 0.05$ then $Z_{\alpha/2} = 1.96$.)

Z_{β}:   this is the value of the Normal distribution which cuts off an upper tail probability of β. (For example, if $\beta = 0.2$, then $Z_{\beta} = 0.84$.)

We are now in a position to consider the (approximate) formula for sample size, which is

$$n = 2(Z_{\alpha/2} + Z_{\beta})^2 \sigma^2 / \Delta^2. \tag{13.1}$$

(N.B. This is the formula which is appropriate for a two-sided test of size α. See chapter 12 for a discussion of the issues.)

Power: That which statisticians are always calculating but never have.

Example 13.1

It is desired to run a placebo-controlled parallel group trial in asthma. The target variable is forced expiratory volume in one second (FEV_1). The clinically relevant difference is presumed to be 200 ml and the standard deviation 450 ml. A two-sided significance level of 0.05 (or 5%) is to be used and the power should be 0.8 (or 80%). What should the sample size be?

Solution: We have $\Delta = 200$ ml, $\sigma = 450$ ml, $\alpha = 0.05$ so that $Z_{\alpha/2} = 1.96$ and $\beta = 1 - 0.8 = 0.2$ and $Z_\beta = 0.84$. Substituting in equation (13.1) we have $n = 2(450\,\text{ml})^2(1.96 + 0.84)^2/(200\,\text{ml})^2 = 79.38$. Hence, about 80 completing patients per treatment arm are required.

It is useful to note some properties of the formula. First, n is an *increasing* function of the standard deviation σ, which is to say that if the value of σ is increased so must n be. This is as it should be, since if the variability of a trial increases, then, other things being equal, we ought to need more patients in order to come to a reasonable conclusion. Second, we may note that n is a *decreasing* function of Δ: as Δ increases n decreases. Again this is reasonable, since if we seek a bigger difference we ought to be able to find it with fewer patients. Finally, what is not so immediately obvious is that if either α or β decreases n will increase. The technical reason that this is so is that the smaller the value of α, the higher the value of $Z_{\alpha/2}$ and similarly the smaller the value of β, the higher the value of Z_β. In common-sense terms this is also reasonable, since if we wish to reduce either of the two probabilities of making a mistake, then, other things being equal, it would seem reasonable to suppose that we shall have to acquire more information, which in turn means studying more patients.

In fact, we can express (13.1) as being proportional to the product of two factors, writing it as $n = 2F_1 F_2$. The first factor, $F_1 = (Z_{\alpha/2} + Z_\beta)^2$ depends on the error rates one is prepared to tolerate and may be referred to as *decision precision*. For a trial with 10% size and 80% power, this figure is about 6. (This is low decision precision). For 1% size and 95% power, it is about 18. (This would be high decision precision.) Thus a range of about 3 to 1 covers the usual values of this factor. The second factor, $F_2 = \sigma^2/\Delta^2$, is specific to the particular disease and may be referred to as *application ambiguity*. If this factor is high, it indicates that the natural variability from patient to patient is high compared to the sort of treatment effect which is considered important. It is difficult to say what sort of values this might have, since it is quite different from indication to indication, but a value in excess of 9 would be unusual (this means the standard deviation is 3 times the clinically relevant difference) and the factor is not usually less than 1. Putting these two together suggests that the typical parallel-group trial using continuous outcomes should have somewhere between $2 \times 6 \times 1 = 12$ and $2 \times 18 \times 9 \approx 325$ patients per arm. This is a big range. Hence the importance of deciding what is indicated in a given case.

In practice there are, of course, many different formulae for sample size determination. If the trial is not a simple parallel-group trial, if there are more than two treatments, if the outcomes are not continuous (for example, binary outcomes, or length of survival or frequency of events), if prognostic information will be used in analysis, or if the object is to prove equivalence, different formulae will be needed. It is also usually necessary to make an allowance for drop-outs. Nevertheless, the general features of the above hold.

A helpful tutorial on sample size issues is the paper by Steven Julious in *Statistics in Medicine* (Julious, 2004); a classic text is that of Desu and Raghavarao (1990). Nowadays, the use of specialist software for sample size determination such as NQuery, PASS or Power and Precision is common.

We now consider the issues.

13.2   ISSUES

13.2.1   In practice such formulae cannot be used

The simple formula above is adequate for giving a basic impression of the calculations required to establish a sample size. In practice there are many complicating factors which have to be considered before such a formula can be used. Some of them present severe practical difficulties. Thus a cynic might say that there is a considerable disparity between the apparent precision of sample size formulae and our ability to apply them.

The first complication is that the formula is only approximate. It is based on the assumption that the test of significance will be carried out using a *known* standard deviation. In practice we do not know the standard deviation and the tests which we employ are based upon using an estimate obtained from the sample under study. For large sample sizes, however, the formula is fairly accurate. In any case, using the correct, rather than the approximate, formula causes no particular difficulties in practice.

Nevertheless, although in practice we are able to substitute a sample estimate for our standard deviation for the purpose of carrying out statistical *tests*, and although we have a formula for the sample size calculation which *does* take account of this sort of uncertainty, we have a particular practical difficulty to overcome. The problem is that we do not know what the sample standard deviation will be until we have run the trial but we need to plan the trial before we can run it. Thus we have to make some sort of guess as to what the true standard deviation is for the purpose of planning, even if for the purpose of analysis this guess is not needed. (In fact, a further complication is that even if we knew what the sample standard deviation would be for sure, the formula for the power calculation depends upon the unknown 'true' standard deviation.) This introduces a further source of uncertainty into sample size calculation which is *not* usually taken account of by any formulae commonly employed. In practice the statistician tries to obtain a reasonable estimate of the likely standard deviation by looking at previous trials. This estimate is then used for planning. If he is cautious he will attempt to incorporate this further source of uncertainty into his sample size calculation either formally or informally. One approach is to use a range of reasonable plausible values for the standard deviation and see how the sample size changes. Another approach is to use the sample information from a given trial to construct a Bayesian posterior distribution for the population variance. By integrating the conditional power (given the population variance) over this distribution for the population variance, an unconditional (on the population variance) power can be produced from which a sample size statement can be derived. This approach has been investigated in great detail by Steven Julious (Julious, 2006). It still does not allow, however, for differences from trial to trial in the true population variance. But it at least takes account of pure sampling variation in the trial used for estimating the population standard deviation (or variance) and this is an improvement over conventional approaches.

The third complication is that there is usually no agreed standard for a clinically relevant difference. In practice some compromise is usually reached between 'true' clinical requirements and practical sample size requirements. (See below for a more detailed discussion of this point.)

Fourth, the levels of α and β are themselves arbitrary. Frequently the values chosen in our example (0.05 and 0.20) are the ones employed. In some cases one might consider that the value of β ought to be much lower. In some diseases, where there are severe ethical constraints on the numbers which may be recruited, a very low value of β might not be acceptable. In other cases, it might be appropriate to have a lower α. In particular it might be questioned whether trials in which β is lower than α are justifiable. Note, however, that β is a theoretical value used for planning, whereas α is an actual value used in determining significance at analysis.

It may be a requirement that the results be robust to a number of alternative analyses. The problem that this raises is frequently ignored. However, where this requirement applies, unless the sample size is increased to take account of it, the power will be reduced. (If power, in this context, is taken to be the probability that *all* required tests will be significant if the clinically relevant difference applies.) This issue is discussed in section 13.2.12 below.

13.2.2   By adjusting the sample size we can fix our probability of being successful

This statement is not correct. It must be understood that the fact that a sample size has been chosen which appears to provide 80% power does not imply that there is an 80% chance that the trial will be successful, because even if the planning has been appropriate and the calculations are correct:

(i)   The drug may not work. (Actually, strictly speaking, if the drug doesn't work we wish to conclude this, so that failure to find a difference is a form of success.)
(ii)   If it works it may not produce a clinically relevant difference.
(iii)   The drug might be better than planned for, in which case the power should be higher than planned.
(iv)   The power (sample size) calculation covers the influence of random variation *on the assumption* that the trial is run competently. It does not allow for 'acts of God' or dishonest or incompetent investigators.

Thus although we can *affect* the probability of success by adjusting the sample size, we cannot *fix* it.

13.2.3   The sample size calculation is an excuse for a sample size and not a reason

There are two justifications for this view. First, usually when we have sufficient back-ground information for the purpose of planning a clinical trial, we already have a good idea what size of trial is indicated. For example, so many trials now have been conducted in hypertension that any trialist worth her salt (if one may be forgiven for mentioning salt in this context) will already know what size the standard trial is. A calculation is hardly necessary. It is a brave statistician, however, who writes in her trial protocol, 'a sample size of 200 was chosen because this is commonly found to be appropriate in trials of hypertension'. Instead she will usually feel pressured to quote a standard deviation, a significance level, a clinically relevant difference and a power and apply them in an appropriate formula.

The second reason is that this calculation may be the final result of several hidden iterations. At the first pass, for example, it may be discovered that the sample size is higher than desirable, so the clinically relevant difference is adjusted upwards to justify the sample size. This is not usually a desirable procedure. In discussing this one should, however, free oneself of moralizing cant. If the only trial which circumstances permit one to run is a small one, then the choice is between a small trial or no trial at all. It is not always the case that under such circumstances the best choice, whether taken in the interest of drug development or of future patients, is no trial at all. It may be useful, however, to calculate the sort of difference which the trial is capable of detecting so that one is clear at the outset about what is possible. Under such circumstances, the value of Δ can be the determined function of α, β, σ and n and is then not so much the *clinically relevant* as the *detectable* difference. In fact there is a case for simply plotting for any trial the power function: that is to say, the power at each possible value of the clinically relevant difference. A number of such functions are plotted in Figure 13.1 for the trial in asthma considered in Example 13.1. (For the purposes of calculating the power in the graph, it has been assumed that a one-sided test at the 2.5% level will be carried out. For high values of the clinically relevant difference, this gives the same answer as carrying out a two-sided test at the 5% level. For lower values it is preferable anyway.)

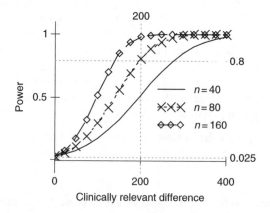

Figure 13.1 Power as a function of clinically relevant difference for a two-parallel-group trial in asthma. The outcome variable is FEV_1, the standard deviation is assumed to be 450 ml, and n is the number of patients per group. If the clinically relevant difference is 200 ml, 80 patients per group are needed for 80% power.

13.2.4   If we have performed a power calculation, then upon rejecting the null hypothesis, not only may we conclude that the treatment is effective but also that it has a clinically relevant effect

This is a surprisingly widespread piece of nonsense which has even made its way into one book on drug industry trials. Consider, for example, the case of a two parallel group trial to compare an experimental treatment with a placebo. Conventionally we would use a two-sided test to examine the efficacy of the treatment. (See Chapter 12 for a discussion. The essence of the argument which follows, however, is unaffected by whether one-sided or two-sided tests are used.) Let τ be the true difference (experimental treatment–placebo). We then write the two hypotheses,

$$H_0 : \tau = 0 \qquad H_1 : \tau \neq 0. \tag{13.2}$$

Now, if we reject H_0, the hypothesis which we assert is H_1, which simply states that the treatment difference is *not* zero or, in other words, that there is a difference between the experimental treatment and placebo. This is not a very exciting conclusion but it happens to be the conclusion to which significance in a conventional hypothesis test leads. As we saw in Chapter 12, however (see section 13.2.3), by observing the sign of the treatment difference, we are also justified in taking the further step of deciding whether the treatment is superior or inferior to placebo. A power calculation, however, merely takes a particular value, Δ, within the range of possible values of τ given by H_1 and poses the question: 'if this particular value happens to obtain, what is the probability of coming to the correct conclusion that there is a difference?' This does not at all justify our writing in place of (13.2),

$$H_0 : \tau = 0 \qquad H_1 : \tau = \Delta, \tag{13.3}$$

or even

$$H_0 : \tau = 0 \qquad H_1 : \tau \geq \Delta. \tag{13.4}$$

In fact, (13.4) would imply that we knew, before conducting the trial, that the treatment effect is either zero or at least equal to the clinically relevant difference. But where we are unsure whether a drug works or not, it would be ludicrous to maintain that it cannot have an effect which, while greater than nothing, is less than the clinically relevant difference.

If we wish to say something about the difference which obtains, then it is better to quote a so-called 'point estimate' of the true treatment effect, together with associated confidence limits. The point estimate (which in the simplest case would be the difference between the two sample means) gives a value of the treatment effect supported by the observed data in the absence of any other information. It does not, of course, have to obtain. The upper and lower $1 - \alpha$ confidence limits define an interval of values which, were we to adopt them as the null hypothesis for the treatment effect, would not be rejected by a hypothesis test of size α. If we accept the general Neyman–Pearson framework and if we wish to claim any single value as the proven treatment effect, then it is the lower confidence limit, rather than any value used in the power calculation, which fulfills this role. (See Chapter 4.)

13.2.5   We should power trials so as to be able to prove that a clinically relevant difference obtains

Suppose that we compare a new treatment to a control, which might be a placebo or a standard treatment. We could set up a hypothesis test as follows:

$$H_0 : \tau < \Delta \qquad H_1 : \tau \geq \Delta. \tag{13.5}$$

H_0 asserts that the treatment effect is less than clinically relevant and H_1 that it is at least clinically relevant. If we reject H_0 using this framework, then, using the logic of hypothesis testing, we decide that a clinically relevant difference obtains. It has been suggested that this framework ought to be adopted since we are interested in treatments which have a clinically relevant effect.

Using this framework requires a redefinition of the clinically relevant difference. It is no longer 'the difference we should not like to miss' but instead becomes 'the difference we should like to prove obtains'. Sometimes this is referred to as the 'clinically irrelevant difference'. For example, as Cairns and Ruberg point out (Cairns and Ruberg, 1996; Ruberg and Cairns, 1998), the CPMP guidelines for chronic arterial occlusive disease require that, 'an irrelevant difference (to be specified in the study protocol) between placebo and active treatment can be excluded' (Committee for Proprietary Medicinal Products, 1995). In fact, if we wish to prove that an effect equal to Δ obtains, then unless for the purpose of a power calculation we are able to assume an alternative hypothesis in which τ is greater than Δ, the maximum power obtainable (for an infinite sample size) would be 50%. This is because, in general, if our null hypothesis is that $\tau < \Delta$, and the alternative is that $\tau \geq \Delta$, the critical value for the observed treatment difference must be greater than Δ. The larger the sample size the closer the critical value will be to Δ, but it can never be less than Δ. On the other hand, if the true treatment difference is Δ, then the observed treatment difference will less than Δ in approximately 50% of all trials. Therefore, the probability that it is less than the critical value must be greater than 50%. Hence the power, which is the probability under the alternative hypothesis that the observed difference is greater than the critical value, must be less than 50%.

The argument in favour of this approach is clear. The conventional approach to hypothesis testing lacks ambition. Simply proving that there is a difference between treatments is not enough: one needs to show that it is important. There are, however, several arguments against using this approach. The first concerns active controlled studies. Here it might be claimed that all that is necessary is to show that the treatment is at least as good as some standard. Furthermore, in a serious disease in which patients have only two choices for therapy, the standard and the new, it is only necessary to establish which of the two is better, not by how much it is better, in order to treat patients optimally. Any attempt to prove more must involve treating some patients suboptimally and this, in the context, would be unacceptable.

A further argument is that a nonsignificant result will often mean the end of the road for a treatment. It will be lost for ever. However, a treatment which shows a 'significant' effect will be studied further. We thus have the opportunity to learn more about its effects. Therefore, there is no need to be able to claim on the basis of a single trial that a treatment effect is clinically relevant.

13.2.6   Most trials are unethical because they are too large

The argument is related to one in Section 13.2.5. If we insist on *'proving'* that a new treatment is superior to a standard we shall study more patients than are necessary to obtain some sort of belief, even it is only a mere suspicion, that one or the other treatment is superior. Hence doctors will be prescribing contrary to their beliefs and this is unethical.

I think that for less serious non-life-threatening and chronic diseases this argument is difficult to sustain. Here the patients studied may themselves become the future beneficiaries of the research to which they contribute and, given informed consent, there is thus no absolute requirement for a doctor to be in equipoise. For serious diseases the argument must be taken more seriously and, indeed, sequential trials and monitoring committees are an attempt to deal with it. The following must be understood, however. (1) Whatever a given set of trialists conclude about the merits of a new treatment, most physicians will continue to use the standard for many years. (2) In the context of drug development, a physician who refuses to enter patients on a clinical trial because she or he is firmly convinced that the experimental treatment is superior to the standard treatment condemns *all* her or his patients to receive the standard. (3) if a trial stops before providing reasonably strong evidence of the efficacy of a treatment, then even if it looks promising, it is likely that collaborating physicians will have considerable difficulties in prescribing the treatment to future patients.

It thus follows that, on a purely logical basis at least, a physician is justified in continuing on a trial, even where she or he believes that the experimental treatment is superior. It is not necessary to start in equipoise (Senn, 2001a, 2002). The trial may then be regarded as continuing either to the point where evidence has overcome initial enthusiasm for the new treatment, so that the physician no longer believes in its efficacy, or to the point at which sceptical colleagues can be convinced that the treatment works. Looked at in these terms, few conventional trials would be too large.

13.2.7   Small trials are unethical

The argument here is that one should not ask patients to enter a clinical trial unless one has a reasonable chance of finding something useful. Hence small or 'inadequately powered' trials are unethical.

There is something in this argument. I do not agree, however, that small trials are uninterpretable and, as was explained in Section 13.2.2, sometimes only a small trial can be run. It can be argued that if a treatment will be lost anyway if the trial is not run, then it should be run, even if it is only capable of 'proving' efficacy where the treatment effect is considerable. Part of the problem with small trials is, to use Altman and Bland's memorable phrase, that 'absence of evidence is not evidence of absence' (Altman and Bland, 1995) and there is a tendency to misinterpret a nonsignificant effect as an indication that a treatment is not effective rather than as a failure to prove that it is effective. However, if this is the case, it is an argument for improving medical education, rather than one for abandoning small trials. The rise of meta-analysis has also meant that small trials are becoming valuable for the part which they are able to contribute to the whole. As Edwards *et al.* have argued eloquently, some evidence is better than none (Edwards *et al.*, 1997). See Bachetti *et al.* (2005) for a criticism of the view that small trials are unethical.

> **Clinically relevant difference**: Used in the theory of clinical trials as opposed to *cynically* relevant difference, which is used in practice.

13.2.8 A significant result is more meaningful if obtained from a large trial

It is possible to show, with an application of Bayes' theorem, that if we allow a certain prior probability that a product is effective, then the posterior probability of the effectiveness of the product, given a significant result, is an increasing function of the power of the test. Suppose, for example, that the prior odds for a given alternative hypothesis against the null hypothesis are pr_1/pr_0. Let L_1 be the likelihood of observing a given piece of evidence under H_1 and L_0 be the likelihood under H_0. Let po_1/po_0 be the posterior odds. Then Bayes' theorem implies (see Chapter 4) that

$$\frac{po_1}{po_0} = \frac{pr_1}{pr_0}\frac{L_1}{L_0}. \tag{13.6}$$

If the evidence is that a result is significant at level α and the power for the given alternative is $1 - \beta$, then these are the two likelihoods associated with the evidence and we may write

$$\frac{po_1}{po_0} = \frac{pr_1}{pr_0}\frac{1-\beta}{\alpha} \tag{13.7}$$

Now, from (13.7) for given prior odds and fixed α, the posterior odds are greater the smaller the value of β, which is to say the greater the power of the test. But the power increases with sample size. Hence, other things being equal, significant results are more indicative of efficacy if obtained from large trials rather than small trials.

Although it is technically correct, one should be *extremely careful* in interpreting this statement, as will be shown below.

13.2.9 A given significant *P*-value is more indicative of the efficacy of a treatment if obtained from a small trial

The surprising thing is that this statement can also be shown to be true given suitable assumptions (Royall, 1986). We talked above about the power of the alternative hypothesis, but typically this hypothesis includes all sorts of values of τ, the treatment effect. One argument is that if the sample size is increased, not only is the power of finding a clinically relevant difference, Δ, increased, but the power also of finding lesser differences. Another argument is as follows.

In general, we do not merely observe that a trial is significant or not significant. To do so is to throw information away. We shall observe an exact *P*-value. For example we might say that the results were significant at the 5% level but in fact know that $P = 0.028$. Hence, although (13.6) gives a general expression for the posterior odds, the particular application of it given by (13.7) is irrelevant. Instead of using the likelihood of significance we need to use the likelihoods $L_1(P)$ and $L_0(P)$ associated with the observed P-value. Hence we may write

$$\frac{po_1}{po_o} = \frac{pr_1}{pr_0} \frac{L_1(P)}{L_0(P)} \qquad (13.8)$$

Now, whereas $(1 - \beta)/\alpha$ is a monotonically increasing function of the sample size n, $L_1(P)/L_0(P)$ is not. It may increase at first, but eventually it will decline. The situation is illustrated in Figure 13.2, which takes the particular example of the trial is asthma considered in section 13.1 above and shows the likelihood for the null hypothesis (scaled to equal 1 in the case where the observed treatment difference is zero) for all possible observed treatment differences and also for the alternative hypothesis where the true treatment effect is equal to the clinically relevant difference. The situations for trials with 10 and 200 patients per group are illustrated. The critical value of the observed treatment difference for a two-sided test at the 5% level is marked in each case. For the smaller trial, a larger difference is required for significance. In the larger trial, a smaller difference is adequate.

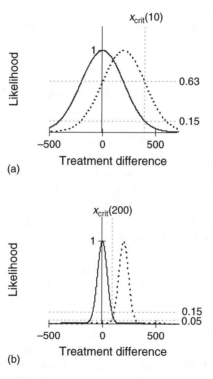

(a)

(b)

Figure 13.2 Scaled likelihood for null and alternative hypotheses for trials with (a) 10 and (b) 200 patients per group. Under the alternative hypothesis the clinically relevant difference obtains.

Note that the scaled likelihood for H_0 is the same in both cases and approximately equal to 0.15. However, in the first case the likelihood is more than four times as high under H_1, being equal to 0.63, and in the second case only a third as high under H_1, being equal to 0.05. Hence a given P-value of exactly 0.05 would provide evidence in favour of the alternative hypothesis in the first case and against it in the second. Thus, on this interpretation, moderate significance from a large trial would actually be evidence for the null hypothesis. (Note that if one is told only that the result is significant, it is the area under the curve to the right of the critical value which is relevant, and this is much higher in the larger trial. This was the situation considered in section 13.2.8 but is not the situation here.)

The fact that a conventionally significant result can give evidence in favour of the null hypothesis is known as the Jeffreys–Lindley paradox (Bartlett, 1957; Lindley, 1957; Senn, 2001b). In practice, such a situation would hardly ever arise. This is because a significant P-value is not very likely given the null hypothesis (this is the basic idea behind the significance test) and it is even less likely given the sort of alternative hypothesis illustrated. The point is rather that, given that this unusual situation has occurred, it actually gives more evidence in favour of the null hypothesis. It is one argument, once a trial has reached a certain power, to reduce the level of significance required.

Again, however, one has to be very careful in interpreting this result. The diagram only illustrates the alternative hypothesis corresponding to the clinically relevant difference. But if this is the difference we should not like to miss, it does not follow that it is the only difference we should like to find. There may be lower values of the treatment effect which are of interest and these will produce higher likelihoods.

13.2.10   For a given P-value, the evidence against the null hypothesis is the same whatever the size of the trial

This has been referred to as the *alpha postulate*. There is a sense in which this is true also! Look at Figure 13.3. Here, instead of displaying the scaled likelihood for that alternative hypothesis which corresponds to the clinically relevant difference, the alternative hypothesis for which the true treatment effect corresponds to the critical value is illustrated. For $P = 0.05$, the ratio of this likelihood is the same for the trial with 10 patients per group as for the trial with 200 as, indeed, it is for any trial whatsoever. But we do not know which value of the alternative hypothesis is true if the null hypothesis is false. It thus follows that for a P-value of exactly 0.05, there is always one value of the alternative hypothesis for which the likelihood is 1/0.15 or more than six times as high as for the null hypothesis. The evidence in favour of *this* alternative hypothesis (which hypothesis changes according to the size of the trial) is always the same.

This is one interpretation of the significance test. It is the sceptic's concession to the gullible. The sceptic asserts the null hypothesis, because he doesn't believe in the efficacy of treatment. The gullible believes exactly whatever the data tell him. He thus adopts as his presumed treatment effect whatever the observed mean difference is. Since the ratio of likelihoods in favour of this hypothesis will always be greater than 1, he will always obtain evidence in favour of his hypothesis. All that the sceptic can do is

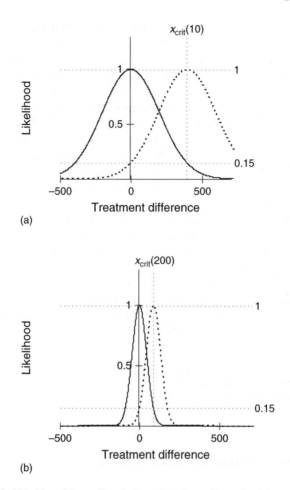

Figure 13.3 Scaled likelihood for null and alternative hypotheses for (a) 10 and (b) 200 patients per group. Under the alternative hypothesis the difference corresponding to the critical value of the test obtains.

counter this by explaining what the consequences of this sort of behaviour are. 'If you regard odds of 6 to 1 for the best supported difference compared to the null hypothesis as being evidence in favour of a treatment effect, then in at least 1 in 20 trials where the treatment is useless you will conclude it is effective.' On this interpretation, a conventionally significant result then becomes a *minimal* requirement for concluding efficacy of a treatment.

In my opinion, this is, the way that drug development usually works. Treatments are not registered unless a significant result is obtained. This is, however, generally a minimal requirement. Other information (treatment estimates, confidence intervals, the analyses of other outcomes, the results of further trials) is presented and unless this is favourable, the drug will not be registered.

The above discussions should serve as a warning, however: the evidential interpretations of *P*-values is a delicate matter (Senn, 2001b).

13.2.11   The effect of the two-trials rule on sample size

If we are required to prove significance in two trials, as is usually believed to be necessary in phase III for a successful NDA application, then from the practical point of view it may be the power of the combined requirement which is important, rather than that for individual trials. On the assumption that the trials are competent and that the background planning has been carried out appropriately and that trial by treatment interactions may be dismissed, then the power to detect the clinically relevant difference in both of two trials, each with power 80%, is 64% since $0.8 \times 0.8 = 0.64$. This means that $1 - 0.64 = 0.36$, or more than one-third, of *such* drug development programmes would fail in phase III for failure of one or both clinical trials on this basis. (This does not mean that one-third of drug developments will fail in phase III, since many drugs which survive that far may, indeed, have an effect which is superior to the clinically relevant difference. On the other hand, there may be other reasons for failure.) If it is desired to have 80% power overall, then it is necessary to run each trial with 90% power since $0.9 \times 0.9 \cong 0.80$.

As explained in Chapter 12, however, the two-trials rule is not particularly logical. The alternative pooled-trials rule would actually require only 4/5 of the number of patients of the two-trials rule for an overall power of 80% and an overall size of 1/1600, which is what, effectively, the two-trials rule implies.

> **Clinically relevant difference**: That which is used to justify the sample size but will be claimed to have been used to find it.

13.2.12   The effect of multiple requirements

Cairns and Ruberg point out that the FDA requires that for registration of treatments for senile dementia, both global cognitive function and overall assessment by physician must be significantly superior to placebo (Cairns and Ruberg, 1996). In Europe, a third additional requirement for 'activities of daily living' is made. This means that to plan a trial of adequate sample size to meet these requirements one would need to use two (three in Europe) clinically relevant differences. One would also have to know the correlation between the repeat measures. A conservative approach would be to assume independence. In that case a sample size determination could be made for each measure for 90% power (USA) or 93% power (Europe) and the largest of all of these determinations taken. (The European requirement would arise because $0.93 \times 0.93 \times 0.93 \cong 0.80$). Comparing the resulting sample size to the largest that would be required for any one of the outcomes taken singly with 80% power, this leads to a 31% increase for the USA and a 46% increase for Europe. Of course, this is extreme. In practice these outcomes will be correlated and better approaches can be used. Nevertheless there will be an increase in sample size required. This issue is discussed in some detail by Kieser *et al.* (2004).

Most statisticians are, of course, aware of the point and will be concerned about requirements for multiple outcomes. What is sometimes overlooked, however, is that a similar point arises if conclusions are required to be robust to a number of analyses: the Mann–Whitney–Wilcoxon test as well as the *t*-test, for example, or including or omitting various covariates. Such multiple requirements also lead to an increase in the sample size needed. (Although, at a guess, the problem will not be as severe as for multiple outcomes.)

Such multiple requirements seem from one point of view to be a good thing. A stronger standards of evidence overall is implicit and in the end we shall have greater confidence in the value of a registered drug. By the same token, however, the ethical problems which arise through sample size requirements can be aggravated by such requirements. In any case, the practical consideration is that the pharmaceutical statistician has to become aware of the requirements of **conjunctive power**, (Senn and Bretz, 2007) that is to say the need for test 1 *and* test 2 *and* test 3, etc. (hence conjunctive) to be significant.

There is also one technical matter which is worth comment. Suppose we require that a *t*-test and a Mann–Whitney–Wilcoxon test both be significant at the 5% level. Let us call this the two-test procedure. These two tests are certainly highly correlated so that the overall type I error rate will be somewhere between 0.05 (the value were they perfectly correlated) and 0.0025 (the value were they independent). Suppose, for argument's sake, that the value is 0.01. I suspect that for moderately sized trials the loss in power as a result of the double requirement, where Normality applies and either test could be used, will be small. Nevertheless, there will be some loss. Of course, there is the gain that a higher standard of evidence of efficacy is required. However, a higher standard of efficacy could be obtained simply by requiring that a *t*-test on its own be significant at the 1% level. It would be interesting to see this requirement compared formally with that of the two-test procedure.

For further discussion of the effect of multiple outcomes on power see Chuang-Stein *et al.* (2007), Offen *et al.* (2007) and Senn and Bretz (2007).

13.2.13   In order to interpret a trial it is necessary to know its power

This is a rather silly point of view that nevertheless continues to attract adherents. A power calculation is used for planning trials and is effectively superseded once the data are in. For an impression of the precision of the result, one is best looking at confidence intervals or standard errors. If the result is significant, then to the extent that one accepts the logic of significance tests, there is no point arguing about the result. An analogy may be made. In determining to cross the Atlantic it is important to consider what size of boat it is prudent to employ. If one sets sail from Plymouth and several days later sees the Statue of Liberty and the Empire State Building, the fact that the boat employed was rather small is scarcely relevant to deciding whether the Atlantic was crossed.

Retrospective power calculations are sometimes encountered for so-called failed trials, but this seems particularly pointless. The clinically relevant difference does not change as a result of having run the trial, in which case the power is just a function of the observed variance. It says nothing about the effect of treatment.

Some check-lists for clinical trials seem to require evidence that a power calculation was performed, but this surely can have very little relevance to the interpretation of the final result. At best it can be a very weak indicator of the quality of the study.

For a trenchant criticism of the use of retrospective power calculations see Hoenig and Heisey (2001).

13.2.14   The dimension of cost

A very unsatisfactory feature of conventional approaches to sample size calculation is that there is no mention of cost. This means that for any two quite different indications with the same effect size, that is to say the same ratio of clinically relevant difference to standard deviation, the sample size would be the same whatever the cost or difficulty of recruiting and treating patients. This is clearly illogical and trialists probably manage this issue informally by manipulating the clinically relevant difference in the way discussed in Section 13.2.3. Clearly, it would be better to include the cost explicitly, and this suggests decision-analytic approaches to sample size determination. There are various Bayesian suggestions and these will be discussed in the next section.

13.2.15   Bayesian approaches to sample size determination

A Bayesian approach to sample size determination may be discussed in terms of a rather artificial and not very realistic case, namely that where a single phase III study must be run in a nonsequential manner and on the basis of this the treatment will be registered or not. Now consider a trial of a given sample size and suppose that a decision will be made on the basis of a statistic from such a trial. Suppose that it is known for every value of the statistic whether the regulator will register the drug or not and that a loss may be associated with failing to register. Of course, the regulator's decision might itself be based on a suitable loss function and prior distribution, but from the sponsor's point of view this does not matter provided only that the decision that will be taken is known.

Now, given a suitable prior distribution (which does not have to be the same as the regulator's), the sponsor can calculate the predictive distribution for the test statistic and hence the expected loss for any given sample size, including the cost of experimentation. The optimal sample size is then the one with the smallest expected loss. This is a double optimization procedure: the optimal decision (minimum loss) for a given value of the test statistic and sample size must be determined and then the sample size which yields the smallest minimum loss is chosen (Lindley, 1997).

Various Bayesian approaches that have been suggested are variants of this. For example, Lindley's approach (Lindley, 1997) involves a sophisticated use of loss functions and is fully Bayesian but applies when regulator and sponsor have the same beliefs and values. That of Gittins and Pezeshk is a hybrid Bayes-frequentist system in which it is supposed that eventual sales of a pharmaceutical are a function of how impressive the trial results are (measured by conventional significance) but that in planning, prior distributions and a Bayesian approach are used (Gittins and Pezeshk, 2000a,b; Pezeshk and Gittins, 2002). For an implementation in SAS of a simpler approach with costs per patient but a single reward for a significant trial, see Burman *et al.* (2007). This uses a prior distribution on the treatment effect. Application of this in a hybrid Bayesian/frequentist approach is discussed in Section 13.2.16.

13.2.16   An appropriate approach to sample size determination is to calculate assurance

Even closer to a frequentist approach than the methods of Section 13.2.15 is that of calculating what O'Hagan *et al.* call **assurance** (O'Hagan *et al.*, 2005). This is the

Bayesian probability of a clinical trial yielding a significant result. Rather than being conditional on a particular posited clinically relevant difference, it uses a prior distribution for the treatment effect and integrates the conventional frequentist power over this distribution to obtain an unconditional expected power, assurance. If this approach alone is used for sample size determination it means that the clinically relevant difference has no role whatsoever in determining how large the trial should be. As suggested in Section 13.2.14, conventional power calculations are already unsatisfactory in that they treat identically two indications with differing costs but identical effect sizes. Assurance, however, seems to take this one stage further. Provided that the prior distributions for treatment effects for two indications are the same and the precision is the same, then if assurance is to be the guide, the sample sizes will be the same, even if in terms of practical interest the prior distributions are quite different.

For this and other reasons, I am not particularly keen on the use of assurance as the primary criterion for designing a clinical trial, although it may well be useful to calculate it in addition. My own view is that if I am going to be Bayesian about sample size calculation I would rather be hanged for a sheep than a lamb and use the methods of section 13.2.15.

References

Altman DG, Bland JM (1995) Absence of evidence is not evidence of absence. *British Medical Journal* **311**: 485.

Bacchetti P, Wolf LE, Segal MR, McCulloch CE (2005) Ethics and sample size. *American Journal of Epidemiology* **161**: 105–110.

Bartlett MS (1957) A comment on D.V. Lindley's statistical paradox. *Biometrika* **44**: 533–534.

Burman C-F, Grieve AP, Senn S (2007) Decision analysis in drug development. In: Dmitrienko A, Chuang-Stein C, Agostino R (eds), *Pharmaceutical Statistics Using SAS: A Practical Guide.* SAS Institute, Cary, pp. 385–428.

Cairns V, Ruberg S (1996) The confirmatory package of trials–design. In: Jones B, Teather B, Teather D (eds), *Proceedings of Statistical Issues in Biopharmaceutical Environments: USA and European Perspectives*, De Monfort University, Leicester.

Chuang-Stein C, Stryszak P, Dmitrienko A, Offen W (2007) Challenge of multiple co-primary endpoints: a new approach. *Statistics in Medicine* **26**: 1181–1192.

Committee for Proprietary Medicinal Products (1995) *Note for guidance on the clinical investigation of medicinal products in the treatment of chronic peripheral arterial occlusive disease*. EMEA, London. http://www.emea.europa.eu/pdfs/human/ewp/071498eu.pdf.

Desu MM, Raghavarao D (1990) *Sample Size Methodology*. Academic Press, Boston.

Edwards SJ, Lilford RJ, Braunholtz D, Jackson J (1997) Why 'underpowered' trials are not necessarily unethical [see comments]. *Lancet* **350**: 804–807.

Gittins J, Pezeshk H (2000a) A behavioral Bayes method for determining the size of a clinical trial. *Drug Information Journal* **34**: 355–363.

Gittins J, Pezeshk H (2000b) How large should a clinical trial be? *Journal of the Royal Statistical Society Series D–The Statistician* **49**: 177–187.

Hoenig JM, Heisey DM (2001) The abuse of power: the pervasive fallacy of power calculations for data analysis. *American Statistician* **55**: 19–24.

Julious SA (2004) Tutorial in biostatistics–Sample sizes for clinical trials with normal data. *Statistics in Medicine* **23**: 1921–1986.

Julious SA (2006) *Designing clinical trials with uncertain estimates of variability*. PhD, University College London, London.

Kieser M, Röhmel J, Friede T (2004) Power and sample size determination when assessing the clinical relevance of trial results by 'responder analyses'. *Statistics in Medicine* **23**: 3287–3305.

Lindley DV (1957) A statistical paradox. *Biometrika* **44**: 187–192.

Lindley DV (1997) The choice of sample size. *Statistician* **46**: 129–138.

O'Hagan A, Stevens JW, Campbell MJ (2005) Assurance in clinical trial design. *Pharmaceutical Statistics* **4**: 186–201.

Offen W, Chuang-Stein C, Dmitrienko A, *et al.* (2007) Multiple co-primary endpoints: medical and statistical solutions–A report from the Multiple Endpoints Expert Team of the Pharmaceutical Research and Manufacturers of America. *Drug Information Journal* **41**: 31–46.

Pezeshk H, Gittins J (2002) A fully Bayesian approach to calculating sample sizes for clinical trials with binary responses. *Drug Information Journal* **36**: 143–150.

Royall RM (1986) The effect of sample size on the meaning of significance tests. *The American Statistician* **40**: 313–315.

Ruberg S, Cairns V (1998) Providing evidence of efficacy for a new drug. *Statistics in Medicine* **17**: 1813–1823.

Senn SJ (2001a) The misunderstood placebo. *Applied Clinical Trials* **10**: 40–46.

Senn SJ (2001b) Two cheers for *P*-values. *Journal of Epidemiology and Biostatistics* **6**: 193–204.

Senn SJ (2002) Ethical considerations concerning treatment allocation in drug development trials. *Statistical Methods in Medical Research* **11**: 403–411.

Senn SJ, Bretz F (2007) Power and sample size when multiple endpoints are considered. *Pharmaceutical Statistics* **6**: 161–170.

Multicentre Trials

> *. . . every thesis and hypothesis have an offspring of propositions; – and each proposition has its own conclusions; every one of which leads the mind on again into fresh enquiries and doubtings.*
>
> Laurence Sterne, *Tristram Shandy*

14.1   BACKGROUND

A concern in planning clinical trials is the supply of patients. Considerable efforts are made in the planning stage to estimate rates of accrual and later, when the trial is implemented, to see that these rates are achieved. The longer a trial takes the more, other things being equal, it will cost the sponsor: in particular in terms of lost sales. In many trials the time between recruiting the first and last patient is a considerable proportion of the total duration of the trial. For example, a 'three-month' study in asthma might take 15 months to complete owing to 12 months' recruitment. The sample sizes required by most clinical trials – the exceptions being cross-over trials in some specialties – are such that acceptable recruitment times can only be achieved by recruiting patients simultaneously to a number of centres. Hence, although they are regarded by some commentators as being problematical, multicentre trials are nonetheless granted to be an absolute necessity.

A data set consisting of a series of results by treatment for a number of centres is closely analogous to one consisting of a number of results by treatment for a number of trials. Accordingly, many similar issues to those that arise in meta-analysis arise in the analysis of multicentre trials, although traditions in the two cases are rather different. Hence, there may be some value in studying this chapter and Chapter 16 on meta-analysis together.

14.2   ISSUES

14.2.1   Patient numbers per centre should be roughly equal

This point of view is often propounded. It is maintained that it is the sign of a bad trial that the numbers of patients per centre are unequal. There are perhaps two reasons why this is believed to be the case. First, it is argued that we ought to wish to treat centres equally and, therefore, failure to recruit equal numbers of patients to centres indicates either poor planning or poor control in execution. Second, it is argued that trials in which the numbers of patients differ greatly from centre to centre will be inefficient. This latter point will be dealt with below under another heading. The first is considered here.

In contradistinction to many commentators, it is my view that unequal numbers of patients per centre, far from being a sign of poor planning or execution, are an inevitable and logical consequence of a rational approach to clinical trials (Senn, 1995). It is rare, although it is occasionally the case, that the rate-limiting factor for a given centre in treating patients in a clinical trial is resource availability: doctors, nurses and so forth. It is more usually the case that the process as a whole is governed by the rate at which patients arrive who both satisfy the inclusion criteria and are willing to give consent to enter the trial. If one seeks a model to describe the probability of arrival of a given number of patients at a given clinic in a given period (say six months) then the simplest candidate is the Poisson distribution. This is a distribution for which the variance is equal to the mean so that, for example, if the mean number of arrivals were 9 patients per six months, the variance would also be 9. (In practice most real-life distributions of events per time period show more variation than that exhibited by the Poisson but it often provides a useful starting point.)

When describing the relative variability of a distribution, however, it is not the ratio of variance to mean which is important but that of standard deviation to mean. This feature is a useful one which can be exploited given an appropriate attitude. The sum of a number of independent Poisson variables is also a Poisson variable, so that if we had four centres each with a mean (Poisson) arrival rate of 9 patients per six months overall, we should have a trial where arrival was described by a Poisson distribution with mean of 36 per six months. Now, since the standard deviation is the square root of the variance, the ratio of standard deviation to mean for a Poisson with mean 36 is $6/36 = 0.17$, whereas for a Poisson with mean 9 it is $3/9 = 0.33$.

We thus see that there is stability in numbers. But where has this stability come from? It comes from the possibility of mutually (randomly) compensating behaviour of the centres. One centre, by chance, may have a smaller than average influx of patients in the period for which the study is planned to run, but another may, by chance, have a greater than average number of patients. Provided we allow the centres to compensate for each other, this feature may be exploited.

Is there any way in which we can destroy this 'safety in numbers' property? Yes: *we can insist on applying individual identical targets for each centre in order to try to ensure that the numbers recruited per centre are equal.* If we adopt this procedure, then the recruitment rate is determined by the slowest-recruiting centre. Far from having obtained stability through large numbers, we shall have designed a trial where the extremes are important.

Consider, for example, a trial in four centres in which it is determined to recruit 96 patients in total. Suppose that in each centre recruitment follows a Poisson distribution with mean arrival rate of 24 patients per year. Mean inter-arrival time is then 1/24 years or 0.042 year. The time to recruit the 24th patient in a given centre will be given by the gamma distribution with parameters 0.042 and 24. The mean recruitment time for a centre will be 1 year and the median will be 0.986 year. The probability of completing in one year or less in a given centre will be 0.527. (Details of the necessary calculations to support these assertions are not given here. Let us accept that they are true.)

If, however, we have to wait for every centre to complete, then the probability of completing in one year or less is the product of the probabilities that each centre does so and is $(0.527)^4 = 0.077$. Further calculations show that the median time to finish the whole trial is 1.2 and that three-quarters of all trials will take more than 1.1 year to finish. If on the other hand, for the purpose of recruitment, we treated the whole trial as one, simply requiring a total recruitment of 96, then the median recruitment time would be 0.997: nearly two and a half months less.

The above argument shows the minimum likely effect of requiring equal numbers per centre and assumes that true long-term recruitment rates are equal in all centres. If one further supposes that such true rates vary from centre to centre, perhaps because some centres serve a larger population than others, then the requirement for equal numbers per centre becomes even more hopeless. Hence, it is the case that any rational approach to planning and managing multicentre trials must allow for disparity in the number of patients per centre.

As far as I am aware, the above discussion of the effect of centre size distribution on recruitment time in the first edition of this book was the first to treat the issue formally. Since then the matter has been studied in much greater depth and generality by Fedorov and Jones and co-workers in a number of papers. See Fedorov and Jones (2005) for a useful account.

14.2.2 Trials with unequal numbers of patients per centre are inefficient

If it were the case that a trial with very variable numbers of patients per centre were less efficient in terms of the precision of the estimate delivered at the end of the trial than a trial with the same total numbers of patients distributed equally among the centres, then the superiority of the former with respect to recruitment rate might be completely vitiated. We should be able to recruit patients faster but would have to recruit more of them in order to provide an estimate of equal precision. It is thus necessary to consider what effect unequal numbers have on the precision of the treatment estimate.

This turns out to be a rather complex matter because, for any multicentre trial, one can conceive of at least four different sorts of estimate which might be calculated even where the trialist's aim is to allow for differences between centres. Two of these estimates are so-called 'fixed'-effect estimates based on within-centre treatment contrasts, the third is a so-called random effects estimate, and the fourth is one that permits the recovery of between-centre information. (There are various variants on these models and for a fuller account the reader should see Senn (2000).) The nature and properties of these estimators are discussed in further sections of this chapter. It is really only with one of the two fixed-effect estimators that this problem of inefficiency is serious. We shall discuss this point below when comparing 'type II' and 'type III' approaches to inference. For the moment, suffice it to say that it is not true that trials with unequal numbers of patients per centre are inefficient unless we insist on weighting centres equally (the type III approach).

14.2.3 Should we use `type II' or `type III' sums of squares?

The non-statistician will often be mystified by the references which medical statisticians make to sums of squares. Partitioning the total variation in a data set into various sources, for example due to differences between centres, due to treatment and due to random variation, is a standard statistician's strategy for analysis. A common measure of variability is the variance, which is based on the sums of squares of values about their mean. Hence partitioning variability can be an exercise in partitioning sums of squares. **Type II** and **type III sums of squares** are two types of sums of squares associated in particular with proc GLM of SAS. (**Type I** and type IV **sums of squares** are also encountered. The latter need not concern us. The former is discussed briefly in due course.)

SAS is the pharmaceutical standard statistical package and proc GLM is a powerful tool of analysis (a procedure within SAS) which permits the statistician to analyse unbalanced designs. As we have seen, clinical trials are nearly always unbalanced in the sense that we have unequal numbers of patients per centre. Furthermore, we frequently wish to make use of important prognostic covariate information, such as baselines, as part of our strategy for analysis. Such covariate information is always unbalanced in that we should never expect to find that mean covariate values were identical in each treatment group in each centre. ProcGLM can easily handle analyses in which some of the variables are classification variables, such as centre number or treatment given, and others are numerical, such as baseline blood pressure, or height or weight.

When we partition variability into various sources, however, we can get different answers depending on the order in which this is done whenever we have unbalanced experiments. As a simple example, suppose that we run a clinical trial in two centres, in one of which all the patients are male and in the other of which all of the patients are female. In that case there can be no distinction in terms of *observed* values between a difference between centres and a difference between sexes. These factors are confounded (to use statisticians' jargon) and we can only assess the joint effect of them both (short of declaring one of them to be irrelevant). If, however, as a pure exercise in calculation we were to establish how much of the total variability could be explained by putting 'sex' into the model, this could be done. When we came to add 'centre' we should find no further variability explained by it. Similarly, if we fitted 'centre first' we would find some variability associated with it but no further variation explained by sex.

The example above is an extreme one. For a less extreme case, where most but not all of the males were in one centre and most of the females in the other, we would be able to ascribe some variability separately to centres and some separately to sex. If we were interested in the separate effects of these factors, the usual strategy would be to look at 'sex' after having first fitted 'centre' when judging the effect of 'sex', and to look at 'centre' having first fitted 'sex' when judging the effect of 'centre'. In commonsense terms the justification for this strategy is that a scientist should first eliminate other explanations before claiming that a given factor of interest is important. Where sex and centre are heavily confounded, this strategy will lead to neither being declared significant. This is as it should be, for short of using some other (perhaps prior) information or argument to say that one of them must be negligible, if they vary together we cannot tell which is responsible for a change in outcome (although we might conclude that at least one must be important). Actually, in analysing a clinical trial, we are not usually primarily interested in the separate effects of sex or centres, but simply in their joint effects in order to eliminate these from the analysis before looking at the effect of treatment. For this purpose, it makes no difference whether sex or centre is fitted first.

We can apply the general strategy outlined above using so-called 'type I' sums of squares. For type I sums of squares, SAS calculates the residual variability for a given factor having adjusted for all other factors previously specified by the model. The order in which the effects are specified is important so that, for example, if we write:

model OUTCOME = SEX CENTRE TREATMENT,

the type I sum of squares for sex would be adjusted for nothing else, but centre would be adjusted for sex, and treatment would be adjusted for both sex and centre. If however, we had written

model OUTCOME = CENTRE SEX TREATMENT,

although the type I sums of squares for treatment would be as before, that for sex and centre would no longer be the same except in the special case of perfect balance. However, a feature in SAS means that we do not need to continually re-specify the order of the factors in the model in order to study the effect of a given factor with all other factors eliminated. This is where type II and type III sums of squares come in. In the case above, type II and type III sums of squares would be identical and for treatment they would be the same as the type I sum of squares since it is specified last. For sex and centre they would correspond to models in which these factors had been fitted last.

This strategy of fitting all other effects first when attempting to say something definitive about another is generally agreed as sensible by statisticians. There is one exception, however, and that is to do with interactive effects such as sex-by-centre, or centre-by-treatment interaction (the tendency for the actual efficacy of the treatment to be different in different centres). One school maintains that such interactive effects should also be adjusted for (the 'type III' philosophy), another maintains that when looking at the effect of treatment (say) all other effects should be adjusted for *except any interactive effect in which treatment itself is involved* (this is the type II philosophy).

When the first edition of this book appeared in 1997, it was still the case that many statisticians in the pharmaceutical industry adhered to the type III philosophy. Since then the espousal of a type II philosophy seems to have become more common. I would like to think that this book played its part in this evolution. There have, however, been other influential statements in favour of the type II philosophy. A particularly clear account is given by Gallo (2001).

We cannot fruitfully follow this discussion further in terms of sums of squares. It turns out, however, that there are treatment estimators which correspond to the particular approaches for estimating sums of squares and it is easier to see the relative merits of the two approaches in terms of these estimators. We shall explain this by considering a two-group trial comparing an active treatment with a placebo. As regards treatment effects adjusted for the effect of centres, both approaches can be described as follows. First, each approach would first estimate a separate treatment effect in each centre. If no other factors were in the model this would correspond to calculating the difference between the mean value under the active treatment and that under placebo on a centre-by-centre basis. This correspond to adjusting treatment for pure differences between centres. The type III approach would then combine these separate treatment effects by weighting each of these equally. For the type II approach they would be weighted according to the precision with which they had been estimated, so that generally larger centres would receive more weight. (It can occasionally happen that the degree of imbalance between the two treatment groups within a centre is so extreme that a large centre can actually provide a less efficient estimate than a well-balanced small one, but this is rare.) Thus, to make a political analogy, type II sums of squares are like the US House of Representatives, in which states are represented according to their population. On the other hand, type III sums of squares are like the Senate: each state is represented equally. In other words, by weighting centres equally, type III estimates tend to weight patients unequally. Patients in larger centres receive less weight. On the other hand, type II estimates give more weight to larger centres and, where the numbers on the two arms in a centre are balanced, do so in direct proportion to the number of patients. Hence type II estimates tend to give patients equal weight.

The arguments made in favour of type III approaches are as follows. (1) If treatment effects vary from centre to centre then the only interpretable overall treatment effect would be a straightforward average of the centre effects. (2) (A related point) If we use the treatment estimate as the basis of a test of a hypothesis then the hypothesis we test concerns some average of the true treatment effects in each centre. It would be absurd if this hypothesized average itself depended on the numbers of patients we happened to have recruited to the trial.

The type II proponent might argue as follows. (1) We really don't care which centres we recruit to the trial provided they deliver enough information. It is therefore nonsense not to weight them according to the amount of information they provide. (2) If we consider all the centres we might have included but didn't, then the type III approach also depends arbitrarily on the numbers of patients recruited: it depends on whether the centre recruited none or some. (3) Under the null hypothesis of no treatment effect there cannot be any treatment-by-centre interaction anyway and so any weighted combination of the treatment effects by centre forms a valid test of this hypothesis. Why not use the most efficient? The following dialogue dramatizes the argument.

Secundus and Tertius hold a Socratic Dialogue on the Analysis of Multicentre Trials

Secundus: I see, Tertius, that you have weighted all centres equally in your estimate of the treatment effect. Why is that?

Tertius: It is because, Secundus, any other weighting would be entirely *arbitrary*.

Secundus: This does indeed appear to be an excellent reason Tertius. However, I am puzzled to understand one thing, and that is on what basis you chose the centres in your trial?

Tertius: Oh that is quite simple, Secundus. All the physicians concerned have good reputations and promised to deliver an adequate number of patients.

Secundus: These are indeed excellent reasons, O Tertius. However, I cannot help noting that, although some physicians have indeed provided many patients, some seemed to have delivered very few patients at all.

Tertius: Indeed, some of the physicians have disappointed me, but when running trials in future I will not use them.

Secundus: A very wise precaution, Tertius, but it seems to imply that provided centres perform well, you do not mind which centres are in the trial.

Tertius: This is indeed true, Secundus; the main thing is to have enough high-quality data.

Secundus: I see. So provided only that the centres delivered enough patients in total you would be indifferent as to whether the trial were based on, say, centres 1, 3 and 7, or on centres 4, 5 and 8, or on centres 1,2, 8 and 9 or indeed on any set of centres.

Tertius: That is indeed so, Secundus.

Secundus: And suppose for argument's sake that centre 3 could give you all the patients you needed: would you use it alone?

Tertius: (*Smiling*) Indeed I would, Secundus. This would make life much simpler. Unfortunately, clinical trials don't usually work like that.

Secundus. What a pity. And if centre 4 could give you all the patients you needed would you be happy to use that?

Tertius: Of course, Secundus. The centre is unimportant.

Secundus: But this implies, Tertius, that you are quite happy to base your treatment estimate on centre 3 alone, if only it has enough patients and on centre 4 alone, if only it has enough patients, and indeed on any centre at all, provided it has enough patients.

Tertius: (*Impatiently*) Quite so. This is obvious.

Secundus: But then, your only preference amongst centres is based on the precision of the information which they provide, not on any peculiar feature of any given centre and, since you are otherwise indifferent to choices between them, I fail to understand why you insist on weighting them equally and in an inefficient manner.

Tertius: I begin to understand your point, but what is the alternative?

Secundus: The alternative is to weight the centres in such a way that the precision of the treatment estimate is as high as possible.

Tertius: But does that not correspond to the type II philosophy?

Secundus: It does indeed.

Tertius: Then I am sorry, Secundus, but you have been wasting my time. That is a dangerous heresy.

Secundus: Why so?

Tertius: Because the regulator says so.

Secundus: In that case I do indeed apologize for having wasted your time, Tertius. The regulatory argument is transcendental in nature and cannot be defeated by mere logic.

My own view is that, although the type III philosophy seems plausible at first, it is untenable. It leads to paradoxes. For example, given a two-centre trial in which patients are allocated in equal numbers within centres to two treatments but in which the two centres are of different sizes, unless the small centre is at least 1/3 the size of the large centre, the type III treatment estimate will have a larger variance than that based on the large centre alone. Thus more information is worse than less. Figure 14.1 shows the variance of the treatment effect in a two-centre trial as a function of the number of patients in the second centre. The effect is bizarre, to say the least. In this sense,

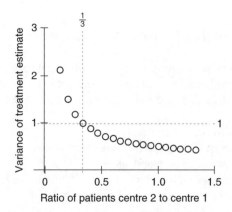

Figure 14.1   Type III efficiency in a two-centre trial. The number of patients in the first centre is fixed. The plot shows the effect on efficiency as more patients are recruited to the second centre.

the general view that trials with variable centre sizes are inefficient is true. However, provided a type II approach is used the problem and paradox disappear.

At the time of the first edition this issue provided a regulatory divide. Virtually the whole of the British school of statistics (including the regulators) disapproved of type III sums of squares (a very influential paper outlining this position was that of John Nelder (Nelder, 1977)). On the other hand, in the USA, there seemed at the time to be less of a consensus. While many statisticians favoured type II sums of squares, the point of view maintained by the FDA had been represented to me as being in favour of type III sums of squares and there had also been some influential theoretical papers promoting this philosophy (Speed *et al.*, 1978).

However, I had *not* heard this directly from the FDA and it should thus only be accorded the status of folklore. Furthermore, since the first edition of this book there has been more US-based support for the type II position. An excellent discussion is given by Gallo (2001). SAS also provides type III as the default rather than type II, and even where type II sums of squares are specifically requested by the user in proc GLM, the estimates it provides seem to correspond to type III. One way around this is not to fit the interactive treatment-by-centre term at all when estimating the treatment effect. This is in fact suggested by the ICH E9 guideline 'Statistical principles for clinical trials' (International Conference on Harmonisation, 1999). The only disadvantage is that the residual mean square may be somewhat higher than it would otherwise be. This can be dealt with by multiplying the standard error for the treatment estimate obtained by not fitting the interactive effects by the ratio of the corresponding root mean square error to the root mean square error when the interactive effect *is* fitted. See also Kallen (1997).

Nevertheless, analyses as carried out by statisticians wedded to the type III philosophy show signs of many concessions to a type II approach. For example, it is a common habit to combine small centres for analysis. This, of course, down-weights their influence on the final result, thus producing an answer more like the type II approach. Furthermore, for meta-analyses, nobody uses an analysis which weights the *trials* equally (Senn, 2000). It is true that a random effects analysis (see below) is sometimes advocated, but where a fixed effects analysis is employed it is essentially a type II analysis which is used. A similar concession is made when fitting baselines and baseline-by-treatment interactions. (The way type II and type III analyses behave where continuous outcomes are fitted will not be obvious from the above discussion and the reader will have to take what follows in the rest of this paragraph on trust.) Most statisticians first subtract the overall mean baseline from the baseline for each patient. This has the consequence that the treatment effect for the *average* patient is estimated whether or not type III or type II sums of squares are used. Not doing this, however, although it has no consequences for the type II approach, has the disastrous effect on the type III approach that the treatment effect is estimated for a patient with baseline 0. (See discussion on baselines.) Such patients may be dead, and so it will be no surprise if the treatment is proved ineffective!

Although the above discussion has been in terms of the linear model and sums of squares, it should be noted that analogous issues apply when using other sorts of models. For example, Chuang-Stein and Tong (1996) consider a case where logistic regression is applied to a trial with two treatments, T_1 and T_2, with two strata, F_1 and F_2, (which could be centres) as given in Table 14.1 (Senn, 2000). Three possible codings of the stratum effect are given, A, B and C. If an interaction is fitted, then depending on how the stratum is coded, quite different estimates (standard errors) of the 'treatment effect' on the log-odds ratio scale will be returned as follows. A, -1.43 (0.528); B, -0.25 (0.703); C, -0.84 (0.440). This is because for coding A the effect is defined as the effect of treatment in stratum F_1, for coding B it is the effect of treatment in stratum F_2, and for coding C it is the unweighted average of the effect in each stratum. Chuang-Stein and Tong recommend coding C, but the unweighted average that this yields is effectively a type III estimate. If the two strata were trials rather than centres or some other factor, then the table has the structure of a meta-analysis and nobody would weight two *trials* of different precision equally. What the meta-analyst would do is give the first stratum (or trial) a bigger weight (Senn, 2000).

Note that whether coding A, B and C is used, the same overall prediction is given when the interaction is kept in the model, it is simply that the labelling of that which is main effect of treatment and that which is interaction changes. The trouble arises because we label something a 'treatment effect' while effectively using a model that recognizes that there is no such thing as a single treatment effect.

In my view, if we wish to retain this single label 'treatment effect' *and* use the model with interaction, the only sensible approach is to regard the model *with* interaction as an elaboration upon the model *without*. In other words, the main effects of treatment and stratum must be as they would be without the interaction and the interactions must be described as a departure from this position. This is effectively the type II philosophy. The reader will perhaps appreciate that there are deep waters here and that the ICH E9

Table 14.1 Summary of results for a binary outcome for a trial with two treatments run in two strata showing three possible codings. Based on an example by Chuang-Stein and Tong (1996).

Treatment	Stratum	Successes	Trials	Coding of covariate		
				A	B	C
T_1	F_1	18	100	0	1	-1
T_2	F_1	5	100	0	1	-1
T_1	F_2	5	50	1	0	1
T_2	F_2	4	50	1	0	1

advice to fit the model without treatment-by-centre interaction first and as primary is wise (International Conference on Harmonisation, 1999).

Having discussed two different approaches to estimation, we now move on to considering a third. This third approach involves a completely different paradigm for considering treatment effects.

14.2.4   What is the difference between fixed- and random-effect estimators?

Before proceeding to discuss this issue, a note on terminology is appropriate. When talking about random effects in connection with multicentre trials, statisticians are usually referring to random variation in the true treatment effect from centre to centre. In other words, they are allowing for the fact that the effect of treatment may be unpredictably (within bounds) different from centre to centre. Such a phenomenon might be referred to also as a random treatment-by-centre interaction. There is, however, another form of random variation from centre to centre that may also occur, namely that the so called main effect of centres may differ randomly from centre to centre. That is to say that one might find, for example, that the true mean under placebo is not the same from centre to centre. Of course, one allows for such variation by fitting the centre effect in the model, but in doing this conventionally, as in section 14.2.3 above, one is fitting centre as a fixed effect. It is also possible, however, to fit centre as a random effect. This will be discussed in section 14.2.8 below. In this section, we do not consider this type of random effect. Instead, when contrasting so-called fixed- and random-effect estimators, we are concerned instead with whether the treatment-by-centre interaction should be regarded as fixed or random.

Choices between fixed- or random-effect estimators arise wherever we have data sets with multiple levels within the experimental units: for example, patients within trials for a meta-analysis, episodes per patient for a series of n-of-1 trials or patients within centres for a multicentre trial. The issue is an extremely complex one and it is difficult to give hard and fast rules as to which is appropriate.

The choice between them has something to do with treatment-by-centre interaction, although (in my view) with our attitude towards it rather than whether its presence is detectable or not. It is a commonplace that patients vary from centre to centre. Provided that the treatment effect is additive on our chosen scale of measurement (in other words whatever the state of patients, it brings the same measured benefit), such differences may be simply eliminated in analysis. Suppose, for example, that in one large centre in an asthma trial the mean value for forced expiratory volume in one second (FEV_1) for patients is 1620 ml whereas that for patients being given active treatment is 1870 ml, but that in another centre the value for placebo patients is 1900 ml whereas that for patients being given active treatment is 2150 ml. Clearly there are important differences between centres: patients on active treatment in the one are apparently worse off than those on placebo in the other! However the difference (active − placebo) is 250 ml in each centre, so that it is conceivable that the treatment is having the same effect (given an appropriate definition of effect). Suppose, furthermore, that we believed that the treatment effect was identical in every centre in the trial (whatever general differences in level there might be) and that it would also be the same in any centre we might study in the future even if the patients there did not fulfill the inclusion criteria of the trial. (Of course, random variation would mean that we would not always observe identical apparent effects as in the above example but we might conceivably believe them to be similar.) In that case the following treatment effects would be the same (Senn, 2004):

(I)   The true mean of the effects for all patients in the trial.
(II)   The mean over all centres in the trial of the true mean effect for each centre.
(III) The true individual effect for any patient in the trial.
(IV)   The true mean effect for all possible selections of patients into the trial *as designed*.
(V)   The true effect for any future patient or centre to which we might wish to apply the results.

This list is by no means exhaustive but shows that very different sorts of treatment effects may be entertained.

Suppose, however, that the treatment effect was not the same from centre to centre. Then not all of the above would be identical. For example, (I) and (II) would be the same if we had equal numbers of patients per treatment group per centre but not otherwise. (This, at least, is one apparent advantage of trials with equal numbers per centre!) In general, therefore (as we saw above), we may have a choice of effects to estimate.

Suppose that we remain very unambitious and adopt as an objective simply to show that the drug had an effect in *these* patients and also to describe what effect we think might have applied. We posit as a null hypothesis that the drug had no effect at all. That being the case it follows that the effect is identically zero in every centre. We adopt as an alternative hypothesis that the drug has an effect somewhere. Under the alternative hypothesis, the effect might well be different in different centres. However, because this is a multicentre trial it follows that the numbers per centre are scarcely adequate to produce a reasonable estimate individually for each centre. Although they are not in themselves valuable, we may nevertheless produce individual estimates per centre with a view to combining them in one overall estimator. Such an estimator, although technically subject to some bias when applied to individual centres or patients, may have a much lower variance and, therefore, nevertheless be more accurate (a justification of the type II attitude). Furthermore, to *test* the null hypothesis, any combination we choose (provided it is prespecified) of the estimates from the individual centres may be employed.

Since we have adopted as our objective the description and detection of treatment effects in *these* patients, there is no need for us to consider patients we *might* have studied and, it thus follows, centres from which we *might* have recruited. This does not mean, however, that chance does not affect our treatment estimate. Ideally, to measure the treatment effect in these patients, we should like to be able to study each twice under *identical* conditions: once under each treatment. In practice, a given patient will have been allocated to a particular treatment (using some form of randomization). This allocation introduces variability. Furthermore, if patients do not react identically to treatment and especially if these effects vary from centre to centre, then what we define as the treatment effect is a partly arbitrary choice. However, if we make this choice (a) taking account of the random variation introduced by allocation of treatment to *these* patients and (b) with a view to describing what happened in *these* patients, and in particular if in calculating standard errors and confidence intervals we regard (a) as being the source of variability, then we have what is known as a fixed-effects approach. As we discussed above, this can still leave us with a choice of estimates. However, my own opinion is that the type II approach is logical.

If instead we consider that we wish to make probabilistic statements about patients in general, including those from centres we did not include, we then have to move to regarding the centres themselves as some realization of a random process. The true difference in treatment effects from centre to centre now becomes a further source of random variation because, although, if we restrict inference to these centres only, this variability is frozen (the differences are what they are and that is an end of it), if we talk about future centres then these might also vary and there is no reason why these other differences should be exactly the same which now apply. If we take account of this further source of variation, not only in forming estimators but also in calculating confidence intervals, then we have a random-effects model.

The technical consequence of the random-effects model as regards its effect on estimates is generally to produce values between those produced by the type II and type III fixed-effects approach. This is because we now have two sources of random variation: random variation within centres and random variation of the treatment effect between centres. The former affects the precision with which we estimate the treatment effect at a given centre. The variability of this estimate is smaller the more patients there are in a given centre. The latter, however, is a measure of how well the true treatment effect from any centre represents that in general, and will not usually be affected by the number of patients in the centre. Therefore, if we weight treatment estimates according to their reliability, this leads only to a partial weighting by number of patients and hence produces an answer between type II and type III. The effect on the estimated variance of the resulting treatment effect and hence on standard errors, confidence limits, tests of hypotheses and *P*-values is more complex and is perhaps most easily explained by considering the case of equal numbers of patients in each treatment group in each centre. Here type II and type III fixed-effects and random-effects approaches produce the same estimate. Estimated variances for type II and type III will also be identical. For the random-effects model they would usually be much higher. This is as it should be, since in the first case we are saying something about what happened in the centres actually studied. In the second case we are attempting to say what might happen in other centres.

14.2.5   Should we use fixed-effect models or random-effect models?

In consider my whether we should we use fixed or random effects, the following points apply.

Pro fixed:

(1)   The approach gives a fairly precise answer to a fairly well defined question.
(2)   It is the only possible approach for a single-centre trial. Many trialists would be quite happy to run a trial in a single centre if only they could, and this implies that there must be an implicit acceptance on their part of the fixed-effect policy.
(3)   It is also the only realistic option when we have very few centres.
(4)   Random sampling of centres does not take place in clinical trials and it is rather hard to define precisely what question the random-effects model is answering.
(5)   The definition of a centre is largely arbitrary. What makes a centre: the patients (who will not be the same tomorrow as they are today)? the doctors and nurses (who may leave to take jobs elsewhere)? The random-effects model involves a degree of 'reification' of the centre, granting it a substantive significance it does

not really have. *Centre* is not a well-defined experimental unit to the same degree as *patient*.

Pro random:

(1) We develop treatments to say things about their effects on patients in general. We should not dodge this issue even if it is difficult to come up with precise answers.
(2) If we attempt to answer this difficult question, the random effects model will almost certainly produce a better approximation.
(3) In practice, confidence limits for random-effect models will be wider than for fixed-effect models and this is a more realistic representation of the true uncertainties if we are interested in prediction. This may accord with our intuition in the sense that in borderline cases where the result was otherwise significant, a large centre-by-treatment interaction might cause us to doubt that it was genuine.
(4) If we *are* interested in saying something about patients in a given centre (see Section 14.2.6 below), the fixed-effect approach leaves little alternative but to use the results from that centre only. The random-effects approach will allow us to combine information with the given centre with information from all centres in a way which may be more appealing and useful.

Unlike for the controversy over type II and type III sums of squares, I have no firm opinion as to which of fixed or random effects is the right approach and consider that both have their place. I would nearly always propose a fixed-effect analysis of a clinical trial. I might also consider that a random-effect analysis would be useful on occasion; especially if there were rather many centres which had been fairly widely selected. I am, however, rather sceptical of some of the enthusiasm which proponents of the random-effect model seem to generate on occasion. There are a number of worrying problems to be addressed when dealing with random-effect models. The definition of the centre, for example, is an important one. Most trials are randomized in subcentre blocks. If we were to apply a random-effect model at that level rather than the centre level, we should end up weighting the blocks approximately equally and, since centres differ according to the number of blocks, move back closer to the type II estimator. Furthermore, if we consider that the reason for a centre-by-treatment interaction is that larger centres tend to produce different results from smaller ones, then centre size becomes a stratum. If the distribution of centres in the trial reflects the distribution in general, then weighting centres more nearly equally will give a misleading position as to what happens on average. Again we should have to move closer to the type II estimator. In short, because centre is not a well-defined experimental unit (the label might sometimes be applied separately to two physicians in the same hospital and sometimes to hospitals in different countries), random-effect models involve a partially arbitrary choice. This does not make them inappropriate, but it means that one should be cautious in the claims made for them.

Further discussion of this issue will be found in papers by Fleiss (1986), Grizzle (1987), Senn (2000, 2004) and Fedorov and Jones (2005) and from a Bayesian perspective in that by Berry (1990).

14.2.6 Should we study effects from individual centres?

It is difficult to think of any objections to this, but if such study is undertaken, caution must be exercised. First, it should be appreciated that results from individual centres are almost never of interest in themselves. However, it may be that if centres can be found which produce a particular type of result then some common factor can be identified. This might be useful knowledge. Furthermore, looking for unusual centres may be part of an approach to detecting fraud (Ward, 1995). The second point is that the precision of centre-specific treatment estimates is very low. It is almost invariably the case that the reason a multicentre trial has been contemplated is that the power of a single-centre trial would be far too low. As a consequence, we may expect considerable chance variation between centres. Consider a placebo-controlled multicentre trial with 80% power in total at the 5% level (two-sided). Suppose that the true treatment effect is identically equal to the clinically relevant difference. It then follows that provided we have at least six centres, there is an odds-on chance that at least one of them will show an 'effect reversal' (the placebo will appear superior). Figure 14.2 provides a plot of the probability of at least one effect reversal as a function of the number of centres. (I first saw a demonstration of this phenomenon from Willi Maurer and Uwe Ferner and it was also subsequently investigated more thoroughly by Robert O'Neill. It was discussed in the first edition of this book and by Senn and Harrell (1997, 1998) and Senn (2001). It has bee treated more recently by Li *et al.* (2007).) Hence the trialist needs to be on guard not to over-interpret results from single centres.

A notorious example in which investigators were misled by looking at effects from individual centres is given by the re-analysis of the beta-blockers in heart attack (BHAT) study by Horwitz et al. (Horwitz *et al.*, 1996). They were struck by the fact that in this 31-centre placebo-controlled trial of propranalol, for which the overall effect of treatment on mortality was significant in 10 centres, the observed survival under placebo was superior to that under active treatment. However, a random-effects analysis by Senn and Harrell showed a surprising result: there was actually slightly less variation in the observed results from trial to trial than one would expect purely by chance (Senn and Harrell, 1997, 1998). The example serves as a warning to the dangers of over-interpretation.

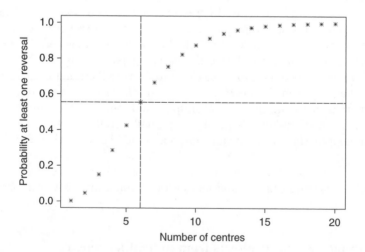

Figure 14.2 Probability of at least one effect reversal as a function of the number of centres given 80% overall power for a two-sided significance level of 5%.

14.2.7   What effect does treatment-by-centre interaction have on the power of multicentre trials?

This issue is not what it seems, since to the extent that treatment-by-centre interaction has an adverse effect on the power of clinical trials it probably has an even worse effect on single-centre trials than on multicentre ones. Consider an extreme case in which only half of all centres would be capable of showing any treatment effect whatsoever. It then follows that the probability of getting a significant result in any of *these* centres if run as a single centre trial is 5%: the type I error rate (assuming the most usual conventional rate is used). At the very best the probability of getting a significant result in one of the other sort of centre must be less than 100%. Hence the overall power of the single-centre trial must be less than $1/2 \times 5\% + 1/2 \times 100\%$ and hence less than 52.5% *however large the centre*. On the other hand, for a multicentre trial, by increasing the number of centres one could continue to increase the power.

   The point about multicentre trials is rather that they cause us to think about the problem of treatment-by-centre interaction. We are thus tempted to believe that such interaction is uniquely a problem for multicentre trials. In fact it is more of a problem for single-centre trials but because there is no way of investigating the phenomenon we assume that it doesn't exist. Figure 14.3 shows the power as a function of the number of centres for a trial designed to have 80% power for a two-sided test at the 5% level given that the treatment effect is believed to be 6 in every centre for a standard deviation of 10 but is, in fact, 8 with probability 1/2 and 4 with probability 1/2.

   The above discussion is of course posited on the assumption that the fact that one has more centres in a trial does not adversely affect the average quality of the centres. If it is possible to identify a centre which is better in terms of quality of work than all others, or if monitoring standards suffer as one includes more centres, then it is possible that a single-centre trial could be at an advantage.

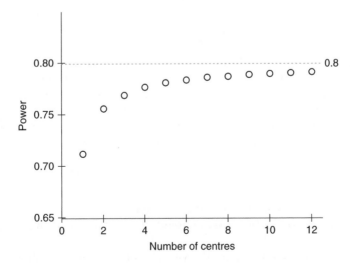

Figure 14.3   Power of a multi-centre trial as a function of the number of centres given treatment by centre interaction. (See text for explanation.)

14.2.8   Should one recover inter-centre information?

We return to an issue we raised briefly in section 14.2.4. If we treat the main effect of centres as fixed, then every time we fit a new centre we fit a new parameter. In producing an estimate of the treatment effect that is unbiased by the presence of such parameters, we have to eliminate them, yet we can only eliminate the parameter for a given centre by using results from that centre. Thus we can regard our estimating procedure as calculating, in a first step, a series of within-centre treatment estimates. For example, in a placebo-controlled trial of an active treatment we produce for each centre an estimate of the treatment effect as the difference between the mean result under the active treatment and that under placebo. Once these within-centre treatment estimates are produced they are averaged. For a type III approach a straightforward unweighted average is produced, whereas for a type II approach the estimates are weighted in inverse proportion to their variance.

Suppose that we have some (small) centres that, by chance, have only patients under placebo or only patients under active treatment. We cannot produce a within-centre estimate of the treatment effect for them. However, suppose that there are a great many such centres and that in fact on studying them we get the impression that those where (by chance) only placebo was given have rather different results than those where (by chance) only active treatment was given. Clearly such centres provide some evidence of the efficacy of treatment that our formal estimation procedure fails to recover.

The way in which we can recover such information is by declaring the main effect of centre to be random. This permits a direct comparison of results between centres in order to compare treatments. In fact, some further information in addition to the within-centre treatment estimates is contained in the average responses over both treatment arms from any unbalanced centres. This is because if the treatment arms are unbalanced, the average response must be influenced by the relative proportions of the two treatments. Thus centres with only one treatment are merely an extreme case of this more general phenomenon.

In practice, estimation proceeds not in this laborious way using within-centre differences and by-centre averages as two sources of information (although in practice it could) but in one (apparent) step using one of the popular approaches to estimation from mixed models. A good account of such approaches is given in the excellent text by Brown and Prescott (1999, 2006) in the same series as this book.

A similar issue arises in the analysis of what are known as incomplete block designs, and in that context fitting a random effect for the block (analogous here to centre) is sometimes referred to as *recovering inter-block information*.

However, we are not concerned here with the technicalities of this but with the pros and cons of treating the main effect of centre as random and the consequent effect on estimation.

14.2.9   We should exploit variation in treatment effects from centre to centre in order to improve predictions for target populations

In section 14.2.4 we drew attention to five different questions that could be asked of a multicentre trial and pointed out that given constancy of the treatment effect they could all be answered with the same analysis. The most ambitious of these is 'What is the effect of treatment likely to be for some future target population?' Fedorov and co-workers have drawn a careful distinction between the treatment effect in what they call the *test ground* (that is to say the trial that is being studied) and the *combined response to treatment* it is desired to estimate (Dragalin *et al.*, 2001; Fedorov and Jones, 2005). For example, if we knew that centres of particular types had been sampled from strata of centres of a particular sort within a population, then we could use the sampling weights to produce an unbiased estimate of the treatment response in that population. They even suggest that the design of the trial could be modified so as to choose the method of sampling of centres in a way that efficiently meets this objective. This is similar in spirit to Longford's suggestion that estimation in clinical trials should take account of the way patients were selected (Longford, 1999).

In my view this proposal, however theoretically desirable, is so far removed from practical reality as to be infeasible. The task of proving that a treatment works at all is so difficult and faces so many ethical, practical and financial constraints that most trialists struggle to design a trial that is adequate to proving that the treatment works in the patients studied. As was explained in Chapter 3, trialists seek not typical patients but suitable patients for their trials. In any case, there is a philosophical problem in that one cannot sample at random from the future. Thus, I maintain that most trialists will continue to be satisfied with the limited aim of proving that the treatment works at all. To the extent that they attempt to answer the more ambitious question of what the effect of treatment will be more generally, they are unlikely to want to move beyond the conventional random-effects estimator. Trying to define more complicated combined responses to treatment is unlikely to be attractive and in particular is unlikely to be reflected in trial design (Senn, 2004).

14.2.10 Bayesian analogues to fixed-effect and random-effect models

Finally, it is perhaps useful to draw attention to Bayesian analogues of frequentist fixed- and random-effect models, not least because more and more statisticians are using Bayesian methods to estimate treatment effects.

From the Bayesian point of view, all effects are random, since parameters have a probability distribution. However, it turns out that various assumptions in terms of prior distribution permit one to mimic the various frequentist approaches. Again we must be careful with terminology since, as mentioned in section 14.2.4, *random effect* can mean that the main effect of centre is random, or that the centre-by-treatment interaction is random, or both. The first of these cases is the one that permits recovery of inter-centre information as outlined in section 14.2.8. The Bayesian analogue is to treat the centre in a hierarchical sense with a single distribution whose mean and variance need estimating. As regards the main effect of centre, only two prior distributions are needed, one for the mean and one for the variance. On the other hand, treating the main effect of centre as fixed corresponds to having a separate 'uninformative' prior distribution for the true mean of each centre.

On the other hand, modelling the treatment-by-centre interaction as can be handled using a hierarchical framework for the treatment effect in each centre. It is assumed that nothing is known about the variability of these effects. Replacing the individual parameters by one common parameter corresponds to using a fixed-effects approach. Equivalently, if the random-effect variance is made vanishingly small (corresponding to a highly informative prior that the effects are the same from centre to centre), the same result can be achieved.

References

Berry DA (1990) Basic principles in designing and analysing clinical studies. In: Berry DA (ed.), *Statistical Methodology in the Pharmaceutical Industry*. Marcel Dekker, New York and Basle.

Brown H, Prescott R (1999) *Applied Mixed Models in Medicine*. John Wiley & Sons, Ltd, Chichester.

Brown H, Prescott R (2006) *Applied Mixed Models in Medicine* (2nd edition). John Wiley & Sons, Ltd, Chichester.

Chuang-Stein C, Tong DM (1996) The impact of parametrization on the interpretation of the main-effect terms in the presence of an interaction. *Drug Information Journal* **30**: 421–424.

Dragalin V, Fedorov V, Jones B, Rockhold F (2001) Estimation of the combined response to treatment in multicenter trials. *Journal of Biopharmaceutical Statistics* **11**: 275–295.

Fedorov V, Jones B (2005) The design of multicentre trials. *Statistical Methods in Medical Research* **14**: 205–248.

Fleiss JL (1986) Analysis of data from multiclinic trials. *Controlled Clinical Trials* **7**: 267–275.

Gallo P (2001) Center-weighting issues in multicenter clinical trials. *Journal of Biopharmaceutical Statistics* **10**: 145–163.

Grizzle JE (1987) Analysis of data from multiclinic trials. *Controlled Clinical Trials* **8**: 392–393.

Horwitz RI, Singer BH, Makuch RW, Viscoli CM (1996) Can treatment that is helpful on average be harmful to some patients? A study of the conflicting information needs of clinical inquiry and drug regulation [see comments]. *Journal of Clinical Epidemiology* **49**: 395–400. [Comment in *Journal of Clinical Epidemiology* **50**(7): 749–751 (1997)].

International Conference on Harmonisation (1999) Statistical principles for clinical trials (ICH E9). *Statistics in Medicine* **18**: 1905–1942.

Kallen A (1997) Treatment-by-center interaction: What is the issue? *Drug Information Journal* **31**: 927–936.

Li ZQ, Chuang-Stein C, Hoseyni C (2007) The probability of observing negative subgroup results when the treatment effect is positive and homogeneous across all subgroups. *Drug Information Journal* **41**: 47–56.

Longford NT (1999) Selection bias and treatment heterogeneity in clinical trials. *Statistics in Medicine* **18**: 1467–1474.

Nelder JA (1977) A reformulation of linear models. *Journal of the Royal Statistical Society A* **140**: 48–77.

Senn SJ (1995) A personal view of some controversies in allocating treatment to patients in clinical trials [see comments]. *Statistics in Medicine* **14**: 2661–2674. [Comment in *Statistics in Medicine* **15**(1): 113–116].

Senn SJ (2000) The many modes of meta. *Drug Information Journal* **34**: 535–549.

Senn SJ (2001) Individual therapy: new dawn or false dawn. *Drug Information Journal* **35**: 1479–1494.

Senn SJ (2004) Added values: controversies concerning randomization and additivity in clinical trials. *Statistics in Medicine* **23**: 3729–3753.

Senn SJ, Harrell F (1997) On wisdom after the event [comment] [see comments]. *Journal of Clinical Epidemiology* **50**: 749–751. [Comments in *Journal of Clinical Epidemiology* **50**(7): 753–735 (1997); **51**(4): 301–303 (1998)].

Senn SJ, Harrell FE, Jr. (1998) On subgroups and groping for significance [letter; comment]. *Journal of Clinical Epidemiology* **51**: 1367–1368.

Speed FM, Hocking RR, Hackney OP (1978) Methods of analysis of linear models with unbalanced data. *Journal of the American Statistical Association* **73**: 105–112.

Ward P (1995) Europe takes tentative steps to combat fraud. *Applied Clinical Trials* **4**: 36–40.

14.A TECHNICAL APPENDIX

14.A.1 Recruitment

It is assumed that each centre contributes patients according to a common stable Poisson process with intensity λ per year. It is required to recruit N patients in total in k centres. Thus inter-arrival times in a given centre are exponential with mean $1/\lambda$ and we require the time, t, to recruit patient number n_i in a given centre i. This is given by the gamma distribution with parameters $B = 1/\lambda$ and $C = n_i$. The probability density is

$$\frac{f(t; \lambda, n_i) = (\lambda t)^{n_i - 1} e^{-\lambda t}}{(n_i - 1)!/\lambda}. \tag{14.1}$$

The distribution function is given by

$$F(t; \lambda, n_i) = 1 - e^{-\lambda t} \sum_{j=0}^{n_i - 1} (\lambda t)^j / j!. \tag{14.2}$$

For strategy 1 there is no individual centre requirement. The time to recruit N patients in k centres is given by the gamma distribution with parameters $B = 1/(k\lambda)$ and $C = N$. The probability density function is

$$\frac{g(t, k\lambda, N) = (k\lambda t)^{N-1} e^{-\lambda k t}}{(N - 1)!/(k\lambda)} \tag{14.3}$$

and the distribution function is

$$G(t, k\lambda, N) = 1 - e^{-\lambda k t} \sum_{j=0}^{N-1} (\lambda k t)^j / j!. \tag{14.4}$$

For strategy 2 each centre must recruit the same number of patients and we have distribution function

$$H(t) = \{F(t, \lambda, N/k)\}^k \tag{14.5}$$

and probability density function

$$h(t) = \frac{\mathrm{d}}{\mathrm{d}t} H(t). \tag{14.6}$$

By setting (14.4) or (14.5) $= 0.5$ and solving for t we can obtain median recruitment times for the two strategies. For $k = 4$, $N = 96$, and $\lambda = 24$ we obtain $G^{-1}(0.5) = 0.99$ and $H^{-1}(0.5) = 1.20$.

14.A.2 Estimators

Assume that we have k centres. The true treatment effect for centre i is τ_i and its estimator is $\hat{\tau}_i$ with variance σ_i^2. An overall treatment effect will be estimated by $\sum_{i=1}^{k} w_i \hat{\tau}_i$

where w_i is the weight for centre i and $\sum_{i=1}^{k} w_i = 1$. The type III approach consists of setting $w_i = 1/k$ for all i so that

$$E(\hat{\tau}_{\mathrm{III}}) = \sum_{1=1}^{k} \tau_i/k = \bar{\tau} \text{ and } \mathrm{var}(\hat{\tau}_{\mathrm{III}}) = \sum_{i=1}^{k} \sigma_i^2/k^2.$$

The type II approaches uses weights

$$w_i = \frac{1/\sigma_i^2}{\sum\limits_{i=1}^{k} (1/\sigma_i^2)}.$$

If the variances within centres are identically equal to σ^2 (this is an assumption which is commonly made and then becomes a theoretical property of the model rather than an empirical fact) and we have n_i patients in total in centre i with $n_i/2$ on each treatment arm, then for the type II approach we have

$$w_i = \frac{1/(4\sigma^2/n_i)}{\sum\limits_{i=1}^{k} \{1/(4\sigma^2/n_i)\}} = \frac{n_i}{\sum\limits_{i}^{k} n_i} \tag{14.7}$$

Hence centres are weighted according to the number of patients. It then follows that under these circumstances expectations and variances of the type II estimator are given by

$$E(\hat{\tau}_{\mathrm{II}}) = \frac{\sum\limits_{i=1}^{k} n_i \tau_i}{\sum\limits_{i=1}^{k} n_i} \quad \text{and} \quad \mathrm{var}(\hat{\tau}_{\mathrm{II}}) = \frac{4\sigma^2}{\sum\limits_{i=1}^{k} n_i}.$$

It is the first of these properties which makes the estimator unacceptable to the type III adherent, but it becomes unobjectionable when one realizes that the individual τ_i are completely without interest.

The random effects estimator, $\hat{\tau}_R$, uses weights

$$w_i = \frac{1/(\gamma^2 + \sigma_i^2)}{\sum\limits_{i=1}^{k} \{1/(\gamma^2 + \sigma_i^2)\}} \tag{14.8}$$

where $\gamma^2 = \mathrm{var}(\tau)$ and the treatment effect is now regarded as random. If γ^2 is large compared to the values of σ_i^2, then (14.8)$\approx 1/k$. On the other hand, if γ^2 is small, then (14.8)$\approx$(14.7). Hence, in practice it will usually be the case that either $\hat{\tau}_{\mathrm{II}} \leq \hat{\tau}_R \leq \hat{\tau}_{\mathrm{III}}$ or $\hat{\tau}_{\mathrm{II}} \geq \hat{\tau}_R \geq \hat{\tau}_{\mathrm{III}}$. Note that if we have equal numbers per centre so that $n_i = n$ for all i, then (14.8)$=$(14.7)$=1/k$ so that all three estimators are identical. Even under these circumstances, however, the variance of the random effects estimator will exceed that of the other two.

14.A.3   Probabilities of effect reversals

The precision ψ (if we take this to be the ratio of clinically relevant difference to standard error) of a trial designed to have a power of $1 - \beta$ for a two-sided test of size of α will be

$$\psi = \Phi^{-1}(1 - \alpha/2) + \Phi^{-1}(1 - \beta),$$

where $\Phi(.)$ is the distribution function of the standard Normal and $\Phi^{-1}(.)$ is its inverse. If patients are equally divided between k centres, then the precision in a given centre will be $\psi / \sqrt{k}$. If we assume that the probability of an effect reversal overall is negligible and suppose that the overall treatment effect is positive, then the probability of not showing a reversal in a given centre is the probability that the estimated treatment effect is positive in that centre which is $1 - \Phi\left(-\psi / \sqrt{k}\right) = \Phi\left(\psi / \sqrt{k}\right)$. Hence, the probability that it is positive in all k centres is $\left[\Phi\left(\psi / \sqrt{k}\right)^{k}\right]$ from which the probability of at least one reversal is

$$1 - \left[\Phi\left(\psi / \sqrt{k}\right)^{k}\right]. \tag{14.9}$$

14.A.4   Power of single-centre and multicentre trials

Assume that centres are of equal sizes and of two sorts: those in which with probability p there is a treatment effect of size τ_1 and those for which with probability $1 - p$ there is a treatment effect of size τ_2. Assume that the variance of individual observations is σ^2, that there are k centres and that the total number of patients is N. Assume that there are equal numbers of patients per group per centre and that this integer number may be approximated by $N/(2k)$.

It is also assumed that the trial has been designed to have a target power $1 - \beta$ for a size α based on a treatment effect of $\Delta = p\tau_1 + (1 - p)\tau_2$, based on the mistaken assumption that the treatment effect is constant from centre to centre but that the analysis employed will eliminate patient-by-treatment interaction. From the power and size requirements we may find N as

$$N = \frac{4\sigma^2\{\Phi^{-1}(1 - \alpha/2) + \Phi^{-1}(1 - \beta)\}^2}{p\tau_1 + (1 - p)\tau_2}. \tag{14.10}$$

The number of centres of one type or another actually chosen is assumed binomial (k, p) and the conditional power given the number of each type chosen is easily calculated. The sum of the product of the marginal and conditional distributions gives the required power, $\pi(k, p)$ as a function of the proportion of centres over all of each type and the number of centres in the trial. Thus

$$\pi(k, p) = \sum_{i=0}^{k} \frac{k!}{i!(k - i)!} p^i (1 - p)^{k-1} \Phi\left[\frac{\{i\tau_1 + (k - i)\tau_2\}/k}{2\sigma\sqrt{N}} - \Phi^{-1}\left(1 - \frac{\alpha}{2}\right)\right]. \tag{14.11}$$

Active Control Equivalence Studies

I own, in one case, whenever a man's conscience does accuse him (as it seldom errs on that side), that he is guilty . . . but the converse of the proposition will not hold true.

Laurence Sterne, *Tristram Shandy*

How have you made division of yourself?
An apple cleft in two is not more twin
Than these two creatures.

William Shakespeare, *Twelfth Night*

15.1 BACKGROUND

A treatment which is no better on average than an existing treatment may nevertheless be useful. It may be that because of individual response to treatment, whether in terms of main effects or side-effects, a given patient may find one or other of apparently equivalent treatments preferable. Obviously, ideally, such differences at the individual level should be explored if at all possible. This is the thinking behind so called n-of-1 trials, and will be dealt with separately. Such investigations, however, are usually best undertaken at a later stage in drug development, once basic efficacy and tolerability of a treatment has been established. Where, however, an effective treatment already exists then, at least for serious diseases, as we discussed in Chapter 6, the withholding of such a treatment is unethical. Hence it is not always possible to run trials with a control group which is either given a placebo or no treatment at all. (It is sometimes possible to run such a trial if all patients are given the standard therapy and then either placebo or experimental as an 'add-on', but this is not practical or desirable in all cases.) Trials are sometimes run, therefore, in which the object is simply to show that the new treatment is at least as good as (no worse than) the existing treatment. Such trials have been called active control equivalence studies (ACES) (Makuch and Johnson, 1989).

Note that not all trials involving active comparators are ACES. For example, the long-acting beta-agonists salmeterol and formoterol were developed by comparing them in therapeutic trials in asthma to the shorter-acting beta-agonist salbutamol (US albuterol) and were able to demonstrate superiority to this control in terms of their bronchodilating effect 12 hours after treatment. To take an indication where such superiority would be unlikely to be proved, however, consider depression. Some authorities are of the opinion that placebos are unethical and most trialists would not be optimistic about being able to prove superiority to a standard therapy. Where both these conditions apply, ACES would seem to be the alternative. (One could, of course argue that where an effective therapy exists all trials are unethical, but in many cases efficacy is only partial and this may open the door for experimentation.) There may also be occasions where it may be desirable to prove that an experimental treatment is neither worse nor better than an existing treatment. For example, we may wish to prove that a generic treatment is equivalent to a branded drug. If it proved to be more efficacious, the suspicion might be raised that it would have worse tolerability and this would raise in turn the issue of carrying out a full development. Such equivalence is usually examined in so-called bioequivalence studies in which the plasma concentration–time profiles of two drugs are compared (see Chapter 22). However, sometimes therapeutic trials are also run as true equivalence trials. Because the technical statistical issues are generally greater when equivalence rather than lack of clinical inferiority is the object of the trial, we shall, except where explicitly stated otherwise, assume in the discussion which follows that equivalence is the object. In practice, trials in which the object is to prove that a new drug is not clinically inferior to a comparator are more usual. The exception is the field of bioequivalence, which is dealt with separately in Chapter 22. The reader should bear in mind, therefore, that equivalence is often used as a confusing synonym for noninferiority and that where noninferiority is the object, one only has to prove that the experimental treatment is not inferior to control and not vice versa. However, in the following paragraph we assume that the more difficult case of true equivalence is what is being considered.

In considering the issues which follow, it may be useful to have Figure 15.1 in mind. This shows a set of the sort of possible estimates and associated confidence intervals which might arise in an equivalence trial. The vertical dashed line is the line of exact equality (treatment difference is zero). The two solid vertical lines are the lines of practical equivalence. If the true treatment difference lies between these lines, the treatments

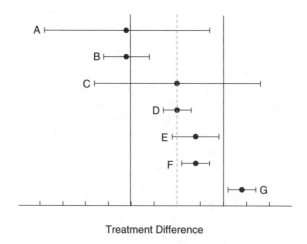

Treatment Difference

Figure 15.1 Possible point estimates and confidence intervals arising from an equivalence trial.

are considered equivalent. In the case of trial A, the treatment estimate lies outside the region of equivalence. However, the confidence intervals are so wide that exact equality of the treatments is not ruled out. In case B exact equality is ruled out (if the conventions of hypothesis testing are accepted), since there is a significant difference, but the possibility that the true treatment difference lies within the region of equivalence is not. In case C, no treatment difference is observed, but the confidence intervals are so wide that values outside the regions of equivalence are still plausible. In cases D, E and F, practical equivalence is 'demonstrated'. However, in case E it corresponds to no observed difference at all, whereas in case F the treatments are significantly different (confidence interval does not straddle zero) even though practical equivalence appears to have been demonstrated (confidence interval lies within region of equivalence). In case G there is a significant difference and equivalence may be rejected.

In the rest of this chapter, it will be assumed that some general approach via classical confidence intervals, one-side for the case of noninferiority and two-sided for genuine equivalence) will be used. In fact, for true equivalence there are various technical controversies surrounding the use of two-sided confidence intervals (Mehring, 1993; Senn, 2001b). These will be taken up in Chapter 22.

Since the first edition of this book there has been much further discussion in the statistical and medical literature of active control equivalence trials. Particularly important in the context of drug development is the International Conference on Harmonisation 'Harmonised tripartite guideline: choice of control group and related issues in clinical trials' (International Conference on Harmonisation, 2000). Also important for revealing regulatory thinking are papers by Röhmel and by Temple and Ellenberg (Röhmel, 1998; Temple and Ellenberg, 2000). Andy Garrett's paper in *Statistics in Medicine* is a very nice investigation of both practical and inferential issues (Garrett, 2003). A standard reference is the book by Wellek (2002).

15.2 ISSUES

15.2.1 'Absence of evidence is not evidence of absence'

This general principle, memorably expressed by Altman and Bland (1995) in the form quoted, is extremely important. At the time of writing the first edition of this book (which was published in 1997), a major public health concern in Britain was that bovine spongiform encephalopathy (BSE) might be transmissible to humans through eating beef and manifest itself as Creutzfeldt–Jakob Disease (CJD). At the time there was little in the way of hard evidence that this could happen. This did not prove, that it couldn't happen and hasn't happened and, indeed, general scientific opinion since, then seems to have switched to thinking that it could and has (Cooper and Bird, 2003). This in turn does not necessarily imply that it is rational to demand evidence that such transmission is *not* possible before agreeing to eat beef. For example, the risk might exist but be extremely small and some risk attends eating all food. Should one refuse to eat rye bread because of the risk of St Anthony's fire (ergotism), which causes madness and gangrene? To take an example of what John Adams has called virtual risk (Adams, 1995), I might claim that cereals are a major cause of cancer, on the grounds that (a) cancer is a disease of civilization, (b) the growing of cereals is associated with the growth of civilizations and (c) the link between cereals and maladies like St Anthony's fire (mentioned above) and coeliac disease is well established, so that the ability of cereals to produce toxins in the body is accepted. The proof that cereals are not a cause of cancer would be difficult to find and, indeed, they may be carcinogenic for all I know. Simply because I have made the claim, are we all required by the so-called precautionary principle to stop eating cereals? Nevertheless, to return to the more general issue of evidence and equivalence, the business of drug development is that of finding evidence about the properties of drugs. Therefore, if equivalence is the aim, evidence of equivalence must be found.

It is not adequate, however, to claim, merely by virtue of having looked for a difference and failed to find it, that two drugs are equivalent (Senn, 1991; Temple, 1982). One may not have looked hard enough. In particular, failure to find a difference in a conventional test of significance is no guarantee that the drugs are equivalent. For example, cases A and C in Figure 15.1 correspond to failing to prove via conventional tests of significance that there is a difference, but the evidence for equality is very weak. Basically, from the technical point of view, what may be done is to replace the conventional hypothesis-testing framework, whereby we test the null hypothesis that the true treatment difference τ is zero, $H_0: \tau = 0$ against the alternative hypothesis that it is not, $H_1: \tau \neq 0$, by one in which we try to reject two null hypotheses (Schuirmann, 1987): the null hypothesis of inferiority and the null hypothesis of superiority. The situation is represented in Figure 15.2. (And where we are interested simply in proving lack of inferiority we only need to reject that hypothesis alone.) If δ represents the degree of difference we wish to rule out, then we test $H_{0A}: \tau \leq -\delta$ against $H_{1A}: \tau > -\delta$ and $H_{0B}: \tau \geq \delta$ against $H_{1B}: \tau < \delta$. Rejection of both null hypotheses leads to the conclusion that the treatment difference is neither less than or equal to $-\delta$ nor greater than or equal to $+\delta$ and, therefore, in absolute terms must be less than δ. If each of the tests is carried out at level α, then under any given value of either of the two null hypotheses the probability of committing a type I error must be less than α. It thus follows that such a procedure, which corresponds to establishing that the $1 - 2\alpha$ confidence limits lie within the region of equivalence $-\delta, \delta$, is conservatively adequate. (Because of

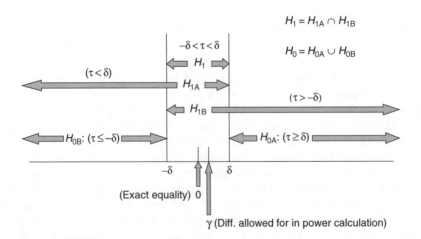

Figure 15.2 Illustration of hypotheses for proving equivalence.

this conservatism various theoretical 'improvements' are possible, but for adequately powered trials they make no practical difference (Senn, 2001b). This issue is further discussed in Chapter 22.)

15.2.2   The competence of equivalence trials

There is a paradox of competence associated with equivalence trials and that is that the more we tend to provide proof within a trial of the equivalence of the two treatments, the more we ought to suspect that we have not been looking at the issue in the correct way: that the trial is incapable of finding a difference where it exists. In other words, there is more to a proof of equivalence than the matter of reversing the usual roles of null and alternative hypotheses. Even if in a given trial the test results indicated that the effects of the treatments being compared were very similar (as, say, in case D) the possibility could not be ruled out that a trial with different patients, or alternative measurements or some different approach altogether would have succeeded in finding a difference. No probabilistic calculation on the data in hand has anything to say about this possibility: it is essentially a matter of data not collected. There is a difference in kind between 'proving' that drugs are similar and proving that they are not similar. This difference is analogous to the difference which exists in principle between a proof of marital infidelity and fidelity. The first may be provided simply enough (in principle) by evidence; the second, if at all, only by a repeated failure to find the evidence which the first demands.

In fact it is possible to show in a Bayesian formulation that if some prior doubt is allowed that the trial may not be competent to find a difference, then although, conditional upon a belief in competence, the posterior probability of equivalence will rise the more patients are studied and the more that prognosis is found to be the same in the two groups, the more the posterior belief must increase that the trial is not competent to find a difference (Senn, 1993). In short, the whole field is summed up by the oxymoron 'equivalence is different'.

Equivalence: Proving that apples are pears by comparing the weight.

15.2.3   Gold-standard trials

In an attempt to deal with the issue of competence, an alternative design (sometimes referred to as the 'gold standard') is sometimes employed. This is a three-arm trial in which, in addition to reference and experimental treatments, a placebo is included. An example is given by Lange *et al.* (1998). This trial should then be in the position of delivering a proof of competence by demonstrating the superiority of experimental and reference treatments to placebo and thus showing that the trial is capable of detecting differences between treatments.

The use of such trials is not unproblematic, however. First, it may be claimed that a trial which is competent to show a difference from placebo is not necessarily competent to detect a difference between active treatments. Thus the initial problem is not completely eliminated by such a design. Second, if the reason for employing an equivalence trial is that the use of a placebo is unethical, then the design is clearly impossible. Third, there is a considerable cost in efficiency since only one-third of all patients receive the experimental treatment.

15.2.4   A proof of exact equality is impossible

Even if we accept the limitations to which equivalence trials are subject, if our purpose is to prove that two treatments are exactly equal it does not matter how weak our standards of 'proof' are, we shall not be able to do so. Consider case D in Figure 15.1. The confidence limits for the true treatment difference lie well within the limits of equivalence but it is clear that we could establish much narrower limits of equivalence which the confidence limits would exceed. One way to deal with narrower limits of equivalence would be to demand lower standards of proof. For example, instead of using 90% confidence intervals we could use less stringent 50% limits in an attempt to match narrower limits of equivalence. Alternatively, we could increase the sample size. However, whatever we do we shall never succeed in shrinking the confidence intervals to a point. Hence a 'proof' of exact equality is impossible.

15.2.5   A clinically relevant difference is not a clinically irrelevant difference

In conventional clinical trials the clinically relevant difference is used for the purpose of sample size determination only. It is sometimes described as the difference we should not like to miss and it must, of course, be understood that where a significant difference is found this does not deliver with it a proof that the clinically relevant difference obtains. (See Chapter 13 for a discussion.) The clinically relevant difference used for planning the trial is not necessary for interpreting its outcome. For that purpose we may use point estimates of the treatment effect and associated confidence limits. The reader is then free to compare these to whatever he or she considers to be the clinically relevant difference and is not bound by our initial choice. Furthermore, this difference plays no part in the interpretation of significance: it is not used in the test of significance. If the reader of a clinical trial report disagrees with the trialist regarding the significance or otherwise of a given test then this is, presumably, a matter of disagreement over the appropriate level of significance. It will have nothing to do with the choice of clinically relevant difference. (Of course, more general hypothesis tests are possible where our ambitions go beyond the simple one of demonstrating that some sort of difference exists, to demonstrating that the difference is useful. This requires a shifted null hypothesis and then some sort of difference must be adopted for the purpose of conducting the test. My own feeling, however, is that this issue is best handled using confidence intervals.)

In a trial of equivalence, however, we must take the issue more seriously. The *null* hypotheses considered under Section 15.2.1 make explicit reference to a difference, δ. Of course, we can still calculate the confidence intervals and leave it up to the reader to determine whether they fall within whatever limits of equivalence are considered appropriate (see section 15.2.9 below), but one would hardly embark on such a trial without having at least some idea as to what constitutes a success. In general, one should not assume that the clinically relevant difference used for planning conventional trials is the same as the equivalent difference. In developing a new treatment for asthma we might be prepared to contemplate losing one which, say, had less than 15% bronchodilation in terms of FEV_1 compared with placebo. However, a much smaller value would still constitute an important difference between treatments. In general, therefore, we must expect that clinically irrelevant differences will be much smaller than clinically relevant differences.

In an extensive survey of the literature, Lange and Freitag identified 332 noninferiority trials (Lange and Freitag, 2005). These, of course, involved a great variety of different indications and outcome measures. In order to provide some sort of a comparison across indications, Lange and Freitag referred the noninferiority margins (whether explicitly or implicitly defined) to the within-treatment between-patient standard deviations. (See Chapter 8 for a discussion of the difficulties with such sigma-divided measures and also Senn (2005) for a general discussion.) They found that in about half the trials a difference of about half a standard deviation or less was taken to be an irrelevant difference. In only about one trial in ten were explicit references to differences from placebo made. (One does sometimes come across the suggestion that the irrelevant difference should be no more than one-third of the usual difference between the active control and placebo. See section 15.2.10.)

As a practical example of the difficulties, consider a useful tutorial paper by Jones *et al.* (1996), which describes a number of statistical issues in proving equivalence. The context is that of asthma and they consider a difference of 15 l/min in peak expiratory flow as providing a limit of equivalence. On this basis, for a particular example comparing two inhalers, they assume that a point estimate of 3, with a 95% confidence interval of −4.8 to 10.8, shows equivalence. The problem is, that given what we know about bronchodilators, it is quite plausible that a doubling of the dose delivered by a given inhaler would not produce a difference of 15 l/min. From that point of view, therefore, the limit is impossibly wide and it raises the issue that within a given trial comparing formulations some sort of parallel assay should be carried out (Kallen and Larsson, 1999; Senn *et al.*, 1997) and indeed that the trial should perhaps demonstrate the ability to distinguish between doses if two different formulations are to be declared equipotent. This is thus a question of competence as discussed in Section 15.2.2. This issue is taken up further in Chapter 22, in the context of bioequivalence. It is raised here simply to illustrate how extremely difficult judgements of equivalence can be.

15.2.6   Sample size determination

Even if the clinically irrelevant difference is the same as the clinically relevant difference and not, as will usually be the case, considerably smaller, it is generally the case that equivalence trials require a larger sample size for the same power as a conventional trial. The general position is illustrated by Figure 15.2. For purposes of sample size determination it will generally be unwise to assume that the treatments are exactly equal. This would be the best possible case and this already shows an important difference from conventional trials. We plan such trials to have adequate power to detect the difference we should not like to miss, but we may of course be fortunate and be faced with an even better drug. In that case the power is better than hoped for. If we are truly interested in showing equality (and not merely that an experimental treatment is not worse than a standard by some amount) then exact equality is the best possible position. In practice, we may suppose that a true difference γ (where $-\delta < \gamma < \delta$) may obtain and plan our trial accordingly.

As an example to help understand the effect of equivalence on sample size, consider a case where we wish to show that the difference in FEV_1 between two treatments is not greater than 200 ml and where the standard deviation is 350 ml for conventional type I and type II errors rates of 0.05 and 0.2. If we assume that the drugs are in fact exactly identical, the sample size needed (using a Normal approximation) is 53. If we allow for a true difference of 50 ml this rises to 69. On the other hand, if we wished to demonstrate superiority of one treatment over another for a clinically relevant difference of 200 ml with the other values as before, a sample size of 48 would suffice. Thus, in the best possible case a rise of about 10% in the sample size is needed (from 48 to 53). This difference arises because we have two one-sided tests each of which must be significant in order to prove efficacy. To have 80% power each must (in the case of exact equality) have approximately 90% power(because $0.9 \times 0.9 \cong 0.8$). The relevant sum of z-values for the power calculation is thus $1.2816 + 1.6449 = 2.93$ as opposed to for a conventional trial $0.8416 + 1.9600 = 2.8$. The ratio of the square of 2.93 to 2.8 is about 1.1 explaining the 10% increase in sample size.

15.2.7   Equivalence studies provide no incentive to excellence

The argument here is that the less you pay attention to details of conduct and control in a clinical trial, the less likely you are to find a difference. Hence, if your object is not to find a difference, there is no good reason to be unduly concerned about these matters. This is a potentially worrying feature of such trials.

I am not completely convinced, however, that the argument is entirely valid. It is true that a sloppily conducted trial will give little chance for treatments to distinguish themselves. But by the same token, the within-group variability is likely to be large and this will have a corresponding effect on the confidence intervals, which will themselves be broad. Hence equivalence is less likely to be 'demonstrated'. Thus, even in ACES, there are some good reasons for doing good work.

> **Equivalence trials**: A means of flooding the market with identical drugs in order to give patients more choice.

15.2.8   Blinding in ACES

The theory we wish to assert in ACES is that two treatments are similar. This corresponds to demonstrating that all the data may be regarded as coming from one distribution and that the labels 'experimental' and 'control' are essentially irrelevant for determining the prognosis of the patients. If this holds, then the treatments are truly equivalent.

The value of blinding in clinical trials, is essentially this: despite making sure that there are no superficial and nonpharmacological differences which enable us to distinguish one treatment from another (the trial is double-blind), the labels 'experimental' and 'control' do have an importance for prognosis. Thus, for a conventional trial where such a difference between groups is observed, because the trial has been run double-blind, we are able to assert that the difference between the groups cannot be due to prejudice and must therefore be due either to pharmacology or to chance. The whole purpose of ACES, however, is to be able to assert that there is no difference between treatment and clearly, therefore, blinding does not protect us against the prejudice that all patients ought to have similar outcomes. The point can be illustrated quite simply by considering the task of a statistician who has been ordered to fake equivalence by simulating suitable data. It is clear that he does not even need to know what the treatment codes are. All he needs to do is simulate data from a single Normal distribution with a suitable standard deviation (Senn, 1994). Whatever the allocation of patients, he is almost bound to demonstrate equivalence. If he is required to prove that one treatment is superior to another, however, such a strategy will not work. He needs to know the treatment codes.

This is not to say that ACES should not be run double-blind. We may, in such a trial, discover a difference and then would like to be reassured that this is not due to prejudice. It is rather that if an ACES achieves its primary purpose, blinding will have achieved little in the way of protecting the result from prejudice.

15.2.9 It is essential that the noninferiority margin be prespecified

This is a general opinion in a regulatory context. In fact at least two 'points to consider' documents issued by the European Medicines Agency stress the importance of a prespecified margin (Committee for Medicinal Products for Human Use, 2005; Committee for Proprietary Medicinal Products, 2000). However, this raises a troubling issue. Suppose it were the case that two sponsors were desiring to show noninferiority of a new bronchodilator when used in asthma, with FEV_1 as the target measure. The first specifies a limit of -10% and the second a limit of -5%. Trials are run and for the first sponsor the lower confidence limit is at -9% and for the second at -6%. If the prespecified limit is what counts, then the first sponsor can claim noninferiority but the second cannot. However, clearly this is absurd. If anything the claim is stronger for the second sponsor.

What this suggests is that it is not prespecification of the interval of equivalence that is important but rather the interval that may be believed to obtain once the data have been analysed. A cynical interpretation of current accepted practice is that the regulators are merely abandoning their obligation to decide what is and what is not equivalent and attempting to hide behind prespecification. To be fair, these guidelines do require that the margin should also be medically justified in some way, but it is not clear why this can be left to the sponsor.

15.2.10 Switching between superiority and noninferiority (and vice versa)

There is no reason why, from the point of view of controlling the type one error rate, one cannot test for noninferiority and superiority in the same trial without having to adjust the individual significance levels. This is because the null hypotheses in question form a nested set. For example, the null hypothesis that the new drug is inferior in terms of effect on mean diastolic blood pressure by at least 2 mmHg logically implies that it is inferior by at least 1 mmHg and that it cannot be better by 3 mmHg and so on (Bauer and Kieser, 1996).

It also makes no difference whether one has the strategy of attempting to prove superiority first and if that fails proving noninferiority or of proving noninferiority first and if successful trying to demonstrate superiority, although the regulator much prefers the latter strategy (Committee for Proprietary Medicinal Products, 2000). In fact, logically, all that is necessary is to calculate the classical confidence interval and see what margin is excluded. In practice the regulator is unlikely to accept this and the 'safe' strategy is for a sponsor to write a noninferiority margin into the protocol first, to proceed to attempt to reject the null hypothesis of inferiority and then to move on to attempting to prove superiority.

15.2.11   Indirect comparison with placebo

One way of interpreting equivalence studies is by trying to construct the indirect comparison with placebo. Consider the set of trials consisting of the current trial comparing an active treatment with a standard registered comparator and the trials that compared the standard treatment with placebo. The data from these trials have the structure of an incomplete blocks design, with trial as the block. The comparison of the experimental treatment with placebo is 'connected' indirectly to placebo via the standard treatment and it is a fairly trivial matter to construct estimates, standard errors of estimates and confidence intervals for the difference of the experimental treatment from placebo. In the general context of experimental design, this is a very old idea, going back at least as far as Yates (1936); however, a couple of papers that appeared in 2001, and which have been cited 30 times each at the time of writing, have specifically considered its application for equivalence studies (Fisher *et al.*, 2001; Hasselblad and Kong, 2001; see also Hirotsu and Yamada (1999)).

The technique is based on the fact that the double contrast of standard minus placebo subtracted from that of experimental minus standard eliminates the effect of the standard. One is thus left with an indirectly established contrast of experimental versus placebo. Assuming a so-called fixed-effects model, its variance is equal to the sum of the variances of the two contrasts used in its construction and it therefore follows that, however large the current trial, its variance cannot be lower that that pertaining to the (historical) comparison of the standard treatment with placebo.

This is one of the practical problems of the method, but it has the very great advantage that the issue of how well the standard treatment performs is addressed formally rather than simply being assumed by default. A further difficulty is that if it were allowed that the effect of the standard treatment varied from trial to trial then some sort of random-effects model would be needed. There has been some confusion over how such a random-effects model needs to be applied. The issue is not estimation of the overall mean effect of the standard treatment compared with placebo. Uncertainty regarding this would go to zero as the number of previous trials comparing the standard treatment with placebo went to infinity. The issue concerns the (unmeasured) effect of the standard treatment compared with placebo in the current trial, that is to say the trial comparing the experimental with the standard treatment. Uncertainty regarding this reflects the way the effect of standard compared with placebo varies from trial to trial and this will not go to zero as the number of trials run increases (Senn, 2005).

15.2.12   Scales of equivalence (in particular where binary and survival outcomes are involved)

Equivalence trials raise an issue that is particularly acute for binary outcomes, and also survival outcomes: that the best scale for statistical modelling may not be the most appropriate one for practical clinical decision making. For example, decision analysis requires inputs on the probability scale since it works by comparing expected, that is to say probability weighted and summed, outcomes. However, logistic regression will yield a treatment estimate on the log-odds scale rather than on the risk-difference scale. This issue was discussed in some detail in Chapter 8, where it was explained that it is logically necessary to separate the two stages of building a model and predicting the consequences. A parameter estimate does not necessarily automatically provide a useful prediction (Lane and Nelder, 1982; Senn, 2004).

It may then become necessary to use some additional information to see what the implications are of applying the treatment in practice in a target population. For example, given a log-odds ratio and a level of background risk one could then calculate the implied risk difference (in giving one treatment rather than another) and see what the implications were for an individual patient. A nice illustration of this is given by Glasziou and Irwig (1995).

However, in a regulatory context, which usually leads to a yes or no decision regarding the acceptability of a product, regulators and sponsors are still stuck with the (unrealistic in my view) idea that a single trial will deliver the answer as to whether equivalence is accepted or rejected without further context or calculation. Thus, sponsors who ignore this reality may be in for a unwelcome surprise at the end of a trial. Suppose, for example, that in a trial of antibiotics noninferiority is defined as a margin of no more than 5% in cure rate. It is expected that the cure rate on the standard comparator will be 80%. If the experimental treatment has a response of 75% (that is to say 5% less) then the odds ratio will be $(0.75/0.25) \times (0.2/0.8) = 0.75$. One interpretation of this requirement might be to show that the lower 95% confidence limit for the odds ratio at the end of the trial is greater than 0.75.

A huge trial with 1500 patients per arm is run with the results given in Table 15.1. If the trial is analysed using StatXact (R), then an exact lower limit for the confidence interval for the odds ratio is 0.7502. However, the problem is that, although this odds ratio corresponds to a risk difference of 0.05 for a control group rate of 0.8, that is not the control group rate in this trial. The control group rate is only 0.51, for this value an odds ratio of 0.7502 corresponds to a risk difference of 0.071 and it is not

Table 15.1   Possible 2×2 table giving patients by treatment and outcome for a trial in antibiotics.

	Treatment		
	Standard	**Experimental**	**Total**
Cure	1 050	1 008	2 058
Failure	490	492	942
Total	1 500	1 500	3 000

Table 15.2 Possible 2 × 2 table giving patients by treatment and outcome for another trial in antibiotics.

| | Treatment | | Total |
	Standard	Experimental	
Cure	1 350	1 335	2 685
Failure	350	165	315
Total	1 500	1 500	3 000

obvious that the regulator will accept the combination of the actual odds-ratio limit of 0.7502 and the theoretical control group rate of 0.8 as being relevant for a decision on equivalence.

Of course, the sponsor faces a game of heads you win, tails I lose. It is conceivable that the results could be the other way around. Consider Table 15.2. Now StatXact (R) produces a lower confidence interval of 0.7064 and nowhere near the value of 0.75 requested. However, the control group rate is 0.9 and, for this rate, the odds ratio of 0.7064 produces a risk difference of 0.027. Similar situations arise with survival analysis where one may be interested regarding decision making in the difference in median or mean survival but the analysis delivers a hazard ratio.

It would be quite wrong in my opinion to conclude that that what therefore needs to be done is to abandon the usual additive scales of analysis, such as log-odds ratios and log-hazard ratios, in favour of risk differences and differences in median survival. There is every reason to suppose that these will not transfer well from one trial to another and hence, of course, from clinical trial to clinical practice.

So what may be done? One solution for the binary case is to calculate what odds ratio can guarantee a risk difference of no more than some specified value irrespective of the control group rate (Garrett, 2003; Senn, 2000). For example, an odds ratio of 0.82 corresponds to a risk difference of at most 0.05, this value being achieved when the control group rate is 0.525. The trouble with this is that it is excessively conservative and could require cripplingly expensive trials to achieve. Another solution is to agree some complex but realistic modelling strategy with the regulator, whereby uncertainties about control group rates in target populations as well as results from the trial are integrated together to see whether agreed objectives are met. It seems that the regulatory environment is not ready for this yet, although regulators in the field of medical device regulation have shown themselves more flexible. Two companion texts in this series give useful examples of Bayesian decision making and of integrating information from different sources (Parmigiani, 2002; Spiegelhalter *et al.*, 2003).

15.2.13   Is the ethical case for active control equivalence trials sound?

In recent years a number of vigorous criticisms have been made of placebo-controlled trials stressing the ethical problems in giving placebo where effective remedies exist (Rothman, 1996; Rothman and Michels, 2000). Anderson has gone so far as to criticize the usual assumption that placebo-controlled trials are more convincing than active controlled equivalence studies, arguing (correctly in my view) that even placebo-controlled trials require external assumptions for their interpretation and therefore concluding (incorrectly in my view) that they are just as problematic as active controlled studies (Anderson, 2006).

In fact, these and other authors, including those who wrote the Declaration of Helsinki (World Medical Association 52nd Assembly, 2000) have, in my opinion, picked up the problem at the wrong end. As regards potential benefit (that is to say, efficacy) it is not what treatments are *given* to patients that needs to be considered, it is rather what treatments are *withheld* (Senn, 2001a, 2002). (Treatments *given* are relevant when issues of harm, that is to say side-effects, are considered.) Looked at in this light, the problem in trials with diseases in which (partially) effective remedies exist is not that of giving placebos but that of withholding standard therapies, and this problem exists for the experimental treatment for any trial in which it is not given in addition to the control treatment.

From this point of view, the ethical solution is to use so-called **add-on trials**–that is, to randomize patients to receive either the new treatment or placebo in addition to standard therapy. In fact, if one studies the field of therapy for HIV infection, which is characterized by the seriousness of the disease and the rapidity of therapeutic progress, then this is exactly what has been done. The trials that have been run have been add-on trials and these are commonly described as placebo-controlled trials. Researchers and clinicians have come to the conclusion that active controlled trials would have been unethical.

References

Adams J (1995) *Risk*. UCL Press, London.

Altman DG, Bland JM (1995) Absence of evidence is not evidence of absence. *British Medical Journal* **311**: 485.

Anderson JA (2006) The ethics and science of placebo-controlled trials: assay sensitivity and the Duhem–Quine thesis. *Journal of Medicine and Philosophy* **31**: 65–81.

Bauer P, Kieser M (1996) A unifying approach for confidence intervals and testing of equivalence and difference. *Biometrika* **83**: 934–937.

Committee for Medicinal Products for Human Use (2005) *Guideline on the choice of the non-inferiority margin*. London, European Medicine Agency.

Committee for Proprietary Medicinal Products (2000) Points to consider on switching between superiority and non-inferiority. Available at: http://www.eudra.org/humandocs/PDFs/EWP/048299en.pdf.

Cooper JD, Bird SM (2003) Predicting incidence of variant Creutzfeldt–Jakob disease from UK dietary exposure to bovine spongiform encephalopathy for the 1940 to 1969 and post-1969 birth cohorts. *International Journal of Epidemiology* **32**: 784–791.

Fisher LD, Gent M, Buller HR (2001) Active-control trials: how would a new agent compare with placebo? A method illustrated clopidogrel, aspirin, and placebo. *American Heart Journal* **141**: 26–32.

Garrett AD (2003) Therapeutic equivalence: fallacies and falsification. *Statistics in Medicine* **22**: 741–762.

Glasziou PP, Irwig LM (1995) An evidence based approach to individualising treatment. *British Medical Journal* **311**: 1356–1359..

Hasselblad V, Kong DF (2001) Statistical methods for comparison to placebo in active-control studies. *Drug Information Journal* **35**: 435–449.

Hirotsu C, Yamada L (1999) Estimating odds ratios through the connected comparative experiments. *Communications in Statistics–Theory and Methods* **28**: 905–929.

International Conference on Harmonisation (2000) *ICH harmonised tripartite guideline: choice of control group and related issues in clinical trials.* Geneva: International Conference on Harmonisation.

Jones E, Jarvis P, Lewis JA, Ebbutt AF (1996) Trials to assess equivalence: the importance of rigorous methods. *British Medical Journal* **313**: 36–39.

Kallen A, Larsson P (1999) Dose response studies: how do we make them conclusive? *Statistics in Medicine* **18**: 629–641.

Lane PW, Nelder JA (1982) Analysis of covariance and standardization as instances of prediction. *Biometrics* **38**: 613–621.

Lange S, Freitag G (2005) Choice of delta: requirements and reality–results of a systematic review. *Biometrical Journal* **47**: 12–27; discussion 99–107.

Lange S, Freitag G, Trampisch HJ (1998) Practical experience with the design and analysis of a three-armed equivalence study. *European Journal of Clinical Pharmacology* **54**: 535–540.

Makuch R, Johnson M (1989) Issues in planning and interpreting active control equivalence studies. *Journal of Clinical Epidemiology* **42**: 503–511.

Mehring G (1993) On optimal tests for general interval hypotheses. *Communications in Statistics: Theory and Methods* **22**: 1257–1297.

Parmigiani G (2002) *Modeling in Medical Decision Making: A Bayesian Approach.* John Wiley & Sons, Ltd, Chichester.

Röhmel J (1998) Therapeutic equivalence investigations: statistical considerations. *Statistics in Medicine* **17**: 1703–1714.

Rothman KJ (1996) Placebo mania. *British Medical Journal* **313**: 3–4.

Rothman KJ, Michels KB (2000) Declaration of Helsinki should be strengthened. *British Medical Journal* **321**: 442–445.

Schuirmann DJ (1987) A comparison of the two one-sided tests procedure and the power approach for assessing the equivalence of average bioavailability. *Journal of Pharmacokinetics and Biopharmaceutics* **15**: 657–680.

Senn SJ (1991) Falsificationism and clinical trials [see comments]. *Statistics in Medicine* **10**: 1679–1692. [Comment in *Statistics in Medicine* **11**(9): 1263–1265 (1992)].

Senn SJ (1993) Inherent difficulties with active control equivalence studies. *Statistics in Medicine* **12**: 2367–2375.

Senn SJ (1994) Fisher's game with the devil. *Statistics in Medicine* **13**: 217–230.

Senn SJ (2000) Consensus and controversy in pharmaceutical statistics (with discussion). *The Statistician* **49**: 135–176.

Senn SJ (2001a) The misunderstood placebo. *Applied Clinical Trials* **10**: 40–46.

Senn SJ (2001b) Statistical issues in bioequivalence. *Statistics in Medicine* **20**: 2785–2799.

Senn SJ (2002) Ethical considerations concerning treatment allocation in drug development trials. *Statistical Methods in Medical Research* **11**: 403–411.

Senn SJ (2004) Added values: controversies concerning randomization and additivity in clinical trials. *Statistics in Medicine* **23**: 3729–3753.

Senn SJ (2005) 'Equivalence is different'–Some comments on therapeutic equivalence. *Biometrical Journal* **47**: 104–107.

Senn SJ, Lillienthal J, Patalano F, Till MD (1997) An incomplete blocks cross-over in asthma: a case study in collaboration. In: Vollmar J, Hothorn LA (eds), *Cross-over Clinical Trials.* Fischer, Stuttgart, pp. 3–26.

Spiegelhalter DJ, Abrams KR, Myles JP (2003) *Bayesian Approaches to Clinical Trials and Health-Care Evaluation.* John Wiley & Sons, Ltd, Chichester.

Temple R (1982) Government view of clinical trials. *Drug Information Journal* **16**: 10–17.

Temple R, Ellenberg SS (2000) Placebo-controlled trials and active-control trials in the evaluation of new treatments. Part 1: Ethical and scientific issues. *Annals of Internal Medicine* **133**: 455–463.

Wellek S (2002) *Testing Statistical Hypotheses of Equivalence.* Chapman and Hall/CRC, Boca Raton, FL.

World Medical Association 52nd Assembly (2000) *World Medical Association Declaration of Helsinki Ethical Principles for Medical Research Involving Human Subjects.* Edinburgh: World Medical Association.

Yates F (1936) Incomplete randomized blocks. *Annals of Eugenics* **7**: 121–140.

15.A   TECHNICAL APPENDIX

15.A.1   Sample sizes for equivalence trials

The argument here is based on Schuirman's approach to equivalence using two one-sided tests (Schuirmann, 1987). Assume that we have a reference product for which the response Y_r is Normally distributed with

$$E[Y_r] = \mu_r \quad \text{and} \quad \text{var}[Y_r] = \sigma^2.$$

Suppose that for the test drug we have a response Y_t which is Normally distributed with

$$E[Y_t] = \mu_t \quad \text{and} \quad \text{var}[Y_t] = \sigma^2.$$

Let $\delta, \delta > 0$, be a 'limit of indifference'. True absolute differences greater than this constitute a nonignorable distinction between drugs. We wish to show that $-\delta < \mu_t - \mu_r < \delta$. An approximately adequate way to do this is to carry out two one-sided tests of significance. Let $\mu_t - \mu_r = \tau$, then we can test:

$$H_{0A}: \tau \geq \delta \quad \text{against} \quad H_{1A}: \tau < \delta$$

and

$$H_{0B}: \tau \leq -\delta \quad \text{against} \quad H_{1B}: \tau > -\delta.$$

We refer to the first of these tests as test A and the second as test B

Now let us assume that the variance is known and that we shall use, as in the usual case of hypothesis testing, the difference between the two sample means for the test. Let $d = \bar{Y}_t - \bar{Y}_r$ and let $\text{SE} = \sigma\sqrt{(1/n_1) + (1/n_2)}$ where n_1 and n_2 are the sample sizes in the two treatment groups. Now suppose that we have $\tau = \delta$ and that we run test A as an α level test. We require a critical value C_A such that $P[d < C_A | \tau = \delta] = \alpha$. Equivalently, we require

$$P\left[Z < \frac{C_A - \delta}{\text{SE}}\right] = \alpha, \tag{15.1}$$

where Z is distributed as a standard Normal.

From (15.1) we have $(C_A - \delta)/\text{SE} = \Phi^{-1}(\alpha)$, where $\Phi^{-1}(.)$ is the inverse distribution function of the standard Normal and hence

$$C_A = \delta + \text{SE}\,\Phi^{-1}(\alpha). \tag{15.2}$$

Similarly, we can show that for test B we have critical value

$$C_B = -\delta - SE\Phi^{-1}(\alpha).$$ (15.3)

For 'significant' equality to be declared, the joint test requires $d < C_A$ and $d > C_B$. Note that for $\alpha < 0.5$, $\Phi^{-1}(\alpha) < 0$. Thus, in practice, $C_A < \delta$ and $C_B > -\delta$. It follows, therefore, that for very small δ and large SE, $C_B > C_A$, in which case it is impossible to satisfy both test requirements. For a reasonably powered test this will not arise. In general, however, the probability associated with satisfying both of these test requirements is slightly less than α (Senn, 2001b). In this sense, from one point of view, the procedure cannot be 'optimal'. In practice, for reasonable cases, this objection may be ignored.

The power function of this test is

$$H(\tau) = P[C_B < d < C_A | \tau],$$

or

$$H(\tau, \delta, SE, \alpha) = P[-\delta - SE\Phi^{-1}(\alpha) < d < \delta + SE\Phi^{-1}(\alpha) | \tau],$$

from which,

$$H(\tau, \delta, SE, \alpha) = P\left[\frac{-\delta - \tau}{SE} - \Phi^{-1}(\alpha) < Z < \frac{\delta - \tau}{SE} + \Phi^{-1}(\alpha)\right].$$ (15.4)

Now, as is usual, this power depends upon the unknown treatment effect. In the best of the cases that comprise H_1 we shall have $\tau = 0$. However, more generally, we might not have exact equality and suppose that $t = \gamma$, $-\delta < \gamma < \delta$, $\gamma \neq 0$, where, for any reasonable hope of success, γ must lie well within the interval.

Thus, to calculate the sample size associated with an equivalence trial we consider (15.4) as a function of γ, substitute the requisite values of $H(\gamma, \delta, SE, \alpha)$, γ, δ, α and solve for SE. Then, with a known value of σ^2, we can solve for n using the standard formula for the standard error of the difference between two means.

16

Meta-Analysis

a wheen o' mickles maks a muckle

Scottish proverb

Little drops of water
Little grains of sand
Make the mighty ocean
And the beauteous land

And the little moments
Humble though they be
Make the mighty ages
Of eternity

Julia Carney, The Home Book of Verse, VI

The drop of rain maketh a hole in the stone, not by violence, but by oft falling.
Hugh Latimer, Seventh Sermon before Edward VI

16.1 BACKGROUND

The world of medical research is full of small studies: taken alone, each may be inaudible but if they are brought to speak together their message can be loud and clear. Even where trials are large, they do not always give exactly the same result, or perhaps they have been large enough to answer general questions but not to study effects in subgroups. A *meta-analysis*, or *overview*, is an attempt to pool the results of individual studies into a single analysis with the intention to produce a message where before there was none, or to make the message clearer, or to resolve an apparent contradiction in messages, or even to assess whether the message changes from subgroup to subgroup.

There are a number of techniques which may be used. If the studies involved have a similar structure and use the same outcome variables and the meta-analyst has access to the original data (which is usually the situation of the drug developer), then an analysis of these raw data is both possible and (almost invariably) desirable. This has been referred to as a *type A* meta-analysis (Senn, 2000b). The situation is then very like that in a multicentre trial, with trials rather than centres forming the strata. In principle all the controversies, issues and difficulties which arise with multicentre trials may be attendant on such an analysis but there is no particular reason why new difficulties should present themselves.

Statistical Issues in Drug Development/2nd Edition   Stephen Senn
© 2007 John Wiley & Sons, Ltd

At the other extreme is the situation where studies have been designed to answer the same general question but used different measures. For example, in a number of trials in asthma, PEF measurements might have been taken and in others FEV_1 might have been recorded. A technique, due originally to Glass (1976), who coined the term 'meta-analysis', is to calculate the apparently unit-free ratio formed by dividing the mean effect by the standard *deviation* of the measure. This has been referred to as a type C meta-analysis (Senn, 2000b). Such a ratio is termed an effect size. Given fairly strong assumptions, it may be assumed that the effect of the treatment acts roughly identically on these ratios, even though the original measures may have quite different units from trial to trial.

In between these two extremes are type B meta-analyses (Senn, 2000b). These, like type C, use summary statistics but, like type A, measure the same outcome variable. Many of the important published meta-analyses that have been carried out in the public sector are of this sort.

It is possible to base a meta-analysis on *P*-values alone (see Sonneman (1991) for an excellent discussion and also Hedges and Olkin (1985)). Fisher himself suggested an approach whereby each *P*-value is transformed to $-2\log(P)$ (Fisher, 1932). Such a value is always positive and is larger the smaller the *P*-value and will, in fact, have a chi-square distribution with two degrees of freedom under the null hypothesis. These chi-square statistics may be assumed independent from study to study and if summed over k studies will, under the null hypothesis that the treatments are identical in every study and by the usual property of chi-square statistics, have a chi-square distribution with $2k$ degrees of freedom. The method takes no account of the direction of the observed treatment difference in any study and is thus equally powerful against some rather strange alternative hypotheses (that the treatment improves prognosis in some trials but makes it worse in others) as it is against some more reasonable hypotheses, but it can be made more sensitive for coherent treatment hypotheses by suitable modification. It also weights large and small studies equally, however, and this is a severe disadvantage.

In some indications, the number of deaths or the frequency of some serious event forms the main outcome. Given that the length of follow-up is the same, or that there is some other suitable standard (for example, we might be observing cases of pre-eclampsia in relation to number of pregnancies), it may then be possible to base an analysis on counting such events (although one might argue that, with pre-eclampsia, a continuous measure – blood pressure – has artificially been turned into an 'event' by dichotomizing it). For such a series of k trials, even though we cannot identify individual patients, we shall have three pieces of information collected on every patient: first, the trial in which he or she was entered; second, the treatment given; and third, a binary outcome. The results can then be summarized in a single $k \times 2 \times 2$ table (or a set of k 2×2 tables) recording how many patients fall into any given cell. Since there is a vast array of techniques available for analysing binary data even for a single 2×2 table, there is an enormous potential choice for ensemble of k such tables. The basic idea, however, is to treat the trial as a stratum, or covariate, and analyse accordingly. Candidate methods include the Mantel–Haenszel procedure, logistic regression and others to be discussed under issues below.

Finally, before proceeding to the issues, it is perhaps appropriate to draw attention to the increasing importance of meta-analysis as a tool to aid medical decision-making. This was already the case at the time (1997) the first edition of this book appeared.

Since then the importance of meta-analysis has grown. Not only has there been an explosion in published analyses over the past twenty years, but initiatives such as that of the Cochrane collaboration of databases as well as the trend towards 'evidence-based medicine' make it both easier to use meta-analysis on the one hand and less acceptable not to do so on the other. In drug development, while being satisfied with an expert's judgement alone in the past, the regulator now expects to see it backed up with a formal overview of all studies. (See, for example, ICH E9 (International Conference on Harmonisation, 1999).) Like them or hate them, meta-analyses are here to stay.

Reviews of various issues and practical matters are to be found in the papers by Peto (1987), Pocock and Hughes (1990), Emerson (1994), van Houwelingen (1995), Geller and Proschan (1996), Normand (1999) and Senn (2000b) and the books by Petitti (2000) and Whitehead (2002), the latter being a volume in this series. For graphical representation of meta-analyses see Galbraith (1988).

16.2   ISSUES

16.2.1   If you need meta-analysis to prove it, you can't believe it

The argument here is that an effect of a reasonable size ought to be demonstrable in a single trial. The counterargument is that in common but serious diseases such as cancer and heart disease, even small treatment effects can be important in terms of their total impact on public health. Moreover, as we cannot reasonably expect dramatic break-throughs in these diseases, we should be looking for small effects. However, investigators are eternal optimists and so plan trials to look for large effects. To make some use of these individually inadequate studies, we need to pool them. Depending upon which side of this argument one stands, one can either regard the proponents of meta-analysis (statisticians in the main, or physicians who think like them) as being like the tailors in the story of 'The Emperor's New Clothes', persuading the gullible to see what isn't there, or as latter-day Galileos making bold discoveries with their brand new telescope but having the greatest difficulty in persuading the obdurate to believe the evidence of their eyes.

The situation in drug development is different from that in public health. Here a sponsor may well be capable of showing effects in a single trial (and after all it is the sponsor who has to run the trials to show it). However, we ought to be interested not only in showing that a treatment works but also how well it works and for whom. For this purpose, pooling results can be invaluable.

> **Medical statisticians** can be divided into two sorts: those who think that sample size determination is the alpha and omega of planning clinical trials and those who think that it is merely the beta.

16.2.2   Meta-analyses do not predict the results of future trials well

This criticism surfaces from time to time. For example, LeLorier *et al.* (1997) carried out a number of meta-analyses and concluded that 'the outcomes of the 12 large randomized, controlled trials that we studied were not predicted accurately 35 percent of the time by the meta-analyses published previously on the same topics'. But as a criticism of meta-analysis this is entirely irrelevant. One has to consider the alternative. If a decision has to be made based on available evidence then it will have to be done either by some process of informal summary of the results of the trials that have been run or by choosing one of the trials run so far as the basis for future decision-making. For the findings of LeLorier *et al.* (1997) to constitute a criticism of meta-analysis they would have to have shown that the meta-analysis of all trials run to date was worse at predicting the trial to follow than was the analysis of the largest trial run to date. This they failed to do.

There is another technical problem to do with P-values and inference generally. There is a tendency to interpret a P-value less than 0.05 as indicating that the treatment is definitely effective and that therefore with high probability another trial should be significant. In fact, this is far from being the case (Goodman, 1992). One tends to forget that even if it were the case that a given P-value indicated that the effect of a treatment was certainly genuine (which can never be the case), a further trial will not have infinite size and hence will not have 100% power (Senn, 2002). See Chapter 12 for a discussion.

More generally, the critics of meta-analysis fail to consider the alternative. For meta-analysis to be useful it simply has to be better than the alternative. It does not have to be perfect. This point is developed further below.

16.2.3　You cannot pool different studies

A criticism of meta-analysis is that apples are mixed with pears. Studies with different protocols and different populations have different messages. It may well be that the studies were too small to deliver these messages clearly, but this does not mean that the result of pooling them will be meaningful.

In my view, however, there is a tendency to confuse imperfections inevitably associated with clinical research in general, with particular difficulties of meta-analysis. Consider the case where two trial protocols (A and B) for a given treatment in a given indication are rather different but each is considered to be a potential solution to the business of studying the treatment and disease in question. However different they are, it is unlikely that they will between them exhaust all possible reasonable ways of studying the performance of the treatment in this indication. We could, for example, have also used protocols C, D, E, F or G but in fact used only A or B. Suppose we take the point of view that where protocols are different, pooling is forbidden. Then, when practising evidence-based medicine, a future prescribing physician will have to choose which of A or B should guide his choice. But if we had studied the drug using D or G instead, he would have to choose between these two trials and neither A nor B would be available to him. It seems rather naive, therefore, to assume that when making decisions about applying the results of research, particular physicians make particular use of specific features of protocols. Even if they wanted to, they would find this rather difficult since the way in which information filters through to the physician rarely includes much in the way of specific details of trials run and in any case physicians have neither the time nor inclination to be involved in such minutiae. One may assume, therefore, that to all intents and purposes the prescribing physician exhibits, in his or her behaviour (within bounds), what might be termed *protocol exchangeability*.

Note also that we should have been no better off as regards the validity of making predictions if we had used two trials with identical protocols A, for the simple reason that we do not restrict prescribing a drug to the exact circumstances which obtain in a clinical trial. (I note, by the by, the illogical practice of some drug developers of insisting that the two protocols for the two trials designed to satisfy the FDA's two-trial rule should be identical.) The fact that the results of the largest trial in a given indication have been less than perfectly predicted by meta-analysis of those that remain is also a red herring. As has been argued elsewhere in this book, the justification of the statistician's methods is not that they are *perfect* but that they are *better*. For this sort of example to be convincing, one would have to show that either the results of the largest trial run to date or the judgement of some expert was better at predicting the results of the next trial one would run than would be a meta-analysis. In short, it is not enough to be squeamish about pooling results. One has to show that the alternative is not worse.

16.2.4   The interpretation of studies that have pooled different treatments

The fact that pooling is often justified does not mean that one does not have to be careful in interpreting the results of meta-analyses that have pooled different treatments. It will be useful to consider a specific example.

Juni *et al.* (2004) carried out a cumulative meta-analysis in which they 'included all randomised controlled trials in patients with chronic musculoskeletal disorders that compared rofecoxib with other non-steroidal anti-inflammatory drugs (NSAIDs) or placebo' (p. 2021). The outcomes targeted were cardiovascular side-effects, in particular myocardial infarctions, and they found that by the year 2000 there was already evidence of a significant effect on rofecoxib on cardiovascular health, which they interpreted as harm compared with placebo. This drew an angry response from Kim and Reicin (2004), who worked for Merck, the makers of rofecoxib, claiming that the approach 'contravenes the basic principle of meta-analyses to combine like with like, and thus arrives at flawed conclusions'.

In my opinion there is no such basic principle, but the conclusions of Juni *et al.* (2004) were, indeed, flawed. Note that two things were not in dispute by either side. The first is that cardiovascular mortality on rofecoxib had been proved to be higher than that on naproxen by 2000 when the VIGOR study reported (Bombardier *et al.*, 2000). (Although the way these results were presented was less than transparent.) The second is that the study reported by Bresalier *et al.* (2005) had shown an excess risk over placebo in 2004, when its results led Merck to pull rofecoxib of the market. The point in dispute is whether the excess risk over placebo had already been shown by the year 2000 or whether a valid interpretation of the VIGOR study at the time was that the difference was due to a beneficial effect of naproxen.

In my view, the meta-analysis conducted by Juni *et al.* (2004) validly tested the null hypothesis: *rofecoxib is no different from any of the comparators included in this meta-analysis as regards effect on cardiovascular events.* If this hypothesis is rejected (and given the direction of rejection) then its logical alternative can be asserted: *rofecoxib is worse than at least one comparator as regards effect on cardiovascular mortality.* This alternative hypothesis is not at all the same as this one: *rofecoxib is worse than all the comparators as regards its effect on cardiovascular mortality.* However, the cumulative meta-analysis to 2000 was driven by the huge VIGOR study, which had shown that rofecoxib was worse than naproxen as regards this outcome. To assert that this proves that it is worse than placebo requires an auxiliary hypothesis that naproxen is the same as placebo.

To simplify things, consider a meta-analysis of a series of trials that are of two sorts, those comparing rofecoxib with naproxen and those comparing rofecoxib with placebo. These have the structure of an incomplete blocks design. If a model is fitted with trial as a factor and treatments as another factor at three levels – rofecoxib, naproxen, placebo – it is actually the rofecoxib results that permit the comparison of naproxen and placebo. To try to use this comparison to justify pooling placebo and naproxen is a hopelessly circular argument. To the extent that the model above is used, all that will happen is that rofecoxib will be separately compared with placebo using those trials in which they appeared.

Thus, the assertion that rofecoxib could have been known to be worse than placebo by 2000 is based entirely on an auxiliary hypothesis that naproxen and placebo are identical. This hypothesis may or may not have been reasonable at the time, but the meta-analysis as carried out by Juni *et al.* (2004) cannot prove it. To be fair to these authors, they did carry out some independent investigation of this hypothesis by looking at studies that had compared naproxen with placebo but here they assumed that absence of evidence was evidence of absence and did not use methods that have been developed for formally incorporating evidence regarding previous trials of comparators. (See the discussion of the approaches of Hasselblad and Kong (2001) and Hirotsu and Yamada (1999) in Chapter 15).

Thus, to sum up, pooling of trials with different treatment arms may well be legitimate but one has to be careful about resulting inferences. Some inferences may require auxiliary hypotheses and this should not be lost sight of. The issue is closely related to Don Rubin's problem of treatment versions (Rubin, 1980) and this is discussed briefly in Chapter 22.

16.2.5   Publication bias

Studies which show a positive result are more likely to be published than those which do not. A meta-analysis which is based on published studies only will therefore tend to be biased in favour of significance.

There are three points to make in connection with this. First, the sponsor in drug development is usually in the fortunate position of having results of all studies available and the regulator is also usually in a position to check that all studies have been presented. In the context of meta-analyses within drug development, this should not be a problem. Second, the bias exists whether or not studies are pooled. It is sometimes mistakenly regarded as being a peculiar difficulty of meta-analysis. In fact, it can cause even more problems for the interpretation of individual studies. The first and second points taken together suggest that, quite apart from any advantages of reduced variability, a meta-analysis of a sponsor's studies will be more reliable than individual published studies. Third, under the null hypothesis of no difference between treatments, a control treatment is just as likely to show spurious significance as an experimental treatment. For there to be bias in the treatment *estimate* where the treatment is ineffective, therefore, requires a bias not only in favour of significant trials but also in favour of studies in which new treatments are 'shown' to be effective. It is true, however, that even a nondirectional bias in favour of significance will invalidate a test of significance in connection with a meta-analysis (especially if Fisher's method is used), but it obviously also has a bad effect on individual trials.

16.2.6 A meta-analysis provides an opportunity for the sponsor to manipulate results

We have now moved to a position in drug development where trial protocols have a detailed description of the intended analysis. (The same high standard does not always apply elsewhere.) This constrains the ability of the sponsor to manipulate the results which are presented to the regulator. However, it is difficult to exert the same degree of control over a drug development programme as a whole (although the European Statistical Guidelines indicate the desirability of doing this and the FDA, has, of course, for years taken an active interest through its approach to regulation in the way that programmes are put together).

If the approach to pooling and analysing data from a drug development programme is not prespecified, then the sponsor has the ability to analyse the data in a number of ways and present the most favourable *a posteriori* rather than the most reasonable *a priori*. This is clearly biasing and in principle it would be desirable to ensure that it does not happen by having a prespecified standard for analysis. (Unfortunately, even if it can be proved that a protocol was agreed upon before starting the meta-analysis, in many cases it will have been determined after individual trial results have been delivered and so conscious or unconscious bias cannot be entirely eliminated.)

Again, however, one must retain a sense of proportion. If the alternative to a meta-analysis is an expert report, then the scope for bias is even greater. The regulator will, after all, have the results of the individual trials. It is hard to believe that an additional meta-analysis can be less useful than the largely subjective opinion of some potentially biased expert who in any case must also – but using some hidden and poorly understood mental processes – make some summary of the data as a whole. This is just another example, in my view, of one of those difficulties which exist anyway but which more formal statistical methods bring to our attention. It is a mistake to regard the general problem of summarizing evidence as a being a particular difficulty of statistical approaches to doing so.

> **Meta-analyst**: One who thinks that if manure is piled high enough it will smell like roses.

16.2.7 Cochrane Collaboration meta-analyses are superior to those carried out by the pharmaceutical industry

This misleading claim is made from time to time by those associated with the Cochrane Collaboration (CC). For example, Jadad *et al.* (2000) carried out a review of 50 meta-analyses in asthma and concluded that 'most reviews published in peer-reviewed journals or funded by industry have serious methodological flaws that limit their value to guide decisions. Cochrane reviews are more rigorous and better reported than those published in peer-reviewed journals' (p. 537). A similar claim was repeated some years later by Jorgensen *et al.* (2006).

However, both sets of authors used for this purpose an index (Oxman and Guyatt, 1991) that placed little premium on correct analysis but a great deal on the extent to which publication bias had been dealt with. Furthermore, the validation of this index employed a very narrow base, involving only colleagues from the same department in McMaster University and involving none based in the pharmaceutical industry. For example, double-counting of trials is a serious error in meta-analysis, and one which the CC has not always avoided (see Kozyrskyj *et al.* (2000) for an example discussed in Senn (2007)), but this is not explicitly mentioned in the index. Nor does it cover whether cross-over trials and parallel group trials had been combined properly (Senn, 2000c). This is a serious issue since the software that the CC used in its earlier versions was incapable of handling anything but a parallel-group trial: cluster-randomized and cross-over trials could not be dealt with, nor could covariates or centres be accounted for. The latter is somewhat ironic since it can be shown that the information contained in baseline values can be regarded as being equivalent to information provided by a further trial (Senn, 2005).

In fact, from a pharmaceutical industry perspective, the Oxman and Guyatt index is very unfair (Senn, 2000c). The thing to which it gives most emphasis, searching for trials, is the one that causes least concern. A sponsor is likely to know the trials that were carried out with its drug, at least until the drug is marketed; hence, identification of studies is an item that is so obvious it may not be reported in detail. On the other hand, where industry is likely to score is on the quality of the statistical analysis, something that receives almost no attention in the Oxman and Guyatt index. This is all that the index has to say about correct analysis:

> Were the methods used to combine the findings of the relevant studies reported?
> Were the findings of the relevant studies combined appropriately?

Since the enthusiasm of meta-analysts frequently exceeds their statistical knowledge, many will be incapable of judging whether these two points are adequately addressed

Ironically, despite the emphasis on finding all studies, in their meta-meta-analysis Jadad *et al.* (2000) did not find the one carried out by Richardson and Bablok (1992). Since Bernhard Bablok worked in my group at CIBA-Giegy and Bill Richardson was a colleague, I am biased, but I think that this is a finer meta-analysis than many in asthma that will appear in the CC.

However, I do not wish to leave this section, with a negative note about the CC. The CC is a force for good in medicine and is doing extremely important work. It is not the work of the CC I object to but biased articles comparing CC analyses with those from the pharmaceutical industry. My main complaint is that this is pointless. I wouldn't dream of using an index to judge the quality of a meta-analysis; I would study it and whether I found it to be of high or low quality, credible or not, the fact that it was a CC meta-analysis or a pharmaceutical industry one would (I hope) play no part in that judgement.

16.2.8   Interpretation of effect sizes

Glass (1976) introduced the term meta-analysis into the literature and was concerned with pooling studies in education where the outcome measures might be different. For a well-planned drug development, this problem should not arise. Occasionally it does, however (an example is given by Richardson and Bablok (1992)) and it can then be appropriate to use the Glass effect size as a means of pooling data. For each study the ratio of the treatment estimate (for example, the difference between means) to the within-group standard deviation is calculated.

Suppose that two treatments A and B are being compared in a parallel-group study, that we calculate the treatment difference in the direction A − B and that high values of the outcome measure are good. It is intuitively reasonable that the higher the effect size the greater the probability that a patient chosen at random from A will have a higher reading than one chosen at random and treated with B. In fact, if the original data are Normally distributed and variances in the two groups are the same, then this probability may be simply calculated as a function of the effect size. A plot of this probability is given in Figure 16.1, which is nothing less than the plot of a suitably scaled cumulative Normal distribution.

For reasons given in Chapters 3 and 8, however, one should be very careful in interpreting effect sizes in this way. For example, in Figure 16.1, we may see that an effect size of 1 corresponds to a probability of observed superiority of 0.76. This does not mean, however, that 76% of all patients will be better off being given treatment A rather than B. The figure is likely to be much higher and depends on the sources of variability within the study. Suppose we were to run a study with much narrower entry criteria. We ought to see similar treatment effects but a much lower variance. Hence, the effect size would be greater. This seems paradoxical at first, but if we remember our key (causal) definition of the true treatment effect – the difference between what happened and what would have happened – the paradox disappears. That a given patient chosen at random is observed to be better on treatment A than a given patient chosen at

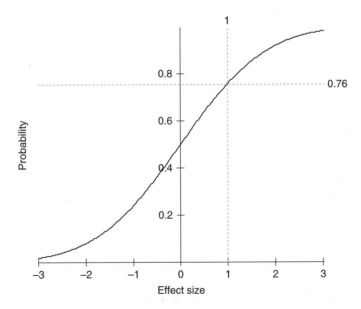

Figure 16.1 Probability that a patient chosen at random from the experimental group will have a higher measured outcome than another chosen at random from the control group.

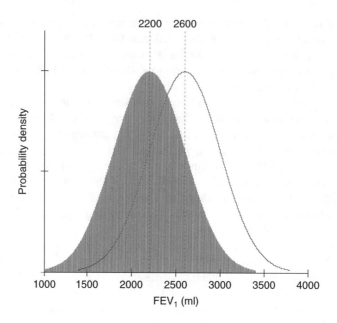

Figure 16.2   Distribution of FEV$_1$ measurements for two treatment groups.

random is observed to be on B does not contradict the possibility that both would be better on A or even (although it is less plausible) that both would be better on B. The probability associated with an effect size calculates the probability of observing such a superiority. However, to know whether a given patient will be better treated with A or with B, or even to know what proportion of patients will be better off is quite another matter. No simple comparison of means whether scaled by the standard deviation or not can answer this question. Consider the two histograms of Figure 16.2, which represent an idealized version of a possible distribution of results from a trial in asthma to compare two treatments. The two histograms overlap. Some patients in the left-hand histogram have higher FEV$_1$ readings than those in the right-hand one. But the right-hand histogram may be obtained from the left-hand one simply by adding 400 ml to each value. It *could* represent a constant benefit for every patient and we would be unable to tell, simply by inspecting two such histograms for different patients, that this had not happened.

This whole matter is complex and difficult. Again, I issue the warning: it is all too easy to over-interpret clinical trials and seek explanations which, while they may be correct, are not needed. One must be very careful in interpreting effect sizes.

16.2.9   Sequential meta-analyses

This is an issue which has received much attention elsewhere but which is generally seen to be less relevant within the context of drug development. If one performs regular meta-analyses of clinical trials and then stops doing clinical trials if or when the result of the meta-analysis becomes significant, then such a procedure is subject to the general bias to which (unadjusted) sequential clinical analysis of ordinary clinical trials is liable.

Thus, some sort of adjustment for sequential analysis would be indicated. In medical statistics, or indeed in statistics generally, this is an extremely controversial topic (see Chapter 19). Sequential methods is the field in which the distinction between Bayesian methods and frequentist approaches is sharpest. Bayesian approaches do not appear to require adjustment for repeated testing, whereas frequentist approaches do.

The difficulty within the context of drug development is that if some adjustment is indicated it is not at all clear what it should be. It is rarely the case that an ongoing sequential meta-analysis itself drives the decision-making process. It might seem, therefore, that once a development programme has reached a conclusion, a meta-analytic summary of results would not require an adjustment. The fact is that results along the way of individual trials do, of course, influence the decision to continue. Phase III trials will not take place unless phase II trials have been successful to some degree. Thus, one view of a phase III programme might be that it ought to be an independent confirmation that a hypothesis developed within phase II was justified. As such, it should not be combined in any formal way with phase III results. (And by extension, this purist view could be applied to any trials carried out as a result of a decision to continue.) This might seem to form an argument either in favour of developing formal stopping rules to be used in connection with meta-analyses or for being circumspect as to which trials may be pooled, or perhaps for using some other approach to inference altogether (say the Bayesian approach). It should be noted, however, that these difficulties are there whether or not the pooling mechanism is formal. Thus, expert opinion suffers potentially from the same difficulties.

16.2.10   Bayesian meta-analysis

Some of these difficulties could perhaps be overcome by Bayesian meta-analysis. In fact, any Bayesian analysis of clinical trials is, or ought to be, a meta-analysis. Yesterday's posterior becomes today's prior to which tomorrow's data are added. The result is a posterior which is available to serve as a prior for the day after tomorrow, and so on. This model can be represented schematically as $P_{n-1} + D_n \rightarrow P_n$. With this model, there is no question of performing an explicit meta-analysis: the analysis of the latest trial already incorporates a prior which itself reflects all data from previous trials. Hence, there is nothing left to add.

In practice, a problem arises with what might be called 'the date of information problem' (DIP). Other trials may report before a trial is finished but after it was planned. Hence the prior used for planning is not the same as that to be used for analysis. It thus becomes important to know what was known and by whom and when. Otherwise there is a danger of counting information twice on the one hand or overlooking it on the other.

A particular dilemma exists for any Bayesian called in during the middle of a drug development programme at a time at which certain data (say D_1) have been collected but before further data (say D_2) have been obtained. If she elicits a prior from a subject-matter expert for the purpose of preparing an analysis, he (the expert) will already have been exposed to D_1. Should she now regard the prior she obtains as excluding the data (say P_0) or as including the data (say P_1)? If she takes the former course, then she assumes that she will be performing an analysis of the form Step 1: $P_0 + D_1 \rightarrow P_1$, Step 2: $P_1 + D_2 \rightarrow P_2$, or equivalently in a single step: $P_0 + D_1 + D_2 \rightarrow P_2$. If, however, the expert's opinion *does* include D_1, then the Bayesian has instead performed the illegitimate Step 1: $P_1 + D_1 \rightarrow P'_1$, where P'_1 is now a pathological prior (potentially as misleading as a pathological liar) in which the same information D_1 is included twice. (This would be as wrong as, say, taking a contingency table in which the frequencies added up to 50 and analysing the *percentages* using the chi-square test!) On the other hand, if the Bayesian decides that the prior given to her by the expert already includes P_1 and therefore proceeds to step 2, then if it does not include P_1 she will have ignored D_1, a course of action which seems less serious than counting it twice but runs contrary to the principle of total information accepted by most Bayesians. (Here the analogy would be to taking a contingency table where the totals were 200 and analysing the percentages.) Furthermore, she has just done herself out of a job, for if the expert's prior represents a true updating of all available information, then it follows that he is a natural Bayesian in no need of her advice.

A further difficulty arises in deciding whose priors to use. As argued in Chapter 6, the ethics of clinical trials may require that the participating physicians have prior belief in the efficacy of the experimental treatment. If it is their priors which determine when the sequence of trials will terminate, it will terminate without convincing other physicians. A good discussion of the issues involved in determining priors will be found in the paper by Spiegelhalter *et al.* (1994), and there is also further useful discussion in the book in this series by Spiegelhalter *et al.* (2003).

16.2.11 Prior distributions for random-effect variances

An increasingly employed approach to conducting meta-analyses is to perform a Bayesian analysis. In fact, the most commonly employed analysis is not fully Bayesian but a hybrid. That is because, although prior distributions are employed for the treatment parameters, the nuisance parameters themselves are treated as fixed (Senn, 2007). That is to say that the variances of the treatment contrasts from various trials are treated as if they were known. This means that such analyses do not avoid many of the problems associated with frequentist approaches outlined in section 16.2.14.

However, Bayesians do commonly put a prior distribution on the treatment effect variance, that is the variance of the extent to which the true effect varies from trial to trial. The precision with which this is estimated depends largely on the number of trials in the meta-analysis. If this is large, then the Bayesian analysis is likely to produce similar results to the frequentist one.

If the number of trials is small, however, then the Bayesian inferences are likely to be highly dependent on choice of prior. An extensive investigation of this by simulation was carried out by Lambert *et al.* (2005). However, simulating from some supposed reality is really irrelevant. The real issues are, first, to what extent different priors produce results that differ from each other and, second (and more important), to what extent the prior used reflects what one truly believes, since this is the purpose of a prior in a Bayesian analysis (Senn, 2007).

Here there is a delicate issue that is not easy to deal with. It is difficult to believe in a large random effect if the effect of treatment itself is negligible. Hence what is really required is a joint specification of treatment and random-effect variance, and this is not easy. See Senn (2007) for further discussion.

16.2.12   Fixed- versus random-effect meta-analyses

An almost identical issue with respect to centres was touched upon when discussing multicentre trials. Within drug development, however, the almost uniform practice is to fit fixed-effect models for treatments within *centres*. (Elsewhere it is not unusual to ignore centres altogether!) Outside of drug development, and in the context of meta-analyses, there has been an extremely vigorous debate between the proponents of fixed-effect and random-effect models for treatment effects within *trials*.

The proponents of fixed-effect models can claim (a) that this is the only technique suitable for analysing a single trial, a practice which almost nobody considers illegitimate; (b) that '*protocol*' is a partly artificial label and should not be reified; and (c) that if we wish to discover whether a treatment can have an effect (as opposed to whether it will), then the approach is both logically indicated and powerful. The proponents of random-effect models might reply (d) that treatment effects *do* differ from trial to trial; (e) that if we wish to take account of the effect of this source of variability for the purposes of prediction, then we need to use a random effects model; and (f) that the fact that we have difficulty in answering an important question (what effect may we reasonably expect future patients will have from a given treatment?) is no excuse for answering a simpler but less relevant question instead.

I do not wish to add anything to the discussion already given on this subject in the context of multicentre trials, except to state that this issue has little if anything to do with whether treatment-by-trial interaction is detected by some formal test. The choice between models has to do with the purpose to which the model is being put.

16.2.13   Estimates from random-effect analyses

Conventionally, a random-effect analysis predicts the response in the average future trial. Provided that responses vary randomly from trial to trial in a way that is unassociated with any observed features of trials, this might also be a reasonable prediction for a randomly chosen future patient. If, however, the fixed- and random-effect analyses differ markedly in terms of their predictions of average future response, this may be an indication that the effect of treatment varies according to the size of trial. After all, if all trials have equal precision, they will be given equal weight, whether a fixed-effect or random-effect approach is used. As such, the two estimates will be the same. Similarly, if all estimates of treatment effects are similar then it makes no difference to the average how they are weighted. Thus the combination is needed of different weights (when moving from fixed- to random-effect analysis) and a correlation between weights and estimate effects for the two systems to produce different estimates.

Suppose that the estimates are different and that we wish to estimate the effect in the average future patient. We might argue that, most patients having been recruited on large trials, most future patients are of the sort who would be recruited on large trials. We therefore wish to give more weight to large trials, which is exactly what a fixed-effect analysis does. The point here is that an estimate is not the same as a prediction (Lane and Nelder, 1982; Senn, 2004). Even if a random-effect analysis is considered appropriate it may also be appropriate to go beyond the estimate of the response in the average future trial, which is what such an analysis conventionally delivers, in order to make a useful prediction.

A similar issue was discussed in Chapter 14 in connection with estimates from multicentre trials, which the reader may wish to consult.

16.2.14   Weighting studies in fixed-effect meta-analyses

It is a remarkable fact that whereas the industry default standard appeared for many years to have been to weight centres equally in analysing multicentre trials (in the context of continuous outcomes, this is the type III sums of squares approach), for fixed-effect meta-analyses carried out elsewhere this approach is almost never used. There the general approach is to weight trials according to the information they may provide (analogous to type II sums of squares). It was argued in Chapter 14 that the type II approach of giving larger centres more weight is logical and, by extension, the same should apply for trials also.

Note that a false analogy with least squares has been made more than once in the statistical literature and it has been claimed that the meta-analytic approach is equivalent to the linear model without trial-by-treatment interaction (Mathew, 1999; Olkin and Sampson, 1998). This is not true, because in the linear model without interaction, the trial by treatment interaction makes a contribution to the residual sum of squares, which it does *not* make in a fixed-effect meta-analysis although it is used in a random-effect analysis. It is easy to see this by noting that if there are N patients in k trials comparing two treatments, then two degrees of freedom must be lost for variance estimation from each trial, meaning that in total $N - 2k$ are available. However, a linear model without interaction would remove, from the $N - 1$ available, one for the effect of treatment and $k - 1$ for the effects of the main effects of trials, leaving $N - 1 - 1 - (k - 1) = N - k - 1$. In fact, the equivalence is to a particular version of the model with interactions. If a further $k - 1$ degrees of freedom are removed for trial-by-treatment interaction, we have $N - 2k$ left for variance estimation as before.

However, the point is that as soon as an interaction is included the parameterization of the main effect is arbitrary. If the minimum variance parameterization is used then this is the type II approach and also the meta-analysis approach. Hence a fixed-effect meta-analysis is analogous to a least-squares model including interaction but using a type II weighting. Further discussion of this will be found in Senn (2000b).

Of course the analogy is not perfect, since in a meta-analysis the weights depend on the observed variances from trial to trial and the weights are, therefore, random variables. In a linear, model, however, the assumption of homoscedasticity is imposed. This means that the weights are fixed. This point is taken up in the next section.

16.2.15   Weighting used observed variances

If we use empirical estimates of the weights to be used, say by using the data themselves from a given trial to determine the weight given, we shall bias the estimate of the variance of the treatment estimate downwards. (Note that for binary outcomes the variances of the common treatment estimates, whether differences in probability, relative risks, odds ratios or log-odds ratios, depend upon the unknown parameters and are commonly estimated from the data.) Hence significance tests associated with such a meta-analysis will be too liberal. The problem is usually not too serious provided that the number of patients in a given trial is not too small. (The problem gets better not as the number of trials increases but as the number of patients per trial increases.) The problem can be avoided altogether by using independent weights for the trial and if, for example, an analysis of raw continuous data is carried out using the general linear model this can be done automatically. Alternatively, if a true meta-analysis is performed on summary results from trials, we may weight trials by the number of patients rather than by using some function of the observed variance of the treatment estimate.

It is interesting to note that this problem was recognized in an early paper on meta-analysis by Yates and Cochran (1938). They considered pooling estimates from series of agricultural trials and proposed equal weighting to avoid the dangers of weighting by observed precision. However, the context in which they were working was one of experiments of similar size with few degrees of freedom for error. This is usually not the case in a clinical context (Senn, 2000b, 2004).

16.2.16   We should use meta-analytic techniques for analysing multicentre trials

This was proposed by Salsburg (1999). He claimed that when many small centres were included in a clinical trial they affected the efficiency of the resulting treatment estimate because of lower quality. A least-squares approach would impose an assumption of homoscedasticty and give them too much weight. Using a meta-analytic technique would down-weight centres with large variances and hence be more efficient.

In fact, the sort of variation in variances one can see randomly in clinical trials from centre to centre, even when the true variance is the same, is enormous. A variation of 10 to 1 is easily achievable by chance alone (Senn, 2000a). This means that, for reasons well known to Yates and Cochran (1938) and discussed in Section 16.2.15, such meta-analytic weighting is generally a bad idea. In theory an ideal compromise would be possible by putting a random effect on the variance estimates and hence shrinking them towards some average variance. Bayesian methods would be ideally suited for this although in practice, when performing meta-analyses, Bayesians tend to treat the trial variances as if they were known parameters (Senn, 2007). The double-hierarchical generalized linear models of Lee and Nelder (2006) would also provide a suitable approach (Senn, 2006).

16.2.17   Quality indices

This topic is perhaps more important outside drug development than within. Meta-analysts who pool published studies often encounter very great variation in apparent quality. The reported precision of a trial may not then give a very good impression of its reliability. One approach is to produce quality indices for trials and use these to modify the weights they are given in the overall analysis.

The argument for this approach is obvious. If we knew that a study was completely fraudulent we would exclude its results. In extreme cases, therefore, we are prepared to use 'quality' of evidence as a means of weighting it. A quality index simply uses a graduated rather than an all-or-nothing scale. The arguments against using a quality index include that such an approach gives the meta-analyst an unwelcome flexibility to influence the results. He may be tempted to weight results according to outcome rather than according to standards of design, conduct and reporting.

16.2.18   Baseline risk

Because meta-analysis is such a powerful technique it invites us to go beyond the simple task of studying an overall treatment effect to studying the way in which the effect may vary according to demographic or other baseline characteristics. A good example of what may be achieved here is given by Thompson (1993, 1994). A question which has received some attention is whether the treatment is more effective (in the sense of providing a bigger difference) where the patients are more severely ill. It is tempting to classify the trials by severity using the 'response rate' (however defined) in the control group. One has to be extremely careful, however, as such an approach will be subject to a form of regression to the mean (Senn, 1994). This can be seen simply by considering the case where there is no true difference in risk from trial to trial and where the true treatment effect is constant. Because of random variation, the observed risk will vary from trial to trial and, of course, those trials where just by chance the risk is high in the control group will have a tendency to produce a more impressive difference from control for the experimental group. There will thus be a correlation between control group risk and treatment effect, which will invite us to believe that the true treatment effect varies according to risk.

It is more sensible either to classify trials by some measure of the baseline risk (that is to say, in terms of measures taken before treatment) of all patients or, even better, to classify patients individually in this way. Note that even if a statistically sound way could be found of estimating the treatment effect in a series of trials as a function of the response in the placebo group, this information would be of no direct use to prescribing doctors. Not only is such information related to a trial aggregate, while what is important is individuals, but to make use of it inorder to prescribe effectively a prescribing physician would have to know the response a patient *would* have under placebo were he or she to be entered into a trial. There is no such problem if the relationship between the treatment effect and an individual baseline measurement can be established.

Since the note by Senn (1994), this topic has continued to attract considerable attention. Unfortunately, not all proposals for dealing with it are sound. A valuable investigation is provided by Arends *et al.* (2000).

16.2.19   The principle of concurrent control and random main effects of trial

The basic idea behind a conventional meta-analysis is that it is based on within-trial contrasts. This eliminates the main effect of trial and such elimination corresponds to declaring the main effect of trial as fixed in a linear model. In this way the idea of concurrent control, which randomized trials themselves espouse, is observed in the meta-analysis.

For certain purposes it may be desirable to have the main effect of trial as random. This particular approach was used, for example, by vanHouwelingen *et al.* (1993).

Essentially they treat the results from each arm as defining a joint occurrence from a bivariate distribution. This approach may be desirable, indeed necessary, for certain purposes, for example studying the relationship between treatment effects and 'baseline risk' as discussed in Section 16.2.18. Such an approach will also be particularly natural to the Bayesian.

What has not always been appreciated, however, is that treating the main effect of trial as random permits the recovery of inter-trial information and thus abandons the principle of strict concurrent control. Usually, it is true, such information will be minimal and in any cases differences between trials may well be random, so that little bias may occur. A problematic case would be one where a few trials have been run and unequal randomization was been employed in some. I do not wish to exaggerate the problem with this, simply raise it to point out that it is an issue often overlooked but worth a second thought. See Senn (2000b) for further discussion.

16.2.20   The two-trials rule

The general requirement that scientific results have to be repeatable has been interpreted by the FDA to mean that two well-controlled studies are required to support a claim. This requirement is not uncontroversial and has a relationship to meta-analysis; it will therefore be discussed as an issue here. (See also Chapters 12, 13 and 19.)

One interpretation of the two-trials rule is that it simply reflects a more stringent standard of significance. If we regard the standard placebo-controlled clinical trial as conventionally operating with a type I error rate of 1 in 40 (see Chapter 12), then the probability that two such trials will be significant is 1 in 1600. The objection to this interpretation would seem to be that a single trial with a P-value less than 1 in 1600 ought to be equally acceptable. Also, the two-trials requirement does not seem to specify a limit to the number of nonsignificant studies there may be.

An efficient meta-analysis is supposed to summarize and use all the information from a series of trials. If this claim is true, then once the meta-analysis is available the results from the individual trials are no longer relevant. Suppose now that we have two meta-analyses each based on two trials and that the P-values in each case are highly significant and that the point estimates and confidence intervals are identical. Does it make any difference to know that in the one case (case A) both contributing trials were just significant and that in the second case (case B) one trial was more highly significant but the other not quite? If not, then the two-trials rule is superfluous.

An argument in favour of having two significant trials can be made in terms of a random-effects model. If it is possible, say, that a treatment might be effective in one population and not another, then the results from case A may be more impressive than those from case B. Similarly, if the trial protocols are different, case A is more impressive than case B: a demonstration has been given that the findings are fairly robust to the design used. However, the standard practice within the industry seems to be to carry out two identical trials in identical populations. That being so, it is hard to see what value the two-trials rule can have. Since the first edition of this book, a number of authors have carried out further investigations on the losses associated with the two-trials rule. The interested reader is referred to Darken and Ho (2004), Fisher (1999), Maca *et al.* (2002) and Rosenkranz (2002).

References

Arends LR, Hoes AW, Lubsen J, Grobbee DE, Stijnen T (2000) Baseline risk as predictor of treatment benefit: three clinical meta-re- analyses. *Statistics in Medicine* **19**: 3497–3518.

Bombardier C, Laine L, Reicin A, *et al.* (2000) Comparison of upper gastrointestinal toxicity of rofecoxib and naproxen in patients with rheumatoid arthritis. *New England Journal of Medicine* **343**: 1520–1528.

Bresalier RS, Sandler RS, Quan H, *et al.* (2005) Cardiovascular events associated with rofe-coxib in a colorectal adenoma chemoprevention trial. *New England Journal of Medicine* **352**: 1092–1102.

Darken PF, Ho S-Y (2004) A note on sample size savings with the use of a single well-controlled clinical trial to support the efficacy of a new drug. *Pharmaceutical Statistics* **3**: 61–63.

Emerson JD (1994) Combining estimates of the odds ratio: the state of the art. *Statistical Methods in Medical Research* **3**: 157–178.

Fisher LD (1999) One large, well-designed, multicenter study as an alternative to the usual FDA paradigm. *Drug Information Journal* **33**: 265–271.

Fisher RA (1932) *Statistical Methods for Research Workers*. Oliver and Boyd, Edinburgh.

Galbraith RF (1988) A note on graphical presentation of estimated odds ratios from several clinical trials. *Statistics in Medicine* **7**: 889–894.

Geller NL, Proschan M (1996) Meta-analysis of clinical trials: a consumer's guide. *Journal of Biopharmaceutical Statistics* **6**: 377–394.

Glass GE (1976) Primary, secondary and meta-analysis of research. *Educational Research* **5**: 3–8.

Goodman SN (1992) A comment on replication, p-values and evidence. *Statistics in Medicine* **11**: 875–879.

Hasselblad V, Kong DF (2001) Statistical methods for comparison to placebo in active-control studies. *Drug Information Journal* **35**: 435–449.

Hedges L, Olkin I (1985) *Statistical Method for Meta-analysis*. Academic Press, Orlando.

Hirotsu C, Yamada L (1999) Estimating odds ratios through the connected comparative experiments. *Communications in Statistics – Theory and Methods* **28**: 905–929.

International Conference on Harmonisation (1999) Statistical principles for clinical trials (ICH E9). *Statistics in Medicine* **18**: 1905–1942.

Jadad AR, Moher M, Browman GP, *et al.* (2000) Systematic reviews and meta-analyses on treatment of asthma: critical evaluation. *British Medical Journal* **320**: 537–540.

Jorgensen AW, Hilden J, Gotzsche PC (2006) Cochrane reviews compared with industry supported meta-analyses and other meta-analyses of the same drugs: systematic review. *British Medical Journal* **333**: 782.

Juni P, Nartey L, Reichenbach S, Sterchi R, Dieppe PA, Egger M (2004) Risk of cardiovascular events and rofecoxib: cumulative meta-analysis. *Lancet* **364**: 2021–2029.

Kim PS, Reicin AS (2004) Rofecoxib, Merck, and the FDA. *New England Journal of Medicine* **351**: 2875–2878; author reply 2875–2878.

Kozyrskyj AL, Hildes-Ripstein GE, Longstaffe SE, *et al.* (2000) Short course antibiotics for acute otitis media. *Cochrane Database Systematic Review*:CD001095.

Lambert PC, Sutton AJ, Burton PR, Abrams KR, Jones DR (2005) How vague is vague? A simulation study of the impact of the use of vague prior distributions in MCMC using WinBUGS. *Statistics in Medicine* **24**: 2401–2428.

Lane PW, Nelder JA (1982) Analysis of covariance and standardization as instances of prediction. *Biometrics* **38**: 613–621.

Lee Y, Nelder JA (2006) Double hierarchical generalized linear models. *Journal of the Royal Statistical Society Series C – Applied Statistics* **55**: 139–167.

LeLorier J, Gregoire G, Benhaddad A, Lapierre J, Derderian F (1997) Discrepancies between meta-analyses and subsequent large randomized, controlled trials. *New England Journal of Medicine* **337**: 536–542.

Maca J, Gallo P, Branson M, Maurer W (2002) Reconsidering some aspects of the two-trials paradigm. *Journal of Biopharmaceutical Statistics.* **12**: 107–119.

Mathew T (1999) On the equivalence of meta-analysis using literature and using individual patient data. *Biometrics* **55**: 1221–1223.

Normand SL (1999) Meta-analysis: formulating, evaluating, combining, and reporting. *Statistics in Medicine* **18**: 321–359.

Olkin I, Sampson A (1998) Comparison of meta-analysis versus analysis of variance of individual patient data. *Biometrics* **54**: 317–322.

Oxman AD, Guyatt GH (1991) Validation of an index of the quality of review articles. *Journal of Clinical Epidemiology* **44**: 1271–1278.

Petitti DB (2000) *Meta-Analysis, Decision Analysis and Cost-Effectiveness Analysis.* Oxford University Press, Oxford.

Peto R (1987) Why do we need systematic overviews of randomized trials. *Statistics in Medicine* **6**: 233–244.

Pocock SJ, Hughes MD (1990) Estimation issues in clinical trials and overviews. *Statistics in Medicine* **9**: 657–671.

Richardson W, Bablok B (1992) Clinical experience with formoterol in adults. In: Holgate ST (ed.), *Formoterol: Fast and Long-Lasting Bronchodilation.* Royal Society of Medicine Services, London.

Rosenkranz G (2002) Is it possible to claim efficacy if one of two trials is significant while the other just shows a trend? *Drug Information Journal* **36**: 875–879.

Rubin DB (1980) Randomization analysis of experimental data – the Fisher randomization test – Comment. *Journal of the American Statistical Association* **75**: 591–593.

Salsburg D (1999) Why analysis of variance is inappropriate for multiclinic trials. *Controlled Clinical Trials* **20**: 453–468.

Senn SJ (1994) Importance of trends in the interpretation of an overall odds ratio in the meta-analysis of clinical trials [letter; comment]. *Statistics in Medicine* **13**: 293–296.

Senn SJ (2000a) Letter to the Editor: In defence of the linear model. *Controlled Clinical Trials* **21**: 589–592.

Senn SJ (2000b) The many modes of meta. *Drug Information Journal* **34**: 535–549.

Senn SJ (2000c) Review is biased. *British Medical Journal* **321**: 297.

Senn SJ (2002) A comment on replication, p-values and evidence, S.N.Goodman, Statistics in Medicine 1992; 11: 875–879. *Statistics in Medicine* **21**: 2437–2444.

Senn SJ (2004) Added values: controversies concerning randomization and additivity in clinical trials. *Statistics in Medicine* **23**: 3729–3753.

Senn SJ (2005) An unreasonable prejudice against modelling? *Pharmaceutical Statistics* **4**: 87–89.

Senn SJ (2006) Double generalized linear models – Discussion. *Journal of the Royal Statistical Society Series C – Applied Statistics* **55**: 2006.

Senn SJ (2007) Trying to be precise about vagueness. *Statistics in Medicine* **26**: 1417–1430.

Sonneman E (1991) Kombination unabhängiger Tests. In: Vollmar J (ed.), *Biometrie in der chemisch-pharmazeutischen Industrie 4.* Fischer Verlag, Stuttgart.

Spiegelhalter DJ, Abrams KR, Myles JP (2003) *Bayesian Approaches to Clinical Trials and Health-Care Evaluation.* John Wiley & Sons, Chichester.

Spiegelhalter DJ, Freedman LS, Parmar MKB (1994) Bayesian approaches to randomized trials. *Journal of the Royal Statistical Society Series A – Statistics in Society* **157**: 357–387.

Thompson SG (1993) Controversies in meta-analysis: the case of the trials of serum cholesterol reduction. *Statistical Methods in Medical Research* **2**: 173–192.

Thompson SG (1994) Systematic review – Why sources of heterogeneity in metaanalysis should be investigated. *British Medical Journal* **309**: 1351–1355.

van Houwelingen H (1995) Meta-analysis, methods, limitations. *Biocybernetics and Biomedical Engineering* **15**: 53–61.

vanHouwelingen HC, Zwinderman KH, Stijnen T (1993) A bivariate approach to metaanalysis. *Statistics in Medicine* **12**: 2273–2284.

Whitehead A (2002) *Meta-analysis of Controlled Clinical Trials.* John Wiley & Sons, Ltd, Chichester.

Yates F, Cochran WG (1938) The analysis of groups of experiments. *Journal of Agricultural Science* **28**: 556–580.

16.A TECHNICAL APPENDIX

16.A.1 Interpreting effect sizes

Consider a parallel-group trial. Let values for patients in the experimental group be $Y_e \approx n(\mu_e, \sigma^2)$. Let values for patients in the experimental group be $Y_c \approx n(\mu_c, \sigma^2)$. The probability that a patient drawn at random form the experimental group has a measured value greater than that from the control group is $P[Y_e > Y_c] = P[Y_e - Y_c > 0]$. However, $(Y_e - Y_c) \approx n(\mu_e - \mu_c, \ 2\sigma^2)$. Hence we may write

$$P\left[\frac{(Y_e - Y_c) - (\mu_e - \mu_c)}{\sigma\sqrt{2}} > \frac{0 - (\mu_e - \mu_c)}{\sigma\sqrt{2}} \right] = P\left[z > -\frac{\xi}{\sqrt{2}} \right]. \qquad (16.1)$$

where z has the standard Normal distribution and ξ is the expected value of the effect size. Hence there is a simple relationship between the expected effected size and the probability of *observing* superiority of a patient under one treatment rather than another. Note, however, that this probability is a property not only of the treatment but of our method of observation. If we use a cross-over trial rather than a parallel group trial, then (if we can ignore potential difficulties with carry-over to be discussed in the next chapter) the value of $\mu_e - \mu_c$ is unaffected but σ will be much smaller. The effect size will now be larger. If we treat patients a number of times with each treatment and use the average, then the relevant standard deviation will be even smaller and effect size will be even larger. Hence the probabilities associated with effect sizes must not be interpreted as providing the proportion of patients who are better treated under the experimental than under the control.

16.A.2 Why using empirical weights biases the estimated variance of the treatment estimate

Given a series of k trials with treatment estimates, $\hat{\tau}_1, \hat{\tau}_2, \ldots, \hat{\tau}_k$, and variances, $v_1, v_2, \ldots, v_k$, then if we wish to construct a combined weighted estimator, $\hat{\tau}$, using weights $w_1, w_2, \ldots, w_k$ so that

$$\hat{\tau} = \sum_{i=1}^{k} w_i \hat{\tau}_i \qquad (16.2)$$

then (given the constraint that these weights must sum to 1), the variance of $\hat{\tau}$ is minimized if $w_i \propto 1/v_i$. In other words, to combine trials efficiently we should weight proportionately to the reciprocal of their variances. If we do this we obtain

$$\text{var}(\hat{\tau}) = \frac{1}{\sum\limits_{i=1}^{k}(1/v_i)}. \tag{16.3}$$

Since the smaller is reciprocal of the variance, the larger is the variance, and vice versa, the consequence is that trials for which the treatment estimate has a smaller variance should be given more weight. Suppose we have a series of perfectly balanced trials, so that for trial i we have n_i patients in the experimental and n_i in the control group. If we perform a meta-analysis of continuous outcomes using original data and the standard linear model, then we conventionally assume that variances within strata are equal. Where that is so, the variance of the ith treatment estimate is

$$\text{var}(\hat{\tau}_i) = \frac{2\sigma^2}{n_i}. \tag{16.4}$$

Hence, weighting by $1/v_i$ is equivalent to weighting by n_i (since $1/(2\sigma^2)$ is simply an irrelevant constant). This weighting does not involve the unknown parameter, σ^2, and is thus exact (subject to the model being correct). This would not be the case, however, where we did not believe that the within-trial variances were equal: the optimal weighting would then depend not only on the sample sizes but also on the individual variance terms σ_i^2. These, however, are unknown parameters and have to be estimated, say, using the sample variances. This will introduce a bias in the estimate of the variance of the overall treatment estimate, as may be seen quite simply by considering the case where all trials are of equal size and (unbeknown to us) the within-strata variances are also equal. Under those circumstances, the optimal weight for each trial is $1/k$ (since all trials have equal size and there are k of them). However, because the observed variances in individual trials will be subjected to random variation, we shall weight them unequally, and since this is not the optimal weighting scheme we shall produce an estimator with a true variance which is *higher* than that for the optimal scheme. When we come to estimate this variance, however, we shall produce a lower estimate than by simply weighting each trial equally. But the variance produced by weighting each trial equally would be unbiased for the optimal estimator. Hence, we shall produce a treatment estimate which has higher variance than the optimal estimator but lower estimated variance. Thus the estimated variance will be too low and in consequence the significance test based upon it too liberal.

16.A.3　Baseline risk and regression to the mean

Let R_c be the measure of risk in the control group and R_e be the measure in the experimental group. Let $\hat{\tau} = R_e - R_c$ be the estimate of the treatment effect. Let

$\mathrm{var}(R_c) = \sigma_c^2$, $\mathrm{var}(R_e) = \sigma_e^2$ and $\mathrm{cov}(R_e, R_c) = \sigma_{e,c}$, then $\mathrm{var}(\hat{\tau}) = \sigma_c^2 + \sigma_e^2 + 2\sigma_{e,c}$ and $\mathrm{cov}(\hat{\tau}, R_c) = -\sigma_c^2 - \sigma_{e,c}$, from which

$$\rho_{\hat{\tau}, R_c} = \frac{-\sigma_c^2 - \sigma_{e,c}}{\sqrt{(\sigma_c^2 + \sigma_e^2 + 2\sigma_{e,c})(\sigma_c^2)}}. \tag{16.5}$$

If we define the baseline risk to be the observed risk in the control group, then expression (16.5) gives the correlation between the estimated treatment effect and the 'baseline risk'. However, this expression has a negative correlation even where the treatment effect is constant from trial to trial. For example, where this is the case and where in addition the true baseline risk is the same from trial to trial we have, $\sigma_e^2 = \sigma_c^2 = \sigma^2$ and $\sigma_{e,c} = 0$ so that

$$\rho_{\hat{\tau}, R_c} = \frac{-\sigma^2}{\sqrt{(2\sigma^2)\sigma^2}} = -\frac{1}{\sqrt{2}}. \tag{16.6}$$

Hence, an observed correlation from trial to trial between the estimated treatment effect and the 'baseline risk' is no guarantee that the treatment effect truly varies according to the risk of patients.

17

Cross-over Trials

So shall I wait his will, the neck stroke welcome
If some great heart can hold fast, strike a hero's blow
Let him stride forward sprightly, this steel clasp boldly
This weapon once he's wielded, glad shall I forswear
Foursquare his blow I shall not fend, but meet unflinching
If he'll but pledge a prize, redeem his promise:
                                  when kept

And year and day are by
I'll meet with this adept
And then his neck I'll try
Who dares this doom accept?

Anon, *Sir Gawain and the Green Knight*

17.1 BACKGROUND

Cross-over trials are trials in which patients are allocated to sequences of treatment with the purpose of studying differences between individual treatments. For example, in a study to compare two doses of diclofenac (D1 & D2) with placebo (P), patients might be allocated at random and perhaps in equal numbers to sequences as follows:

Sequence	Period 1	Period 2	Period 3
I	D1	D2	P
II	P	D1	D2
III	D2	P	D1

The patients thus receive each of the three treatments in a different period. In this design each treatment also appears in each period. This property that the treatments are chosen so that treatments appear once in each period and once in each sequence means that the design is a **Latin square**. Another Latin square in three periods would be given by:

Sequence	Period 1	Period 2	Period 3
IV	D1	P	D2
V	D2	D1	P
VI	P	D2	D1

and in some designs in three periods and three treatments, all six sequences (for which each patient receives each treatment once) would be used. The most studied design is the so-called AB/BA cross-over comparing two treatments ('A' and 'B') in two periods in which patients are allocated at random to one of the two sequences which give the design its name.

As we have seen above, designs are possible in which there are more sequences than treatments. It is also not necessary for the number of periods to equal the number of treatments. For example, in a trial comparing two treatments we might decide to use four periods and two sequences as follows: ABBA/BAAB. Here, each patient would receive each treatment for two periods. In a so-called incomplete blocks design we might have more treatments than periods. For example, we could have compared the doses of diclofenac to placebo using the sequences

Period 1	Period 2
P	D1
D1	D2
D2	P
P	D2
D2	D1
D1	P

Obviously, cross-over designs can only be used in chronic diseases. If cure or death is a likely outcome of treatment, designs in which patients are to be treated more than once become unsuitable. (In this respect the meeting of Sir Gawain and the Green Knight which forms our chapter quotation is somewhat unusual. Each took an axe to the other's head in turn and each survived! It is also unusual for the subjects in a cross-over trail to treat each other!) Other problems will be discussed as issues below. The main advantages of cross-over designs are efficiency and the ability to study individual reaction to treatment.

An Arthurian Cross-over Trial

	First New Year	**Second New Year**
Gawain	Beheads	Is Beheaded
The Green Knight	Is Beheaded	Beheads[†]

[†] Intention to treat only.

The reader who is interested in looking at this subject in more depth should look at either Senn (2002) for a practical treatment or Jones and Kenward (2003) for a more mathematical one. Encyclopedia review articles will be found in Senn (1998), Senn (2000b) and Senn (2005b) and a review of article on cross-over trials in *Statistics in Medicine* in its first 25 years in Senn (2006).

17.2   ISSUES

17.2.1   The problem of carry-over

Most experimental designs rely on an assumption that there is no interference between units: in particular that units assigned one treatment are not affected by treatments assigned to other units. For example, in growing crops in a field, examination and interpretation of results will become extremely complex if the treatment applied to one plot could also affect growing conditions in another. Clinical trials also rely on the 'no-interference' assumption. In a parallel group trial, however, the units of the experiment are patients and it is usually difficult to suppose that treatments applied to one patient could have an affect on another. There are some exceptions. Suppose that in a trial of a psychiatric disorder patients are in the same hospital and have frequent contact with each other. It is conceivable that effecting a change on the mental condition of one patient might, through some social interaction, bring about a change in the state of another. Similarly, in a trial of prophylactic education in AIDS, it is possible that the control group may receive some of the benefit intended for the experimental group: either through secondary imparting of information or through reduction in infection rates among potential contacts. These sorts of effects might reasonably be supposed to be rare and unimportant for most indications. In a cross-over trial, on the other hand, the experimental units are not patients but episodes and it is quite easy to imagine how episodes might interfere with each other: subsequent periods of treatment for a given patient could be affected by previous treatments. This potential problem is that of *carry-over*, which has been defined as, 'the persistence (whether physically or in terms of effect) of a treatment applied in one period in a subsequent period of treatment' (Senn, 1993, 2002).

The problem of carry-over is that when we come to study results from a given period of treatment for a given patient, the results may reflect not only the effect of the current treatment but also the effect of previous treatments. This may make the disentangling of one effect from another extremely difficult. The problem can be simply illustrated with a numerical example.

Consider an AB/BA cross-over trial in extremely stable asthmatic patients who in the absence of treatment will show no change over time. The trial is to compare a beta-agonist with placebo. Suppose that the outcome measure is forced expiratory volume in one second (FEV_1) and suppose that the patients in the two groups are the same on average and that FEV_1 under placebo is 2000 ml and that the treatment effect is 300 ml. In that case the results (mean FEV_1) that we expect to see are given in Table 17.1, in which the results for the beta-agonist have been set at 2300 ml so that the difference from placebo, recorded in the final column, recovers the treatment effect of 300 ml, not only when averaged over both sequences, but individually in each sequence also.

Table 17.1 FEV_1 readings in ml for patients in a cross-over trial.

Sequence	Period 1	Period 2	Treatment difference
Placebo/beta-agonist	2000	2300	300
Beta-agonist/placebo	2300	2000	300
MEAN			300

Table 17.2 FEV_1 readings in ml for patients in a cross-over trial. The case where there are differences between sequences.

Sequence	Period 1	Period 2	Treatment difference
Placebo/beta-agonist	2350	2650	300
Beta-agonist/placebo	2300	2000	300
MEAN			300

Now let us relax the assumption that the patients were identical while retaining our other assumptions and suppose that patients in the first sequence have an FEV_1 reading which is 350 ml higher under identical circumstances to those in the second sequence. We thus need to increase the readings in the first sequence of Table 17.1 by 350 ml to reach the position in Table 17.2. Of course, although the individual readings are affected, the differences are recovered as before.

Now suppose, however, that there is a secular trend causing treatment values to increase by 100 ml in the second period compared with the first. We then need to take the values in the second period in Table 17.2 and add 100 to reach the position in Table 17.3. We see that the treatment effect of 300 ml (which still applies) is not recovered from each sequence. However it *is* recovered from the average of the two sequences, so that the cross-over trial is still capable of being used in these circumstances.

Now suppose, that the beta-agonist is still completely effective in the second period despite being discontinued and replaced by placebo, which would be an extreme form of carry-over. This will not affect results from the first sequence because the patients receive the beta-agonist second. However, for the second sequence it means that the results in period 2 must be increased by 300 compared with the position in Table 17.3. The results are given in Table 17.4.

We see that the treatment effect is no longer recovered, the mean of the differences over the two sequences being 150 ml. In fact, the apparent treatment effect has been

Table 17.3 FEV_1 readings in ml for patients in a cross-over trial. The case where there are differences between sequences and periods.

Sequence	Period 1	Period 2	Treatment difference
Placebo/beta-agonist	2350	2750	400
Beta-agonist/placebo	2300	2100	200
MEAN			300

Table 17.4 FEV_1 readings in ml for patients in a cross-over trial. The case where there are differences between sequences and periods and also a carry-over effect.

Sequence	Period 1	Period 2	Treatment difference
Placebo/beta-agonist	2350	2750	400
Beta-agonist/placebo	2300	2400	−100
MEAN			150

halved for the simple reason that because the treatment effect is permanent, the sequence beta-agonist – placebo yields no information about the effect at all. The only information comes from the other sequence. However, this sequence on its own would also not yield a valid estimate of the treatment effect as the secular change of 100 ml has inflated the difference.

We thus see that carry-over is a potential problem for cross-over trials.

17.2.2   Is carry-over uniquely a problem for cross-over trials?

Carry-over can also pose a problem for parallel-group trials, but less plausibly so. Consider a parallel-group trial in asthma of a new beta-agonist (let us call it *lasterol*) against salbutamol (known as albuterol in the USA), a well established beta-agonist. Most patients recruited to the trial will have been taking salbutamol for many years. If tachyphylaxis affects these patients they will no longer achieve the same relief with the salbutamol (this may of course be misinterpreted as a secular worsening of their asthma). It may be that lasterol is similarly effective to salbutamol and would also show tachyphylaxis in the course of time but that this will not set in during the course of the trial. In that case, because none of the patients has been treated with lasterol before, it will be shown in a rather flattering light. The experiment would then be biased by a form of carry-over which only affected the patients randomized to salbutamol. Lasterol would falsely be regarded as being superior to salbutamol and in the course of time (once lasterol had become the standard) it would be possible to repeat the experiment, proving that salbutamol was superior after all.

Nonetheless, the conclusion that lasterol was superior for *these* patients under *these* circumstances *would* be correct and, of course, the potential for this sort of problem is less with the parallel-group trial than for cross-over trials. It is probably fair to say that carry-over can be ignored for most parallel-group trials but that the possibility of the phenomenon must be taken seriously in planning cross-over trials.

17.2.3   Can we test for carry-over?

In principle it is *possible* to test for carry-over; the issue is rather whether the test is *useful* (see also below). There are two principal difficulties. For the simple AB/BA design, a test is available but it has extremely low power. Thus appreciable carry-over could occur without our being able to detect it. For more complex designs such as the AABB/BBAA design (a design in two sequences and four periods), a more powerful test is available but at the expense of assuming that carry-over can only be of a particular form. We now proceed to discuss both of these cases in more detail.

In the case of the AB/BA cross-over, a test for carry-over is possible if the totals (or equivalently the mean) responses for the two sequences are compared. The argument can be put like this. (1) In constructing totals for a given patient in a given sequence, the effects of both periods and both treatments must be reflected since each patient is studied in each of two periods and each patient is given each of the two treatments. (2) Therefore, if these totals are found to be different from one sequence to another, this cannot be because of treatment or period effects. (3) If, however, carry-over occurs, then the order in which drugs is given will be important (see the example in section 17.2.1 above), and hence the totals could differ from sequence to sequence as a result of carry-over. (4) It is true that in comparing one sequence with another we are comparing different patients, but this sort of comparison is made all the time in parallel randomized clinical trials and there is no reason (provided we have randomized) why the comparison should not be made here. (5) Hence, if we observe that the extent to which such totals differ from one sequence to another is rather improbably large, then either a rare event has occurred or carry-over has caused a difference between sequences. We thus we have the basis of a test of significance.

This test has very low power, however, for three reasons. (1) It is a between-patient test for a trial which has been designed to use within-patient differences to detect treatment effects. (2) The carry-over effect where it occurs is likely to be somewhat smaller than the pure effect of treatment. (3) The carry-over is in any case only manifested in the second period. Therefore, although it is necessary to use the totals to compare sequences to account for other effects that might bias the test of carry-over, the direct information for carry-over comes only from the second period and the effect of this is diluted. In short, although a test of carry-over is available it is too weak to be of much use.

When we move to designs in more than two periods the position is more complicated. There, more powerful tests for carry-over are available but usually only at the expense of making what are (in my view) quite unreasonable assumptions about the form that carry-over will take. We shall not treat this issue directly here but cover the related one of eliminating carry-over in order to illustrate the problem.

17.2.4   Can we eliminate the effect of carry-over?

A simple solution for the AB/BA cross-over is simply to ignore the second-period values, treating the whole as if it were a parallel-group trial. But this is effectively no solution at all, since it destroys the whole purpose of running a cross-over trial. Hence, it is, in my view, inadmissible. For more complex designs other approaches have been advocated.

Consider, for example, the design in four periods, two treatments and two sequences: AABB and BBAA. Table 17.5 gives weights which have been proposed for estimating the treatment effect.

Table 17.5   Weights for an AABB/BBAA cross-over.

Sequence	Period 1	Period 2	Period 3	Period 4
AABB	A 6/20	A a 4/20	B a $-$ 7/20	B b $-$ 3/20
BBAA	B $-$6/20	B b $-$ 4/20	A a 7/20	A a 3/20

The purpose of these weights may be explained as follows. With two sequences and four periods we shall be able to calculate eight 'cell means': means for all the patients in a given sequence in a given period. Our treatment estimate will simply be a weighted combination of these cell means, which is to say that we shall take these cell means, multiply them by the weights, and add the results together. If we study the weights in Table 17.5 we see that they have the following properties: (1) they add to zero in any row, thus eliminating any pure differences between patients; (2) they add to zero in any column, thus eliminating any pure differences between periods; (3) they add to 1 over the cells labelled A and to -1 over the cells labelled B, thus estimating the treatment effect $(A - B)$. They are not, of course the only weights which have this property. For example, the weights $1/4$, $1/4$, $-1/4$ $-1/4$ for the first sequence and $-1/4$, $-1/4$, $1/4$, $1/4$ for the second sequence would also have these three properties. The supposed advantage, however, of the weights in Table 17.5 is that over the cells labelled a and b they add to zero. Now if it were the case that carry-over lasted only for one period and depended only on the previous treatment and we were to use the label a for carry-over from A and b for carry-over from B, we should find that the cells so labelled would be the ones where these carry-over effects occurred. Hence, the scheme of weights would eliminate this form of carry-over.

Unfortunately, however, although this form of adjustment for carry-over has enjoyed a considerable vogue among statisticians, it is not very reasonable when examined in the light of theories of pharmacology (Senn, 1993, 2002; Sheiner *et al.*, 1991). Consider a multiple-dose trial comparing an active treatment A with a placebo B. For example, we might divide a trial in rheumatism into four fortnightly periods in which twice-daily doses of either diclofenac (A) or placebo (B) were given. We should usually hope that after a few doses the active treatment will have reached steady state. There can thus be no or little carry-over from the first A to the second A. Hence, the value of a in the second period for sequence AABB would be very small. On the other hand, carry-over after two periods of A into B might be appreciable. Hence the value of a in the third period of the same sequence might much larger. If this were the case, far from eliminating carry-over, the weights given in Table 17.5 might make matters worse. For this reason I am convinced that this mathematical approach to carry-over is not effective.

> Some drug developers are convinced that clinical trials should be like skiing: stick to the parallels and avoid the cross-overs.

This does not mean that carry-over cannot be eliminated (or at least rendered innocuous). Consider, for example, the trial comparing diclofenac to placebo just discussed. As regards eliminating the effect of carry-over, using the weights 0, $1/2$, 0, $-1/2$ for the first sequence and 0, $-1/2$, 0, $1/2$ for the second sequence must be at least as successful as the scheme of weights in Table 17.5. This is because in multidose trials we are interested in estimating the steady-state effects of treatment. Hence, where carry-over occurs, we would be more interested in estimating the difference $(A + a) - (B + b)$. (Of course, in a placebo-controlled trial we would expect b to be zero but this does not really affect the argument.) By studying these new weights and Table 17.5, it will be seen that this difference is in fact recovered and, furthermore, that the only assumption about carry-over required is that it lasts one period as defined (the other assumption that it depends only on the engendering and not the perturbed treatment is not required). However, since the results at the end of periods 1 and 3 are irrelevant if this scheme of weights is used, then we might as well redefine the cross-over as an AB/BA cross-over with periods twice as long as previously. This appears to have got us back to square one.

If this apparent paradox is considered carefully, however, it will be seen to arise from the arbitrary nature of 'periods'. One of the tasks of physician and statistician in planning a clinical trial is that of determining the length of the period of study (this is true even for a parallel-group trial). Therefore, it is inappropriate to regard the period as being 'given' and consider how the trial may be accommodated to this constraint. The period is also up for discussion and, once this is appreciated, it can easily be understood that models which rely on the carry-over lasting for one 'period' are not credible. What is needed is to consider the *time* for which carry-over is likely to last and plan the trial accordingly. The nature of periods in cross-over trials will be discussed further in section 17.2.9

Thus, the best approach to planning cross-over trials is to consider carefully, in the light of pharmacokinetic and general pharmacological theories, what wash-out period is required. Such wash-out periods can either be *passive*, in that no treatment is given, or *active*. Active wash-out periods are used either instead of or as well as passive wash-outs and are periods of treatment during which no measurements are taken (or, if taken, are not used for analysis). Of course such an approach can offer no guarantees, but neither can any other. It is always conceivable that some mistake can be made regarding the necessary wash-out period. Indeed, there are famous cases in medical research where extreme forms of carry-over have occurred. An interesting example cited by Nelson (1959) concerns Pasteur's investigation of chicken cholera. Some chickens were accidentally inoculated with a weak culture; when they recovered and, to all apparent intents and purposes, were as before, Pasteur used them again so as not to waste them. However, they then proved to be resistant to an inoculation that would have killed an ordinary chicken.

We can never guarantee that such extreme cases might not occur. A drug which was believed to be palliative might actually be curative. Or a drug might potentiate some extreme reaction for good or ill of another. What is required, however, is a mature and realistic approach to drug development. This recognizes that (a) pharmacology is the thread that links drug development, (b) some assumptions are necessary to make any progress and (c) perfection is impossible.

17.2.5   Carry-over and the two-stage procedure

For many years it was supposed that an appropriate way to analyse AB/BA cross-over trials was to use the so-called 'two-stage procedure' originally described in detail by Grizzle (Grieve, 1982; Grizzle, 1965, 1974) and also clearly illustrated by Hills and Armitage (Hills and Armitage, 1979). This proceeded via a preliminary test for carry-over as defined in Section 17.2.3. Because of its low power, a test at the 10% level of significance was usually proposed. If this was significant, then the second-period data were discarded and the treatment effect was judged using the first-period data only, as if they had come from a parallel-group trial. Of course, the trialist would hope that the

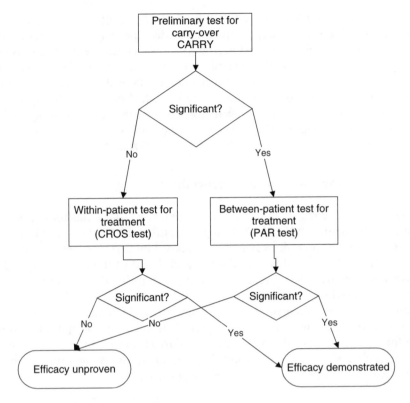

Figure 17.1   The two-stage procedure.

preliminary test for carry-over would not be significant, as this would then be taken to justify using the data from both periods, thus exploiting the precision of the cross-over trial. The procedure is illustrated in Figure 17.1, where the three tests potentially involved are labelled CARRY (for the test for carry-over), CROS (for the hoped for within-patient test of the treatment effect) and PAR (for the fall-back parallel-group test using first-period data only).

However, in a very important investigation, Freeman (1989) was able to show that this procedure, far from dealing with the bias due to carry-over, actually made it worse. The exact reason for this is too technical an issue to deal with thoroughly in this book but has been dealt with at length elsewhere (Senn, 1993, 1995a,b, 2002). Statistical screening procedures potentially suffer from the same disadvantages as medical screening procedures: what at first sight may appear beneficial may, when examined carefully, turn out to be harmful. Whether a medical screening procedure turns out to be beneficial depends on many things: the sensitivity and specificity of the test, the prevalence of disease and the consequences of treating the well as if they were ill and the ill as if they were well. When looked at in these terms, the two-stage procedure is indefensible.

The reason has to do with the conditional behaviour or the PAR test given that significance has been found. If by chance, the random allocation is such that the patients happen to be rather different between the two sequences, we will tend to conclude that there is a carry-over effect. However, under such circumstances, the two-stage procedure invites us to abandon the CROS test, which (being a within-patient test) is not affected by differences between patients, and use instead the PAR test, which is affected by differences. Hence, looked at from this perspective the procedure is back to front. The net consequence is that overall, the procedure is too liberal. For the case where there is in fact no carry-over, at a nominally claimed significance level of 5%, the type I error rate for the test of the treatment effect is, in fact, between 7% and 9.5%. Conditionally, the situation is even worse. Given that one has proceeded down the right-hand arm of Figure 17.1 (an event which will occur in at least 10% of all cases), the type I error rate lies somewhere between 25% and 50%.

17.2.6   Correcting the two-stage procedure

It is, in fact, possible to reform the two stage procedure so that it has the correct overall type I error rate (Senn, 1996, 1997; Wang and Hung, 1997). One way of doing this is to use the two-stage procedure exactly as proposed by Grizzle except to carry out the PAR test at the 0.5% level rather than the 5% level. The PAR test then has a conditional type I error rate which lies between 2.5% and 5% and this then ensures that overall the two-stage procedure has correct size.

Although (as far as I am aware) I was the first to draw attention to how this might be done, I do not recommend it. Quite apart from all the philosophical objections I have to this approach, once the two-stage procedure is corrected in this way, its power advantage compared with always using CROS seems to disappear under all plausible circumstances. Thus, I recommend always using CROS.

17.2.7   Cross-over trials and patient-by-treatment interaction

This is an issue which places cross-over trials in a more positive light. There is one particular task for which they are supremely useful and for which no parallel-group trial, however many patients are recruited on to it, can match them. Because the cross-over paradigm permits one to study patients on all treatments being compared, it is possible to use such designs to identify individual reaction to treatment. The ideal device for such an investigation is, in fact, a trial in which each patient receives each treatment more than once. It is then possible to compare the extent to which differences between different treatments given to the same patient vary from patient to patient with the extent to which the results for the same treatment vary when given to the same patient. This enables one to isolate a component of variation due to treatment-by-patient interaction (Senn, 2001, 2003).

This topic will not be considered further here but is dealt with separately in Chapter 18 on *n*-of-1 trials and also in Chapter 25 on pharmacogenetics.

17.2.8   Attitudes to carry-over in single dose and multidose cross-overs

Many cross-over trials are carried out in early phases of drug development or in order to investigate rather specialist questions such as, the bioequivalence of two formulations. (This particular topic is covered in detail in Chapter 22.). Most such studies are single-dose studies. The subject is given a single dose of a treatment in a given period and then the pharmacokinetic or pharmacodynamic effects of the treatment are studied over time. Concerns about carry-over in such cases are largely artificial. It is usually possible to arrange for a wash-out period that is many times the presumed duration of action of the drug. In any case, whatever effects will be found will receive their ultimate validation in the phase III therapeutic studies that will be run and these will hardly ever be cross-over studies.

There is also some empirical evidence that for such single-dose studies the wash-out period is generally successful. In a large series of bioequivalence studies carried out in 20 drug classes over a 10-year period, consisting of 324 and 96 three period designs, D'Angelo *et al.* (2001) reported the results of test for significance in carry-over for both area under the curve (AUC) and concentration maximum (C_{max}). The resulting distributions of *P*-values were indistinguishable from that of a uniform distribution (Senn *et al.*, 2004), which is what one would expect if the null hypotheses of no carry-over were true. Of course, these are a rather special class of study and one should be cautious about extending the results to single-dose studies generally. Nevertheless, it is my personal opinion that the usual concern regarding studies of this sort is somewhat exaggerated.

Somewhat rarer than single-dose studies are multidose studies. Here, during a given treatment period the patients will be dosed using the sort of regular dosing schedule, for example twice daily, that it is intended will be used when and if the drug is on the market. The period will have to be chosen to be of sufficient length for the treatment to reach steady state. It is more likely to be the case – although it is by no means regularly the case – that the outcome being studied will be therapeutic. Concerns about potential carry-over are more serious for this sort of study, although it should be appreciated that the judgement about how long it takes for the treatment to reach steady state in its effects is one that is no different in kind from the judgement about how long it takes to wear off and that the former is required for any parallel-group trial also. The strategy of an active wash-out period discussed in section 17.2.4 is often used for such studies.

17.2.9   The meaning of period

Some rather bizarre recommendations have been made in the statistical literature by statisticians who are unfamiliar with the way cross-over trials are actually run. For, example, both Jones and Donev and John *et al.* (John *et al.*, 2004; Jones and Donev, 1996) have considered the possibility of modifying the subsequent schedule of treatments in a multiperiod design once the results from the first two periods (say) have been studied.

This is a logistic impossibility, since patients are recruited for a clinical trial when they fall ill and they do not fall ill simultaneously (Senn, 2005c). In practice, by the time all patients have received the second period of treatment, most will have completed the trial. The misunderstanding arises through a misunderstanding of the term *period*. This has a relative not an absolute significance. Thus, period 2 is not a given calendar period in which all patients receive treatment but simply the second course of treatment for each patient, the actual calendar time depending on when the patient was recruited. One occasionally sees *order* used instead of *period* as a term, although period is more usually employed by medical statisticians who are generally so familiar with the practical realities of trial design that they risk no danger of being confused about this.

In general far too little attention has been paid to practical reality by those working on design theory for cross-over trials. Another issue regarding periods to which attention has already been drawn in section 17.2.4 is that for a multidose trial the length of the period has to be determined by the trialist. Thus the total time under observation may be the more natural primitive constraint than the the number of periods. Two different statisticians, for example, might divide four available months of observation into different numbers of periods, for example, two periods of 2 months' duration or four of 1 month's duration.

The reader should be warned that much of the extensive literature on 'optimal' design of cross-over trials is extremely impractical (Senn, 2005a, 2006).

17.2.10   A Bayesian approach can deal with the problem of carry-over

In theory this is correct. The problem in practice is that of determining a suitable joint prior for carry-over and the treatment effect. Establishing the priors independently can lead to contradictions. Consider, for example, an AB/BA cross-over trial reported by Martin and Browning, (1985) for which a Bayesian analysis was produced by Racine *et al.* (1986). The uninformative priors used imply that it was just as likely, *a priori* that the carry-over would exceed the treatment effect in magnitude as that the treatment effect would exceed the carry-over. The direct effect of treatment was measured only 4–8 hours after treatment, whereas the wash-out period was 6 weeks or more than 125 times as long. Given these details of the trial, the implied prior joint distribution of carry-over and treatment is most implausible (Senn, 2000a). In my opinion, if a Bayesian approach is to prove useful in this context it will have to be grounded in the sort of realistic mechanistic pharmacokinetic and pharmacodynamic tradition for which carry-over is analysed as a time-modified phenomenon that has is explained by the same sort of model that explains the direct effect of treatment. An example of this approach is the paper of (Sheiner *et al.*, 1991).

References

D'Angelo G, Potvin D, Turgeon J (2001) Carryover effects in bioequivalence studies. *Journal of Biopharmaceutical Statistics* **11**: 27–36.

Freeman P (1989) The performance of the two-stage analysis of two-treatment, two-period cross-over trials. *Statistics in Medicine* **8**: 1421–1432.

Grieve AP (1982) The two-period changeover design in clinical trials [letter]. *Biometrics* **38**: 517.

Grizzle JE (1965) The two-period change over design and its use in clinical trials. *Biometrics* **21**: 467–480.

Grizzle JE (1974) Correction to Grizzle (1965). *Biometrics* **30**: 727.

Hills M, Armitage P (1979) The two-period cross-over clinical trial. *British Journal of Clinical Pharmacology* **8**: 7–20.

John JA, Russell KG, Whitaker D (2004) CrossOver: an algorithm for the construction of efficient cross-over designs. *Statistics in Medicine* **23**: 2645–2658.

Jones B, Donev AN (1996) Modelling and design of cross-over trials. *Statistics in Medicine* **15**: 1435–1446.

Jones B, Kenward M (2003) *Design and Analysis of Cross-over Trials*. Chapman and Hall, London.

Martin A, Browning RC (1985) Metoprolol in the aged hypertensive: a comparison of two dosage schedules. *Postgraduate Medical Journal* **61**: 225–227.

Nelson R (1959) The simple economics of basic scientific research. *Journal of Political Economy* June:297–307.

Racine A, Grieve AP, Fluhler H, Smith AFM (1986) Bayesian methods in practice – experiences in the pharmaceutical industry. *Journal of the Royal Statistical Society Series C – Applied Statistics* **35**: 93–150.

Senn SJ (1993) *Cross-over Trials in Clinical Research*. John Wiley & Sons, Ltd, Chichester.

Senn SJ (1995a) Cross-over trials at the cross-roads? *Applied Clinical Trials* **4**: 24–31.

Senn SJ (1995b) Some controversies in designing and analysing cross-over trials. *Biocybernetics and Biomedical Engineering* **15**: 27–39.

Senn SJ (1996) The AB/BA cross-over: how to perform the two-stage analysis if you can't be persuaded that you shouldn't. In: Hansen B, de Ridder M (eds), *Liber Amicorum Roel van Strik*. Erasmus University, Rotterdam, pp. 93–100.

Senn SJ (1997) The case for cross-over trials in phase III [letter; comment]. *Statistics in Medicine* **16**: 2021–2022.

Senn SJ (1998) Cross-over trials. In: Armitage P, Colton T (eds), *Encyclopedia in Biostatistics*. John Wiley & Sons, Inc., New York, pp. 1033–1049.

Senn SJ (2000a) Consensus and controversy in pharmaceutical statistics (with discussion). *The Statistician* **49**: 135–176.

Senn SJ (2000b) Crossover design. In: Chow SC, Liu JP (eds), *Encyclopedia of Biopharmaceutical Statistics*. Marcel Dekker, New York, pp. 142–149.

Senn SJ (2001) Individual therapy: new dawn or false dawn. *Drug Information Journal* **35**: 1479–1494.

Senn SJ (2002) *Cross-over Trials in Clinical Research* (2nd edition). John Wiley & Sons, Ltd, Chichester.

Senn SJ (2003) Author's Reply to Walter and Guyatt. *Drug Information Journal* **37**: 7–10.

Senn SJ (2005a) At cross-purposes: cross-over trials in theory and practice. *International Chinese Statistical Association Bulletin* 50–53.

Senn SJ (2005b) Cross-over trials. In: Everitt BS, Palmer CR (eds), *Encyclopaedic Companion to Medical Statistics*. Hodder Arnold, London, pp. 88–91.

Senn SJ (2005c) Letter to the editor: Misunderstandings regarding clinical cross-over trials. *Statistics in Medicine* **24**: 3675–3678.

Senn SJ (2006) Cross-over trials in statistics in medicine: the first '25' years. *Statistics in Medicine* **25**: 3430–3442.

Senn SJ, D'Angelo G, Potvin D (2004) Carry-over in cross-over trials in bioequivalence: theoretical concerns and empirical evidence. *Pharmaceutical Statistics* **3**: 133–142.

Sheiner LB, Hashimoto Y, Beal SL (1991) A simulation study comparing designs for dose-ranging. *Statistics in Medicine* **10**: 303–321.

Wang SJ, Hung HM (1997) Use of two-stage test statistic in the two-period crossover trials. *Biometrics* **53**: 1081–1091.

18

n-of-1 Trials

No man is an island entire in it self

John Donne, *For whom the Bell Tolls*

There are probably no two men in existence on whom the drug acts in exactly the same manner.

Wilkie Collins, *The Moonstone*

If we could, this year, exactly reproduce, in your case, the conditions as they existed last year, it is physiologically certain that we should arrive at exactly the same result. But this – there is no denying it – is simply impossible.

Wilkie Collins, *The Moonstone.*

18.1 BACKGROUND

One man's meat is another man's poison. Simple and common medicines such as penicillin and aspirin are notorious for their ability to cause adverse reactions in a minority of patients. If their side-effects vary from individual to individual, might their main effects not also be expected to do so, and is this not something which we should expect of all medicines? Patients come in different ages, sexes and sizes. They differ with respect to their ability to absorb, metabolize and eliminate drugs. They may have differing co-morbidity. Some may lack enzymes which most possess. The more we learn about genetics, the more we identify factors which can have an effect on health. Patients also differ with respect to lifestyles and severity of disease. These are all reasons to suspect that, when it comes to therapy, 'one size fits all' may be an inappropriate philosophy.

On the other hand, there appears to be a near-universal human tendency to underestimate the effects of chance. Two apparently identical light-bulbs may have very different lifetimes. There may be nothing predictable about the eventual difference between the two yet, due to something we have little choice but to label 'chance', this may be large. In a similar way, with patients we find that they may differ considerably from day to day, even when given the same treatment. We should be cautious, therefore, when comparing two patients given the same treatment, in ascribing to individual factors a difference which may be transient and due to chance.

Both of these two opposing considerations are reflected in our chapter quotations from *The Moonstone* concerning the effect of opium. The plot of that novel hinges on the

Statistical Issues in Drug Development/2nd Edition   Stephen Senn
© 2007 John Wiley & Sons, Ltd

fact that the hero Franklin Blake takes a diamond, the Moonstone of the story, while under the influence of a dose of opium administered to him without his knowledge, and one of whose effects appears to be to erase all memory of the incident. In order to stage a reconstruction of his actions on the fateful night, he is to be given a second dose of opium. It is known from a physician's notes that he was given 'five and twenty minims of laudanum' on the night in question. However, various circumstances have changed in the meantime and there is no certainty that the same dose will reproduce the same effect, even though given to the same person. (In the end it is decided to give him 40 minims and this does the trick.)

These two features are at the heart of this chapter. The fact that different patients respond differently to treatment suggests that individualizing therapy may increase the utility of treatments considerably; that patients vary in their response from occasion to occasion suggests that establishing which treatments are best for which patients may be extremely difficult. For example, in a clinical trial we generally need a large sample of patients just in order to be able to say something about treatment effects in general. As we saw in Chapter 9, even our ability to say something about the effect of treatments on subgroups is limited. One might suppose, continuing the argument, that to say something definitive about an individual patient is almost impossible. There are exceptions, however. The first is where the course of the untreated disease is so predictable that there is little difficulty in establishing in a given patient whether the treatment has worked or not by comparing the state of the patient after treatment to that which would have occurred. (Note the importance of our general notions of causality in all this.) However, very few treatments fall into this category. A famous candidate, perhaps, is rabies, where the efficacy of Pasteur's vaccine was dramatically demonstrated in 1885 by treating a single boy. (Although note that not all who are bitten by rabid dogs and are untreated develop rabies, so that the demonstration is short of being perfect.) A second approach, which is possible for chronic diseases, is to turn the mechanism of the clinical trial inwards. Just as we repeatedly study different patients to determine the effects of treatments in general, so we study repeated episodes of treatment in a given patient in order to establish the effects of treatment for him or her.

Such trials are extremely old. In fact, examples pre-date the modern era of randomized clinical trials. An early example is the trial in 11 inmates of the Insane Asylum of Kalamazoo carried out by Cushny and Peebles at the beginning of the 20th century and used by Student to illustrate the *t*-test (Cushny and Peebles, 1905; Senn and Richardson, 1994; Student, 1908). In modern times, such trials have been referred to as '*n*-of-1' trials (Guyatt *et al.*, 1990; Johannessen, 1991) and may be defined as follows. *An 'n-of-1' trial is a trial in which a number of episodes of treatment are studied in a single patient, usually with a view to making inferences about the effect of treatment on that patient.* We shall now discuss some of the issues, but before we do we so draw attention to some important links with other chapters. In Chapter 8, 'The Measurement of Treatment Effects', we covered matters to do with patient-by-treatment interaction. Where we run series of '*n*-of-1' trials, we may regard ourselves as having run one experiment on at least two levels (patients and episodes). This means that many of the issues to do with *n*-of-1 trials are similar to those encountered in analysing muticentre trials (Chapter 14), where the levels are centres and patients, or in carrying out a meta-analysis of a series of trials (Chapter 16), where the levels are trials and patients. By virtue of the fact that *n*-of-1 trials are within-patient studies, they also share many of the features of cross-over trials (Senn, 2002) discussed in Chapter 17.

18.2   ISSUES

18.2.1   At which stage of drug development should *n*-of-1 trials be used?

There is an opinion that *n*-of-1 trials should only be employed late in drug development (Lewis, 1991). Indeed, it is an opinion I have expressed myself (Senn, 1993). Essentially the argument is that establishing the effect on individual patients of treatment is a refinement of a more important question: 'Does the treatment work?' If that is so, the broader question should be answered first. Furthermore, for reasons given in Chapter 9, even where individuals react differently to treatment there is usually some value in using to some extent the results of others to predict the effects. Of course, given a large amount of data on a given patient we do not need results from others. However, even where we run *n*-of-1 trials it is rarely the case that we have very large amounts of data on individual patients. For example, in a series of trials run by March *et al.* each of a number of patients suffering from osteoarthritis was randomly allocated to receive either diclofenac or placebo in three pairs of periods (March *et al.*, 1994). However, the individual trials had little power to detect appropriate treatment differences and it was necessary to look at the results in totality in order to interpret the trial correctly (Senn *et al.*, 1995). In fact, it is a classic use of random effect models to 'shrink' individual effects closer to the overall mean.

Furthermore, where there are true differences between patients, a more efficient way to gain information about the effect of a treatment with the object simply of establishing that it works would be to run an AB/BA cross-over. There is more information to be gained about the average effects of treatment under such circumstances by adding more patients rather than more periods. Hence in phase II there is generally little point in running *n*-of-1 trials.

The above argument presupposes, however, that more patients can be obtained. For rare diseases, for example Gilles de la Tourette syndrome, this may not be possible. (I am grateful to Arend Heyting for pointing this out to me.) Under such circumstances (and given that the condition is chronic), repeatedly treating the few patients available may be the only way to gain experimental material.

18.2.2   *P*-values and *n*-of-1 trials

It is almost never the case that we run a single *n*-of-1 trial. Usually we run a series using a number of patients. It has been suggested that such a series may be adequately analysed by calculating the *P*-value for the treatment effect for each patient and noting in which cases the treatment was significant and in which it was not.

Of course, many statisticians (notably, but not exclusively, the Bayesians) think that *P*-values are generally inappropriate, whatever the context. There are, however, further reservations which may be applied to *n*-of-1 trials. First, there is the same problem which arises in trials of equivalence. Failure to find a significant difference does not imply that none exists. Many *n*-of-1 trials will have rather low power for individual patients. Therefore, there will be many false-negative results. Figure 18.1 illustrates the distribution of a one-sided *P*-value for different *n*-of-1 trials on the assumption that the test statistic has a Normal distribution. The case where the treatment is ineffective is illustrated. This leads to a uniform distribution. Cases are also illustrated where the

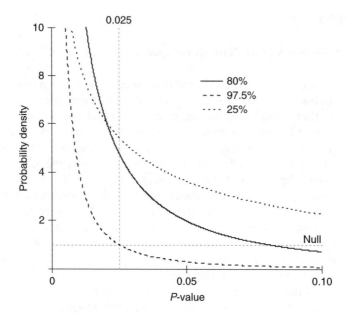

Figure 18.1   Distribution of a one-sided *P*-value given as a function of power given a nominal size of 0.025. (The range of *P*-values illustrated is restricted to 0.1 or less in order to produce a more readable graph.)

power to detect a genuine treatment effect is respectively 0.25, 0.8 and 0.975. Second, we also have the general problem of multiplicity of *P*-values. Even where the treatment is ineffective it is likely that the odd patient will have a low *P*-value if we are treating many. Third, treating information on patients as completely independent is inefficient and runs contrary to general medical practice: how could we have medical handbooks describing the therapeutic effects of any treatments if we had to start from scratch with every new patient? Fourth, it is not clear what we should adopt as the null hypothesis. Consider a series of *n*-of-1 trials where there is overwhelming evidence that on average the experimental treatment is superior to the control. Is it then logical to accept as the null hypothesis for individual trials that the treatment effects are the same?

18.2.3   Random-effects analysis

A way to use information from other patients together with information from an individual patient, in a way which weights the two appropriately, for the purpose of producing treatment estimates for him or her is to construct a random-effect model (Senn, 1991). An alternative reason for using such a model might be to describe the true distribution of treatment effects in patients not studied. A fixed-effects model cannot do this since either it makes the assumption that all patients react identically to treatment or it can be regarded as a means of testing whether there is a treatment effect in at least some patients. (See Chapter 14 for a discussion.) If it is truly desired to say something about the distribution of treatment effects in patients in general, then the combination of a series of *n*-of-1 trials together with a random-effects model is the most powerful available.

Table 18.1 Number of pairs of periods Y in which patients preferred amitriptyline to placebo as a ratio of the number n of pairs of periods tested for 23 subjects. The number of patients exhibiting the given pattern of response Y/n is given by f.

Y/n	0/3	1/3	2/3	3/3	3/4	4/4	4/6	Total
f	1	6	5	5	3	2	1	23

In fact, one can go further than this and suggest that unless a series of n-of-1 trials is conducted and analysed appropriately using a random effects model, it will generally not be possible to tease out the differential sources of variation in a trial: between-patient, within-patient and treatment-by-patient interaction. This point, for example, was misunderstood by Guyatt *et al.* (1998). See (Senn, 2001, 2003, 2004) for a discussion.

As an example of the sort of thing that can be done, consider data from the series of 23 placebo-controlled n-of-1 trials of amitriptyline in fibromyalgia originally reported by Jaeschke *et al.* (1991) as reported by Schluter and Ware (2005). These data show the number of preferences Y expressed in n pairs of periods by the 23 patients. In Table 18.1 the data are given in the form $Y/n, f$, where f is the number of patients who expressed Y preferences in n periods.

Analysing these data using the hierarchical generalized approach (HGLM) of Lee and Nelder (1996) in GenStat or using proc nlmixed of SAS produces extremely similar results. For both approaches, it is assumed that each patient has his or her own probability P of preferring active treatment in a pair of periods. The number of preferences, Y in n pairs of periods is binomially distributed (n, P). Finally it is assumed that the logit $\theta = \log\{P/(1-P)\}$ is distributed Normally over all patients with mean μ and variance σ^2. The effect of fitting is shown in Figure 18.2. (For the sake of brevity only the HGLM results are given here; the proc nlmixed results are almost identical.)

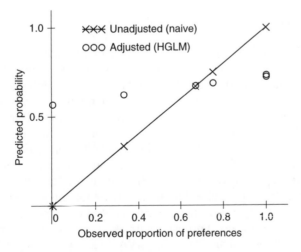

Figure 18.2 Raw and shrunk probabilities of preferring treatment to placebo for the trial reported in Jaeschke *et al.* (1991) using the approach of Lee and Nelder (1996).

The figure plots the adjusted 'shrunk' probabilities under the model against the raw probabilities, Y/n. For comparison, the raw probabilities are plotted against themselves. Note that although there are 23 patients, as can be seen from Table 18.1, there are only seven different types of results and these yield only five different raw probabilities since $3/3 = 4/4$ and $2/3 = 4/6$. What is noticeable is how strong the shrinkage is. In fact, the shrunk prediction for $4/6$ is nearly indistinguishable from $2/3$ because the shrinkage is so strong. The analysis suggests that there is very little true variation between patients.

18.2.4   Correlated observations

Any decent model used to analyse a series of *n-of-1* trials will allow for at least three sources of variation: pure between-patient variability, within-patient variability and a random effect for patient-by-treatment interaction. Since a series of measurements are being obtained, however, it may be inappropriate to assume that within-patient errors are independent (or more formally that the correlations between measures are equal). If patients are subject to spells of illness for example, then two measurements taken during two administrations of the same drug are more likely to be similar if the administrations are close together rather than far apart. This phenomenon can be referred to as serial correlation and is potentially a problem for the analysis of *n-of-1* trials. (It would also be a problem for multiperiod cross-overs, the standard analysis of which, however, ignores the even more serious problem of patient-by-treatment interaction.)

The practical experimenter's way to deal with this will include randomizing the order of treatment given to the patient. An alternative approach, which exploits the correlation, would be to allocate the two treatments being compared in pairs but randomize the order within pairs. The paired differences can then be analysed using an appropriate random-effects model. The alternative would be to introduce an explicit model for the correlation structure of repeated measures, but this is unlikely to be simple.

18.2.5   Blinding

The problems with blinding *n-of-1* trials are particularly acute if the object is to say something about an individual patient. This is because the number of observations available for him or her alone will usually be small. Hence the probability of the patient's correctly guessing the complete sequence used will be relatively large (Senn, 1994). For example, if two treatments are to be allocated at random in three pairs using sequences such as AB AB BA, or AB BA AB and so forth, then there are only $2^3 = 8$ possible sequences in total. Hence, the probability of the patient's correctly guessing a random sequence is 1/8. If all possible sequences are used, subject only to the restriction that each treatment will appear three times, then there are $6!/(3!3!) = 20$ possible sequences. If the patient has a strong prejudice that one of the treatments is effective, and a strong belief (however irrationally based) that a particular sequence will be used, then he may guess and report a series of biased numbers corresponding to the believed sequence. For example, the following visual analogue scale (VAS) pain scores might be reported in a trial in arthritis in which patients received treatment A three times and treatment B three times in random order and the patient assumed that the sequence actually used was A

A B A B B and wrongly believed B to be more effective: 63, 66, 24, 61, 27, 23. Now, there is a 1 in 20 chance that the patient guessed correctly, and if he did then the mean difference between the two groups will be $(63 + 66 + 67)/3 - (23 + 24 + 27)/3 \cong 29$ and the t-statistic will be 20.5 on 4 degrees of freedom corresponding to a P-value of 0.000033, which does not at all represent the true probability involved. Of course, a nonparametric test would get around the difficulty, but these lack power for very small samples. As the sample size gets larger and larger, the problems caused by this sort of guessing strategy get less. The relevant sample size, however, is that of the episodes given to each patient. Increasing the number of patients will deal with this problem as regards the overall estimate of the treatment effect, but individual patient estimates may still suffer and this will have an effect on the estimate of the variability of the treatment effect from patient to patient.

These problems should not be exaggerated, but n-of-1 trials exemplify with respect to blinding a particular general problem regarding blinding, randomization and control which is often overlooked in clinical trials. The fact that these elements have been used in designing and running a clinical trial does not means that any conceivable analysis of the data is afforded the sort of protection they are designed to offer.

References

Cushny AR, Peebles AR (1905) The action of optimal isomers. II. Hyoscines. *Journal of Physiology* **32**: 501–510.

Guyatt GH, Heyting AH, Jaeschke R, Keller J, Adachi JD, Roberts RS (1990) N of 1 trials for investigating new drugs. *Controlled Clinical Trials* **11**: 88–100.

Guyatt GH, Juniper EF, Walter SD, Griffith LE, Goldstein RS (1998) Interpreting treatment effects in randomised trials [see comments]. *British Medical Journal* **316**: 690–693. [Comment in *BMJ* **317**(7157): 537–538 (1998)].

Jaeschke R, Adachi J, Guyatt G, Keller J, Wong B (1991) Clinical usefulness of amitriptyline in fibromyalgia: the results of 23 N-of-1 randomized controlled trials. *Journal of Rheumatology* **18**: 447–451.

Johannessen T (1991) Controlled trials in single subjects: 1 value in clinical medicine. *British Medical Journal* **303**: 173–174.

Lee Y, Nelder JA (1996) Hierarchical generalized linear models. *Journal of the Royal Statistical Society Series B – Methodological* **58**: 619–656.

Lewis JA (1991) Controlled trials in single subjects: 2. Limitations of use. *British Medical Journal* **303**: 175–176.

March L, Irwig L, Schwarz J, Simpson J, Chock C, Brooks P (1994) n of 1 trials comparing a non-steroidal anti-inflammatory drug with paracetamol in osteoarthritis. *British Medical Journal* **309**: 1041–1045; discussion 1045–1046.

Schluter PJ, Ware RS (2005) Single patient (n-of-1) trials with binary treatment preference. *Statistics Medicine* **24**: 2625–2636.

Senn SJ (1991) Controlled trials in single subjects [letter; comment]. *British Medical Journal* **303**: 716–717.

Senn SJ (1993) Suspended judgment n-of-1 trials. *Controlled Clinical Trials* **14**: 1–5.

Senn SJ (1994) Fisher's game with the devil. *Statistics in Medicine* **13**: 217–230.

Senn SJ (2001) Individual therapy: new dawn or false dawn. *Drug Information Journal* **35**: 1479–1494.

Senn SJ (2002) *Cross-over Trials in Clinical Research*. John Wiley & Sons, Ltd, Chichester.

Senn SJ (2003) Author's reply to Walter and Guyatt. *Drug Information Journal* **37**: 7–10.

Senn SJ (2004) Individual response to treatment: is it a valid assumption? *British Medical Journal* **329**: 966–968.

Senn SJ, Bakshi R, Ezzet N (1995) n of 1 trials in osteoarthritis. Caution in interpretation needed [letter; comment]. *British Medical Journal* **310**: 667.

Senn SJ, Richardson W (1994) The first t-test. *Statistics in Medicine* **13**: 785–803.

Student (1908) The probable error of a mean. *Biometrika* **6**: 1–25.

19

Sequential Trials

'Where shall I begin please your Majesty?' he asked.
'Begin at the beginning,' the King said, gravely, 'and go on till you come to the end: then stop.'
Lewis Caroll, *Alice in Wonderland*

19.1 BACKGROUND

But what is the *end* and can we recognize it when we get there? In the standard clinical trial, the end is defined by the number of patients we intended to recruit and the length of the trial by the time it takes to recruit them. But in running a clinical trial it is conclusions that we are interested in and not patients per se. Results are what we are looking for, not numbers, and this raises the possibility that we can run trials until a useful result is reached. This result may be either the conclusion that one of the treatments is indeed superior, or that nothing is to be gained by studying the treatments further. Such trials are known as sequential trials. This is a rather confusing name since nearly all trials, even those with a fixed sample size, recruit patients sequentially. However, in such trials we do not analyse the results sequentially and, if we are to use information on results as they accrue to determine the point at which the trial will stop, this is what is necessary.

   We have already touched on some of the issues which affect sequential trials when considering treatment allocation in general in Chapter 6. In this chapter we shall mainly consider the issue of deciding when to stop a trial on the basis of results. **Adaptive designs** of the bandit and play the winner form, will not be covered but were considered briefly in Chapter 6. However, another sort of adaptive design introduced in the 1990s by Bauer and Kohne (1994) and also independently suggested by Proschan and Hunsberger (1995) and then again by Fisher (1998), but which were not covered in the first edition of this book, will be discussed briefly here.

   Looked at in terms of the number of *trials* that are run by the pharmaceutical industry, sequential trials are relatively unimportant. However, since such trials are often run where the number of patients needed is suspected to be great, they are relatively more important in terms of numbers of *patients* and also of cost. Nevertheless, it remains true that there are many indications in drug development where such trials are never or rarely used and I think it is only fair that I should warn the reader that in all my time in the pharmaceutical industry I never designed or analysed one myself. But since leaving

Statistical Issues in Drug Development/2nd Edition   Stephen Senn
© 2007 John Wiley & Sons, Ltd

the pharmaceutical industry in 1995, I have frequently been a member of data-safety monitoring committees. I consequently feel that I know rather more about this topic than when I wrote the first edition. It is still the case, however, that it is one in which I do not count myself as an expert. As a consequence, this chapter still owes a lot to the work of others, in particular the excellent discussion of various approaches in John Whitehead's companion book in this series *Sequential Clinical Trials* (Whitehead, 1997) as well as some very useful notes of Laurence Freedman's (Freedman, 1996) and an article by Robert O'Neill outlining regulatory viewpoints (O'Neill, 1993). I have also used Sue Todd's very helpful review of papers on sequential methodology in the first 25 years of *Statistics in Medicine* (Todd, 2007).

For reasons which will be discussed in due course, sequential analysis (like survival analysis) is a topic which is less important in the particular context of drug development than in medical statistics in general. Nevertheless, from time to time it is *extremely* important, and since the related issues are complex, they merit an airing. Furthermore, some of the issues affecting sequential designs have to be understood when designing fixed-sample-size studies. Before going on to discuss the various issues, we describe the most common approaches. We shall consider four common frequentist approaches first and then discuss some Bayesian techniques. In the discussion which follows, it will be assumed that two-arm parallel-group trials only are being considered, that a one-sided test is to be used and that a one-to-one treatment allocation between the two arms will be employed. (These restrictions are not necessary to the theory but make our description of it easier and we shall assume that at any moment that we choose to look at the trial the same number of patients will have been treated in each arm.)

The method, which is first from the point of view of history if not of frequency of use, is also the frequentist one which (as an outsider) I find most appealing. It is the so-called **boundary approach** (Whitehead, 1997), based on the work on sequential testing in an industrial context developed independently by Barnard and Wald in the 1940s (Barnard, 1946; Wald, 1947), and its main proponent in its modern version as applied to clinical trials has been John Whitehead and colleagues who developed the PEST (planning and evaluation of sequential trials) software at Reading University, England. A detailed description of this is beyond the scope of this book but it has the following general features.

1. It is assumed that a number of inspections may be made of the trial results as they accrue.
2. In the light of the type of measurement to be taken and using the likelihood under a suitable model, a statistic Z_i is defined which summarizes the treatment difference at inspection i. (This statistic is related to the cumulative treatment difference.) For example, for a binary outcome, the statistic would be $(S_E - S_C)/2$ where S_E and S_C are the successes in experimental and treatment arms, respectively.
3. A further statistic, V_i, is defined which measures the variability of Z_i under the null hypothesis of no treatment effect. For the binary example, this statistic is $SF/(4n)$ where S, F and n are the total number of successes, failures and patients, respectively.
4. Two theoretical boundaries are calculated, on the assumption that data monitoring will be continuous. In a common approach, these define a triangular continuation region against which the test statistic Z is to be plotted. (See Figure 19.1, which is based on Whitehead, (1997).) Other boundary shapes are also possible. The peregrinations of Z define what is called a *sample path*. The vertical axis is

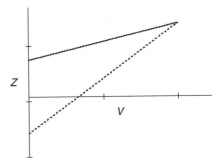

Figure 19.1 Continuous framework for a triangular test.

measured in terms of Z and the horizontal axis in terms of V. The upper boundary is chosen in such a way that when it is crossed the trial is ended with a conclusion that the experimental treatment is superior. The lower boundary is chosen so that when it is crossed the trial is ended for lack of evidence of efficacy. The underlying theory of the test is based on the assumption that monitoring is continuous. Progress on the horizontal axis is plotted in terms of information V rather than the number of patients recruited. The two are closely but not absolutely related.

5. Because, in practice, the sample path is inspected only at discrete intervals, an adjustment is made and inner boundaries, referred to as *Christmas tree boundaries* (owing to their shape), which are related to the triangular *continuous framework*, are used for actual stopping. The classic text on the boundary approach is the companion volume in this series by Whitehead mentioned above (Whitehead, 1997).

The boundary approach starts with the theory for continuous monitoring and adjusts it for the fact that monitoring is in fact discrete: that perhaps only a few inspections are made during the course of a trial. The method of repeated significance tests, used in connection with **group sequential trials** starts from the opposite end. (We shall use the term *group sequential trials* in a rather restricted sense here. In some usages, trials run according to the boundary approach would also be included.) It assumes, essentially, that what will be performed at the end of the trial is the sort of conventional analysis which would be used for a trial of fixed sample size and then considers what adjustment is necessary if a number of such tests have been made along the way. The basic theory has its origin in work by Armitage *et al.* (1969), was developed by Pocock (1977) in an influential paper, and has since been refined extensively by others. Consider a case where in theory we can take three *looks* at a trial. The trial will stop if the result of the first, second or third look is significant. Therefore, other things being equal, we shall conclude that the treatment is significant at least as often as if we performed the third look only. But if we carry out the third look at the conventional 5% level, this means that where the null hypothesis is true, by taking three looks we shall conclude significance in more than 5% of the cases. Hence, the type I error rate for the procedure will be larger than planned. A way to deal with this is to carry out significance tests at each look using a lower nominal level, rather in the same spirit that adjustments can be carried out for multiple outcomes. However, because information

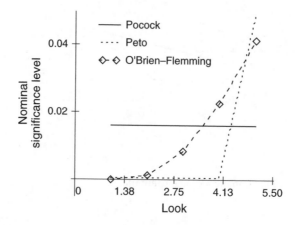

Figure 19.2   Nominal significance level at each look for three group sequential schemes.

generally arises in independent increments (as, say, further patients are studied), the correlation between tests to date and the latest test can be explicitly allowed for and more precise adjustments than the conservative Bonferroni approach are possible. Various schemes are possible. Pocock (1977) originally considered the case where each look was at the same nominal level. Peto *et al.* (1976) had earlier proposed an informal scheme whereby early looks were made at extremely low nominal levels of significance and the final look was made at the originally intended level. (This leads to a slight but unimportant inflation of the type I error rate.) O'Brien and Fleming (1979) proposed a scheme which has proved very popular, whereby the nominal significance level required gradually decreases with each look. In Figure 19.2, which is based upon a discussion of Demets and Lan (1994), these schemes are illustrated for a trial with five looks at equal intervals.

A third approach, the **alpha-spending approach**, is due to Lan and Demets (1983) (but similar work had been carried out by Slud and Wei (1982).) Group-sequential boundaries are established as for the group-sequential approach above in such a way that the overall type I error rate is at the predetermined level. These boundaries are then expressed in terms of the actual cumulative type I error rates as opposed to the nominal type I error rate. So, for example, corresponding to Figure 19.2 we would have another figure consisting of increasing curves converging at the end on 5 per cent. The situation is illustrated in Figure 19.3, which gives simple approximations proposed by Lan and Demets (1983) to the Pocock and O'Brien–Fleming rules. If an interim look takes place at some other moment than originally planned, then the nominal test is fixed at the level which ensures that the total amount of alpha spent to date corresponds to the spending curve. This gives the alpha-spending approach a flexibility in operation which the standard repeated significance tests approach to group sequential trials does not have. However, it is now almost universally the case that group-sequential designs are implemented using alpha-spending approaches so that the two techniques are seen as inextricably entwined. For example, Todd (2007) reviews the two under the same group-heading *alpha-spending functions approach*. For in-depth discussion of group-sequential and alpha-spending approaches, a key text is Jennison and Turnbull (2000).

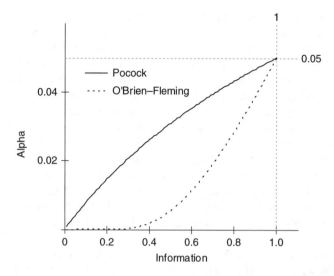

Figure 19.3 Alpha-spending functions for Pocock and O'Brien–Fleming approaches.

The fourth frequentist approach is known as **stochastic curtailment**. This was proposed by Lan *et al.* (1982) and has its origin in quality control inspection schemes. These sometimes require that a batch be rejected if a certain number of defective items are found. However, if and when this total number defective is reached, the batch may be rejected without inspecting the rest of the items since it is already known that the limit of acceptability has been reached. In clinical trials a similar situation could arise where we have historical controls. Suppose, for example, we know that only about 19% of the patients suffering from a particular disease survive to one year when given a standard treatment and intend to study 10 patients on a new treatment for one year each. Each patient can be either dead or alive at the end of one year's follow-up. On the assumption that the new treatment has the same efficacy as the standard treatment, the probability of having 4 or more survivors is about 0.025 and so can be regarded as being conventionally significant. Now suppose that at the point at which the fourth patient recruited has been treated for one year all 4 patients are alive. We shall then know that whatever happens to the next 6, the results of the trial as a whole will be significant. Hence we could stop the trial. (This could actually be bad news for future patients since, without special arrangements, they would now be have to be given the conventional treatment!) Furthermore, in likelihood terms, the evidence in favour of the new treatment is actually greater than if we stopped after 10 patients with 4 alive and 6 dead. Hence, if evidence of efficacy alone is what concerns us, there would seem to be no reason not to stop.

For a conventional trial, with concurrent controls, things would be a little more complex. Here we would have to judge the efficacy of the treatment compared with the control group being studied at the same time. Nevertheless, a point can be reached in a conventional trial at which, whatever the future results are, the trial will be significant. However, most trialists would want to stop a trial even if statistical significance at the end was a theoretical but remote probability. If the trial is stopped or extended on the basis of some calculation of what the likely conclusion might be, then this approach is referred to as stochastic curtailment.

In practice, stochastic curtailment is often used in connection with stopping for **futility**. That is to say, the trial is stopped because there is little hope of obtaining a significant result if the trial is continued to conclusion. Consider, for example, the CARDS study, a placebo-controlled of atorvastatin in diabetes (Colhoun *et al.*, 2004). I was the statistician on the data-safety monitoring board. We used an O'Brien–Fleming rule for judging efficacy of atorvastatin. In other words, we required stringent levels of significance to stop the trial early in favour of atorvastatin. However, we did not think it was appropriate to insist on similar standards to stop early in favour of placebo because, if placebo were the better treatment, then stopping the trial early would ensure that all patients immediately got the better treatment. Hence we had an asymmetric strategy whereby it would have been much easier for us to stop had placebo seemed better. This was a stopping for futility provision. (In the end this was not needed as the trial concluded early with evidence in favour of atorvaststin.) In fact, stopping for futility is probably one of the most important uses of sequential analysis in drug development.

A fifth frequentist approach, that of flexible designs (Bauer and Kohne, 1994; Gallo *et al.*, 2006; Proschan and Hunsberger, 1995), has a rather different flavour and will be considered after looking at Bayesian approaches.

Sequential analysis: A means of stopping a trial before it becomes useful.

There are various **Bayesian** alternatives to the frequentist approach. A fully Bayesian procedure would establish not only a prior distribution for the treatment effect but also the utilities associated with each effect. A random-effect model for the treatment effect would be used and (to be fully Bayesian) one would also have to use a random-effect model for the utilities of potential future patients and also some trade-off function between interests of current and future patients. Randomization would not be equally to the two groups but according to some trade-off between information gained for future patients and using what is currently believed to be the best treatment for a current patient. (See discussion of bandits in Chapter 6.) It would also be necessary to establish how many future patients are likely to be treated before an even better treatment emerges. In theory, such a procedure dictates what treatment the next patient should be given, so that the distinction between trials and general medical care simply disappears. There is thus no question of stopping the trial as such, although, I suppose, it could be deemed stopped once it seems very unlikely that a future patient will ever be allocated to either the control treatment or the experimental treatment, as the case may be. This procedure seems to be almost impossible to apply, not least because it is generally impossible to coordinate treatment of all the patients in the world suffering from a disease and (as far as I am aware) no one does so.

However, not being able to determine the perfectly appropriate loss function does not necessarily mean that it might not be appropriate to design a trial using a simpler, less realistic loss function. A Bayesian approach including explicit use of loss functions is described by Cheng and Shen (2005). The authors of this paper also show how this general approach can be combined with frequentist requirements regarding control of the type I error rate and claim favourable properties in terms of expected run-length for their method. However, they fall short of actually providing a real-life example except to reanalyse some already published data. For a Bayesian approach with a practical illustration in an AIDS trial, see Carlin *et al.* (1998). For further discussion and SAS code illustrating how such approaches can be implemented, see Burman *et al.* (2007).

In practice, a simpler Bayesian approach, pioneered by Spiegelhalter and co-workers, seems more practical (Spiegelhalter *et al.*, 1994). (Like the paper by Bauer and Kohne (1994), which appeared in the same year, this also had been cited nearly 200 times by September 2007.) This approach is to define a region of practical equivalence using the opinion of experts. Such experts also provide priors for the effects of treatments and some approach to combining these is employed. Patients are randomized in equal numbers to control and experimental treatments as in a conventional trial. Monitoring takes place at various times. These may be either at predetermined intervals or as decided during the trial. At any given analysis the previous posterior distribution is used as a prior distribution, which is then updated, by the operation of Bayes' theorem, using the additional information which has accrued since the previous analysis. (Equivalently, the total information in the trial can be added to the original prior.) The trial continues until there is a reasonable degree of belief that the difference between the treatments lies outside the region of equivalence.

The above discussion has classified methods according to the major division Bayesian or frequentist and then according to various approaches within these two categories. Freedman (1996) offers an alternative classification into three major approaches: *estimative*, *predictive* or *hypothesis testing*. Under hypothesis testing he includes Whitehead's triangular test and Wald's sequential probability ratio test. Under predictive are included stochastic curtailment and a Bayesian approach based on the predictive distribution. Under estimative he includes his own Bayesian approach of using the posterior distribution, as well as group-sequential methods and the alpha-spending approach. (Although one might argue that these two are also partly in the hypothesis testing camp.)

Some mention should also be made of sequential analysis of clinical trials in which no use is made of information regarding the treatments given but, nonetheless, the results are used to decide when to terminate the trial. Such analyses are sometimes referred to as *sample size reviews* and the trials are sometimes described as having an *internal pilot trial*. For example, Gould (1992) considers the problem of planning trials with a binary outcome. The clinically relevant difference might be postulated on the log-odds scale. If the effect sought is additive on this scale, then it does not depend on the number clinical outcomes. However, the variance of this statistic *does* depend on the number of outcomes. If, for example, the population recruited into the trial is much healthier than we thought, we shall have to study rather more patients to demonstrate the value of the drug. Various methods are available for monitoring such trial without unblinding in order to determine when sufficient information has been gathered.

Sample size reviews can be regarded as a form of sequential design modification: a crucial planned aspect of the trial (the sample size) is modified as a result of information that has accrued. Shortly before the first edition of this book appeared, the field of sequential design modification received an influential impetus through the work of Bauer and Kohne (1994), a paper which had attracted 200 citations by September 2007. They pointed out that by judging the overall significance of a trial in terms of suitable combinations of *P*-values of individual stages that had been separately analysed, provided that due care was taken, an overall type I error rate could be controlled at some desired level. (The issue of combining *P*-values was considered in connection with meta-analysis in Chapter 16.) This possibility gives the trialist considerable flexibility since it would in principle be perfectly acceptable to use different outcome measures for different stages of the trial. Other adaptions could see arms of the trial being dropped. This general area has come to be known as that of adaptive analysis.

A useful article in the *Journal of Biopharmaceutical Statistics* provides a summary of a Pharmaceutical Research and Manufacturers of America (PhRMA) 'white paper' and discusses some issues in using 'adaptive designs' in drug development (Gallo *et al.*, 2006).

Before leaving our background discussion we consider some more practical matters to do with data-monitoring. A sequential trial requires a considerable amount of organization. Freedman (1996) points out that it is essential to have an experienced but independent data-monitoring board (DMB) with well defined rules of procedure as well as a suitable stopping rule. It is a grave mistake not to have such rules, but also unwise to think that they can always be slavishly adhered to. One can only go so far in imagining what might be a problem and writing rules to cover it. As Kipling puts it, 'a policy is the blackmail levied on the Fool by the Unforeseen'. Other pitfalls to avoid are stopping too early for efficacy, using a different outcome for monitoring than was used to design the trial, using an outcome of little clinical relevance, and having only one boundary. (The ability to stop for lack of efficacy or worse, should be there.) Further useful practical material can be found in Simon (1994) and a medical perspective is given by Souhami (1994).

As regards the composition of such DMBs, Ellenberg (1996), writing from an FDA perspective, suggests that they should have both medical clinical experts in the indication and biostatisticians. It might be appropriate also to have someone with a training in ethics as well as experts in the basic science and pharmacology. Some monitoring boards will also include epidemiologists and even lawyers and possibly 'lay persons'. Ellenberg's view is that independence requires the following. First that there will be no financial advantage to the members if the product proves effective. (She also mentions that they should not have an interest in a competing product.) Second, that 'they are not involved with entering or treating patients on the study' (p. 554). A third point which needs to be watched, in my opinion, is that members do not have an interest in significance per se because of involvement in publication. Herson (1993) also gives a useful discussion looking at such boards from an industry point of view.

For the reader who wishes to know more, there is an excellent book devoted to practical, ethical and methodological aspects of data-monitoring written by three experts in the field, and published in the same series as this one (Ellenberg *et al.*, 2003).

19.2 ISSUES

19.2.1 Adjusting for repeated testing is nonsense

This is certainly the Bayesian point of view, although, effectively, it is not so much a specific criticism of frequentist approaches to sequential analysis but a general criticism of frequentist methods, which reveal their weaknesses most fully in the sequential context.

The following is an argument I first heard from Don Berry. Suppose that two physicians run a clinical trial of an experimental treatment to be compared with a control with a ceiling of 100 patients and that the outcome for each patient is success or failure.

Dr A decides to look at his results and carry out some 'test' after 50 patients have been treated. If the result is significant he will stop. If not he will continue. Dr B decides that she will treat 100 patients and then stop. There will be no interim analysis. Both physicians run their trials. Because he fails to obtain significance with 50 patients, Dr A continues to the end. When the final results are examined, it is seen that the results are identical: identical in *every* detail. Thus, it is not only the case that the numbers of successes and failures cross-classified by treatment group are the same for the 100 patients in each trial but it is also the case that if (say) patient 23 in A's trial received the experimental treatment, then so did patient 23 in B's trial and if patient 42 had a successful outcome in B's trial, then so did patient 42 in A's trial and so forth. Thus, if Dr B had looked at her data after 50 patients according to A's strategy she would also have continued.

A and B now perform an analysis of their respective trials (which, but for the inspection strategy, are identical). As it turns out, the results for B's trial are significant. However, A, faced with the same data, has to pay a penalty for having looked and (as it turns out) when this penalty is paid, his results are not significant. The fact that A and B come to different conclusions based on the same data violates what is called the **likelihood principle**, and in any case (without having to refer to statistical principles) seems to many intuitively quite unreasonable. On the other hand, if one does carry out repeated hypothesis tests at (say) the 5% level and one does stop as soon as a result is significant, then the type I error rate associated with this strategy will be in excess of 5%. Hence, if one regards the combination of hypothesis tests and controlled type I error rates as being the essence of the frequentist approach to statistics, then either one must accept it that *is* reasonable for A and B to come to different conclusions after all, or one must accept that that frequentist approach is unreasonable.

I will now discuss why this Bayesian argument is not quite as water-tight as it seems. In doing this I am not attempting to deny its importance: it *is* important and it ought to be more widely appreciated by frequentists. Let us return to the two physicians. If we consider that they *ought* to come to the same conclusion under all circumstances in which the trial results are identical, whatever the trial results might be, and that, since the frequentist approach lets them down in this respect, they ought therefore to be Bayesians (if this is the only alternative), then it follows that they must have the same posterior distribution and also the same utilities. However, since they have seen the same data, they must have had the same prior distribution to have reached the same posterior distribution. Although there is now no difficulty in explaining their posterior distributions, there is no means of explaining their differing behaviour. Two Bayesians with the same prior distribution and the same utilities *ought* to design the same experiment. The fact that A was prepared to stop the trial under certain circumstances, whereas B would have continued regardless cannot now be explained.

It should also be stressed that frequentists are not alone in thinking that *formal* stopping rules are important. Many Bayesians can be found who think this also. For example, Freedman (1996) describes failure to have a formal stopping rule as being one of the ten pitfalls to be avoided in conducting sequential trials, and Kadane (1996) have devoted a whole book to expounding a formal ethical approach to conducting clinical trials which determines whether the next patient can be randomized or not. For Bayesians, such rules, of course, must reflect priors and utilities as well as evidence.

It thus seems that it is difficult to phrase the paradox in a way which makes it perfect. Either we have to accept that Bayesians who had behaved differently *would* come to different conclusions also (thus arguing that, although this is an unreasonable feature of frequentist statistics, it is fine for Bayesian statistics), or we are left with a Bayesian paradox of behaviour. Thus the frequentist can reply that since the Bayesians argue that beliefs *ought* to affect conclusions then, since intentions are the links between beliefs and actions, it is hardly surprising that when intentions differ, conclusions may do so also. Furthermore, Bayesian rules can be produced which are not radically different from the frequentist ones. For example, Freedman and Spiegelhalter (1989) showed that certain sceptical priors produce behaviour in sequential trials which is similar to some frequentist approaches (in fact closer to some frequentist alternatives than they are to each other). It is important to understand, however, that this does not quite let the frequentists off the hook, the reason being that it is of course a natural consequence of the Bayesian position that two persons having seen the same data ought not necessarily to come to the same conclusion. What the frequentist must do to defend his position is to accept that there is a subjective element to it after all, but in that case a standard objection to the Bayesian approach – that it is subjective – is no longer valid. That would amount to the pot calling the kettle black.

Sit by a sequential trial long enough and significance will come floating by unless you take steps to sink it.

19.2.2   Sequential trials are not generally relevant to drug development

It is the case for many indications that the number of patients needed to prove efficacy is actually less than the number who must be exposed to the new treatment to assess its safety. Furthermore, for most treatments under study, once the trial is finished, if it is successful, there will be a period of time before the drug will be generally available. The first reason makes stopping boundaries for efficacy irrelevant. The second reason means that there is no good reason for stopping because the experimental treatment has proved itself more effective than the control treatment since it will not be possible to switch all future patients onto this treatment. The second reason does, of course, leave the door open for stopping trials for lack of efficacy of an experimental treatment but this, in any case, does not raise quite the same number of issues which are attendant upon early stopping for proven efficacy.

It is perhaps also worth noting that the fact that experimental treatments are not generally available to physicians means that it is not necessary for a physician to be in equipoise for it to be practically ethical for him to participate in a randomized clinical trial. Indeed, it is simply necessary for him not to believe in the inferiority of the experimental treatment. As long as he believes that the experimental treatment is superior, by refusing to randomize and not participating in the trial he condemns all of his patients to receive the treatment he believes is inferior. His participation in the trial is therefore logical until the moment when the new treatment is proved inferior (Senn, 2001, 2002). Thus, without some special arrangement to continue to receive the experimental treatment, there is never any reason for him to withdraw his patients because the experimental treatment is apparently superior. Even where he did negotiate some deal with the sponsor by which, with the regulator's approval, he would be allowed to obtain further material on a **named-patient basis** once he was so convinced that he felt no further evidence was needed, nothing would stop the sponsor from recruiting another centre to replace him on exactly the same grounds on which he was recruited in the first place.

This is an important contrast to clinical trial work outside of drug development because this, of course, cannot (by definition) involve drugs which are not yet developed. Hence both treatments being compared are (in principle) available to all physicians. Thus, stopping for proven efficacy becomes important. Even here, however, matters are complicated. It would be interesting to know, for example, whether more or fewer physicians are taking aspirin prophylactically than when the Physician's Health Study was still running (Steering Committee of the Physicians' Health Study Research Group, 1989). This trial was stopped because efficacy was proved. If the answer is 'fewer', then this is rather ironic.

Of course, one could argue, and no doubt some would, that this is the fault of the drug regulatory set-up, which is ethically deficient in this respect. If regulations make it necessary to run trials which are larger than are strictly needed for efficacy, or if regulations forbid new drugs from being instantly available, then this is a fault of 'the system', which should be changed to make the ethically superior sequential trial a practical proposition. While not pretending that the current regulatory set-up is ideal, I think that these sorts of criticisms are ill-founded. To pursue this argument to its logical conclusion would require many more radical changes than simply re-writing the rules under which the FDA, the MHRA and so forth operate. We also require, for instance, that pharmaceutical companies gear themselves up in such a way that they have sufficient manufacturing capacity to instantly satisfy all future patients if the drug proves successful, having braced themselves, of course, for the possibility that the plant in which they have heavily invested will be redundant. And we must go further. If we insist on occupying such high moral ground, is a sponsor not under an obligation to press on full steam ahead with *any* development once it is suspected in the company that it *might* be effective, even if the outside world is yet to be convinced, even if maximum haste may not make economic sense? (See Chapter 24 for a discussion of economic issues.) And is the sponsor, or the government, or somebody, not morally obliged to make sure that such treatments are available in the third world also, despite the fact that they cannot be paid for?

I neither believe that the world is perfect nor that it would not be a good idea to attempt to improve it, but I believe, by and large, that drug developers have to take the world as it is and make a good job given the existing constraints. And I have nothing but contempt for the cant of certain critics of the clinical trial.

So, if there is a place for sequential analysis of drug-development trials, monitoring and so forth, it is either for safety and/or lack of efficacy reasons, or for economic reasons. The latter can be important for some indications. There may be cases where the sponsor realizes that the number of patients needed to prove efficacy may, for a fixed trial, exceed those which need to be studied for registration. Under such circumstance, the possibility of early stopping, either for proven efficacy or lack of efficacy (what was referred to in section 19.1 as *futility*), may be attractive. The expected run length will be less than the fixed sample size required, the costs of the trial may be less, and the time to registration if the trial is successful will probably be reduced.

19.2.3 Conflicts between sponsor and independent monitoring committees

Because of the ethical dimension it is important to have independent monitoring committees. Freedman (1996), speaking essentially of nonindustry trials, regards not having a monitoring committee independent of the chief investigator as one of the 10 pitfalls to be avoided of sequential trials. By extension, the same applies to industry trials, substituting 'sponsor' for 'chief investigator'. The fact that part of the conduct of a trial has been given over to others while the costs are borne by the sponsor is a potential source of friction. As Herson (1993) puts it, 'pharmaceutical firms are reluctant to give up total control to DMBs because the research is so specifically directed by internal development programmes...' (p. 557). For a more recent discussion of potential conflicts see Hilbrich and Sleight (2006).

It is my opinion that the reason some sponsors have had unhappy experiences in running sequential trials with independent monitoring committees is that neither side has realized that the other had different expectations in monitoring. The sponsor will have an eye on the economic consequences. There may be no particular value in continuing to the end of the trial unless a reasonable commercial result is in sight. The members of the monitoring committee may be more used to nonindustry trials, where two readily available therapies are compared. They may feel that as long as the new therapy has not been proved worse than the standard and as long as some reasonable possibility of a significant result remains, it may be worth continuing. Thus, it is extremely important for both sides to state their positions honestly before starting the trial and to agree the monitoring rules beforehand. (As Freedman points out, however, the point of having a board is that human imagination is insufficient to envisage all possible occurrences during a trial and that therefore human judgement is needed in addition to algorithms. It is inevitable, therefore, that these rules will be broken from time to time. In the much-quoted words of Emerson, 'A foolish consistency is the hobgoblin of little minds'.) It is also important that, where the trial is being run by one of the various clinical trial organizations which now exist, the monitoring committee be independent not only of the sponsor but of this organization also.

Useful practical advice on organizing the running of data monitoring boards will be found in Ellenberg *et al.* (2003).

19.2.4 The two-trials rule

It is a general requirement of the FDA that two well-controlled trials demonstrating efficacy are needed to make a given claim which will lead to approval. The ethical argument for conducting a sequential trial, however, is hard to maintain if it will not be the last trial conducted to investigate the particular question it was designed to investigate. We can hardly stop a trial because we feel that it is unethical to continue to randomize patients to a treatment we believe to be inferior but then either proceed to start a second trial where we do just that or continue with another trial which is currently running.

However, just such a situation did arise on a trial I was involved in. This was the CARDS study (Colhoun *et al.*, 2004) of atorvastatin referred to in section 19.1. I was the statistician on the data-safety monitoring board and we called a halt to the trial two years earlier than expected as a result of a significant difference using an O'Brien–Fleming boundary. However, another trial, the ASPEN study, of similar design in the same indication using the same drug, was underway and this carried on. This trial went to its planned conclusion and did not have a significant result (Knopp *et al.*, 2006). This is a rather unsatisfactory state of affairs and in general matters are best organized to avoid it.

It would thus seem that the sort of serious and life-threatening diseases where sequential trials are run ought to be an exception to the two-trials rule. However, this raises a problem with the standard of evidence. As we saw in Chapter 12, one interpretation of the two-trials rule is that it reflects the fact that higher standards of evidence are required in practice than suggested by the conventional 5% significance level. If we do not have a two-trials rule, then it simply means that our standards of evidence are lower for the sorts of indications in which sequential trials are run than for other areas of drug development. This may seem to be appropriate for serious diseases, where more is at stake and we intuitively feel that it is unreasonable to carry on in the search for 'proof' of efficacy where belief is already strong.

There are some problems with this. The first is that the disparity in proof is actually greater than might appear at first sight. For a treatment in chronic disease, even after registration, trials will continue to be run and in general randomized trials are still possible. For example, the well-known beta-agonist salbutamol (US albuterol) was developed in the 1960s to treat asthma yet, at a guess, dozens of trials are still run every year using salbutamol and placebo as comparators for new treatments. Hence we are still able to learn more in an efficient way about this drug. The same will not be true for any drug for which a sequential trial has been run. Thus the irony is that, where two trials are required for registration, this is unlikely to be the last word, whereas it may well be where one trial is accepted.

The second problem is that the trialists may convince themselves that a treatment is effective by stopping at a conventional 5% level of significance (suitably adjusted for repeated testing) but fail to convince their medical colleagues elsewhere. Thus a deadlock would be reached where randomized trials would no longer be possible because the medicine had been 'proved' to be effective but the medicine was not being used because the proof had had no impact.

19.2.5 Adjustment for bias (shrinkage)

Naive estimators associated with sequential tests may also be biased in the sense that the expectation of standard fixed trial estimators taken over all possible trials run to the same stopping rule may not be equal to the true treatment effect. Adjustments for estimators and associated intervals are possible but raise similar issues to those discussed under section 19.2.1. For example, suppose that we have a fixed parallel-group trial and calculate, as a conventional treatment estimate, the difference between the mean outcomes in each group. Suppose we then notice, however, on looking at the results for the patients ordered over time, that had we run this trial as a given sequential trial with three looks at equal intervals, then we would have stopped exactly at the point dictated by the fixed trial, which happens to correspond to the second look of the sequential trial. Had we carried out the sequential trial we should have adjusted the treatment estimator, but since we have carried out a fixed trial we shall not.

The Bayesian, of course, will also wish to adjust naive treatment estimates. This is because the posterior estimate at any point must reflect not only what the data say about the model ('the likelihood') but prior belief. This sort of adjustment is sometimes referred to as *shrinkage*. The posterior estimate 'shrinks' the naive estimate towards the prior estimate. The more data available the less the shrinkage that takes place but, in the Bayesian scheme, there is no *direct* dependence on the stopping *rule*. As discussed in section 19.2.1, there is an indirect dependence, since the stopping rule itself will depend on the prior distribution.

19.2.6   Over-running

A source of potential embarrassment with sequential trials is that having decided on the basis of results to date to stop the recruitment of patients because the results are convincing, further information will continue to accrue. For example, in a trial where survival is the main outcome we will continue to follow up patients we have treated. Those recruited most recently will usually still be alive and thus have, at the time of stopping, censored and relatively uninformative survival times. In such a trial it is actually the number of deaths which affects the power of the study, rather than the number of patients per se. Thus, as time goes on, further information will be obtained and it is always theoretically possible that this will tend to contradict results to date, so that once the further information is received we are no longer as convinced as when we stopped that the treatment is efficacious.

As Whitehead (1997) points out, this can even occur with fixed sample size studies of survival analysis. For example, consider a fixed sample size trial with a recruitment over one year. We may have determined to analyse the results once the last patient recruited has been followed up for one year. This means, though, that patients recruited earlier in the trial will have been followed up longer: those recruited at the beginning will, in fact, have been followed up for two years. Often this extra information will also be included in the analysis, which thus reflects a mixture of follow-up times from one to two years. However, once this analysis is complete it will still be possible to obtain further data and in a year's time an analysis of patients with 2 – 3 years' follow up could be carried out. I think it is fair to say, however, that it is more likely to be a problem which makes itself known in a sequential rather than a fixed trial framework. Nevertheless, it is a potential feature of all forecasting systems that they are hostages to the future: further information which embarrasses us can always arise.

This feature seems to be embarrassing for frequentist systems where there seems to be no formal way of declaring a hypothesis 'not rejected' once it has been rejected. It does not appear to be a reversible process. However, this is not the only interpretation of what goes on in a sequential analysis with over-running. One view is that the only analysis which counts is the final one, once the further information has been collected. The trial has been stopped earlier on the practical grounds that it seems as if a decision of efficacy is now possible. There is no question of 'unrejecting' H_0. It was not rejected in the first place. After all, in a fixed sample size trial, we would have made a decision when to stop the trial and then some time later we would either have found that the result would or would not have been significant. The only difference with the sequential trial is that the decision when to stop has made some use of the results.

It would also be wrong to think that this sort of thing is not a worry for Bayesian systems. For example, assuming a Normal prior and likelihood and defining the precision to be the inverse of the variance the following relationships hold (Lee, 1989, p. 38).

1. Posterior precision = prior precision + sample precision.
2. Posterior mean = weighted mean of prior mean and sample precision, the weights being proportional to the respective precisions.

Now, the sample precision simply increases with the size of the sample; thus as more information accrues we *must* become more confident in our beliefs. However, there is no *guarantee*, that the sample mean will be the same as or even similar to what it was before more information has accrued. (Although, of course, previous results will be included as a subset of the total.) Hence our beliefs do *not* have to remain the same, or even similar. Thus it is theoretically possible to move from being extremely confident that the treatment effect is in one region to being even more confident that it is in another, without ever having exhibited any doubt en route.

The Bayesian can reply, of course, that this is very unlikely. Future results are unlikely to be inconsistent with those of the past. This is often a reasonable hope but, it seems to me, no more of a defence than the frequentist's claim that the Jeffreys–Lindley paradox (see Section 13.2.9) is unlikely to occur. In fact, this sort of result is a necessary consequence of what is known technically as *exchangeability*. This is an assumption of indifference to the order in which results arrive. Thus, for example, a trial in which for the first half of the trial the treatment effect was +4 and in the second half was −6 is equivalent (other things being equal) in terms of inference to one in which the observed effect was close to $(4-6)/2 = -1$ more or less at any time during the conduct of the trial. This is not necessarily illogical, but it shows that Bayesians, just like frequentists, can be embarrassed by any predictions they make. Of course the Bayesian can always say 'So I was wrong but I was right to be wrong,' but users of his forecasts may not be so impressed with this argument. That forecasts may be wrong is, therefore, a general problem of being prepared to make them. Hindsight, however, is an exact science and foresight is all we are left with. Statistical approaches to evaluating evidence are not perfect. They are just better than the alternatives.

19.2.7 Decisions versus information

Quite apart from the usual ethical justification for running sequential trials, a practical justification is that, for given power, clinically relevant difference and significance level, the expected number of patients will be smaller than for a corresponding fixed sample size. We do not get something for nothing, however. By the same token, the expected amount of information obtained from the trial is less, so that having stopped the trial because we have just convinced ourselves that the treatment is effective, we shall be very much in the dark as to *how* effective it is. This is especially true of the triangular test, where sampling continues until either significance has just been demonstrated or we stop for lack of efficacy. In theory this can be dealt with by using stopping rules which require a given degree of proven equivalence. Spiegelhalter *et al.* (1994) have actually incorporated the notion of a region of practical equivalence into their Bayesian approach to running sequential trials. Frequentist approaches are also possible.

Furthermore, he who plans a fixed sample size clinical trial may be embarrassed by later discoveries about precision. For example, we may plan a trial on the assumption that the variance is fairly small but discover once the trial has completed that it is much larger than we thought. Or, in a trial where events are important, we may discover that the background event rate is actually less than we though. Under such circumstances the information provided by the trial is less than intended. This sort of thing can be avoided by a sequential approach. Even if results are not unblinded as we go along, we can monitor the information provided in the way suggested, for example, by Gould (1992). Flexible designs, including but not limited to those that permit sample size re-estimation, are discussed in Section 19.2.9 below.

19.2.8   Concerns about un-blinding

If it is considered desirable and feasible to run a double-blind trial in a given indication, the fact that a sequential trial is being run with repeated looks at accumulating data has the capacity, as O'Neill (1993) puts it, 'to influence parts of the trial conduct such as types of patients entered, definitions of endpoints, exclusion criteria etc.' (p. 606). Sometimes the data-monitoring board is kept in the dark as to which treatment is which and results are presented to it without revealing the treatment labels. This is not always possible: for example, where an asymmetric stopping rule is being used, as may be the case when trials can be stopped for lack of efficacy.

Even where the treatment labels are not revealed it is a mistake to think that the blind has been maintained. The fact that analysis is only possible by grouping results from patients by treatment given, even if the treatment has not been identified, means that to a large extent the trial is un-blinded. For example, in a conventional fixed-size clinical trial, if a physician were to know which patients had received the same treatment even if he did not know which it was, he could exaggerate any apparent difference. Although in the case of an ineffective treatment this would work against the sponsor's drug as often as in favour of it, it would not maintain the type I error rate at 5%. In the extreme case it would inflate this to 100% two-sided or 50% one-sided in favour of the experimental treatment. Thus un-blinding is a potential concern. One safeguard is to make sure that the standard operating procedures of the DMB and the sponsor prevent bias from influencing the results. Here formal rules of procedure are extremely valuable.

19.2.9   Controversies regarding flexible designs

There is considerable and growing interest in the class of so-called flexible designs introduced by Bauer and Kohne (1994). A similar suggestion regarding sample size review was made independently by Proschan and Hunsberger (1995) and Fisher (1998), who referred to such designs as being *self-designing*. In his interesting review and discussion of issues, Emerson (2006) lists the sort of things that might be changed as a result of interim review of clinical trials as follows:

- *The scientific hypothesis of interest.* For example, one might change inclusion criteria or doses of the treatment.
- *The statistical hypotheses of interest.* For example, changing the measure used to compare treatment arms.

- *The randomization scheme.* For example, one might adjust the allocation ratio in favour of one of the treatments.
- *The rule for determining the maximal statistical information to be accrued.* One might decide to enroll fewer or more patients than planned.
- *The rule determining the schedule of analysis.* For example, changing the timing or frequency of individual looks.
- *The rule determining the conditions for early stopping.*
- *The inferential methods that will be used when reporting the results.* For example, switching from chi-square to Fisher's exact test.

Not all of the above are equally easily incorporated into the framework of flexible designs, which in the original Bauer and Kohne (1994) recommendation required weighted combinations of *P*-values from each stage. This implies, for example, that you could switch from a chi-square analysis of one stage to logistic regression for another; you would combine the results in terms of *P*-values as is sometimes done for a meta-analysis (see Chapter 16) but would not be carrying out a logistic regression of both stages.

Burman and Sonesson, in their thought-provoking and critical discussion of flexible designs (Burman and Sonesson, 2006a,b) describe the approach clearly. First, we have a series of nonnegative weights with the weight for stage k as v_k defined independently of the data from stage k and all future stages. (This condition is easily satisfied, for example, if the weight is specified in advance of obtaining data from that stage). The weights eventually used must sum to 1 so that $\sum_k v_k = 1$. but the number of stages, m does not have to be specified in advance. However, one must take care in assigning weights as one goes along that they do not sum to more than 1, and when the last stage has been reached one then assigns the remaining weight to that stage so that $v_m = 1 - \sum_{k=1}^{m-1} v_k$. Next we will test the joint null hypothesis $H = H_1 \cap \cdots \cap H_m$ using the *P*-values for each stage, One approach is to transform the *P*-values to *Z*-scores using the inverse cumulative density function of the Normal distribution $\Phi^{-1}(\cdot)$ to obtain $Z_k = -\Phi^{-1}(p_k)$ and then construct the weighted statistic $Z* = \sum_{k=1}^{m} \sqrt{v_k} Z_k$, which under the null hypothesis H and given the other conditions above will be distributed $N(0, 1)$.

Burman and Sonesson (2006a) point, however, to some disturbing features of such designs and give some examples that strongly exhibit undesirable behaviour. A particular example is extremely striking, which is perhaps understood best in terms of sampling items from a production line, although the extension to clinical trials is obvious. Suppose we intend to examine 1000 items for which we are to obtain measurements Y to test at level $\alpha = 0.05$ the null hypothesis that the mean $E[Y]$ for the population of measurements from which they are drawn is $\mu \le 0$ against the alternative that it is $\mu > 0$. Suppose we know that the variance of Y is σ^2. In standardized terms, the critical value $C_\alpha = 1.645$. If, in fact, the true value of μ is 0.08, then the power of the resulting one-sided test is 81%. Now suppose, in fact, that we plan to look after $N_1 = 100$ observations using a statistic to which we quite naturally assign a weight $v_1 = 0.1$. However, the result is disappointing with $\bar{Y} = -0.03$. We decide to take only one further observation, Y_{101}, which turns out to be 2.5. We now construct our weighted statistic as $Z* = \sqrt{0.1} \times -0.03 + \sqrt{0.9} \times 2.5 \approx 2.28$, which is significant. However, the unweighted mean would be $(100 \times -0.03 + 2.5)/101 = -0.5/101 \approx 0.005$ and so clearly not significant.

Table 19.1 Allocation of subjects in a smoking cessation trial

	Treatment group		
	---	---	---
Cohort	Intervention	Control	Total
First	60	120	180
Second	291	291	541
Total	351	411	762

The problem is that the requirement we put on weighting data in order to control the type I error rate is quite different from what we feel is instinctively appropriate for weighting the data as information. One should be careful, however, in assuming that the solution to the issue raised is to rush to the other extreme of ignoring the adaptive nature of such designs and pooling all the data in a 'natural' fashion. To demonstrate this we shall discuss a genuine example.

In a smoking cessation trial in Glasgow, pregnant smokers were randomized to two groups. One group (the control group) received standard health promotion literature and the other (the intervention group) received motivational interviewing at home. It was planned to recruit 310 women to the intervention group and 620 to the control group (Tappin et al., 2005). There may have been economic reasons for this choice (Dumville et al., 2006). After six months the recruitment ratio was modified from 2:1 to 1:1. In the end, 351 women were recruited to the intervention group and 411 in the control group. More precise details are not given but randomization could have been as in Table 19.1.

As far as I am aware, the authors did not consider a potential problem with their analysis. The analysis simply compared the 351 intervention patients with the 411 control patients. This is, in fact, the efficient analysis if one can assume that there are no trend effects. However, there is a potential bias in such an analysis in that one is not comparing like with like. The proportion of intervention patients treated in the first cohort was about 60/351 or about 17%, whereas the corresponding proportion in the control group is $120/411 = 29\%$. Hence, if there were a trend effect the naive comparison would be biased. On the other hand, the sort of comparison that would be made using the method of Bauer and Kohne (1994) would be sound.

One way out of this sort of situation, where we fear the efficient analysis might be biased but find the 'flexible' analysis not entirely convincing either, is, as Jonathan Denne proposed, to require that dual criteria be satisfied: our testing procedure should be significant not only in terms that satisfy the requirements of flexible designs but also in fixed sample size terms (Denne, 2001). This is a solution that Burman and Sonesson (2006a) endorse, although they point out that there will be some inevitable loss of power. For comments on their paper see Bauer (2006), Frisen (2006), Jennison and Turnbull (2006), and Proschan (2006), and for a rejoinder see Burman and Sonesson (2006b).

As regards more practical matters concerning implementation of adaptive designs, issue four of the *Drug Information Journal* in 2006 has a special section devoted to designs reporting a Pharmaceutical and Research Manufacturers of America (PhRMA) working group's 'white paper' on the subject Gallo and Krams (2006). The white paper is split into articles on terminology (Dragalin, 2006), operational considerations (Quinlan and

Krams, 2006) confidentiality and integrity issues (Gallo, 2006), dose-finding studies (Gaydos *et al.*, 2006), so-called seamless phase II/III studies (Maca *et al.*, 2006) and sample size re-estimation (Chuang-Stein *et al.*, 2006).

References

Armitage P, McPherson CK, Rowe BC (1969) Repeated significance tests on accumulating data. *Journal of the Royal Statistical Society A* **132**: 235–244.

Barnard GA (1946) Sequential tests in industrial statistics. *Journal of the Royal Statistical Society, Supplement* **8**: 1–26.

Bauer P (2006) Are flexible designs sound? Discussion. *Biometrics* **62**: 676–678.

Bauer P, Kohne K (1994) Evaluation of experiments with adaptive interim analyses. *Biometrics* **50**: 1029–1041.

Burman CF, Sonesson C (2006a) Are flexible designs sound? *Biometrics* **62**: 664–669.

Burman CF, Sonesson C (2006b) Are flexible designs sound? Rejoinder. *Biometrics* **62**: 680–683.

Burman C-F, Grieve AP, Senn S (2007) Decision analysis in drug development. In: Dimitrienko A, Chuang-Stein C, Agostino R (eds), *Pharmaceutical Statistics Using SAS: A Practical Guide*. SAS Institute, Cary, NC, pp 385–428.

Carlin BP, Kadane JB, Gelfand AE (1998) Approaches for optimal sequential decision analysis in clinical trials. *Biometrics* **54**: 964–975.

Cheng Y, Shen Y (2005) Bayesian adaptive designs for clinical trials. *Biometrika* **92**: 633–646.

Chuang-Stein C, Anderson K, Gallo P, Collins S (2006) Sample size reestimation: a review and recommendations. *Drug Information Journal* **40**: 475–484.

Colhoun HM, Betteridge DJ, Durrington PN, *et al.* (2004) Primary prevention of cardiovascular disease with atorvastatin in type 2 diabetes in the Collaborative Atorvastatin Diabetes Study (CARDS): multicentre randomised placebo-controlled trial. *Lancet* **364**: 685–696.

Demets DL, Lan KKG (1994) Interim Analysis – the alpha-spending function approach. *Statistics in Medicine* **13**: 1341–1352.

Denne JS (2001) Sample size recalculation using conditional power. *Statistics in Medicine* **20**: 2645–2660.

Dragalin V (2006) Adaptive designs: terminology and classification. *Drug Information Journal* **40**: 425–435.

Dumville JC, Hahn S, Miles JNV, Torgerson DJ (2006) The use of unequal randomisation ratios in clinical trials: A review. *Contemporary Clinical Trials* **27**: 1–12.

Ellenberg SS (1996) The use of data monitoring committees in clinical trials. *Drug Information Journal* **30**: 553–557.

Ellenberg S, Fleming T, DeMets D (2003) *Data Monitoring Committees in Clinical Trials: A Practical Perspective*. John Wiley & Sons, Ltd, Chichester.

Emerson SS (2006) Issues in the use of adaptive clinical trial designs. *Statistics in Medicine* **25**: 3270–3296.

Fisher LD (1998) Self-designing clinical trials. *Statistics in Medicine* **17**: 1551–1562.

Freedman LS (1996) Sequential methods. In: Henry Stewart Conference, Washington. Henry Stewart Conference Studies, London.

Freedman LS, Spiegelhalter DJ (1989) Comparison of Bayesian with group sequential-methods for monitoring clinical trials. *Controlled Clinical Trials* **10**: 357–367.

Frisen M (2006) Are flexible designs sound? Discussion. *Biometrics* **62**: 678–680.

Gallo P (2006) Confidentiality and trial integrity issues for adaptive designs. *Drug Information Journal* **40**: 445–450.

Gallo P, Krams M (2006) PhRMA Working Group on Adaptive Designs: Introduction to the full White Paper. *Drug Information Journal* **40**: 421–423.

Gallo P, Chuang-Stein C, Dragalin V, Gaydos B, Krams M, Pinheiro J (2006) Adaptive designs in clinical drug development – an Executive Summary of the PhRMA Working Group. *J Biopharm Stat* **16**: 275–283; discussion 285–291, 293–278, 311–272.

Gaydos B, Krams M, Perevozskaya I, *et al.* (2006) Adaptive dose-response studies. *Drug Information Journal* **40**: 451–461.

Gould AL (1992) Interim Analyses for monitoring clinical trials that do not materially affect the type-I error rate. *Statistics in Medicine* **11**: 55–66.

Herson J (1993) Data monitoring boards in the pharmaceutical industry. *Statistics in Medicine* **12**: 555–561.

Hilbrich L, Sleight P (2006) Progress and problems for randomized clinical trials: from streptomycin to the era of megatrials. *European Heart Journal* **27**: 2158–2164.

Jennison C, Turnbull B (2000) *Group Sequential Methods with Applications to Clinical Trials* (Interdisciplinary Statistics) Chapman and Hall/CRC, London and Boca Raton.

Jennison C, Turnbull BW (2006) Are flexible designs sound? Discussion. *Biometrics* **62**: 670–673.

Kadane J (1996) *Bayesian Methods and Ethics in Clinical Trials Design*. John Wiley & Sons, Inc., New York

Knopp RH, d'Emden M, Smilde JG, Pocock SJ (2006) Efficacy and safety of atorvastatin in the prevention of cardiovascular end points in subjects with type 2 diabetes: the Atorvastatin Study for Prevention of Coronary Heart Disease Endpoints in non-insulin-dependent diabetes mellitus (ASPEN). *Diabetes Care* **29**: 1478–1485.

Lan KKG, Demets DL (1983) Discrete sequential boundaries for clinical trials. *Biometrika* **70**: 659–663.

Lan KKG, Simon R, Halperin M (1982) Stochastically curtailed tests in long term clinical trials. *Sequential Analysis* **1**: 207–219.

Lee PM (1989) *Bayesian Statistics: an Introduction*. Edward Arnold, London.

Maca J, Bhattacharya S, Dragalin V, Gallo P, Krams M (2006) Adaptive seamless phase II/III designs – background, operational aspects, and examples. *Drug Information Journal* **40**: 463–473.

O'Brien PC, Fleming TR (1979) A multiple testing procedure for clinical trials. *Biometrics* **35**: 549–556.

O'Neill RT (1993) Some FDA perspectives on data monitoring in clinical trials in drug development. *Statistics in Medicine* **12**: 601–608.

Peto R, Pike MC, Armitage P, *et al.* (1976) Design and analysis of randomized clinical trials requiring prolonged observation of each patient. I. Introduction and design. *Br J Cancer* **34**: 585–612.

Pocock SJ (1977) Group sequential methods in design and analysis of clinical trials. *Biometrika* **64**: 191–209.

Proschan MA (2006) Are flexible designs sound? Discussion. *Biometrics* **62**: 674–676.

Proschan MA, Hunsberger SA (1995) Designed extension of studies based on conditional power. *Biometrics* **51**: 1315–1324.

Quinlan JA, Krams M (2006) Implementing adaptive designs: logistical and operational considerations. *Drug Information Journal* **40**: 437–444.

Senn SJ (2001) The misunderstood placebo. *Applied Clinical Trials* **10**: 40–46.

Senn SJ (2002) Ethical considerations concerning treatment allocation in drug development trials. *Statistical Methods in Medical Research* **11**: 403–411.

Simon R (1994) Some practical aspects of the interim monitoring of clinical trials. *Statistics in Medicine* **13**: 1401–1409.

Slud E, Wei LJ (1982) 2-Sample repeated significance tests based on the modified Wilcoxon statistic. *Journal of the American Statistical Association* **77**: 862–868.

Souhami RL (1994) The clinical importance of early stopping of randomized trials in cancer treatments. *Statistics in Medicine* **13**: 1293–1295.

Spiegelhalter DJ, Freedman LS, Parmar MKB (1994) Bayesian approaches to randomized trials. *Journal of the Royal Statistical Society Series A – Statistics in Society* **157**: 357–387.

Steering Committee of the Physicians' Health Study Research Group (1989) Final report on the aspirin component of the ongoing Physicians' Health Study. Steering Committee of the Physicians' Health Study Research Group. *New England Journal of Medicine* **321**: 129–135.

Tappin DM, Lumsden MA, Gilmour WH, *et al.* (2005) Randomised controlled trial of home based motivational interviewing by midwives to help pregnant smokers quit or cut down. *BMJ* **331**: 373–377.

Todd S (2007) A 25-year review of sequential methodology in clinical studies. *Statistics in Medicine* **26**: 237–252.

Wald A (1947) *Sequential Analysis.* John Wiley & Sons Inc., New York

Whitehead J (1997) *The Design and Analysis of Sequential Trials*, revised 2nd edition. John Wiley & Sons, Ltd, Chichester.

20

Dose-finding

Like other parties of the kind, it was first silent, then talky, then argumentative, then disputatious, then unintelligible, then altogethery, then inarticulate, and then drunk.

Lord Byron, *Letter to Thomas Moore*

A little Learning is a dang'rous Thing;
Drink deep, or taste not the Pierian Spring
There shallow Draughts intoxicate the Brain
And drinking largely sobers us again

Alexander Pope, *An Essay on Criticism*

20.1 BACKGROUND

A usable treatment is not just an effective molecule but also a formulation, a unit dose and a dosing interval. Dose-finding is difficult, essential and often badly done. It is a safe bet that many a potentially useful drug has been lost by failing to establish an appropriate dose. If the dose is set too high, the result may be problems with safety and tolerability. If the dose is set too low, the drug will fail for lack of efficacy. In this chapter, various issues to do with dose-finding will be considered. Because dose-finding has, or ought to have, a close relationship to pharmacokinetics, some of these issues will be considered in the next chapter. Before proceeding to the issues, however, some background matters will be discussed.

Two concepts often used in dose-finding are those of the **maximum-tolerated dose** and of the **minimum effective dose** (Pledger, 2001). There is no absolute definition of these and they may, of course, vary from individual to individual. If the maximum tolerated dose is higher than the minimum effective dose, then we have a treatment! The difference between them is the **therapeutic window**. Thus dose-finding studies are carried out for tolerability and for efficacy. In a sense, tolerability is always studied in all clinical trials including dose-finding. The same is not true of efficacy and dose-finding studies are unusual, in this respect, in that they may be carried out to study tolerability only. This is often done on healthy volunteers and for many drug development programmes the first studies will be pharmacokinetic and tolerability studies in healthy volunteers. (There are exceptions, however. For example, cytotoxic drugs will be studied on patients directly because of the toxicity of these treatments, which are designed for severely ill patients.)

With some drugs, the point at which efficacy fails to improve is reached before the maximum tolerated dose is reached. In that case, the concept of the **maximum useful dose** (International Conference on Harmonisation, 1995) may be relevant, although this concept can also be ambiguous as it may be the dose for which some utility reflecting a trade-off between efficacy and tolerability is a maximum. (See section 20.2.13 for a discussion.)

A central assumption in much of drug development is that the effects and side-effects of a treatment are related to the concentration of the treatment in the blood. An important concept in this respect is that of **steady-state concentration** (see also Chapter 21): the concentration eventually reached after regular therapy. It becomes important, therefore, to study the effects and side-effects of a treatment not only after a single dose but also over a period of time when given regular treatment. Note that a dose which is tolerated as a single dose will not necessarily be tolerated if given repeatedly. (Alcohol provides an extreme example!) Similarly, a dose which is in ineffective in a single administration may be highly effective when given repeatedly. Thus both single-dose dose-finding and multiple-dose dose-ranging studies are carried out. (Here 'single-dose' refers to the fact that, although a number of different doses are being studied, either a given subject or patient is given a single dose, or, if the patient is given a further dose, this is after a suitable wash-out, so that this further dose may be regarded as a single dose.) Except where specifically stated otherwise, it will be implicitly assumed in the discussion which follows that a single-dose study is being discussed.

Some rather special designs are used in dose-finding. For example, **dose-escalation designs** are common. These are designs in which the dose is gradually increased throughout the experiment until either some desired response or unwanted side-effect is encountered. These may be between-patient group escalations, where the first group receives the lowest dose, the next group the next highest, and so forth until the trial stops, or may be within-patient titrations.

The difference between **direct** and **indirect assays** is relevant here (Finney, 1978). In a direct assay a given response is targeted and the dose is adjusted until it is reached. In indirect assays the response is studied as a function of the dose and in consequence a useful dose is chosen. An issue that then arises is whether the dose that is eventually chosen should be limited to being one of those that has been studied or whether interpolation (or even extrapolation) can be considered. This relates to issues regarding the way that dose-response is modelled, which are covered in Section 20.2.1.

Sometimes dose-finding involves more than one drug and the designs may be rather complex. An example is the so -called **parallel assay** design. This compares the potency of (usually) closely related drugs. For example, one trial in asthma that I was involved in designing was a single-dose study in which three doses of a new formulation of a bronchodilator were compared with three doses of a standard formulation of the bronchodilator and placebo. This was run as an incomplete-blocks cross-over design using 21 sequences in which each patient received five treatments (Senn, 2002b; Senn *et al.*, 1997). Sometimes a **free combination therapy** is involved and dose-finding may be run as a **factorial design** in which different, doses of each of the two treatments are tried together (Byar, 1990). More complex explorations of the effect of doses in combination may be carried out as so-called **response surface designs**. Usually where this is done a model of at least quadratic complexity is fitted, which is to say that linear and quadratic terms in each dose, together with an interaction term, will be allowed for. However, such designs are rarely used in clinical trials. For an example in a pre-clinical context see Machado and Robinson (1994) and Tam *et al.* (2004).

Since dose-finding studies almost always have more than two treatment groups, they also involve multiple comparisons and there is a choice of comparisons to make (Bauer, 1991). For example, if we have a trial with a number of doses of an experimental drug as well as some comparator, either a placebo or some standard alternative, we might be interested in comparing each dose with the control. Alternatively, we may wish to compare neighbouring doses. If we wish to control the type I error rate, various schemes of differing power and with alternative properties have been proposed.

A special approach to dose-finding was introduced in cancer trials by O'Quigley *et al.* (1990). This is the **continual reassessment method**. In phase I cancer studies, patients are the subjects for study rather than healthy volunteers. It is usually assumed that there is a narrow therapeutic window and that the dose should be established as high as possible given the constraints impose by the dangers of toxicity. Patients are entered sequentially and the dose they are given is determined using a suitable algorithm and depending on the number of toxicities seen to date.

A useful concept in dose–response studies is that of the **dose metameter** (Wong and Lachenbruch, 1996). This is that function of the dose, say $g(d)$ used for studying response. For example, for a trial in which doses were $d = 4$, 8, 16, 32 and 64 mg, one might decide to study response as function of log-dose. Since the doses are at constant log-intervals, one could then code the doses using the transformation $g(d) = \left[\log_2 (d/4)\right]/4 = \log_{16} (d/4)$ to create values 0, 0.25, 0.5, 1.0 on a standard 0 to 1 scale.

Two useful books on dose-finding in clinical medicine are that edited by Ting (2006) and the one in this series edited by Chevret (2006). In the latter, the chapter by Hemmings (2006) provides a regulatory perspective. Regulatory guidance is provided by International Conference on Harmonization (1995). As regards practical implementation of dose escalation schemes in phase I in cancer, such as are discussed in Sections 20.2.7 to 20.2.9, some freely available software, Escalation With Overdose Control (EWOC) 2.0, is available from Emory University and is described by Xu *et al.* (2007).

20.2 ISSUES

20.2.1 Regression versus disconnected treatment models

In a parallel-group dose-finding study involving two doses (and no placebo), the dose-response can either be modelled as the straight line going through the two group means or as the difference between the two treatment means. These two approaches are effectively equivalent. Where there are three or more doses, however, there are different ways of approaching the modelling problem. One general approach, the regression approach, regards the dose as being a (potentially) continuously variable quantity and the actual doses studied as having no substantive interest of their own but merely as points we have chosen to help us determine the dose-response. An alternative approach, which, for want of a better term, I shall call the *disconnected treatment* approach, regards the doses as being treatments in their own right and the task of the trialist to be that of making precise statements about the effects of the actual doses studied.

For example, given two doses and a placebo, one could compare the two doses with each other and separately with placebo (or perhaps compare their average with placebo). This would be the disconnected treatments approach. Alternatively, one could fit a straight line response to the doses. This would be the regression approach. If the lower dose is half-way between placebo and the higher dose, then it will actually play no part in determining the slope of this line, which will simply be a function of the difference between the upper and lower doses. For this function, an optimal design would actually dispense with the lower dose group altogether. On the other hand, the quadratic term in a model of three doses would compare the lower dose with the average of placebo and the higher dose. In the end, then, given a model of adequate complexity, the two approaches amount to the same thing.

Nevertheless, the two approaches are somewhat different in spirit and this difference is worth commenting on. In some cases in drug development it is quite possible to regard a dose as being infinitely variable. This is more likely to be the case early in development. Here, in the particular dose range being considered, any dose may be a potential option and it is of interest to be able to predict dose-response at any point in the range. Furthermore, it is ludicrous to suppose that the dose-response cannot be reasonably well approximated by some sort of smooth function. If this were not the case we should have to rely on pure luck in having hit a useful part of a discontinuous function. However, if the function is not too complex, then design theory suggests that it can be adequately, and indeed in some cases optimally, studied by using a very few doses. Hence the fact that a few rational doses have been used is not incompatible with wishing to estimate a smooth function, and this in turn will enable one to predict the response at any point in the range. At a certain stage of pharmaceutical development, however, dose options become more limited. This is because capsules, tablets or whatever must be finalized and a given strength must be chosen. There may be a selection of strengths, but the lowest strength available then defines the minimum dose step which is possible. Once this stage has been reached, it could be argued that the performance of individual rational doses is all that matters and the potential continuity of the dose-response is irrelevant. (Of course it is still possible that one could consider the results under neighbouring doses as contributing to one's inferences about a given dose being examined.)

Thus, there may be a case for saying that in early drug development the regression approach is appropriate whereas in phase III studies comparing (say) two doses with placebo the disconnected treatment approach may be relevant. Compromise positions are also possible; for example, there is a long tradition of studying dose-response simply using order relationships. The paper by Bretz (2006) considers some alternatives to the classic approach of Williams (1972). Some of these intermediate approaches will be discussed in due course below.

20.2.2   Random-effect models

Given individuals may have different dose–response curves which may, however, bear some similarity to each other. It does not follow, though, that the global dose–response formed by averaging these dose–response curves at each dose will, in fact, resemble the individual dose curves (Hemmings, 2006). The average dose-response is not the same as the dose–response curve of the average person. Furthermore, if we wish to predict what the response will be of a patient who has been observed to fail at a given dose when given a higher dose, we need to study individual response curves and make a judicious balance between using global and local information. (See Chapter 18 on *n*-of-1 trials.) In order to examine the way in which individual dose-responses vary, two things are necessary: first, a design in which different doses are measured within the same person and, second, a random-effects model. Obviously, not all therapies and diseases are suitable for studying more than one dose in the same individual. In general, progressive diseases are not suitable and diseases in which survival is the only endpoint of interest cannot be studied in this way at all. (We can, however, as very much a second best, group patients according to some covariates of interest.)

On the other hand, even where within-patient dose-finding is a theoretical possibility, some trialists are wary of using such studies because of the danger of carry-over. In general, two forms of within-patient studies are advocated: dose-escalation and cross-over. We have already covered the controversies surrounding the latter design in Chapter 17. The late Lewis Sheiner, an important pioneer of nonlinear random-effect models, was an extremely enthusiastic proponent of dose-escalation studies, which are designs in which the doses are given in ascending order. These studies thus have the same potential problem as cross-over designs with respect to carry-over, with the additional difficulty that dose and period effects are confounded. This can be dealt with either by having an accompanying group, which is escalated on placebo, or by having a randomly intervening placebo in the dose-escalation sequence. Neither of these approaches is as efficient as using a cross-over trial (Senn, 1997).

Thus, there is a point at issue here between those who believe that the problem of carry-over is potentially so devastating as to preclude within-patient studies and those who think that the predictive power of random-effect models in conjunction with appropriate within-patient designs is so great that the opportunity to conduct them must not be passed up.

My sympathies are mainly with the latter school (Senn, 2006). In a simulation study, Sheiner *et al.* (1991) compared dose-escalation, cross-over and parallel-group studies and came to the conclusion that the two within-patient designs perform much better than the parallel-group trial, even in the presence of carry-over. On the other hand, one must be cautious. In a famous paper, Temple (1982) discusses the problems with dose-escalation studies and takes the example of captopril and hypertension. He points out that the original dose established for captopril was far too high and speculates that a combination of delayed response and dose escalation might be responsible: what was judged to be the response on the higher doses was in fact a delayed response to the lower doses and hence the dose was set too high.

A possible ethical advantage for dose-escalation studies is that escalation can stop once a patient has reached an optimal dose, and this is often coupled with the practical argument that this is how the drug will be used in practice. This argument is very attractive but not quite as strong as it appears. If it is possible to establish for a given patient his or her own ideal dose by an individual escalation, and if this is the way in which the drug will be used in practice there is no need to establish the ideal target dose for an individual: every individual will start on the minimum and proceed to a satisfactory response. What is then needed is a pragmatic trial in which it is shown that the policy of escalating on this treatment is superior to that of escalating on another.

Furthermore, if individuals stop once a given dose has been reached, special methods of analysis are needed. This can be understood by considering two simple analyses of such data, each with its own bias. Suppose that many patients do discontinue before reaching the highest dose but some do not. If we simply compare the mean response of all patients at each dose, we shall not be comparing like with like. The lowest dose will have information on all patients, the highest only on patients who have failed to respond on the lower doses. These may be the most difficult patients. Thus, we shall bias against the highest dose. Suppose, on the other hand, that we only analyse data from patients who have completed and suppose that, unbeknown to us, the doses are identical but there is considerable variation between occasions for given patients. Any patient who has a random high response on a lower dose will not be escalated further. Therefore, we shall be left with analysing patients who by definition never had such a response on a lower dose. But some of these may, by chance, now have such a response on the highest dose. Therefore, this form of analysis will bias slightly in favour of the highest dose. (However, the general problem of selecting values to be studied precisely because they are extreme is one that produces notoriously different solutions depending on the inferential framework employed and readers who are interested in challenging their intuition are recommended to read Phil Dawid's penetrating and challenging piece on selection paradoxes (Dawid, 1994).)

The moral is, therefore, that dose-escalation studies require complex modelling (nonlinear random-effect models which allow for drop-out are to be used) and this is a price which *must* be paid. I was once a member of working-party on asthma and was delighted to discover a physician colleague who was an enthusiast for Sheiner's approach to dose escalation. I asked him how he managed the modelling. He replied that that was where he parted company with the statisticians. As far as he was concerned, all that was necessary was some simple summaries! Of course, it is not right to avoid using a powerful investigational tool simply because some have misused it. Dose-escalation studies appropriately analysed can be extremely powerful. Where it is ethically possible to run them, cross-over trials are even better.

However, it should not be forgotten that a prescribing doctor, for reasons of time, skill and constraints imposed by dosage strengths available, may not be in the position to vary the patient's dose infinitely, still less to apply the results of random effect modelling for the purpose of adjusting the dose for a given patient. It then becomes important for him or her to have a statement about the expected effect of a limited number of doses available. For this pragmatic purpose, parallel group trials may, after all, be adequate.

20.2.3   Multiple testing schemes

If a number of doses are included in a trial and the approach to estimation is not a regression modelling one, then a number of contrasts may be of interest: either between individual doses or between doses and placebo. This raises the issue of adjusting for repeated testing. (See also Chapter 10). Various schemes have been proposed. Good discussions for the particular context of dose-finding are given by Budde and Bauer (1989) and Bauer (1997) and, in a useful more general discussion of multiplicity, by Bauer (1991).

For dose-finding, such approaches will exploit the dose ordering, at least if we are prepared to assume that the dose-response is monotonic. (Our two chapter quotations give examples where the response, conversation in the one case and intoxication in the other, is *not* a monotonic function of the dose, but dose-finding is often performed in the hope that this sort of response is rare.) An early example of a nonparametric test which tests the hypothesis of equality of all treatments against an ordered alternative is the Terpstra–Jonckheere test (Jonckheere, 1954; Terpstra, 1952). The Williams test (Williams, 1971) is a popular one for comparing doses with placebo to establish the minimum effective dose. Consider, following Bauer (1991) who followed Marcus et al. (1976), the case where we have four doses, with perhaps the lowest as a placebo, and we wish to compare neighbouring doses. The global hypothesis is

$$H_{0,1234} : \mu_1 = \mu_2 = \mu_3 = \mu_4$$

and the alternative hypothesis, if we are prepared to assume monotonicity, is

$$H_1 : \mu_1 \leq \mu_2 \leq \mu_3 \leq \mu_4,$$

with at least one of the $\leq$ being a strict inequality, $<$. The only pair-wise comparisons we are interested in testing are

$$H_{0,12} : \mu_1 = \mu_2, \quad H_{0,23} : \mu_2 = \mu_3, \quad H_{0,34} : \mu_3 = \mu_4.$$

The other three comparisons are not of direct interest. Consequently the only intersection hypotheses we need to look at are

$$H_{0,123} : \mu_1 = \mu_2 = \mu_3, \quad H_{0,12\cap34} : \mu_1 = \mu_2 \cap \mu_3 = \mu_4 \quad \text{and} \quad H_{0,234} : \mu_2 = \mu_3 = \mu_4.$$

Hence, examination of these seven hypotheses (one global, three intersection and three individual) is all that is necessary to investigate the questions of interest and control the type I error rate.

Accompanying such a closed test procedure one then needs to nominate a testing strategy. Budde and Bauer consider two alternatives and investigate their power. For example, one approach is to use some test which is designed to consider ordered hypotheses, such as the Terpstra–Jonckheere test, for each of the seven hypotheses (Jonckheere, 1954; Terpstra, 1952). The only one which causes a problem is $H_{0,12\cap34}$. Here some approach like taking as a test statistic the sum of the test statistics for the individual parts can be considered. Or, because of the independence of the constituent parts, a test can be based on the product of the individual P-values. Each test in this procedure can be carried out at level α.

Alternatively, the higher-level tests can actually be investigated using the lower-level ones, given a suitable strategy. In this example, we would carry out the three individual tests at the level $\alpha/3$. Rejection of any one of these allows us to reject the intersection hypotheses involving it and the global hypothesis. This permits us to consider a reduced set of hypotheses for which we are entitled to use the level $\alpha/2$. We can now revisit our lower-level tests and see whether any of these which were not rejected previously would now be rejected and so forth.

Such schemes *appear* to suffer from a number of difficulties. (I say *appear* because one interpretation is that the difficulties are features of the underlying complexity of the problem, rather than of the scheme.) One problem is to do with the interpretation of significance. There is, of course, a long-standing Bayesian (and also a Neyman–Pearson frequentist) objection to interpreting P-values evidentially. (See, for example Goodman (1992) and Senn (2002a) for a comment.) With such schemes, however, the difficulties seem even greater than usual. For example, in the second of the two schemes considered by Budde and Bauer (1989) and described above, suppose that the apparently most significant contrast is that used for examining $H_{0,12}$ with an uncorrected P-value of 0.015 which is compared with $0.05/3 = 0.0167$ to judge significance and is thus significant, and that the second most significant, that for $H_{0,23}$, has an uncorrected P-value of 0.018 which, while not significant when compared with $0.05/3 = 0.0167$, is significant when compared with $0.05/2 = 0.025$, which is the value we are now entitled to use. What P-values should we now claim when reporting these figures? Are we entitled to leave them as they are? Or should we perhaps multiply them both by 3, in which case the second is not significant? Or should we now multiply the first by 3 and the second by 2, in which case they become 0.045 and 0.036 respectively, so that the second contrast is now actually more significant than the first? Similarly, as we usually are in dose-finding, we are interested in estimation. How should we calculate the confidence intervals associated with the point estimates?

With so many schemes to choose from, which shall we choose? Is the sponsor entitled to choose any scheme at all provided that it is declared in the protocol beforehand? Consider the general framework proposed by Budde and Bauer (1989). One might argue that the comparison of neighbouring doses is actually of no interest. It corresponds to measuring a dose-response as a function of the dose interval but this interval will depend on the number of doses studied and is thus not a fundamental feature of the drug. Of more practical interest might be to establish the minimum effective dose and the minimum dose with maximal efficacy. For example, a scheme which controls the error rate (but is no doubt conservative) tests the hypotheses $H_{0,14}$, $H_{0,13}$, $H_{0,12}$ in order each at level $\alpha/2$, proceeding only if there is significance and then perhaps testing $H_{0,23}$ and $H_{0,34}$ in order, also at level $\alpha/2$ (although for the latter question some sort of equivalence approach might be desirable). Many such schemes could be devised and I am not suggesting that this is a good one. (Peter Bauer has pointed out to me that if monotonicity is accepted, then rejection of $H_{0,1234}$ implies that dose 4 at least is effective, rejection of $H_{0,123}$ implies that dose 3 and 4 are effective, and rejection of $H_{0,12}$ implies that doses 2, 3 and 4 are effective. Hence, if dose 1 is a placebo we have a means of determining the minimum effective dose for free. See Bauer (1997), for a discussion.) However, whatever scheme is eventually regarded as being of interest, it raises the issue whether the regulator is bound to accept any scheme which controls the type I error rate provided it has been specified in the protocol. If one argues that dose-finding studies are not the regulator's concern because final doses will be investigated in phase III, why is it necessary to use such schemes anyway? Is the sponsor trying to protect himself from rash conclusions and if so is this the way to do it?

20.2.4   Cumulative dose studies

A 'quick and dirty' way of establishing potency of a drug is quite often used in asthma (Senn, 1993). For all I know, similar approaches may be applied in other indications as well. The approach is to give patients within one day at short intervals (perhaps half an hour) various doses of (say) a new bronchodilator or, on another day, doses of a standard bronchodilator. Often a scheme is used whereby cumulative doses are doubled, so that one again one, then two and then four unit doses are used, supposedly corresponding to 1, 2, 4 and 8 cumulative unit doses. The effect on FEV_1, or some other measure of lung function, is recorded after each dose and the relative potency of the new bronchodilator compared with the standard is then established by comparing cumulative dose–response curves, usually having plotted dose on a log scale.

In my opinion this is potentially misleading since not only does this strategy confound dose and time, but the importance of this confounding is difficult to assess. Responses to a treatment will vary over time and the dosing interval is usually chosen so that the effect will have reached its maximum by about the time the next dose is given. Since some proportion of a dose must be eliminated, the total reached by the end of the exercise is not, in fact, 8 unit doses but something less than this. How much less depends on the rate of elimination and, if this is different for the two drugs, the number of units cumulated will not be the same. In fact, in pharmacokinetic terms this form of dose–response, which compares maximum effect (the pharmacodynamic analogue of C_{max}), is rather unusual since this is more sensibly done by comparing areas under the curve, although for certain simple types of pharmacodynamic response the two approaches are equivalent.

This form of dose–response study is, of course, quick to run, since all the doses are delivered in one day. However, because of the extreme difficulty in saying anything sensible about the effect of the doses over time, I do not recommend it.

20.2.5 Accompanying-placebo designs

In certain dose-finding studies, because of fears for safety, an escalation of doses by group takes place. Thus, the first dose will be examined in one group of patients (or sometimes healthy volunteers) before proceeding to study the next dose, and so forth. The dose is then confounded with a period effect and if subject recruitment changes over time, or if systems of measurement (such as assays) change, or if external conditions change, then estimates produced from such a trial will have a bias. Furthermore, such trials are not fully blind but **veiled**, since, although the subjects will not know whether they are being given an active treatment or placebo, they do know, to the extent that informed consent has been observed (and in any case they may guess), to which group they belong (Senn, 1995).

Sometimes placebo patients are included with each dose group. This permits a controlled comparison to be made. It also makes it possible to compare different doses in a way that eliminates the trend effect. Each dose is compared with its own placebo first and these contrasts are then compared with each other. Such indirect comparisons are less precise, involving as they do four groups to compare two doses, than would be direct comparison of the doses. We then have another example of a **bias–variance trade-off**. The direct comparison is potentially biased but efficient. The indirect comparison is inefficient but unbiased (Senn, 1997).

I once helped to design such a trial involving four doses and 36 subjects for which the physicians involved proposed having a 6:3 split between active and placebo subjects for each dose level. I pointed out that for four fewer subjects altogether, a 4:4 split would be just as efficient. For example, for the purpose of comparing active with placebo, the variance would be proportional to $(1/4 + 1/4) = 1/2$ and thus the same as for the proposed design where it would be proportional to $(1/6 + 1/3)$ which is also equal to $1/2$. Of course, a 5:4 split would be more efficient and would use exactly the same number of subjects as originally proposed.

The physicians argued, however, that in the end, since there were four groups, we would have 12 patients on placebo, twice as many as on each dose. I pointed out that pooling the placebo patients would only make sense if (a) we considered that blinding was not a problem and (b) there was no trend effect. For example, subjects in the highest dose would know that they were either receiving the highest dose or placebo. If they were nervous about adverse reactions as a consequence, this sort of bias would only be eliminated by comparing each dose with its accompanying placebo (see Senn (1995) for a discussion of this issue). The physicians countered by saying that the most important measures were objective and that in any case trend effects were completely unimportant. I accepted this argument and had the proposed analysis (that is to say without adjustment for trend) written into the protocol together with the justification.

Unfortunately, by the time the trial came to be run, the physicians had completely changed their minds about trend effects. Whereas before they considered they were completely unimportant, they now considered that it was essential to eliminate them. The trial was in a respiratory indication and a delay in starting meant that it now straddled the hay-fever season. For the purpose of eliminating such a trend, we now had an inefficient design.

I leave it to the reader to draw the necessary morals.

20.2.6 Pooling variances

A general problem arises in trials with more than two treatment groups regarding the estimation of variances, but it is particularly acute for dose-finding studies. The general habit appears to be to pool the variances from all the treatment groups even when comparing only two treatments and, indeed, it is more or less automatically assumed that this is desirable by many computer packages for which this is the standard analysis.

As far as I am aware, this widespread habit first arose in the analysis of agricultural experiments where residual degrees of freedom were generally few. For example a 5×5 Latin square would leave 12 residual degrees of freedom for error altogether. In the context of a clinical trial, however, we commonly have more than 20 patients per group (often many more) and cases where we have fewer than 40 degrees of freedom for error, even if we only choose to base our estimate for a given contrast on the two groups concerned, are rare. (In fact, trials with hundreds of degrees of freedom are not uncommon.) As regards power, there is little to be gained by pooling across all groups. For instance, the variance of a t-distribution with 40 degrees of freedom is only 1.05, 5% higher than the value for a standard Normal.

The downside of pooling can be considerable. Consider a case where we are comparing three doses with placebo. If we have treatment-by-patient interaction, then the variance in the highest-dose group might be considerably higher than, say, that in the placebo group. If we compare the lowest-dose group with placebo but use a variance pooled over all groups, this variance may be inappropriately large and we shall lose power. On the other hand, when we come to compare the second-highest dose with the highest, which might in fact be equivalent in effect, if we use a variance pooled over all groups, this may be inappropriately small and we shall have an inflation of the type I error rate.

Under such circumstances little seems to be gained by pooling and much may be lost (Julious, 2005; Senn, 2000, 2004a). Pooling does appear to have one advantage, however. It tends to keep statistical significance in line with estimated differences.

(Whether this is important or not is debatable.) If this approach is not used, then even for a case where the observed treatment means are monotonic, we may conclude that the highest dose is not significantly different from placebo but that a lower dose is.

It must also be conceded that where regression modelling approaches are used, some sort of pooling is almost inevitable, since one is willing to estimate dose-response and produce an estimate of its precision even though one might have no replicated doses. (In theory every patient could be on a different dose.) This raises the issue of joint modelling of mean and variance. This is currently a live topic and in particular has been extensively developed in connection with hierarchical generalized linear models by Youngjo Lee and John Nelder; see, for example, Lee and Nelder (2006), Nelder and Lee (1998).

20.2.7 O'Quigley's Continual Reassessment Method

In a series of papers with various co-workers, O'Quigley proposed a method for dose-finding in phase I studies in cancer (O'Quigley and Chevret, 1991; O'Quigley *et al.*, 1990; O'Quigley and Shen, 1996). (For a full description of the design see Chevret and Zohar (2006) in the book on dose-finding (Chevret, 2006) in the same series as this one.) For chemotherapy in cancer, as the dose of a drug is increased then eventually toxic side-effects are produced. It is generally the case, however, that doses which are well below those which produce toxicity are commonly ineffective. Thus one would ideally like to raise the dose to a level just short of that which will produce serious toxicity. One way of managing dose-finding, therefore, is by controlling the probability of toxicity. For example, one might be looking for the dose which will produce toxicity with probability 20%.

In O'Quigley's approach, the probability of toxicity is modelled using working regression functions. As discussed by Chevret and Zohar (2006), in the original paper (O'Quigley *et al.*, 1990) a hyperbolic tangent was used and subsequently a logistic function (O'Quigley and Chevret, 1991). The dose given to the current patient, together with his or her observed result (toxicity or not), is used to update the function in a way which is (effectively) Bayesian. (However, further development has abandoned the requirement for a Bayesian approach except for the first few patients (Chevret and Zohar, 2006).) Thus, at any point in the study, the predicted response is a function of all the results to date. This is then used to determine the dose for the next patient. If the decision is completely given over to the algorithm, then a given sequence of toxicities simply defines the next dose. Provided only that a series of treatments can be ranked in terms of presumed toxicity (which is assumed to be the reveres ranking in terms of efficacy), the algorithm can be applied even where different molecules are involved. An interesting feature of the algorithm is that, if strictly applied, it defines a 'dose path' in terms of a toxicity sequence. Thus, for example, if T is *toxicity* and N is *not* then, given a particular prior, the sequence of observed results NNNTNNT defines the next dose to be given. Hence, for n patients there are *at most* 2^n possible paths. This means that in principle dose tables can be prepared for a trial in advance before carrying it out.

The algorithm is good at establishing the dose with target efficacy. It is not good at learning about the whole of the dose–response function. It thus comes down firmly on the side of what is sometimes called 'individual ethics' as opposed to 'collective ethics'. (See the chapter by Whitehead (2006) in Chevret (2006) for a discussion.) In fixing a dose for a patient, the algorithm used only has his or her interests in mind. This is different from bandit designs, where we are also considering optimizing therapy for future patients, in which we might be prepared to consider giving a patient a dose which has a predicted probability of toxicity that is somewhat different from the target toxicity, in the interests of learning more about the dose–response curve as a whole.

A further problem with the O'Quigley design is that in the very early stages the dose-step indicated can be rather larger than one might wish if a step-up is indicated. Simply making the prior more informative to deal with this might prohibit an adequate step downwards. Whether this is a true difficulty, and if so what should be done about, it is not clear to me.

20.2.8   Working-dose models for the continual reassessment method

The continual reassessment method (CRM) approach consists of the following elements: a set of doses, a definition of toxicity, a target level of toxicity, a working-dose model and a prior distribution for the parameter(s) of the model. John O'Quigley himself has generally used a one-parameter working-dose response model. Others, for example Whitehead (2006) and Whitehead and Brunier (1995), have used two-parameter models. If we are modelling response on the log-odds scale with $p(d)$ as the probability of toxicity at dose d, $\eta(d)$ as the linear predictor on the log-odds scale and $g(d)$ some transformation used to create the dose metamater, so that

$$\log\left[\frac{p(d)}{1-p(d)}\right] = \eta(d),$$

then the choice might be between $\eta(d) = \theta_1 g(d)$ or perhaps $\eta(d) = \theta_0 + \theta_1 g(d)$ but with θ_0 fixed and treated as known, as used by O'Quigley and co-workers, or the latter function with not only θ_1 but also θ_0 treated as unknown and to be estimated, as favoured by Whitehead and co-workers.

At first sight it might appear that the apparently more flexible two-parameter approach is superior. Consider, however, that an infinity of curves go through a point defined by the desired dose and the target response. Of course these dose–response functions do not generally agree as regards their predicted response *except* at the desired dose. However, to the extent that the design delivers its objective, most patients are treated around this dose, so that the question arises whether one can, in fact, identify models with more than one parameter. John O'Quigley has suggested to me that two-parameter models are inconsistent in that the variances of the parameter estimates do not approach zero as the number of patients approaches infinity. Note that this is not the same as saying that the predictions from such models are inconsistent, since even where the variances $\mathrm{var}[\hat{\theta}_0]$ and $\mathrm{var}[\hat{\theta}_1]$ of the individual parameter estimates remain 'large', the variance of the linear combination

$$\mathrm{var}\left[\hat{\eta}(d)\right] = \mathrm{var}\left(\hat{\theta}_0\right) + \{g(d)\}^2 \,\mathrm{var}\left(\hat{\theta}_1\right) + 2g(d)\,\mathrm{cov}\left[\hat{\theta}_0, \hat{\theta}_1\right]$$

might be small given that $\mathrm{cov}\left[\hat{\theta}_0, \hat{\theta}_1\right]$ will be negative.

Personally, however, I am rather sceptical about the value of two-parameter models. Since this is a point about which many eminent researchers disagree, this is very much a live 'issue' in drug development.

20.2.9   Starting doses for the continual reassessment method

Some researchers consider there is an ethical imperative to start subjects off at the lowest dose envisaged, as any other strategy would be unethical. Since the CRM proceeds by starting off at intermediate doses, this is sometimes presented as an ethical drawback of the CRM. This position is absurd, however. Consider a researcher who has designed a study with doses 8, 16, 32 and 64 mg. He intends to treat the first patient with the dose of 8 mg, saying that any higher starting dose is unethical. A proponent of the CRM accepts this but suggests adding doses 1, 2 and 4 mg to the design. The first patient will now be treated at 8 mg as before but this is now the middle dose of all the doses envisaged and not the lowest. However, the risk run by the first patient is just the same as if the doses of 1, 2 and 4 mg were not present but the design now permits a de-escalation of dose for the second patient should there be a toxicity for the first patient (which is, of course, not expected). Thus, the design for which 8 mg is the middle dose cannot be ethically inferior to the design where it is the lowest dose.

Looked at in this light it is clear that the real (and difficult) ethical issue is what in real terms, that is to say on the 'milligram' scale, the starting dose should be – not what it should be on the ordinal scale of doses to be included in the design.

20.2.10   Response-surface methods

Where combination therapies are being investigated it can be argued that dose-finding should take place in two 'dimensions' (Hemmings, 2006). What is being investigated in that case is a response surface. Often, one of the justifications made for combination therapies is in terms of risk–benefit trade-off. For example, to show that it is logical to give a combination of one dose of A and one dose of B it is necessary to show advantages compared not only with the policies of giving one dose of A on its own or one dose of B on its own but also with giving higher doses of A alone or higher doses of B alone. Sometimes the standard doses of A or B are close to the maximum tolerated and it is believed that there will be a synergy of efficacy but not a synergy of side-effects. This, then, is the justification for developing a combination approach. As in all drug development, however, the task is to prove the validity of the assertion. Hence designs are needed in which the response of both efficacy and tolerability to different combinations of drug are investigated.

In the setting of industrial production, such designs have been developed extensively, often to cope with multiple factors, and an elaborate theory of fractional factorials, star designs, Taguchi methods exists. The main differences with the clinical context are that, although it is usually possible to obtain many replicates (patients) for a given combination of factors, there are often ethical constraints in exploring the whole response surface and practical considerations limit the number of dose combinations which can be investigated.

Such an investigation is rarely concluded as a result of running a single trial. Many of the problems which apply to drug-finding in general apply *a fortiori* to this particular field. Other matters are also important. For example, one problem which occurred when we considered demographic subgroups and again when discussing multicentre trials, was how to deal with interactive terms. Simply including such terms in the model has an unwelcome effect on variances of predicted responses. Excluding them can lead to bias. Since response-surface methods are used to investigate drug interactions, this is potentially a problem here also.

In the first edition of this book, I wrote of response surface designs as applied in clinical research that 'the field is still in its infancy'. In the second edition I am tempted to report, flippantly, that the infant in question does not seem to have grown much. However, an interesting paper that reports an actual clinical trial is that by Tangen and Koch (2001). They consider an example of a 3×4 factorial trial in hypertension in which on average 43 patients were randomized to each of 12 possible combinations of three levels of hydrochlorothiazide (placebo, low, high) and four levels of an ACE inhibitor. (For a remarkably similar trial reported in the medical literature, see the 3×4 factorial trial of felodipine and ramipril in 507 patients reported by Scholze *et al.* (1999).)

In their paper, Tangen and Koch (2001) concentrate primarily on the analysis of contrasts of particular interest. The approach is thus in the spirit of that described as the *disconnected treatment approach* in Section 20.2.1. For an alternative regression approach, an extremely interesting paper is that of Pool et al. (1997). This reports and analyses a 4×4 factorial trial of hydrochlorothiazide and fosinopril in hypertension in 550 patients. They fit a quadratic surface model in both doses to the

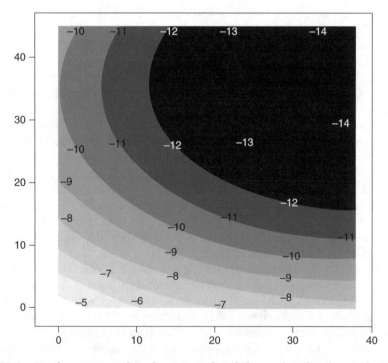

Figure 20.1 Fitted response surface showing predicted change from baseline in diastolic blood pressure in mmHg for the data reported in Pool *et al.* (1997) as a function of dose. The *X* axis gives dose of HCTZ in mg and the *Y* axis dose of fosinopril.

response and report results in some detail. They do not include a linear interaction term for the two doses, although one could argue that it would be natural to do so. Figure 20.1 shows a quadratic response fit, including interaction, for difference from baseline in diastolic blood pressure (DBP) for this trial in order to give an illustration of the sort of information that can result from a response surface fit. (Ideally, baseline DBP should have been fitted as a covariate but this was not possible using the published data.)

20.2.11 Minimum effective dose

A common aim of dose-finding studies is to establish the so-called minimum effective dose. The conceptual difficulty associated with this is that it is not well defined. If we simply use hypothesis tests of contrasts of dose against placebo to establish this, then the minimum effective dose depends on the sample size (Filloon, 1995). Larger trials will have more power to detect smaller differences and so, other things being equal, larger trials will tend to conclude that lower doses are effective. This problem is related to one which was discussed in Chapter 13 where we considered whether trials should be powered to prove that a clinically relevant difference obtains.

Note also that the requirement of finding a minimal dose that is 'proved' to be efficacious is rather different from what is often required of the maximum tolerated dose. Here a dose is likely to be abandoned, if some tolerability problems emerge, even if the dose cannot be proved to be worse by the standard of statistical significance than a dose that is retained. For example, the CRM methods discussed in Sections 20.2.7 to 20.2.9 do not use the notion of statistical significance. Of course, one reason for this is that the primary object of interest is selecting a correct dose for the next patient rather than for all future patients. Nevertheless, the difference in attitude to minimum effective and maximum tolerated (or maximum acceptable) doses is striking.

The moral ought to be that it takes more than a significance test to investigate the minimally effective dose. Consideration of this particular problem suggests that a modelling (regression type approach) to dose-response may be more appropriate, with minimum effective dose established according to some reasonable target and the probability of obtaining it. This sort of objective fits in best within a predictive Bayesian framework. This does not mean that, even if one chooses to stay within a frequentist framework, choosing the lowest dose at which a conventional test of the difference to placebo is significant is the best that can be done.

20.2.12 Parallel assay

When introducing new formulations of a drug we may have considerable information already available on a standard formulation. It may thus be of interest to establish what dose of the new formulation has the same response as the standard. In some cases this can be handled in a way similar to that conventionally used for bioequivalence. That is to say, the bioavailability of the standard formulation and an assumed dose form for the new formulation can be established by studying the concentration–time profiles. The bioavailability of the new formulation can then be adjusted according to these results.

In some cases, however, this approach is not possible. For example, with inhaled preparations for treating asthma, 90% of the preparation may be swallowed rather than inhaled, but it is the inhaled fraction which is important. Under such circumstances it becomes important to compare the pharmacodynamic response of reference and test formulations.

This is a controversial matter, since two doses of the reference formulations might have similar pharmacodynamic responses as regards the target parameter (which will usually be an efficacy parameter) but might have different effects in terms of tolerability, or indeed exhibit different concentrations at the effect site (which will, however, usually not be measurable). Hence, one might find that the test formulation is apparently 'equivalent' to the standard reference formulation but could equally well be 'equivalent' to different doses of the reference formulation. Since the purpose of such equivalence trials is to obviate the requirement for an extensive development which would include long-term studies addressing tolerability, it can be dangerous to naively assume equivalence under such circumstances.

One way to deal with this is to carry out a parallel assay comparing at least two doses of the test with two doses of the reference formulation. Ideally one should show that the two formulations exhibit equivalent dose-response. An example of such a study (Senn, 2002b; Senn et al., 1997) was mentioned in the introduction, where two forms of dry-powder inhaler were compared. The idea, essentially, is to show that the test formulation is equivalent at the same nominal dose as the standard but also *not* equivalent to higher or lower doses of the standard. This is not at all a foregone conclusion and one of the problems has to do with limits of equivalence, which will vary from pharmacodynamic parameter to parameter.

Such studies also share not only many of the difficulties of dose-finding studies in general but also those which attend bioequivalence and equivalence studies. See Kallen and Larsson (1999) for further discussion and also Chapter 15.

20.2.13   Assumptions of monotonicity

Many approaches to dose-finding exploit the usually reasonable assumption that higher doses have greater effects. Of course, it is recognized that this only applies provided one considers the effect of dose on efficacy and tolerability separately. It is the object of dose-finding in drug development to find the most *useful* dose and usefulness involves a trade-off between tolerability and efficacy. Thus *usefulness* (or net benefit) is not monotonic. For an effective remedy it is likely to increase at first with rising doses but then decline. This situation is illustrated in Figure 20.2, which shows efficacy and tolerability or harm measured on some common 'utility' scale as a function of dose (between 0 and 1) with net benefit the sum of the two. The net benefit originally rises above zero, with the optimal dose of about 0.2 at which a maximum net benefit of about 0.5 is reached. It then falls back to zero, which it reaches at about 0.5 (labelled 'zero') on the graph and beyond this point the net result is negative or harmful.

However, under some circumstances, even efficacy can show a nonmonotonic relationship. Suppose that the drug has a beneficial effect on efficacy via one mechanism and a deleterious effect via another. For example, the desirable outcome of a cholesterol-lowering drug is a reduction in cardiovascular events, but this is mainly achieved through lowering of bad cholesterol, or low-density lipids (LDL) (Law et al., 2003)

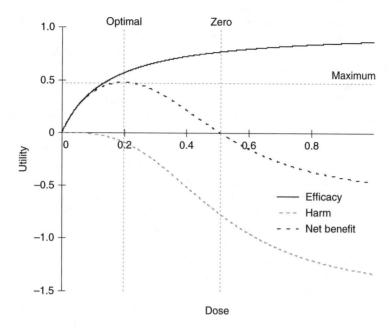

Figure 20.2 Efficacy, harm and net benefit as a function of dose.

whereas the drug might also affect 'good cholesterol, or high-density lipids (HDL). If the dose-response is initially steeper in terms of the positive effect, which, however, eventually tends towards some plateau, but is then subsequently steeper in terms of the negative effect, then a parabolic response will result. In other words, we would now have the sort of situation illustrated in Figure 20.2 but applying to net efficacy.

The fact that this sort of phenomenon cannot be dismissed entirely as impossible but is nevertheless unlikely places the statistician in something of a quandary. Failure to model the dose-response as monotonic will lose power if monotonicity is, in fact, the case. On the other hand, constraining the response to be monotonic may do violence to the facts.

Under certain circumstances, compromises between the two extreme positions of assuming monotonicity and assuming nothing would seem desirable. This is in fact what Frank Bretz, Jose Pinhero and Mike Branson have proposed in an approach that controls the type I error rate while allowing various contrasts, each of which would be optimal for various supposed dose–response relationships, to be tested (Bretz *et al.*, 2004, 2005). In their approach it is possible to take account of the extent to which each of these is believed plausible *a priori*.

20.2.14   Definition of a dose

Many dose-finding studies define the dose in terms of the quantity of the treatment given to the patient. This has the conceptual advantage of being easy to define and the practical advantage of corresponding to that which is prescribable. However, if our objective is to understand the scientific effect of the drug and if we believe that it is the concentration achieved which is important, then this may not be the most useful way to study it, for two reasons. First, patients of different body mass would, other things being equal, achieve different blood levels if given the same dose. Second, since rates of absorption, elimination and possibly distribution will differ from patient to patient, then even where patients have the same body mass they will differ in terms of concentration–time profiles. As a consequence, it has been suggested that dose-response should be studied as a function of concentration achieved or at the very least that dose-finding can be improved by using additional pharmacokinetic measurements, even where therapeutic outcomes are the main focus (Colburn, 1996; Piantadosi and Liu, 1996). A more radical proposal is to randomize patients to a given serum concentration of drug rather than a dose per se (Sanathanan and Peck, 1991). This matter will be considered in Chapter 21. Even where concentration is not measured, however, a source of variation can be taken into account by including the patient's body weight in the model for response. Although clearance is generally considered to be weakly correlated with body weight, volume of distribution may show a stronger relationship.

More controversial, perhaps, is how to use such information. For example, should we recommend to prescribing doctors that they should adjust the dose according to the body weight of their patients? How practical would such a recommendation be? Even if a single dose for adults is chosen, this does not mean that information linking dose and weight might not be useful. We might use it, for example, to predict the probability of certain types of response in a target population whose distribution with respect to weight may be rather different from patients in the trial. It is my impression, however, that this sort of trial is rarely done. A technical question is whether we should actually randomize to dose/weight groups or randomize patients to a dose group simply accepting and observing their weight. Theoretically, randomization to dose/weight groups could be used to increase the efficiency of such an investigation. It would almost certainly involve a central telephone- or web-based randomization in which the prescribing doctor, having entered the weight of her next patient, was informed which pack to pick up.

Note also that there is a general reluctance in pharmaceutical marketing departments to have drugs that are dosed by body weight. The added complication makes implementation of dosing – and hence selling – difficult. In view of the relative availability and ease of use of bathroom scales compared with DNA profiling, the enthusiasm shown by such departments for pharmacogenomics is all the more bizarre (Senn, 2004b).

References

Bauer P (1991) Multiple testing in clinical trials. *Statistics in Medicine* **10**: 871–890.

Bauer P (1997) A note on multiple testing procedures in dose finding. *Biometrics* **53**: 1125–1128.

Bretz F (2006) An extension of the Williams trend test to general unbalanced linear models. *Computational Statistics & Data Analysis* **50**: 1735–1748.

Bretz F, Pinheiro JC, Branson M (2004) On a hybrid method in dose finding studies. *Methods of Information in Medicine* **43**: 457–460.

Bretz F, Pinheiro JC, Branson M (2005) Combining multiple comparisons and modeling techniques in dose – response studies. *Biometrics* **61**: 738–748.

Budde M, Bauer P (1989) Multiple test procedures in clinical dose finding studies. *Journal of the American Statistical Association* **84**: 792–796.

Byar DP (1990) Factorial and reciprocal control designs. *Statistics in Medicine* **9**: 55–63; discussion 63–54.

Chevret S (ed.) (2006) *Statistical Methods for Dose-Finding Experiments.* John Wiley and Sons, Inc., Hoboken.

Chevret S, Zohar S (2006) The continual reassessment method. In: Chevret S (ed.), *Statistical Methods for Dose-Finding Experiments.* John Wiley and Sons, Inc., Hoboken, pp. 133–148.

Colburn WA (1996) Phase I and II trials: designs and strategies. *Drug Information Journal* **30**: 573–582.

Dawid AP (1994) Selection paradoxes of Bayesian inference. In: Anderson TW, Fang Ka-ta, Olkin I (eds), *Multivariate Analysis and its Applications,* vol. 24. Institute of Mathematical Statistics, Hayward, CA.

Filloon TG (1995) Estimating the minimum therapeutically effective dose of a compound via regression modelling and percentile estimation. *Statistics in Medicine* **14**: 925–932; discussion 933.

Finney DJ (1978) *Statistical Methods in Biological Assay.* Griffin, London.

Goodman SN (1992) A comment on replication, *P*-values and evidence. *Statistics in Medicine* **11**: 875–879.

Hemmings R (2006) Philosophy and methodology of dose-finding – a regulatory perspective. In: Chevret S (ed.) *Statistical Methods for Dose-Finding Experiments.* John Wiley and Sons, Inc., Hoboken, pp. 19–57.

International Conference on Harmonisation (1995) *ICH Topic E4 Step 5 Dose-response information to support drug registration.* EMEA, London.

Jonckheere AR (1954) A distribution-free k-sample test against ordered alternatives. *Biometrika* **41**: 133–145.

Julious SA (2005) Why do we use pooled variance analysis of variance? *Pharmaceutical Statistics* **4**: 3–5.

Kallen A, Larsson P (1999) Dose response studies: how do we make them conclusive? *Statistics in Medicine* **18**: 629–641.

Law MR, Wald NJ, Rudnicka AR (2003) Quantifying effect of statins on low density lipoprotein cholesterol, ischaemic heart disease, and stroke: systematic review and meta-analysis. *British Medical Journal* **326**: 1423.

Lee Y, Nelder JA (2006) Double hierarchical generalized linear models. *Journal of the Royal Statistical Society Series C – Applied Statistics* **55**: 139–167.

Machado SG, Robinson GA (1994) A direct, general approach based on isobolograms for assessing the joint action of drugs in pre-clinical experiments. *Statistics in Medicine* **13**: 2289–2309.

Marcus R, Peritz E, Gabriel KR (1976) On closed testing procedures with special reference to ordered analysis of variance. *Biometrika* **63**: 655–660.

Nelder JA, Lee YG (1998) Joint modeling of mean and dispersion. *Technometrics* **40**: 168–171.

O'Quigley J, Chevret S (1991) Methods for dose finding studies in cancer clinical trials – a review and results of a Monte-Carlo study. *Statistics in Medicine* **10**: 1647–1664.

O'Quigley JO, Shen LZ (1996) Continual reassessment method: a likelihood approach. *Biometrics* **52**: 673–684.

O'Quigley J, Pepe M, Fisher L (1990) Continual reassessment method: a practical design for phase-1 clinical trials in cancer. *Biometrics* **46**: 33–48.

Piantadosi S, Liu G (1996) Improved designs for dose escalation studies using pharmacokinetic measurements. *Statistics in Medicine* **15**: 1605–1618.

Pledger G (2001) Proof of efficacy trials: choosing the dose. *Epilepsy Research* **45**: 23–28; discussion 29–30.

Pool JL, Cushman WC, Saini RK, Nwachuku CE, Battikha JP (1997) Use of the factorial design and quadratic response surface models to evaluate the fosinopril and hydrochlorothiazide combination therapy in hypertension. *American Journal of Hypertension* **10**: 117–123.

Sanathanan LP, Peck CC (1991) The randomized concentration controlled trial – an evaluation of its sample-size efficiency. *Controlled Clinical Trials* **12**: 780–794.

Scholze J, Bauer B, Massaro J (1999) Antihypertensive profiles with ascending dose combinations of ramipril and felodipine ER. *Clinical and Experimental Hypertension* **21**: 1447–1462.

Senn SJ (1993) Statistical issues in short term trials in asthma. *Drug Information Journal* **27**: 779–791.

Senn SJ (1995) A personal view of some controversies in allocating treatment to patients in clinical trials [see comments]. *Statistics in Medicine* **14**: 2661–2674. [Comment in *Statistics in Medicine* **15**(1): 113–116 (1996)].

Senn SJ (1997) Statisticians and pharmacokineticists: what can they learn from each other? In: Aarons L, Balant LP, Danhof M, *et al.* (eds), *COST B1 medicine. The Population Approach: Measuring and Managing Variability in Response, Concentration and Dose.* European Commission Directorate-General Science, Research and Development, Geneva, pp. 139–146.

Senn SJ (2000) Consensus and controversy in pharmaceutical statistics (with discussion). *The Statistician* **49**: 135–176.

Senn SJ (2002a) A comment on replication, *P*-values and evidence, S.N.Goodman, Statistics in Medicine 1992; 11: 875–879. *Statistics in Medicine* **21**: 2437–2444.

Senn SJ (2002b) *Cross-over Trials in Clinical Research* (2nd edition). John Wiley and Sons, Ltd, Chichester.

Senn SJ (2004a) Added values: controversies concerning randomization and additivity in clinical trials. *Statistics in Medicine* **23**: 3729–3753.

Senn SJ (2004b) Individual response to treatment: is it a valid assumption? *British Medical Journal* **329**: 966–968.

Senn SJ (2006) Cross-over trials in Statistics in Medicine: the first '25' years. *Statistics in Medicine* **25**: 3430–3442.

Senn SJ, Lillienthal J, Patalano F, Till MD (1997) An incomplete blocks cross-over in asthma: a case study in collaboration. In: Vollmar J, Hothorn LA (eds), *Cross-over Clinical Trials.* Fischer, Stuttgart, pp. 3–26.

Sheiner LB, Hashimoto Y, Beal SL (1991) A simulation study comparing designs for dose-ranging. *Statistics in Medicine* **10**: 303–321.

Tam VH, Schilling AN, Lewis RE, Melnick DA, Boucher AN (2004) Novel approach to characterization of combined pharmacodynamic effects of antimicrobial agents. *Antimicrobial Agents and Chemotherapy* **48**: 4315–4321.

Tangen CM, Koch GG (2001) Non-parametric analysis of covariance for confirmatory randomized clinical trials to evaluate dose – response relationships. *Statistics in Medicine* **20**: 2585–2607.

Temple R (1982) Government view of clinical trials. *Drug Information Journal* **16**: 10–17.

Terpstra TJ (1952) The asymptotic normality and consistency of Kendall's test against trend, when ties are present in one ranking. *Indagationes Mathematicae* **14**: 327–333.

Ting N (ed.) (2006) *Dose Finding in Drug Development.* Springer, Berlin, New York.

Whitehead J (2006) Using Bayesian decision theory in dose-escalation studies. In: Chevret S (ed.), *Statistical Methods for Dose-Finding Experiments.* John Wiley and Sons, Inc., Hoboken, pp. 149–171.

Whitehead J, Brunier H (1995) Bayesian decision procedures for dose determining experiments. *Statistics in Medicine* **14**: 885–893; discussion 895–889.

Williams DA (1971) A test for differences between treatment means when several doses are compared with a zero dose. *Biometrics* **37**: 589–594.

Williams DA (1972) The comparison of several dose levels with a zero dose control. *Biometrics* **28**: 519–531.

Wong WK, Lachenbruch PA (1996) Tutorial in biostatistics. Designing studies for dose response. *Statistics in Medicine* **15**: 343–359.

Xu ZH, Tighiouart M, Rogatko A (2007) EWOC 2.0: Interactive software for dose escalation in cancer phase I clinical trials. *Drug Information Journal* **41**: 221–228.

Concerning Pharmacokinetics and Pharmacodynamics

What three things doth drink especially provoke?

William Shakespeare, *Macbeth*

Blood will have blood

Ibid.

21.1 BACKGROUND

Together with statistics, clinical **pharmacokinetics** can claim to be a core science of drug development. Statistics can make this claim because, at all stages, the evidence produced is quantitative in nature and highly variable. Thus, statistical insights are needed to interpret it. The claims of clinical pharmacokinetics are just as obvious. A successful drug is not just a molecule and a formulation but a unit dose and a dosing regimen. To establish these, it is necessary to know at what rates the drug is absorbed and eliminated from the body and what the therapeutic window is for plasma concentration. It is necessary to undertake studies early in drug development to establish this. However, in all phases of clinical development it is necessary to keep in mind the dosing regime and the pharmacokinetic/pharmacodynamic features of the treatment in order to plan appropriately which measurements should be taken when. Hence, clinical pharmacokinetics is a thread that runs through drug development.

This chapter will deal with various statistical issues to do with pharmacokinetics (PK) and (to some degree) **pharmacodynamics** (PD). The former is often described as being 'what the body does to the drug', the latter as 'what the drug does to the body'. Clinical pharmacokinetics is a science I admire and also consider extremely important for the statistician working in drug development. Unfortunately, although many statisticians working on phase I and early phase II (both inside and outside the industry) have acquired a good understanding of it and made useful statistical contributions to it (for instance, developing techniques for analysing nonlinear random-effect models), statisticians working in later phases of drug development seem to have made little use of its theories. I have already explained in Chapter 17, for example, that the standard model for carry-over employed for decades by statisticians working in design theory for cross-over trials can be shown to be quite ridiculous on the basis of an elementary appreciation of pharmacokinetics and pharmacodynamics.

When I come to consider my own limited knowledge of this subject, however, all I can say is 'I wish I knew *much* more'. The reader should bear this in mind. This chapter is also not about pharmacokinetics in general, which not only makes extensive use of biological theory but also of mathematics. For readers who wish to know more about these two aspects of pharmacokinetics I recommend the excellent books by Rowland and Towzer (1995) (with the stronger accent on biology) and the classic text by Gibaldi and Perrier (1982) (with the accent more on mathematics). For a brief introduction to analysis of pharmacokinetic studies using SAS, Patterson and Smith (2007) is very useful and readers might be interested in my own essay on differences in attitudes of pharmacokineticists and statisticians (Senn, 1997). Instead, I shall cover a few issues in which the statistician is more directly concerned, simply with the object of illustrating what sort of questions can arise in drug development. There are many I shall not cover. Nevertheless, a brief introduction to one or two terms and ideas is perhaps called for and some of these are also important for the chapter which follows on bioequivalence. The exposé which follows is very much indebted to the book by Rowland and Towzer (1995).

Pharmacokinetic studies in humans are among the first to be performed in phase I and are usually initiated in healthy volunteers. A basic idea behind such studies is that effects and side-effects of a drug are a function of the concentration achieved at various sites of action within the body. However, drugs are rarely administered directly to the site of action and must therefore move from a site of administration to a site of action to be effective. From the site of administration, some fraction of the dose delivered finds its way into the blood. In many cases it may be supposed that within a fairly short time some sort of equilibrium is set up between concentration at the site of action and concentration in the blood. Since concentration can rarely be studied at the site, it is studied in the plasma instead. The drug, of course, is distributed to other tissues as well as those of the target organs, in particular to the liver and kidneys, which are involved in metabolism and excretion. Changes in the plasma concentration over time thus reflect **absorption, distribution** and **elimination**, and it is the task of pharmacokinetic studies to examine this. Figure 21.1 shows a typical sort of concentration – time curve over 24 hours for a single dose of an oral preparation. To measure such profiles involves, of course, taking regular blood samples to establish what the concentration is as a function of time. (Sometimes urine samples are also taken.) The situation is also complicated by **protein binding**: the fact that the drug can bind to various proteins in the plasma. Usually only unbound drug can pass through membranes. Thus, unbound plasma concentration would actually be more closely related to effect-site concentration than total plasma concentration, although it is, in fact, more usual to measure the latter. However, plasma binding can be an important factor to keep track of. For example, if most of the drug is bound, then freeing of it through some other process or interference of even a modest fraction of the bound drug can soon lead to overdosing.

Pharmacokinetics: One of the magic arts of divination whereby needles are stuck into dummies in an attempt to predict profits.

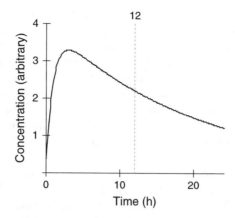

Figure 21.1   Concentration–time profile for a single dose of an oral formulation.

Two important pharmacokinetic concepts are that of (apparent) **volume of distribution** and that of **clearance**. Volume of distribution is the ratio of the amount of the drug in the body to the plasma drug concentration. This is affected by the equilibrium between the concentration in the plasma and other sites in the body. Knowledge of this is necessary in order to relate the amount of drug in the body to the site (the blood) at which it can be measured. This is one reason why intravenous studies are important, since for these it is possible to say exactly how much drug has been delivered. Clearance is the volume of blood cleared of the drug per unit time (Birkett, 1988) and is measured in units of volume per time, for example litres per hour or millilitres per minute. Birkett (1988) gives the following example. If the blood flow through the liver is 1500 ml/min and clearance through the liver is 1000 ml/min, thus means that $1000/1500 = 2/3$ of the drug entering the liver is cleared in a single pass. This fraction is the *extraction ratio*.

Drugs are eventually metabolized – converted into other molecular species. Since it is important to keep track in terms of mass-accounting of the dose originally absorbed, it is sometimes necessary to measure metabolites also. For some drugs the metabolites are effective, and for some of these the original molecule is not. Such drugs are referred to as **pro-drugs**. For other drugs, the metabolites can be toxic. This is potentially serious and can be difficult to handle.

Few drugs are given intravenously. This means that for most drugs the fraction which is absorbed intact into the circulation is often very much less than unity. This fraction, F, is referred to as the **bioavailability**. The bioavailability of oral formulations is often established in special studies (usually cross-over studies in healthy volunteers) in which the area under the plasma – concentration time curve (**AUC**) of the oral formulation is compared with that of an intravenous formulation. The bioavailability can then be calculated as the ratio of AUC to dose delivered for the oral formulation to the corresponding ratio for the intravenous formulation. Since the total amount eliminated from the body is equal to the clearance times the AUC, and since the total amount eliminated equals the amount absorbed, which is simply the dose times the bioavailability, so dose, AUC, bioavailability and clearance are linked by the formula, $F \times \text{Dose} = \text{Clearance} \times \text{AUC}$. For many drugs the bioavailability and clearance are independent of the dose administered. This property is referred to as **dose-proportionality** and is an important one. Under such circumstances, the bioavailability is proportional to the AUC. Since AUC is easily measurable, it is an important parameter of pharmacokinetics.

When plasma concentration, unbound concentration, the amount of drug and metabolite excreted and so forth all increase in proportion to dose, then the **superposition principle** applies. This means that concentration over time of a multidose treatment schedule can be calculated as the sum of the concentrations which would be observed from the individual doses were they given alone. For such drugs, the pharmacokinetics are said to be dose-independent or **linear**. Drugs which do not exhibit dose-proportionality can be difficult to manage. (A notorious example is alcohol.)

An illustration of the superposition principle is given in Figure 21.2. The figure shows the same drug as was represented in Figure 21.1. The thick solid line represents the concentration–time profile of a single dose administered at the start of a treatment. The dashed line represents the profile which would be observed for a second dose given 12 hours later, were it given on its own. In fact, the actual concentration achieved is the sum of the two single-dose profiles and is represented by the dotted line.

With many drugs with reversible actions the effect of the drug at any time is not cumulative but related to the current (or recent) concentration of the drug. It thus becomes important to study the concentration over time. This can be important for maintaining the drug inside its therapeutic window. Figure 21.3 illustrates the concentration–time profile for repeated administrations of the treatment shown in Figure 21.1. Initially the concentration levels are always below the minimum effective level given by the lower dashed line. Eventually, as repeated doses are given, more and more time is spent above the minimum effective level. In this case this is achieved without ever going above the maximum tolerated level, which is illustrated by the upper dashed line. The object of a dosing schedule is then to maintain the patient between the limits. (However, as Holford (2001) points out, these two limits are not necessarily very accurately established for many drugs.) Sometimes a larger so-called **loading dose** may be given initially to bring the patient more rapidly to the desired concentration levels.

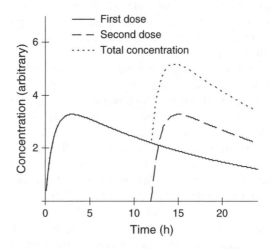

Figure 21.2 Illustration of the superposition principle.

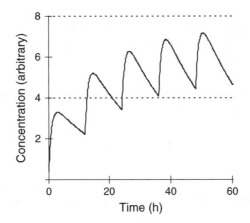

Figure 21.3 Illustration of iteration towards steady-state pharmacokinetics.

Here, the rate of elimination is extremely relevant. In standard pharmacokinetic models, this is governed by the **elimination rate constant**, which is often popularly expressed in terms of the **half-life**: the time it takes for the concentration to reduce by a half. The part of the concentration–time curve where the concentration declines is sometimes referred to as the elimination phase, although in fact elimination starts almost immediately. It is rather that this later period is *not* the absorption phase. For linear kinetics the log-concentration shows a constant decline, so that the elimination rate constant can be estimated as the slope of the log-concentration over this period. (Of course, more sophisticated approaches are available.) Clearance and the dosing schedule together determine the **steady-state** concentration, which, for linear kinetics, is eventually independent of the total dose administered to date but simply reflects the rate at which it is administered. In practice, as illustrated by Figure 21.3, concentrations vary in a saw-tooth manner at steady state with (intravenous treatments excepted) a maximum usually some time after treatment and a minimum usually around about the time of treatment. The maximum concentration reached (especially in connection with single-dose studies) is often given the symbol C_{max}. The time to reach the maximum is known as T_{max}.

Ultimately, it is the therapeutic effects of drugs we are interested in, not the plasma concentration per se. Understanding the effect of dose on the concentration is a step towards the goal of describing the response as a function of dose. A further step which is necessary is to describe the effect of concentration on physiological responses. Such studies are usually carried out in phase II of drug development. For this, a pharmacodynamic model is needed and, of course, appropriate measurements must be taken. Often 'hard' – either biochemical or physiological – measurements such as, cyclic-AMP, glucose, QT_c, blood pressure, FEV_1, cholesterol levels, and so forth are chosen. Later still, in phase III, by which time the effect of dose is better appreciated, these will be supplemented by therapeutic measures such as strokes, asthma attacks, survival, quality of life and so forth. Whereas considerable understanding of pharmacokinetics can be gained for most drugs by studying healthy volunteers, for many drugs it is necessary to carry out pharmacodynamic studies in patients. With many treatments the effect has a sigmoid response showing initially little response to dose, then a greater dose-response and finally reaches some sort of a plateau. A commonly used model to describe this is the so called E_{max} model, or Hill equation (Hill, 1910), where E_{max} stands for effect maximum. This model has three parameters, the maximum possible effect, E_{max}, the concentration which produces 50% of this maximum, EC_{50}, and a shape parameter, γ, the latter often being assumed equal to 1 in simpler applications. (Sometimes the term 'E_{max} model' is reserved for this case only.) The intensity of effect, R (for response), is then described by the relationship

$$R = \frac{E_{max} \cdot C^{\gamma}}{EC_{50}{}^{\gamma} + C^{\gamma}}, \tag{21.1}$$

where C is the concentration. Figure 21.4 is based on figure 20-2 of Rowland and Towzer (1995) and shows response as a function of concentration for different values of the shape parameter.

If we attempt to put response and concentration models together then we have what is sometimes referred to as an integrated pharmacokinetic and pharmacodynamic model (PK/PD). To the extent that the model is fully causal (there is no random element), dose determines concentration, which in turn determines response. Hence, dose determines response and in theory all of the necessary parameters could be estimated by studying dose and response only, omitting concentration. In practice this is usually rather difficult. For example, Figure 21.5 shows the response profiles which result from applying the response function of the sort illustrated in Figure 21.4 with shape parameter of 2 to concentration – time profiles of similar (but not identical) sort to that illustrated in Figure 21.1. The maximum response for each dose occurs at 2.5 hours, illustrating the linear kinetics. It is also possible to deduce from the curves that the concentration reduces to half of its maximum value by 13 hours, which is thus the half-life. (Of course, in practice, estimation would not proceed in this simple way, which does not make efficient use of all the measurements, but it suffices to illustrate that it is possible in principle.)

Sometimes the response being studied is not continuous (graded) but dichotomous (all or none). In such cases it is not possible to apply the E_{max} model directly, since the output from the model will be a continuous quantity and not a 0 or 1 variable. One can suppose, instead that the probability of a given result is what is affected. Modelling

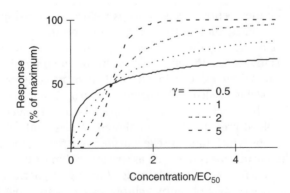

Figure 21.4 Pharmacodynamic response as a function of concentration for various values of the shape parameter, γ of the Hill equation.

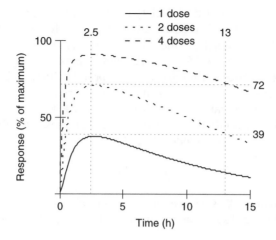

Figure 21.5   Pharmacodynamic time profiles as a function of dose.

can then proceed by transforming this onto a suitable scale, for example the logit scale, and then assuming that this has the E_{max} type response.

There are many other interesting features of PK/PD modelling which we cannot cover here. An excellent reference discussing many aspects and issues of this field is Holford and Sheiner (1981).

We now proceed to consider various issues. These are not all directly related to pharmacokinetics and pharmacodynamics, but in some cases simply illustrate that it is necessary to have good background knowledge of these processes, at least in general terms, in order to make sense of particular clinical requirements or phenomena.

21.2   ISSUES

21.2.1   Nonlinear models

Much analysis of continuous outcomes in drug development takes place using models of the general form

$$Y = \beta_0 + \beta_1 X_1 + \beta_2 X_2 + \cdots + \beta_k X_k + \varepsilon, \tag{21.2}$$

where Y is an outcome measure, ε is a disturbance term, β_0, β_1, ... are parameters to be estimated, and X_1, X_2, ... are explanatory variables. For example, X_1 may be a dummy variable taking on values 0 for placebo and 1 for active treatment, X_2 might be a covariate such as weight and so forth. Often it is assumed that the probability distribution of ε does not depend on the X variables and is Normal. This is an example of an ordinary linear regression model (sometimes referred to as the *general* linear model) and it is in turn a member of a wider class of family known as *generalized* linear models, a term introduced in a key paper of 1972 (Nelder and Wedderburn, 1972). This wider family includes, for example, logistic regression models and Poisson regression models. Thanks to the general fitting algorithm outlined by Nelder and Wedderburn, and in particular implementation through GLIM, a programming language developed in the 1970s by the Royal Statistical Society to fit generalized linear models (hence the acronym GLIM), fitting of such models has been relatively straightforward for many years. This general approach has since been implemented in many other packages such as GENSTAT, R, SPlus, SPSS, and SAS, where this is done using the GENMOD procedure. Other procedures within SAS such as proc LOGISTIC, also enable one to fit special cases of generalized linear models if one so prefers.

If we stick with the ordinary linear regression model, we can, in fact, turn many apparently different models into the same form as (21.2) using a suitable transformation. For example suppose we have a model of the form

$$Y = AX^\beta \varepsilon, \tag{21.3}$$

where Y is an outcome, X is an explanatory variable, β is a parameter and ε is a log-Normally distributed disturbance term. By taking logs we obtain an equation of the form

$$\log(Y) = \log(A) + \beta \log(X) + \log(\varepsilon), \tag{21.4}$$

where $\log(\varepsilon)$ is now Normally distributed and (21.4) now has the same general form as (21.2). Hence, by regressing $\log(Y)$ on X we may use the approach standardly used for ordinary linear regression. Although (21.3) is not linear in the sense that (21.2) is, it is, by virtue of being transformable to the same form, what is called *linear in the parameters*. Not all models are linear in this sense, however. For example, the sine-wave model

$$Y = \alpha + \delta \sin\left(\frac{X+\beta}{\gamma}\right) + \varepsilon \tag{21.5}$$

is not linear in the parameters unless γ is a known constant. In that case, by expressing (21.5) in the form

$$Y = \alpha + \delta \cos\frac{\beta}{\gamma} \sin\frac{X}{\gamma} + \delta \sin\frac{\beta}{\gamma} \cos\frac{X}{\gamma} + \varepsilon \tag{21.6}$$

and regressing Y on the two known variables $\sin(X/\gamma), \cos(X/\gamma)$, the model may be linearized. Models which are nonlinear in the parameters are usually just called *nonlinear* for short.

Now, it is the case, that in PK/PD most models are nonlinear. For example, although the model commonly used to describe plasma concentration after an intravenous bolus injection is linear (although even here the form of the distribution of the disturbance terms might cause problems), more complicated models for oral pharmaceutical preparations are not. Furthermore, the standard $E_{\max}$ response model is also not linear. This means that modelling problems are encountered in PK/PD analysis not usually encountered in drug development. Of course, various packages for estimating nonlinear models are also available and, indeed, SAS includes a routine proc NLIN and the dedicated PK/PD package NONMEM is designed to do these sorts of analyses. Other packages, for example, GENSTAT also include curve fitting routines which will do this, but nevertheless the field is difficult, both in practical terms and in terms of interpretation.

The sorts of difficulties which are associated with nonlinear models are as follows. (1) Fitting: this is more difficult than for linear models. (2) Identifiability: it may not be possible to estimate all parameters of the model from the data and it is sometimes difficult to anticipate this problem. (3) Interpretation: omitting a parameter, say for a covariate, may have a larger effect on the values of other parameters than it does on the fit of the model as a whole. It thus becomes difficult to compare parameters for the two models. (This can also be a problem in generalized linear models, such as logistic regression.) This is rarely a problem in ordinary regression models for clinical trials, where most covariates are reasonably orthogonal to the treatment effect. (4) Models in which we allow random effects for individual patients may not summarize to be equivalent to models in which we don't. (This is because the expectation of a nonlinear function is not the same as the function of the expectation.) (5) Results which are obtained for a given set of patients may be less easily generalizable to others. (6) Finding good designs to estimate parameters of such models efficiently can be more difficult. In general the 'optimal' design depends on the values of the unknown parameters (Atkinson and Donev, 1992). Consider, by comparison, the case for linear models with independent and homoscedastic errors, where the generalized variance – covariance matrix for the vector of estimated parameters $\hat{\beta}$ for the equation $\mathbf{Y} = \mathbf{X}\boldsymbol{\beta} + \boldsymbol{\varepsilon}$ is

$$\text{var}\left(\hat{\beta}\right) = \left(\mathbf{X}'\mathbf{X}\right)^{-1}\sigma^2. \tag{21.7}$$

Here σ^2 is the conditional variance of the response given the *model* and does not depend on the design, so that to the extent the variance in (21.7) depends on the design it depends only on $\mathbf{X}$, the so-called design matrix. That is to say, it depends on the chosen pattern of the values of the variables represented by $\mathbf{X}$. Hence, in principle, optimal designs can be chosen in advance of running the experiment. For nonlinear models, however, the variance of the parameter estimates depends on the parameters themselves. Hence some information about the parameters is needed to find a good design.

   It should be understood, however, that some of these are problems of the complexity of the underlying process, not of nonlinear models per se. For example, using a polynomial model as an alternative to a 'correct' nonlinear model will make it easier to deal with problem (1) above but will make problem (5) worse.

21.2.2   Dose-proportionality

It makes the task of drug development much simpler if a drug exhibits dose-proportionality. Not only does it become easier to calculate the steady-state concentration for a given regime but the effects of changing doses and regimes to ones not yet studied are easy to predict. A type of trial which is run in early in drug development, therefore, is to compare different doses to see whether the concentration AUCs exhibit dose-proportionality. This would most usually be run as a multiperiod cross-over in which each of a number of healthy volunteers would receive each dose being investigated. (A minimum of two doses would be studied.) In the discussion which follows it will be implicitly be assumed that this sort of study is being considered.

   If dose-proportionality does apply, the plot of AUC against dose should be a straight line through the origin. There has, however, been some controversy as to how to examine departure from dose-proportionality. For example, it is evident that a zero dose must produce a zero concentration. Hence, one approach would seem to be to fit a regression model through the origin involving linear and quadratic terms. If the test of the model shows that the quadratic term is redundant, then this suggests that proportionality applies. Another approach which has been suggested would be to fit a straight line through the points in the usual way and prove that the intercept was redundant. (As far as I can tell, these two approaches are equivalent for the case with two doses.)

Ezzet and Spiegelhalter (1993), following Troy *et al.* (1991), have proposed instead that the model

$$AUC_{ij} = \alpha \left(Dose_j\right)^{\beta} \varepsilon_{ij} \qquad (21.8)$$

should be used, where AUC_{ij} is the AUC observed for subject i when given dose j. If dose-proportionality applies, then β in (21.7) should be equal to 1. Equation (21.8) can be log-transformed to

$$\log\left(AUC_{ij}\right) = \log\left(\alpha\right) + \beta \log\left(Dose_j\right) + \log\left(\varepsilon_{ij}\right), \qquad (21.9)$$

which can be then fitted as a linear regression model using ordinary least squares. (Although, unless the variance of $\log\left(\varepsilon_{ij}\right)$ is independent of the dose, this will not be optimal.)

A number of issues arise in connection with this sort of model. An extremely important one concerns the assumptions regarding the distribution of $\log\left(\varepsilon_{ij}\right)$. It might usually be implicitly assumed that $\log\left(\varepsilon_{ij}\right)$ has a Normal distribution. More important, however, would be the assumptions made about the correlation structure of these disturbance terms and also the variances. Discussion of correlations is deferred until considering random-effect models. However the variance has some relevance to a planning issue below.

As concerns planning such trials, for the purpose of estimating β, unless we believe that proportionality can apply when comparing extreme doses while not applying in between, two doses are sufficient. Indeed, if this is the only purpose of the trial, such a design is 'optimal' and it would be best to use doses at the extreme limits of the ranges of interest. What the upper dose should be is not so difficult to imagine. In the interests of reconciling efficiency and safety it should be close to the maximum tolerated dose. When we consider the lowest dose, however, this seems rather puzzling. A first sight it would appear that this ought to be as low as possible, although of course it cannot be zero since we have a regression equation which involves the log-dose. This is because the general form for the variance of a slope estimate from a regression equation estimated by ordinary least squares is

$$\frac{\sigma^2}{\sum (X_j - \bar{X})^2}, \qquad (21.10)$$

where σ^2 is the variance of a disturbance term and the X_i terms are the values of the linear predictor. In this case, the X_i terms are the log doses and, for a given number of observations, the denominator of (21.10) will be maximized if we divide the measurements to be taken equally between two value of X as far apart as possible. However, a very low dose would lead to blood concentration levels below the limit of detection. This implies, in turn, that variances in log-AUC are in fact greater for lower doses than for higher ones, so that the correct model is not in fact the ordinary linear regression model we supposed. (Hence ordinary least squares will not be optimal.) In practice, for these and other reasons, it would seem appropriate to have a lower dose which is at least equal to the minimum effective dose. Furthermore, if, in fact, we find that dose-proportionality does not apply we shall not be in a position to say much about the response of AUC to dose if we have only observed two doses. Thus it would seem to be wise to study at least three doses.

A further point has to do with the sort of inferential procedures we bring to bear in analysing dose-proportionality. The issues raised are similar to those which occur in bioequivalence. It will presumably not be adequate simply to test the null hypothesis that β is equal to 1. In many applications we shall wish to be able to show that β is sufficiently close to 1, perhaps by demonstrating that the confidence limits lie within some suitable range.

For strategies for modeling dose proportionality, including implementation of analysis in SAS, see Patterson and Smith (2007), who, rather surprisingly, do not cite the key paper of Troy *et al.* (1991).

21.2.3 Defining effects for the purpose of PD modelling

It has been a constant theme of this book that one has to be extremely careful in defining and calculating effects. A naive approach to this is to calculate the difference from baseline. However, as was pointed out in Chapters 3 and 7, although it may occasionally be useful to *estimate* treatment effects by a difference from baseline, this difference cannot be used to *define* effects. That definition has to be in terms of what has happened as a result of treatment and what would have happened otherwise and it is nearly always the case that a superior estimate of this is given by comparing the outcome in the treatment effect with that in the control group. Even where such a comparison is ultimately intended, simply calculating difference from baselines to produce change-scores, which will subsequently be compared between groups, is an inefficient way to take account of the information contained in the baselines. Analysis of covariance is superior.

For most purely pharmacokinetic purposes, this causes no difficulty. This is because the relevant blood level measures are absolute. The molecules we are detecting can only have come from the treatment. The baseline measurement is thus zero and completely irrelevant. There are some exceptions to this and they do cause difficulty. For example, when the therapy is a supplement to naturally occurring substances, (an example is hormone replacement therapy) then the effect of the drug is to produce an increase in the naturally occurring substance.

When it comes to PD modelling, however, equation (21.1) is a model for the effect and the effect is not the same as the measure. For example, patients have a blood pressure in the absence of treatment. It is the effect on blood pressure which is to be modelled by (21.1), not the blood pressure itself. Various approaches are employed for dealing with this. The first is, indeed, to define the effect as the difference from baseline. Quite apart from the difficulties with this which we have discussed, one problem can be that for a given patient, measurement error can sometimes produce an impossible value for the effect. For example, blood pressure can appear to increase momentarily. Another problem arises where the placebo effect is strong. We may completely mistake the effect of the treatment. An example is given in section 21.2.6 below. Another possibility is placebo correction, to define the effect at each time point as the difference from placebo.

In a cross-over trial, this can be done individually for each patient, although again apparent negative effects are possible. In a parallel-group trial, the mean PD response over time can be corrected at each time point by the placebo value. This may be adequate for crude estimation, but makes it difficult to establish the precision of the estimates, since individual estimates per patient are not available for analysis.

Better, in principle, is to use a model which formally incorporates the placebo effect over time. For example, a simple fixed-effects approach would be to define a model for the outcome for patient i at time t as follows:

$$Y_{i,t} = \mu_t + \frac{E_{max} \cdot C_{i,t}{}^{\gamma}}{EC_{50}{}^{\gamma} + C_{i,t}{}^{\gamma}} + \varepsilon_{i,t}, \qquad (21.11)$$

where μ_t is a secular trend over time, assumed identical for all patients, and $\varepsilon_{i,t}$ is a disturbance (or 'error') term. In a placebo-controlled study, since the concentration of the placebo at any time is zero, the second term in the model disappears for the placebo group; this permits one to correct the outcome at time t for other groups by that in the placebo group.

21.2.4   Random-effect models and repeated measures

Consider the dose-proportionality case we considered under Section 21.2.2. Ezzet and Spiegelhalter (1993) include an example of a cross-over trial in 4 periods, 4 doses and 16 subjects. (The treatment is not named but the doses are 10, 50, 100 and 200 mg.) If we ignore period and carry-over effects – the latter on the grounds that since serum concentration is being measured it can be established absolutely that carry-over has not occurred (Senn *et al.*, 2004, 2005) and the former on the grounds that period effects can be dealt with but that it will add nothing to the *essence* of the discussion to consider them – there are a number of ways in which we can model the treatment and subject effects which remain. These can be discussed by considering model and error degrees of freedom. A number of possible models (by no means exhaustive) are considered in Table 21.1, some of which are also covered by Ezzet and Spiegelhalter (1993).

Table 21.1 Models and degrees of freedom for dose-proportionality example of Ezzet and Spiegelhalter (1993).

Model	Type	Parameters	Model degrees of freedom	Residual degrees of freedom	Total
A	Fixed	α, β	2	62	64
B	Fixed	α_i, β	17	47	64
C	Fixed	$\alpha_i, \beta, \gamma, \delta$	19	45	64
D	Fixed	α_i, β_i	32	32	64
E	Summary	(α)	(1)	(15)	(16)
		β	1	15	16
F	Random	level 1: α_i, β_i	NA	NA	NA
		level 2:			
		$\mu_\alpha, \mu_\beta,$			
		$\sigma_\alpha^2, \sigma_\beta^2, \sigma_{\alpha\beta}$			

In total we have $16 \times 4 = 64$ degrees of freedom. If we remain with the basic form of model (21.8) then we could, for example, simply treat the data as 16 replicated measurements on each of four doses and fit a common intercept α and common slope β. This is model A of Table 21.1 and has two model degrees of freedom, leaving 62 error degrees of freedom. Because we have made no attempt to incorporate the information that measurements are made repeatedly on the same subjects, all of the variation between subjects must be contained in these 62 degrees of freedom. Effectively we have the sort of analysis which would be appropriate for a trial in which 64 subjects were split at random into four different doses. If we make a minimal attempt to recognize that four data values are provided by every subject and fit a model with a different intercept for each patient but a common slope, we then have model B. In model C, a quadratic parameter, γ, is fitted as well as a cubic parameter, δ, so that the model is of the form

$$\log\left(\mathrm{AUC}_{ij}\right) = \log\left(\alpha_i\right) + \beta \log\left(\mathrm{dose}_j\right) + \gamma \left\{\log\left(\mathrm{dose}_j\right)\right\}^2$$
$$+ \delta \left\{\log\left(\mathrm{dose}_j\right)\right\}^3 + \log\left(\varepsilon_{ij}\right) \tag{21.12}$$

This model is of interest because it is equivalent in some sense to a standard analysis of cross-over trials and it is included here to make that link. Suppose that we simply regarded the four doses as four different treatments. A standard analysis of cross-over trials would then use 15 degrees of freedom for subjects, three for treatments and one for a grand mean, leaving 47 degrees of freedom for error. This is equivalent to model C. For model D we proceed to fit not only a different intercept for each subject but also a different slope parameter. This leaves 32 degrees of freedom. Note that for this model, unlike for A, B and C, the only reason we have any residual degrees of freedom left is because more than two doses were studied. All of models A, B, C and D fit fixed effect parameters and all have a disturbing feature: the degrees of freedom for error are greater than the number of subjects in the trial. This is a worrying feature since residuals under the model will not stand in the same relationship to each other, some being obtained from the same subject and some from different subjects.

Model E takes a completely different tack and uses the so-called **summary-measures** approach (Senn *et al.*, 2000). Here the problem is tackled in two stages. In the first stage an estimate of β is produced from every one of the 16 subjects by fitting model (21.8) to the four observations for that subject. (Of course, thereby, an estimate of α is also produced from each subject, but this is not of direct interest here.) This means that the problem is reduced to one of analysing the 16 estimates from the 16 subjects. One degree of freedom is used up for the overall estimate of β produced from these 16 estimates and so there are 15 residual degrees of freedom. This approach has the advantage that the issue of correlation between measurements is finessed since the 16 estimates of β are, in fact, independent.

Now suppose that we look at how models D and E compare with respect to estimating (i) the overall value of β and (ii) the value for a given subject. As regards the first of these, the situation for model E is quite simple. Each subject provides an independent estimate of the same β. The most efficient overall estimate of this β is the mean of the 16 values. As regards the second, the situation for model D is quite simple. Each subject is given a different slope parameter. Only data from the given subject have anything to say directly about this parameter and, essentially, our estimate of β_i for subject i is simply based on the four values for that subject. Model D appears to have nothing to say, however, about an overall estimate for β. Such a parameter is not mentioned in the model and it is difficult to know how to interpret it if we attempt to introduce it. We can, of course, estimate any linear combination of the β_i we like. So we can estimate the mean β_i if we want, using simply the mean of the various estimates of the β_i, but it is not clear what interpretation to give this. Alternatively, we could assume that the β_i are all equal, but this really brings us back to model B. When we come to consider what model E has to say about the estimation of effects for individual subjects, however, then we are faced with a puzzle. This is because if the various estimates of β vary from subject to subject, we do not know why. It could be that this is simply because of within-subject error. In that case the overall mean will be the best estimate for every subject. It could be that it has nothing to do with within-subject error but reflects the fact that every subject has a different slope (proportionality) parameter. In that case the individual estimate for that patient will be best.

The truth probably lies between these two extremes, and this is where the random-effects model F is useful. Like the summary-measures approach, with which it has conceptually much in common, this also has two levels. However, these two levels are not treated as two stages but are handled together in one model and fitting process. The individual intercept and slopes, α_i and β_i, form the first level. These are considered to be random drawings from a population with a Normal population of such values with parameters μ_α, μ_β, σ_α^2, σ_β^2 and $\sigma_{\alpha\beta}$, the covariance between slope and intercept. A Bayesian approach to modelling such data would go one stage further and consider that the parameters μ_α, μ_β, σ_α^2, σ_β^2 and $\sigma_{\alpha\beta}$, being unknown, were themselves in need of a probability distribution to describe initial uncertainty about them. Ezzet and Spiegelhalter (1993) illustrate this approach.

This sort of choice between models occurs all the time in PK/PD work. This is because even where, and unlike the example above, a subject or patient is given a single treatment, repeated blood samples are taken and we wish to use the observed concentration – time profiles to estimate particular parameters. We thus have a repeated-measures problem. Often a summary-measures approach is used. For example, in bioequivalence studies AUCs are compared for different formulations. These AUCs are always calculated first for each subject before proceeding to the modelling process. On the other hand, in certain applications it is not possible to cover all desired blood sampling points in all patients. Different times are used for different patients to minimize the number of samples taken. The only way in which this can be drawn together is via a random-effects approach.

The advantages of the random-effect approach are: (1) 'Shrunk' or weighted estimates are possible for individual subjects. The extremes of either using personal values only or global values can be avoided. (2) Efficient use can be made of all observations. For example, a subject studied only on one dose could still contribute some information. (3) As a related point, 'strength can be borrowed from others'. Where, in more complex models, data on individual subjects are insufficient to provide a fixed-effect estimate for that subject alone, some sort of estimation is still possible because estimation is simultaneous over the whole design and values for individuals are linked by virtue of the second-level parameters.

The principal disadvantage is that they can be difficult to fit. (Although sometimes it can be impossible to fit a fixed-effects model.) They also run into conceptual difficulties. The meaning and nature of the second-level parameters is not always clear and often it is the random effects you cannot observe which are of interest. For example, the slope parameters for individuals in the Ezzet and Spiegelhalter (1993) example are of no particular interest. None of the healthy volunteers concerned are ever likely to be given the treatment in question. Similarly, the overall variance parameter σ_β^2 is also of little direct substantive interest. It would be unwise to use it as an estimate of the variability of dose proportionality in patients. On the other hand, it might be assumed to provide some sort of lower limit for this. One might say, of course, that this simply means that healthy volunteers should not be used for this type of study, but one could reply that they certainly provide a powerful test of the hypothesis of proportionality (which was in fact rejected in this case).

In this particular application, the summary-measures approach of model E works very well. There is no problem in fitting it to each subject and the subsequent analysis is simple to apply and interpret and is very powerful. On the other hand, as I have pointed out elsewhere (Senn, 2002; Senn and Hildebrand, 1991), fixed-effect models of type B and C make strong assumptions regarding disturbance terms and can, on occasion, be very misleading. Model D on the other hand, is of little practical use. However, we should perhaps not dismiss fixed effect models entirely. Suppose we had a case where a single subject was studied on a number of doses. We could treat this as a standard regression problem in which we simply fitted α and β. It is perfectly possible to test the hypothesis that $\beta = 1$ as is taught in standard texts on linear regression. If we can show that this hypothesis is not true for this subject, then it cannot be true in general and this may be useful information.

There are, however, other cases where random-effect models are the only sensible option. For example, suppose that we have determined the 'optimal' dose to be given to patients on the basis of a large study in which patients have been given various doses, serum concentration has been measured and the result has been analysed using a fixed-effects model. Suppose that we give this to a new patient and then take a serum concentration measurement and find that this is lower than we intended. We thus propose to give him a larger dose. But if we return to our fixed-effects model, all that this can predict for us is what the concentration will be on average for patients at a higher dose. This average figure is, of course, higher than the target. This is why we started the patient out on the lower dose anyway. Thus it seems that there is no use we can make of information from the trial as a whole and all that we can use is some sort of guess based on the patient's measured value. But this, of course, will not be measured without error. If we wish to use global and local information appropriately then we need a random-effects model (Racine and Dubois, 1989; Wakefield and Walker, 1997). This is essentially the same point that was made in discussing n-of-1 trials in Chapter 18.

Other comments regarding fixed- and random-effect models will be found in Chapter 14 and an excellent discussion of various issues including choice of design will be found in Steimer *et al.* (1994).

21.2.5 Population designs and models

The classic pharmacokinetic trial is carried out in healthy volunteers with frequent blood sample taken at predetermined times. This sort of study gives high-quality data suitable for good basic modelling. It is also usually relatively easy to estimate parameters for each subject so that the generally attractive summary-measures approach described above may be used. Unfortunately, patients often differ from healthy subjects in terms of absorption, distribution and, especially, elimination of pharmaceuticals. Hence, such trials do not work as well as might be hoped in predicting what will happen in the target population.

On the other hand, as Grasela (1994) points out, the sorts of measurements which occur in therapeutic trials are sparse and not necessarily at controlled times. They thus tend to be difficult to estimate using traditional approaches. During the 1970s, the sort of random-effect (or mixed-effect) models discussed above were gradually applied to such PK data. (See, for example, the important papers by Lewis, Sheiner *et al.* (Sheiner *et al.*, 1972, 1977).) A useful review of this work, difficulties attending it and the extent to which they had been overcome by 2005 is given by Nedelman (2005). This general approach of applying random-effect models to usually sparse data obtained in target populations came to be known as the 'population approach'. (Although I admire the field, I think that this term is unhelpful and confusing.) This attracted a lot of criticism from more conventionally minded pharmacokineticists who were, perhaps, suspicious of what they saw as an attempt to make good, by purely statistical means, the deficits in what they regarded as being poor data. Many of the arguments on both sides have been discussed in Section 21.2.4 above already. For further enlightenment the reader should consult the excellent paper by Steimer *et al.* (1994).

In his tribute to the late Lewis Sheiner, who was the key instigator and innovator of the 'population approach', Nedelman (2005) draws attention to four potential 'deficiencies' of the population approach, already identified by Sheiner *et al.* (1977). These are possible biases due to confounding effects, reliability of data, inefficiencies due to correlation of variables and lack of control in design and consequent inefficiencies. The second and fourth of these are *potentially* resolvable through design. That is to say that it is theoretically conceivable that one could organize pharmacokinetic sampling in clinical trials in patients in such a way that timing of measurements was optimal and data quality was excellent. Of course, for nonlinear models optimal timing depends partly on the parameters themselves, as discussed in Section 21.2.1. However, given background knowledge from healthy volunteer studies and sequential design, some progress could be made. Nevertheless, in practice any population pharmacokinetic study is likely to run up against imperfect compliance by patients, imperfect recording of noncompliance, and sparse sampling, so that since it is timing relative to dosing that is important, concerns about this will remain.

On the other hand, deficiency number one, confounding effects, is harder to deal with. Nedelman (2005) gives the example of a trial in which patients were randomized to one of three doses of a drug or placebo. Patients provided trough concentration values and a variable representing the average of these, $C_{\min}$, was calculated. This was thus a measure of drug exposure. (Obviously for all the patients on placebo it was zero). A single univariate therapeutic outcome measure, Y, was taken (with high values bad and low values good) and, as might be expected, the correlation between $C_{\min}$ and Y was negative. The problem in interpreting this is that $C_{\min}$ is an outcome. Nedelman (2005) considers the following possible scenario: patients with poor clearance have worse clinical outcomes. That being so, for any two patients on the same dose, the one with higher $C_{\min}$ would be likely to have an inherently (that is to say, in the absence of treatment) worse clinical outcome. This means that relative to a trial in which patients had been randomized to a given concentration (assuming that were possible, see Section 21.2.7) the concentration – effect relationship would be biased towards zero (Kraiczi *et al.*, 2003; Nedelman, 2005).

The third deficiency, correlation of variables, is inherent to clinical trials generally. This was discussed in Chapter 7, where it was pointed out that if one was only concerned with the effects of treatment, then the correlation of demographic variables amongst themselves was not a concern. With population pharmacokinetics, however, things are not quite so simple. This is because it is usually assumed that demographic variables act as effect modifiers. In other words, that they are involved in *interactions*.

A good case in point would be age, where increasing age might be associated with reduced clearance and hence, for a given dose, with greater concentrations. Where that is the case, interest is at least partly concerned with the treatment – covariate interaction and teasing this out when covariates are partly confounded can be a problem. The extent to which this is a practical problem depends on the future use of the information. It is a well-known fact about multiple regression that (near) multicolinearity leads to poor parameter estimation but not necessarily poor prediction. The key is whether future populations to which the results of a clinical trial are applied show the same degrees of confounding. If so, prediction may not be too bad.

21.2.6 Trough-to-peak ratios, therapeutic regimes and the smoothness index

This is an example of an issue which, while not directly connected to mainstream pharmacokinetics, needs to be understood in PK/PD modelling terms.

Although, for a treatment exhibiting linear kinetics, the clearance and hence the half-life and so forth will be dose-independent, the so-called **duration of action** will not be. This is itself a rather nebulous concept but can perhaps be defined either as the time until the effect is no longer measurable or the time until it is no longer clinically relevant. Obviously, the former will (nearly always) be longer than the latter. The former definition has the advantage that it does not depend on the clinically relevant difference, but it does not entirely escape being arbitrary because it does depend on the sensitivity of measurement. Whatever definition is used, the duration of action can be increased by increasing the dose. Thus, although it is important to compare treatments at the footpoint, the point just before administration of the next dose, using this alone as a basis of comparison can be misleading. As can be seen from Figure 21.3, this time of measurement is useful for establishing that the treatment does not fall out of the therapeutic window because the minimal required effect is not reached. But equally, the figure shows that measurements shortly after the time of administration are needed to establish that there are no tolerability problems.

Now for many treatments and indications, the pharmacodynamic measure of tolerability is not at all the same as the measure of efficacy. For example, for beta-agonists in asthma we would use some measure of lung function, such as FEV_1, for efficacy and some cardiac measure, such as the corrected length of the QT interval of the ECG, as a tolerability measure. However, if we are measuring the effect of ACE inhibitors on blood pressure, then the tolerability problem can be that we have too much of a good thing: the drop in blood pressure is such that we turn hypertension into hypotension. Even where hypotension is not a risk, it can perhaps be taken as an indication that the drug is being given in doses that are too high (and not frequently enough) if the effect varies too much in the dosing cycle. It can thus be useful to study not only the 'trough' effect on hypertension but the 'peak' effect also. (This is slightly confusing since, other things being equal, the peak effect occurs at the trough of blood pressure and vice versa. However, it is troughs and peaks of the effect which are referred to in the definitions.) As Lipicky (1994) puts it, discussing the case of the calcium-channel blocker nicardipine, 'The result was a trough:peak ratio of between 25 and 43%, suggesting that with three doses a day the interval between doses was too long . . . out of the nicardipine case came the rational, but arbitrary, standard that 50 – 75% of the peak effect is desirable at trough. Should more of the effect disappear during dosing, adverse labeling would be highly likely and approval could be in danger' (p. S 18).

Elliott and Meredith (1994) point to a number of methodological difficulties in implementing the trough-to-peak ratio requirements. The first is the presence of placebo effects. Elliot and Meredith point out that defining the effects in terms of difference from baseline will overestimate the effect of the active treatment. Table 21.2 is adapted from table 2 of Elliott and Meredith (1994), which in turn was based on an example of Rose and McMahon (1990) and show the example of felodipine extended release. The placebo effect is considerable, and depending whether the treatment effect is corrected for the placebo effect or not, the trough:peak ratio for 10 mg, for example, is either 33% or 60%.

A second difficulty arises from circadian rhythms. Measurements may fluctuate during the day according to some pattern quite apart from that induced by a dosing schedule. A third problem is that measurement conditions may vary during the course of a trial. A fourth, which Elliot and Meredith do not consider, is regression to the mean (see Chapter 3). All of these phenomena show the value of measuring the effect of a treatment with respect to a control rather than with respect to baseline.

A rather different problem arises with individual calculation. Elliot and Meredith point out that the average trough-to-peak ratio may be 60% but that when this is studied for individual patients, many may not satisfy the requirement. This is similar issue to the requirement for 15% bronchodilation which we discussed in Chapter 8. The danger, here is that we do not make sufficient allowance for within-patient error. Even if the true ratio of long-term trough and peak means for all patients is in excess of 60%, if we have only a limited number of measurements on each patient, we shall inevitably find some who, just by chance, happen to give a large peak reading and a small trough reading. Hence, we shall falsely conclude that many do not satisfy the requirement by failing to identify adequately the components of variation involved. Again the cure is a suitable design and random-effect modelling. Failing that, we have to be satisfied with averages only and, indeed, if random-effect models are not applied, I do not recommend anything other than looking at the mean value.

Table 21.2   Trough-to-peak (T:P) ratios for felodipine for systolic blood pressure.

	Uncorrected			Placebo-corrected		
	Trough	**Peak**	**T:P ratio**	**Trough**	**Peak**	**T:P ratio**
Placebo	−8	−11	70%			
Felodipine						
10 mg	−10	−17	56%	−2	−6	33%
20 mg	−14	−23	61%	−6	−12	50%

It has also been noted that the trough-to-peak ratio may not be dose-independent. There are two obvious explanations. One is that the pharmaceutical is not dose-proportional. The other has to do with the pharmacodynamic response. Consider the case illustrated in Figure 21.5. The drug is dose-proportional. However, because the PD response eventually shows 'diminishing returns to scale' as a function of dose it is clear that the trough-to-peak ratio will be higher for the higher dose. Indeed, one could imagine a case where it might be 1. This shows that simply measuring the trough-to-peak ratio does not, of itself, guarantee that the duration of action of the treatment has not been extended artificially by upping the dose.

Since the first edition of this book, there has been further discussion of suitable indices, with the so-called 'smoothness index' being proposed as an alternative (Parati *et al.*, 1998; Zanchetti, 1997). This is a measure of variation, like the trough-to-peak ratio, but based on the standard deviation of the differences time point by time point of the values at outcome compared with the values at baseline. It really presupposes that ambulatory blood pressure monitoring has taken place and that reasonably frequent measurements can be taken. As described by Aboy *et al.* (Aboy *et al.* 2005; Aboy *et al.* 2006), it is supposed that at each of a number of time points, defined with respect to some repeated 24-hour measurement period, averages of blood pressure readings have been taken. So for example, we might have a baseline observation period of several days and be able to calculate the average value for (say) 15:00. In practice, timings might be somewhat variable and also some values might be missing. We can call the mean of such readings at a given time t of the day, $\bar{X}_t$. Similarly, we might have several values after treatment measured at time t, from which we calculate a mean $\bar{Y}_t$. From these we construct a difference, $d_t = \bar{Y}_t - \bar{X}_t$. We then calculate the mean of these differences for a given individual averaging over the daily sampling points, $\bar{d}$, and also the standard deviation also, s_d. Finally the 'smoothness index' for a given patients is $\bar{d}/s_d$. This is, effectively, a reciprocal of a coefficient of variation.

Compared with the trough-to-peak ratio, the smoothness index has the advantage that it makes use of more of the information. However, it shares many disadvantages. It is attempting to discount the mean treatment effect by the variability in that effect. If two drugs have equal mean effect but different variability, that with lower variability will have the higher smoothness index. Similarly if two drugs have the same variability but one has the higher mean effect, then it will have the higher smoothness index. However, it does not follow that of two drugs, the one with the higher smoothness index is the better treatment: it is conceivable that it could have a modest but very steady effect. Furthermore, it is clear that the index reflects measurement error so that the longer the observation period and the greater the number of observations that go to produce the index, the lower the standard deviation and hence the greater the index.

Since the first edition of this book, my position on such indices has hardened and I now consider that, whether trough-to-peak ratio or smoothness index, they are *ad hoc* and unsatisfactory. It seems to me that there is room for some serious statistical modelling, perhaps using Fourier series. For example, in a sine-wave model, the mean level could tell you something about the overall effect of the treatment and the amplitude about its constancy. For that matter, integrated PK/PD models might be useful. In any case, unless some model of the degree of damage caused by hypertension (and perhaps hypotension) is coupled to the serial blood pressure measurements, no single index will capture the *desirability* of a treatment adequately.

21.2.7   Randomized to concentration trials

The conventional general PK/PD framework implies that, given knowledge of the *true* serum concentration, the dose of a drug given is irrelevant in predicting effect. From the explanatory point of view, therefore, it would appear that a sharper understanding of the dose – response relationship may be obtained by studying pharmacodynamic and even therapeutic effects as a function of serum concentration rather than as a function of dose (Peck, 1990). On the other hand, the conventional phase III analytic framework requires that patients be randomized to the treatments. An observed concentration is not a treatment. It is sometimes possible to arrange matters, however, so that we can randomize patients to a concentration (or range of concentrations or steady-state AUC and so forth) and this was proposed as a possible strategy in a key paper of Sheiner and Tozer (1978), although it does not appear to have been often attempted. In their review paper, Kraiczi *et al.* (2003) identified 23 studies in which randomization to concentration had been carried out. In order implement such trials, it is necessary to use a dose which will be expected to produce the required concentration and then adjust the dose further. This manoeuvre itself can be better performed if appropriate PK studies with random-effect modelling have been carried out beforehand. Where this *can* be done, however, it appears that we have a trial which will satisfy both randomization and PK/PD requirements.

The advantage of this sort of trial for the purpose of understanding the concentration – effect ratio is that it can deal with the concern regarding confounding discussed in Section 21.2.5. In fact, Nedelman *et al.* (2007) used the randomized to concentration trial as a methodological hypothetical device for understanding the relationship between concentration and effect for more conventionally dose-randomized trials and proposing diagnostics and suitable analyses for such conventional trials. They state that 'if. . . the relationship between concentration and effect does not depend on the dose needed to attain the target concentration, such a relationship will be called a true PK/PD relationship' (p. 290). Interestingly, although the authors seem to be unaware of it, this is exactly the same as the famous Prentice criterion for a true surrogate (Prentice, 1989). This, however, raises the practical point: why do we want to understand the concentration – effect relationship? If in practice we will prescribe doses and not concentrations, what is the value of knowing the effect of the latter?

One advantage of such studies can be that we will achieve greater efficiency in studying the PD effects of concentration (Kraiczi *et al.*, 2003; Pledger and Treiman, 1991; Sanathanan and Peck, 1991). For a conventional trial, simply randomizing patients to dose and observing the resulting concentration will not enable the trialist to ensure that the range of concentrations she wishes to study are represented. It is conceivable that, as a result of using a randomized to concentration trial, we might get an indication of a treatment effect with fewer patients (Kraiczi *et al.*, 2003). However, a more important use would be in indications where the actual prescribing of the drug in the future may involve concentration monitoring. (That is to say, that patients will be titrated individually in this way.) Under such circumstances, the trial can even be given a pragmatic interpretation.

Only a few years after the first edition of this book, Nick Holford published an interesting essay on such trials (Holford, 2001), which we now discuss. First, Holford discusses the question of choosing a target concentration. This, as he points out, has nothing to do with pharmacokinetics; it has to do with what we know or believe about the relationship between concentration and effect, that is to say pharmacodynamics. Next he considers the theory as to how we should set about achieving a given concentration. If we knew the volume of distribution and clearance for each patient, we could offer subjects a loading dose that was the product of target concentration and volume of distribution and a maintenance dose that was the product of target concentration and clearance. In practice we do not know the values for a given patient and so a mixed-effects model is necessary in which we update our initial guesses for a patient, which were based using background pharmacokinetic information, with the (usually very limited) observations on concentration we will have. This is most naturally done in a Bayesian framework and Holford refers to this as Bayesian forecasting. He also points out that in practice if we are going to adjust a patient's dose we need to have a target concentration not a range of concentrations in mind.

Of course, choice of given target concentrations, either in a clinical trial or clinical practice, will be guided by what is considered to be an acceptable range of concentration in terms of efficacy and tolerability. As Holford (2001) points out, if true variation from patient to patient in long-term average concentration is small, compared with the acceptable range of concentrations, then little additional value in dosing is achieved by monitoring concentration. Essentially the same dose produces an in-range concentration in everybody. Similarly, if concentration varies considerably from occasion to occasion within individuals, then control of concentration in an individual is impossible.

A further point that Holford (2001) mentions is that there is a danger of confusion about the meaning of *control* in connection with concentration-controlled trials. It refers to the control of the concentration itself, not to trials in which the strategy of adjusting concentration is compared in a controlled manner with more conventional treatment by dosing. Such trials have been fairly rare, an example is given by Fletcher *et al.* (2002), although Holford does draw attention to the spectacular increase in five-year survival rates in acute lymphoblastic leukaemia from 66% to 76% when concentration-controlled methotrexate was compared with standard dosing by Evans *et al.* (1998).

One must be careful, however, in assuming that, even where practical, such trials will always be advantageous. For example, it is theoretically possible to conceive of occasions on which studying the relationship with dose may be far superior, perhaps by using trials in which doses per kg of body weight are defined. Suppose that the variability in absorption and elimination is small between individuals compared with either the variability of measurement of serum concentration or the variability in distribution. In that case, dose delivered may actually correlate better with effect-site concentration than will serum concentration. Indeed, it is even possible that the latter might have a negative correlation with effect-site concentration (patients have low serum concentration because the blood has distributed elsewhere, including to the effect site). Under such circumstances, moving from studying response as a function of dose to response as a function of concentration will bring few advantages. However, this sort of thing on the whole would seem to be unlikely. On the other hand, it will quite often be found that because of within-patient and measurement error, dose will have some predictive effect on response, even where concentration is included in the model.

A further difficulty occurs if it is necessary to blind the study. Obviously, continuous monitoring of concentration levels will render this impossible. A modification is possible, however, if the patients are all given the active treatment in the run-in phase, at the end of which the necessary adjustment to the dose regime is calculated. The patients can then be randomized to receive either active treatment or placebo at the adjusted dose (Pledger and Treiman, 1991). Clearly, this is not always satisfactory; but in any case it would be a mistake to assume that blinding is essential to all clinical trials.

21.2.8   Onset of action. An example of a design issue

For treatments in certain diseases, a rapid onset of action can be extremely important but a placebo effect cannot be ruled out. A good example is inhaled beta-agonists for asthma, for which onset can occur in less than a minute; this rapid effect can be extremely valuable for treatment in an attack, but placebo responses can also be considerable. This means that these trials must be run blind. In many cases blinding will require the double dummy technique so that patients will take either treatment A with placebo to B or treatment B with placebo to A. Suppose, simply to make discussion easier, that treatment A is yellow (yellow pill, yellow aerosol or whatever) and that treatment B is blue. In practice, the patient will have to take one of the treatments first. If, for example, they were instructed to always take yellow (A or the indistinguishable placebo to A) first and blue (placebo to B or active B) second, this would bias the comparison of the onset: whenever it was given, B would be given second. Of course, one could arrange to time onset from the time at which the active component of the pair was given, but this might be difficult to arrange and in any case might not deal with all biases. Thus it may be necessary to balance the trial by using two alternative sequences Yellow–Blue and Blue–Yellow, and in addition to the randomization to the two treatment groups to randomize to the two colour sequences (Senn, 1993).

References

Aboy M, Fernandez JR, Hermida RC (2005) Methodological considerations in the evaluation of the duration of action of antihypertensive therapy using ambulatory blood pressure monitoring. *Blood Pressure Monitoring* **10**: 111–115.

Aboy M, Fernandez JR, McNames J, Hermida RC (2006) The individual RDH index: a novel vector index for statistical assessment of antihypertensive treatment reduction, duration, and homogeneity. *Blood Pressure Monitoring* **11**: 69–78.

Atkinson AC, Donev AN (1992) *Optimum Experimental Designs*. Oxford University Press, Oxford.

Birkett (1988) Clearance. *Australian Prescriber* **11**: 12–13.

Elliott HL, Meredith PA (1994) Methodological considerations in calculation of the trough – peak ratio. *Journal of Hypertension* **12**: S3–S7.

Evans WE, Relling MV, Rodman JH, Crom WR, Boyett JM, Pui CH (1998) Conventional compared with individualized chemotherapy for childhood acute lymphoblastic leukemia. *New England Journal of Medicine* **338**: 499–505.

Ezzet F, Spiegelhalter D (1993) Pharmacokinetic dose proportionality: practical issues on design, sample size and analysis. In: *2nd International Meeting on Statistical Methods in Biopharmacy*. Société Francaise de Statistique, Paris.

Fletcher CV, Anderson PL, Kakuda TN, *et al.* (2002) Concentration-controlled compared with conventional antiretroviral therapy for HIV infection. *Aids* **16**: 551–560.

Gibaldi M, Perrier D (1982) *Pharmacokinetics*. Marcel Dekker, Basle.

Grasela TH (1994) The role of therapeutic drug monitoring in pharmacoepidemiology. In: Strom BL (ed.), *Pharmacoepidemiology*, 2nd edition. John Wiley & Sons, Inc., New York.

Hill AV (1910) The possible effect of the aggregation of molecules of haemoglobin on its dissociation curves. *Proceedings of the Physiological Society* **40**: iv–vii.

Holford NH (2001) Target concentration intervention: beyond Y2K. *British Journal of Clinical Pharmacology* **52**(Suppl 1): 55S–59S.

Holford NH, Sheiner LB (1981) Understanding the dose – effect relationship: clinical application of pharmacokinetic – pharmacodynamic models. *Clinical Pharmacokinetics* **6**: 429–453.

Kraiczi H, Jang T, Ludden T, Peck CC (2003) Randomized concentration-controlled trials: motivations, use, and limitations. *Clinical Pharmacology and Therapeutics* **74**: 203–214.

Lipicky RJ (1994) Trough – peak ratio – the rationale behind the United States Food and Drug Administration recommendations. *Journal of Hypertension Supplement* **12**(8): S17–S19; discussion S18–S9.

Nedelman JR (2005) On some 'disadvantages' of the population approach. *The AAPS Journal* **7**: E374–382.

Nedelman JR, Rubin DB, Sheiner LB (2007) Diagnostics for confounding in PK/PD models for oxcarbazepine. *Statistics in Medicine* **26**: 290–308.

Nelder JA, Wedderburn RWM (1972) Generalized linear models. *Journal of the Royal Statistical Society A* **132**: 107–120.

Parati G, Omboni S, Rizzoni D, Agabiti-Rosei E, Mancia G (1998) The smoothness index: a new, reproducible and clinically relevant measure of the homogeneity of the blood pressure reduction with treatment for hypertension. *Journal of Hypertension* **16**: 1685–1691.

Patterson S, Smith B (2007) Analysis of human pharmacokinetic data. In: Dimitrienko A, Chuang-Stein C, Agostino R (eds), *Pharmaceutical Statistics Using SAS: A Practical Guide*. SAS Institute, Cary, NC, pp. 197–211.

Peck C (1990) The randomized concentration-controlled clinical trial (CCT) – an information-rich alternative to the randomized placebo-controlled clinical trial (PCT). *Clinical Pharmacology and Therapeutics* **47**: 148.

Pledger GW, Treiman DM (1991) Design of an individualized fixed-dose clinical trial to test the antiepileptic efficacy of a plasma flunarizine concentration. *Controlled Clinical Trials* **12**: 768–779.

Prentice RL (1989) Surrogate endpoints in clinical trials: definition and operational criteria. *Statistics in Medicine* **8**: 431–440.

Racine A, Dubois JP (1989) Predicting the range of carbamazapine concentrations in patients with epilepsy. *Statistics in Medicine* **8**: 1327–1338.

Rose M, McMahon FG (1990) Some problems with antihypertensive drug studies in the context of the new guidelines. *American Journal of Hypertension* **3**: 151–155.

Rowland M, Towzer TN (1995) *Clinical Pharmacokinetics: Concepts and Applications*. Williams and Wilkins, Baltimore.

Sanathanan LP, Peck CC (1991) The randomized concentration-controlled trial – an evaluation of its sample-size efficiency. *Controlled Clinical Trials* **12**: 780–794.

Senn SJ (1993) Statistical issues in short term trials in asthma. *Drug Information Journal* **27**: 779–791.

Senn SJ (1997) Statisticians and pharmacokineticists: what can they learn from each other? In: Aarons L, Balant LP, Danhof M, *et al.* (eds), *COST B1 medicine. The population approach: measuring and managing variability in response, concentration and dose*. European Commission Directorate-General Science, Research and Development, Geneva, pp. 139–146.

Senn SJ (2002) *Cross-over Trials in Clinical Research* (2nd edition). John Wiley & Sons, Ltd, Chichester.

Senn SJ, Hildebrand H (1991) Crossover trials, degrees of freedom, the carryover problem and its dual. *Statistics in Medicine* **10**: 1361–1374.

Senn SJ, Stevens L, Chaturvedi N (2000) Repeated measures in clinical trials: simple strategies for analysis using summary measures. *Statistics in Medicine* **19**: 861–877.

Senn SJ, D'Angelo G, Potvin D (2004) Carry-over in cross-over trials in bioequivalence: theoretical concerns and empirical evidence. *Pharmaceutical Statistics* **3**: 133–142.

Senn SJ, D'Angelo G, Potvin D (2005) Rejoinder. *Pharmaceutical Statistics* **4**: 216–219.

Sheiner LB, Tozer TN (1978) Clinical pharmacokinetics: The use of plasma concentration in drugs. In: Melmon KL, Morelli HF (eds), *Clinical Pharmacology: Basic Principles of Therapeutics.* Macmillan, New York, pp. 71–109.

Sheiner LB, Rosenberg B, Melmon KL (1972) Modelling of individual pharmacokinetics for computer-aided drug dosage. *Computers and Biomedical Research* **5**: 411–459.

Sheiner LB, Rosenberg B, Marathe VV (1977) Estimation of population characteristics of pharmacokinetic parameters from routine clinical data. *Journal of Pharmacokinetics and Biopharmaceutics* **5**: 445–479.

Steimer JL, Vozeh S, Racine A, Holford NH, O'Neill RT (1994) The population approach: rationale, methods and applications in clinical pharmacology and drug development. In: Welling PG, Balant LP (eds), *Pharmacokinetics of Drugs.* Springer, New York, pp. 405–441.

Troy SM, Cevallos WH, Conrad KA, Chiang ST, Latts JR (1991) The absolute bioavailability and dose proportionality of intravenous and oral dosage regimens of recainam. *Journal of Clinical Pharmacology* **31**: 433–439.

Wakefield J, Walker S (1997) A population approach to initial dose selection. *Statistics in Medicine* **16**: 1135–1149.

Zanchetti A (1997) Twenty-four-hour ambulatory blood pressure evaluation of antihypertensive agents. *Journal of Hypertension* **15**: S21–S25.

Bioequivalence Studies

Strange! that such high dispute shou'd be
Twixt Tweedledum and Tweedledee

John Byrom

And, which was strange, the one so like the other
As could not be distinguished but by names

William Shakespeare, *The Comedy of Errors*

'You can't really say 'similar' if it's the same again you want. 'Similar' means something different.'
Anthony Burgess, *Enderby Outside*

22.1   BACKGROUND

Twenty-four healthy young medical students spend their day having needles stuck into them. Then they go away only to come back the following week and have it done to them again. What is happening? They are partaking in a particularly common form of cross-over trial known as a **bioequivalence trial** in which a test and a reference product are being compared. Usually these are run as double-blind AB/BA cross-overs. The reference product will (usually) be a registered brand-name drug. The test product will either be a new formulation produced (usually) by the same manufacturer or a generic product produced (usually) by another. The purpose of the trial is to prove equivalence of the test and reference product and so obviate the need for a full clinical development for the new product. This is done by observing the time courses of the concentration of the products in the blood, the argument being that where these are effectively identical, the products must be therapeutically equivalent. (The same basic methodology is also used for certain other studies, for example food interaction studies, in which it may be desired to prove that the circumstance under which a product is administered do not affect its pharmacokinetic characteristics and hence its efficacy.)

Most commonly, a single dose of each of test and reference is given on particular days well separated by a wash-out period of at least five half-lives of the drug and a number of blood (or possibly urine) samples are taken until at least three half-lives of the drug have been passed or sometimes until the concentration has passed the limits of detection. These samples are analysed before breaking the blind and the concentration for a given time point is obtained for each individual. Summary statistics such as the area under

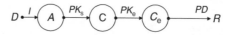

Figure 22.1   Schematic representation of relationship between drug dosage D and response R.

the curve (AUC) concentration maximum (C_{max}) and time to reach a maximum (T_{max}) are calculated. Confidence limits for these are obtained and if they lie within the limits of equivalence, the drugs are declared equivalent.

The basic idea behind bioequivalence studies was well explained by the late Lewis Sheiner and is illustrated by Figure 22.1, which is taken from Sheiner (1992). D is the drug and I is the absorption process. The absorbed drug, A, is then distributed according to some process, PK_s, which produces a concentration in the blood which may be measured. The drug then distributes to and from a site of action according to an effect-site process, PK_e, to produce an effect-site concentration, C_e, which, via the pharmacodynamic response mechanism, PD, leads to a response, R. The arrows are schematic to represent causation rather than to describe mass transfer. The idea behind conventional approaches to bioequivalence is that although it is the response, R, which is of ultimate interest, if formulations are different this will be reflected in the process labelled I rather than any other. The assumption which is made is that, given knowledge of the true value of any particular variable in the diagram, knowledge of any antecedent variable (to the left in the diagram) is irrelevant to predicting any subsequent variable (to the right). (Actually, however, if measurement error is allowed it does not necessarily follow that an equivalent statement can be made in terms of *measured* variables.) A is not generally directly measurable but C is and therefore bioequivalence is used to prove general equivalence, for which purpose it is sufficient. Essentially the blood is regarded as, 'a gate through which the drug must pass'. Equivalence at this point implies equivalence subsequently.

In this chapter, statistical issues to do with bioequivalence are explored. Some of the problems are shared with equivalence trials generally and it may also be relevant to consult Chapter 15. In addition, the problems of attempting to prove bioequivalence without using pharmacokinetic parameters but using pharmacodynamic parameters instead were considered under the section devoted to parallel assay in Chapter 20. See also Senn (2002), Senn *et al.* (1997) and Miller *et al.* (2007). A good practical reference for trial planning is Hauschke *et al.* (1992). There is also a companion book in this series devoted entirely to bioequivalence by Dieter Hauschke, Volker Steinijans and Iris Pigeot (Hauschke *et al.*, 2007), which gives much useful advice on planning and analysis. Other books include those by Patterson and Jones (2005) and Chow and Liu (2000) and the edited collection of articles by Welling *et al.* (1991). The book by Wellek, which treats equivalence more generally is also relevant (Wellek, 2002). A review article on bioequivalence by me (Senn, 2001) appeared in *Statistics in Medicine* in 2001 and a subsequent review on cross-over trials (Senn, 2006) also has a section devoted to bioequivalence.

22.2   ISSUES

22.2.1   The problem of treatment versions

A crucial assumption in the analysis of many experiments is that there are no versions of the treatment (Rubin, 1980); in clinical trials, for example, we assume that a drug is a drug is a drug. Suppose, however, that a drug we investigated had the frightening property that it could actually change the effect it had over time. I do not mean that its effect might change over time as a patient takes it, but that its effect on new patients in 2010 (say) might differ from its effect on very similar patients in 2005. Of course, this possibility is regularly dismissed but it remains a possibility. In fact, the most famous clinical trial of all is Bradford Hill's study of streptomycin in tuberculosis (Medical Research Council Streptomycin in Tuberculosis Trials Committee, 1948), a drug that was proved highly effective at the time but owing to the emergence of resistance no longer is so. There are, in fact, cases where a presumed inconsequential (for efficacy and tolerability) change in manufacturing can have dramatic and unforeseen effects. For instance: the synthesis of a pharmaceutical may be improved and simplified. It is believed that the product should, if anything, be of higher quality; however, there is subsequently an increase in side-effects. Another example: a pharmaceutical company tightens its specification for particle size for an inhaled dry-powder treatment. However, by concentrating the particles towards the average size, it increases the inhalable fraction of product and some patients overdose. Of course, with benefit of hindsight (the most exact of all sciences), an explanation can usually be found. But, if the purpose of drug regulation is to predict effects before they happen, not to explain them once they have happened, such explanations are always too late.

Now suppose that a drug is out of patent and that a generics company wishes to produce its own version of the brand-name pharmaceutical for which registration was originally granted. Is it reasonable to require it to go through a full development? Is it even reasonable to require it to undertake a bioequivalence trial? May it not be assumed, as it will be for the branded product, that there are no versions of the treatment? This depends, of course, by what one means by 'the treatment': an investigation of which has a circular nature and leads nowhere but back to base, for we shall hardly regard a generic and a branded treatment as being the same treatment if their effects are different, but if their effects are identical then it seems obvious that they are the same. In the general spirit of drug development, therefore (where proof is of the essence), it would seem to be necessary to 'prove' that the generic and the branded drug are the same, although even this does not get us out of the philosophical difficulties. For what is it that makes a drug a generic? Is it simply the name, or is it the manufacturing process? Suppose a sponsor wishes to rid itself of a brand-name product because it is currently receiving competition from two generic companies and it prefers to concentrate its efforts on newer patented products. It arranges to sell off the product to a third generic company. Under what circumstances, logically, should the generic company now be required to prove equivalence of the generic product to the brand name? If all the generic company buys is the 'know-how'? If it also buys the manufacturing plant? If it also buys the name?

In fact, this problem arises all the time during drug development since it is nearly always the case that the product undergoes some pharmaceutical development between phase I and final approval. This can range from apparently 'minor' developments involving scaling up manufacture (from plants capable of delivering enough material for clinical trials to those capable of satisfying marketing needs) to major changes in formulations. Thus, drug development may require bioequivalence studies to help bridge gaps caused by changes in formulation, although it is often something of a puzzle to determine whether and when such studies are needed.

The fact that I regard this problem as being difficult and important has been coloured by my experience with two trials which I myself have helped design. Both were to compare different formulations of a bronchodilator. The first, example 7.1 of my book on cross-over trials (Senn, 1993a, 2002) seemed to show that two formulations of the same drug were equivalent. Later studies showed that this was not so. The second (Senn *et al.*, 1997) showed convincingly that two further formulations of the same drug were not equivalent, despite the fact that it had confidently been expected that they would be.

> **Biometrics**: A word increasingly used for the 'science' of uniquely identifying individuals by individuals who couldn't uniquely identify a word for their science.

22.2.2   Limits of equivalence

For many years, many regulatory authorities, following the lead of the FDA (Division of Biopharmaceutics, 1977), required that the limits of equivalence for the ratio of AUCs for test and reference should be 0.8 to 1.2. These limits, however, are not invariant since the reciprocal of 0.8 is 1.25. Furthermore, although the limits appear to be symmetrical, symmetry of the test statistic is actually assumed on the log scale and when log-transformed the limits 0.8 to 1.2 correspond to -0.223 and 0.183, so that their midpoint is not at 0, which is the point on the log scale corresponding to exact equality. Whether two formulations are equivalent may depend, therefore, upon which is declared as test and which as reference. These limits do not exhibit what may be termed 'label invariance', whereby the conduct of the trial and its analysis would be the same if the labels were switched. (Such invariance is a regular feature of many clinical trials and, while it may not be always desirable, it is always useful to consider whether a given analysis observes it.) In a letter to *Biometrics*, Kirkwood (1981) highlighted the anomaly of this asymmetry on the log-scale and pointed out that in another context, that of bioassay, limits symmetrical on the log scale were used. There is now universal agreement among regulatory authorities that the invariant limits 0.8 to 1.25 should be used for AUC. (At the time of writing, the FDA requires these limits for C_{max} also, whereas the CPMP allows that they may have to be wider, for example, 0.75 to 1.33 (Committee for Proprietary Medicinal Products, 2001).) In dealing with this anomaly, however, these are not the only choice one could have made. For example, one could have used the invariant limits 0.83 to 1.2 (to two decimal places 0.83 is the reciprocal of 1.2), or the compromise limits of 0.82 to 1.22, based on the geometric means of these two alternatives, or indeed any other set of limits which are reciprocals of each other.

This raises the issue whether there can be any general standard of equivalence. Two matters which are surely of some relevance are the therapeutic window for treatment and the batch-to-batch variability. Some drugs, such as procainamide, have a very narrow therapeutic window, others such as propranolol have a much wider one (Rowland and Towzer, 1995). On the other hand, for certain products, such as those delivered by transdermal patch or metered-dose inhaler, or generally active at extremely low concentrations, the variability from batch to batch or even from sample to sample may be considerable. As Rhodes (1994) has pointed out, it seems to be unreasonable to require a generic to be equivalent to a brand name if the latter is not equivalent to itself. In particular, the combination of wide therapeutic window and high batch-to-batch variability might imply much less stringent limits, whereas the combination of a narrow therapeutic window and a reference product of low variability would require more stringent limits. Rhodes (1994) has suggested that it would be more logical to have four-period cross-over trials in which two batches of test were compared to two batches of reference.

22.2.3 The power approach

At one time, a popular approach to the statistical testing of bioequivalence was to use a conventional null hypothesis of equality of the two treatments. Since, where this approach is adopted, the type I error is the error in rejecting the null hypothesis of equality when the treatments are, in fact, equal, this approach does not control the error of concluding that the treatments are equivalent when they are in fact different; yet, presumably, this is the error we should like to control. This problem was addressed by requiring that the test used to examine the null hypothesis was of 'adequate' power: say 80%. As Schuirmann showed in a detailed examination (Schuirmann, 1987), this approach is quite inadequate. Not only is the type II error rate 20% but also the sample size is established at the planning stage and depends on the presumed value of the standard deviation rather than the observed precision. Furthermore, two drugs might be slightly different but effectively equivalent. What will then happen with the power approach is that if the sample standard deviation is much less than anticipated, the test will almost certainly reject the null hypothesis. The trouble with the approach is that, whether of high power or not, it remains a means of examining the hypothesis of exact equality of the treatments and, if the logic of hypothesis testing is accepted, is adequate for rejecting this hypothesis but is not for asserting it, nor the hypothesis of approximate equivalence. This approach has now been abandoned.

22.2.4 90% or 95% confidence limits?

For bioequivalence there is now international agreement to calculate 90% confidence limits and see whether these lie within the limits of equivalence. For reasons discussed in Section 15.2.1, this corresponds to carrying out two one-sided tests at the 5% level. However, for tests comparing an active treatment with placebo, the FDA usually requires significance at the 5% level two-sided. For reasons discussed in Chapter 12, it may be argued that the 'regulator's risk' in this circumstance is therefore 2.5%, rather than 5%, since if the drug is significantly worse than placebo it will not be registered. It might thus be argued that 95% limits should be used for bioequivalence to be consistent, since the regulator should require that the risk of registering an inequivalent drug should be 2.5%.

Another argument can be given in favour of conventional 95% confidence limits which removes discussion from the context of formal decision making. Suppose that, with no particular object in mind, we were to assert that the true bioequivalence ratio was some value γ. If we were to test this assertion conventionally we would do so at the 5% level two-sided by adopting the value γ for our true difference under the null hypothesis. The data will either cause us to accept or to reject the hypothesis. By changing the value of γ we can establish all values which are accepted or rejected. The accepted range of values forms a 95% confidence interval and, to use the conventional logic of the confidence interval and its duality with hypothesis testing, any value which lies outside it must be rejected. Now, if the confidence limits lie within the region of equivalence, it then follows that all inequivalent values lie outside the confidence limits and thus that there is no inequivalent value of γ which we would not reject using conventional two-sided tests. Thus, any claim of inequivalence under such circumstances would have to be rejected. Hence we are justified in concluding equivalence.

However, all standards of significance and confidence are in any case arbitrary and, without specific references to losses involved with various decisions, little can be done to remove the arbitrary element. The issue is raised here simply to point to an apparent inconsistency.

22.2.5 C_{max}, T_{max} and possible alternatives

There are good reasons for basing judgements of equivalence on AUC. It measures the extent of absorption, plays a central role in investigations of dose proportionality and makes a fairly efficient use of all of the measurements. (It is closely related to the mean.) Its expected value is also largely independent of the frequency of measurement. However, it is of course, conceivable that two drugs could have identical AUCs but have quite different profiles. One could be extremely peaked and of short duration and the other could have a lower peak but decline more gently. The situation is illustrated in Figure 22.2. The therapeutic behaviour of the two would be quite different.

It is also clear from the diagram that the C_{max} of the two drugs is quite different. This does not mean, however, that it is the most appropriate measure to use in addition to AUC. I have suggested elsewhere (Senn, 1993a, 1993b, 2002) that the difference between the AUC in the first half of the curve and the AUC in the second might be used. For these two drugs, the ratio of this measure is less than the ratio of C_{max} but its variance may also be expected to be lower. There has been quite a lot of discussion

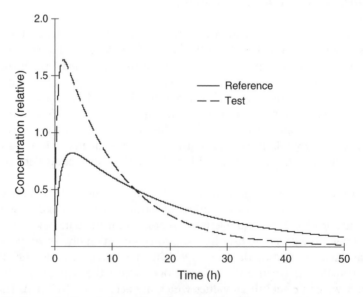

Figure 22.2   Concentration–time profiles for a test and reference product.

of suitable measures and Lacey (1996) have made a detailed evaluation of various alternatives.

Other things being equal, the expected value of C_{max} is higher the greater the frequency of measurement, although this will not necessarily bias any comparison. T_{max} has the further disadvantage that it is a discrete measure dependent on the sampling interval. C_{max}, has the further property that it is highly correlated with AUC. This would appear, on the face of it, to be a disadvantage but the point might be worth investigation. The situation seems to be at the moment that most statisticians are happy with AUC as a measure of bioequivalence but that many are uneasy about the choice and use of further measures.

An investigation of several alternative measures based on direct curve comparisons was undertaken by Polli and McLean (2001). For example, for a cross-over trial they considered the following measure for each subject formed by a weighted sum of relative bioavailabilities over the measurement times i:

$$\rho = \frac{\sum\limits_{i=1}^{n} (R_i + T_i) \, \text{Ratio}_i}{\sum\limits_{i=1}^{n} (R_i + T_i)},$$

where $\text{Ratio}_i = \max(R_i, T_i)/\min(R_i, T_i)$ is the relative bioavailability calculated in such a way that the larger of R_i, T_i is made the denominator at each time point. Other similar measures were defined and the reader is referred to that paper for details.

However, consideration of Polli and McLean (2001) immediately raises the issue whether curves might not be compared using an approach analogous to the Kullback–Leibler (KL) approach (Kullback, 1951) for comparing probability distributions. (Concentrations, like probabilities, are positive. They do not add to 1 but they could be made to do so by dividing by the total of the concentrations, which is extremely closely related to the AUC.) This thus suggests that perhaps as a first comparison one could use AUC, as is commonly done, and then as a second compare normalized curves where each concentration had been replaced by a ratio to AUC. If we let such normalized concentrations be r_i, t_i for test and reference, the KL type measure defined on the reference distribution is then

$$\text{KL}_r = \sum_{i=1}^{n} r_i \log_2 \left(\frac{r_i}{t_i} \right).$$

The same function but defined on the test distribution is

$$\text{KL}_t = \sum_{i=1}^{n} t_i \log_2 \left(\frac{t_i}{r_i} \right)$$

and a label-invariant version is thus

$$\text{KL} = \frac{\text{KL}_r + \text{KL}_t}{2},$$

or more simply just the sum.

Dragalin *et al.* (2003) have applied KL measures to judge individual and population bioequivalence. This, however, is based on applying KL divergence to the distribution of summary measures calculated from the concentration–time curves not to the curves themselves. As the proofs of this edition were being corrected, I became aware of Pereira (2007) which applies the KL measure to concentration–time curves directly.

22.2.6   Log-transformation versus Fieller's theorem

This is an issue where consensus now seems to have been achieved. An ingenious theorem due to Fieller (Fieller, 1940, 1944) enables one to calculate a confidence interval for the ratio of two means. The approach does not require transformation of the original data. (Edgar C. Fieller, 1907–1960, is an early example of a statistician employed in the pharmaceutical industry. He worked for the Boots company in the late 1930s and 1940s.) For many years this was a common approach to making inferences about the ratio of the two mean AUCs in the standard bioequivalence experiment (Locke, 1984).

There is now general agreement that the individual AUCs for each subject on each treatment occasion should be log-transformed and the whole analysis performed on these transformed values. This involves calculating the 90% confidence limits for mean log-AUC and back-transforming them by taking the antilogarithm. (In other words, using the relationship that if log-AUC is the natural logarithm of AUC, then AUC = $e^{\log-AUC}$.) Actually, it is not even necessary to transform back to ratios of AUCs since alternatively the limits of equivalence of 0.8 to 1.25 can be log-transformed to -0.223 and 0.223.

This approach will not give exactly the same result as application of Fieller's method (occasionally a drug might be bioequivalent according to one method but not according to the other) but it has many advantages. It is simpler to apply. In general, once the log-transformation has been made, the standard theory of cross-over trials can be applied. AUC is a measure which is constrained to be above zero. Strictly speaking it cannot be Normally distributed but its logarithm can be. Of course, this applies for many biochemical and clinical variables, but we do not always log-transform them. A case could be made, however, for saying that we should. Where we don't, it is perhaps because we prefer to deal in original units. Since the end inference for a bioequivalence study is a ratio, however, this excuse does not apply here. It should also be noted that the issue whether to carry out a log-transformation is not finessed by using a nonparametric analysis (Keene, 1995). For example, the ranking of differences in AUC is not necessarily the same as the ranking in ratios and even minimalist nonparametric tests, such as the sign test, do not lead to invariant confidence intervals. (See Senn (2002), chapter 4, for a discussion of this point; Hauschke *et al.* (1990) for technical approaches, and Hauschke *et al.* (1999) for sample size determination if Fieller's theorem is used.) A related issue is addressed in the next section.

22.2.7   Means, medians and additivity

It is sometimes said that by log-transforming AUCs we are actually considering the ratios of medians rather than the ratio of means. The argument goes like this. If the log-AUCs are a sample from a Normally distributed population, then the mean and median of this distribution are identical. The AUCs themselves, however, will follow a log-Normal distribution and for this distribution the mean is higher than the median.

However, if μ is the mean (and hence also the median) of the log-AUCs and σ^2 is the variance, then e^μ is the median of the population of AUCs but not its mean, which equals $e^{\mu+\sigma^2/2}$. Hence, an inference about the means of the log-AUCs corresponds to an inference about the medians of AUCs and not directly about their means. Liu and Weng (1992) have suggested that the standard estimator of bioavailability using the log-transformed values is biased and have proposed a correction. However, note that the estimator of log-bioavailability is not biased.

In my view this argument is false or at the very least misleading. Treatments work at the level of the individual, not on populations. Sometimes we may wish to summarize their effects on populations, but I do not think that the bioequivalence experiment can be regarded as a case in point. The volunteers being studied are only 'human test-tubes'. The drug will eventually be used on quite another population. In the analysis of log-AUCs no assumption is necessary about the distribution of the log-AUCs themselves. There is no requirement for these to be Normally distributed. Indeed, we could deliberately have a bimodal distribution. We could, for example, have a trial in which half the subjects were jockeys and half were basketball players. The concentrations would presumably be very different in the one class and the other. The analysis, however, is based on differences between log-AUCs and the only requirement is that these are Normally distributed. Furthermore, we essentially regard ourselves as measuring the same *effect* from each volunteer. No population effect is involved. It is simply that because of random variation we need more than a single difference to make a conclusion. The easiest way to obtain a number of differences is to recruit a number of subjects, and we assume that the treatment effect is additive on the log-AUC scale.

If this is so, it implies that the expected value of the ratio of means will depend on the subjects recruited. This is, however, a quite undesirable property and shows that such a ratio is in fact meaningless. The only sensible thing to do is to measure on the additive scale. There are good reasons for supposing that this is more likely to be log-AUC and not AUC. To sum up, we are not interested in making inferences about ratios of means and medians but in making inferences about means (and medians) of ratios.

22.2.8   Homoscedasticity

Fisher pointed out a long time ago that where we are testing a null hypothesis regarding the equality of two treatments in an experimental setting by examining their means, the equality of the variance belongs to the hypothesis being tested. This is because we have divided the experimental material at random into two groups and under the null hypothesis, and over all randomizations, these two groups must have identical distributions. This is rather different from comparing two samples drawn at random from two populations where we might, conceivably, be interested in seeing whether the population means were equal while accepting that the variances need not be. This is because the inference is directly about the population of units and not about a treatment. These two very different cases are hardly mentioned in standard mathematical approaches to statistics, where the student is introduced to the importance of the assumption of 'homoscedasticity', with little discussion of the circumstances under which it may apply and the seriousness of the consequences where it doesn't.

In equivalence studies in general (see Chapter 15) we are trying to prove that the treatments are not different. Our 'null-hypothesis' is that the treatments are different. Under this null hypothesis the variance can be different. Therefore it may be argued that a stronger assumption is being made in any test which assumes such equality. (As was pointed out in Chapter 15, the confidence interval approach is equivalent to two one-sided tests.) In practice, however, I do not consider that, for bioequivalence studies at least, this is a serious problem. The calculation proceeds on the basis of differences between period 1 and period 2 calculated for every subject. These are compared between the two sequence groups (reference to test and test to reference) and it is the two variances of these groups of differences which are relevant for the comparison. Since we have randomized (usually similar) subjects into two groups, since *each* difference reflects the effect of both treatments and both periods, just about the only systematic difference between the two groups of observations which could have an effect on the variance is the order in which they are administered. This sort of effect seems very far-fetched and, in any case, if this order can have an effect on the variances, it can presumably have an effect on the means, which would be a more serious violation of the assumptions necessary for the analysis of the cross-over trial. So, to sum up, despite the fact that papers have been published describing what to do when variance assumptions are violated in bioequivalence studies, I consider that this topic is of no practical consequence whatsoever. A good discussion is given by Steinijans and Hauschke (1993). See also Hauschke *et al.* (1996).

22.2.9   Variability of formulations and 'prescribability'

To the extent that the homoscedasticity assumption is important, for the conventional test of bioequivalence, as has been explained above, it has an importance at the level of the differences in log-AUC. These differences would have the same variance from one sequence group to another, even if the test and reference product were of quite different variability. However, the fact that these variances might be different, while having no direct impact on the test, might suggest an alternative form of inequivalence and this latter possibility deserves, perhaps, to be taken more seriously. The generic manufacturer might, for example, have a process which, owing to an inferior quality of manufacturing, is much more variable both between and within batches. The mean over all batches or within a given batch might, however, be similar to that for the reference product. Furthermore, as the late Lewis Sheiner pointed out, given sufficient knowledge of a formulation it will in principle be possible to adjust its mean bioavailability to the reference standard (Sheiner, 1992). This would not, of itself, make the *quality* of the formulation adequate. Hence, it is conceivable that variances might be different but means would be the same.

A rather different source of variability may arise if different routes of administration are being compared. Consider a brand-name manufacturer who has a treatment that has been registered as a suppository but now wishes to change the formulation to an oral form. The two formulations will have to interact with different parts of the body and in particular the oral form will have a much longer journey to reach the point of absorption. It may be possible to adjust the dose of the oral form so that it delivers the same average dose into the blood, but it is plausible that the variability will be much greater from patient to patient.

In an influential paper, Anderson and Hauck (1990) referred to the ability of a new formulation to match a test formulation in terms of both mean and variance as *prescribability*, the idea that a formulation that had a higher variance even if it had the same mean might lead both to more side-effects on occasion (too bioavailable) and lack of efficacy on others (not bioavailable enough). Such a formulation would be less prescribable than the reference formulation.

There has been some attention recently in the literature to tests to compare variability of formulations as well as comparing means. (See, for example, Dragalin *et al.* (2003), and Grieve (1998).) A technical difficulty, which has to be dealt with in examining the variances, arises from the correlation of measurements taken on the same individual.

I am however, sceptical about the practical value of all this, for the simple reason that if this is a problem it is far more important to give consideration to the way in which batches, and samples within batches, (if manufacturing variability is suspected as the source of variation) or subjects (if route of administration is varied) are selected for examination, than to devise ways of testing variances. In fact, comparing formulations in terms of variances if human physiology is believed to be part of the source of variation would require testing in patients rather than in healthy volunteers (Senn, 2001). For an extreme espousal of this view see Longford (1999) and Longford and Nelder (1999). Hardly anybody seems to have had anything useful and practical to say on this subject. Rhodes (1994) is an exception.

> **Generic companies**: The Amerigo Vespuccis of drug development: they profit by what others discover.

22.2.10   Individual bioequivalence and switchability

As discussed above, if two products have the same mean bioavailability and the same variability, then they are equally 'prescribable'. A physician faced with a new patient would have no reason (apart from price or prejudice) to prefer one to the other. However, as Anderson and Hauck (1990) pointed out in an influential paper, it does not follow that, given a patient who is already well treated on the one drug, the physician may assume that the patient can be switched to another.

If we retain the additivity assumption – that where there is a difference in the effect of drugs then this is constant on the log-AUC scale – the above problem does not arise. It is at least conceivable, however, that *for a given set of subjects*, two formulations could have the same effect on average but have quite different effects from subject to subject: the reference might be much more bioavailable in some subjects but much less so than the test in others. (Note that this would not at all be a reasonable assumption if *exact* equality of average availability were being postulated. But this is not required for bioequivalence. *Approximate* equality suffices.) The qualification that such a situation can only apply for a given set of subjects is important, for, obviously, if we happen to include in our study only those subjects for whom the reference drug is much more bioavailable, then the mean log-AUC will be much higher for the reference product.

I do not think that there is any value in attempting to answer this question using a traditional AB/BA cross-over. If the matter is at all worth investigating, then a suitable design is a four-period cross-over in which each subject receives each treatment twice. (There has been much discussion in the literature of a three-period protocol in which the reference product is given twice and the test product once. This is more economical of time but does not exhibit label invariance.) This can then be used to resolve the various components of variation: pure between-subject variability, subject-by-formulation inter-action, and random variability within subjects. (See also Chapters 17 and 18.) However, in a similar way to the issue of variability of formulations in Section 22.2.9, as soon as we allow that a treatment may have different effects in different persons, then the issue of sampling is raised. It is reasonable to suppose that if a large interactive effect of the subject-by-formulation sort is found, then 'switchability' in patients will not, in general, apply. The converse does not at all follow, however, and raises the issue discussed above of whether, if we fear this sort of effect, we should be using healthy volunteers at all in bioequivalence studies.

There has been considerable debate in the literature regarding the appropriate analysis of the three-period equivalence protocol. An excellent discussion is given by Steinijans *et al.* (1995). However, I have said elsewhere (Senn, 1991, 1993b) that the most serious problems with equivalence studies in general are not of a technical statistical nature, but are 'philosophical'. Switchability strikes me as being one of these. Sheiner (1992) has also pointed out, quite rightly, that little progress can be made here without clearly describing the clinical context which regulation is trying to address and the consequences of various types of decision.

One problem is that commentators have failed to take account of the fact that bioequivalence is a means to an end and not an end in itself (Senn, 1998, 2001). Suppose a generic manufacturer succeeds in showing that a generic is equivalent to a registered innovator drug in terms of mean and variability but fails to show that it is switchable. (I actually think that this it is fairly unlikely that a formulation is prescribable but not switchable, but unless it is possible there is no point in discussing the issue anyway.) Apart from the financial obstacles there is nothing to stop the manufacturer developing the formulation using a free-standing dossier, without reference to the innovator's marketing licence, but copying the programme of trials that was successful for the innovator. If drug regulation is to mean anything at all, one would have to believe that the generic manufacturer has a high chance of success and would then be given a licence. But nothing would be gained by this for the regulator and a lot would be lost to both the generic manufacturer and society, which has an interest in cheap medicine. And once the generic was registered, switching could take place anyway.

This is not simply a theoretical condition. Formoterol was originally discovered by Yamanouchi, who licensed it to CIBA-Geigy, a forerunner company of Novartis which markets it under the brand name Foradil. The drug has been off-patent for many years and AstraZeneca has its own formulation developed without reference to Foradil and marketed as Oxis. It is not even known whether these formulations are equivalent in a mean sense. Yet patients can be switched from one to the other by their physicians in those markets in which both were licensed. Now suppose a generic manufacturer shows that a new formulation is equally prescribable as Foradil. (Since these formulations are inhaled this would actually be quite difficult.) It would be absurd to object to a licence because switchability was not proved (Senn, 1998, 2001).

22.2.11 The choice of confidence limits

There is no unique set of confidence limits, even for a given level of confidence. We usually calculate limits that are symmetric about the point estimate. For example for 95% confidence limits for the difference between two means, for a large sample, we usually add or subtract 1.96 times the standard error (SE) to/from the observed difference. (We shall discuss this issue in terms of 95% limits rather than the standard limits of 90% now used, but this makes no difference to the essence of the point in question.) This gives limits of $(\bar{X}_1 - \bar{X}_2) \pm 1.96\text{SE}$. However, it is also true that other limits may be calculated. For example, 95% of the Normal distribution lies between limits of -1.76 to 2.3 SE and 95% also lies between -1.85 to 2.1 SE.

In a very influential paper in *Biometrics* in 1976, Westlake suggested that it might be appropriate to calculate limits which were symmetrical about the point of equivalence rather than about the observed difference (see also Westlake, 1979). Since, at the point of equivalence, the ratio is 1 and since Westlake was talking about symmetry on the log scale, he was proposing limits which were symmetrical about $\log(1) = 0$. The way in which this works is best illustrated by example. Suppose, to simplify discussion, that we have a very large bioequivalence study and can therefore use the Normal distribution rather than the t-distribution to calculate a confidence limit and suppose that the observed difference on the log scale is -0.02 and standard error 0.10. If we were to calculate 95% confidence intervals we would use $-0.02 \pm 1.96 \times 0.10$, which gives limits of -0.216 to 0.176. These are symmetrical about -0.02, the observed difference, but not about 0. In order to find limits which are symmetrical about zero, we need two values z_1 and z_2 of the standard Normal distribution such that 95% of the distribution lies between these limits and such that $(z_1 \times 0.10 - 0.02) = -(z_2 \times 0.10 - 0.02)$, or equivalently such that $(z_1 - 0.02/0.1) = -(z_2 - 0.02/0.10)$, or so that $z_1 = -z_2 + 0.4$. (Note that z_1 will be a negative number here.) By suitable manipulation of the Normal distribution (either using some numerical algorithm or trial and error), the values of z_1 and z_2 can be found to be -1.8 and 2.2. Hence the symmetric limits (on the log-scale) are -0.20 and 0.20. On the original scale these limits are 0.819 to 1.221. The situation is illustrated in Figure 22.3, which gives the lower value (z_1) as a function of the upper value (z_2) as well as the sum of the two values. For a sum of zero, the values are -1.96 and $+1.96$. For a sum of 0.4, the values are -1.8 and $+2.2$.

Westlake was a pioneer in bioequivalence, being one of the first to draw explicit attention to the way in which hypothesis testing was being inappropriately used to assert equivalence. (Failure to reject the hypothesis of exact equivalence was being used as a reason for asserting it.) At one time this approach to calculating confidence intervals was widely employed. It soon attracted criticism, however, and was eventually abandoned by Westlake himself, who subsequently recommended the 90% conventional confidence limits symmetric about the point estimate (Westlake, 1981).

22.2.12   Conventional confidence intervals

In a reaction to Westlake's symmetric interval procedure, Kirkwood (1981) proposed using conventional 95% confidence limits and judging the formulations equivalent if these lay within the equivalence bounds. A later proposal by Schuirmann (1987) looked at the issue in terms of using two one-sided tests (TOST) at the 5% level. This procedure, that of requiring each of two null hypotheses, one corresponding to sub-availability and the other to super-availability, to be rejected at the 5% level, is equivalent to requiring that the conventional 90% confidence interval lie within the limits of equivalence. Figure 22.4 gives three critical boundaries for the point estimates

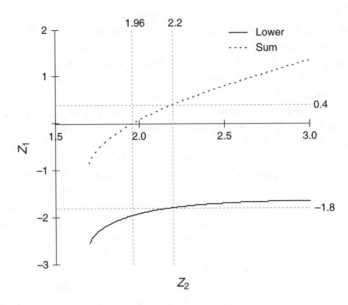

Figure 22.3 Lower value and sum of values as a function of the upper value for 95% confidence for a standardized Normal distribution.

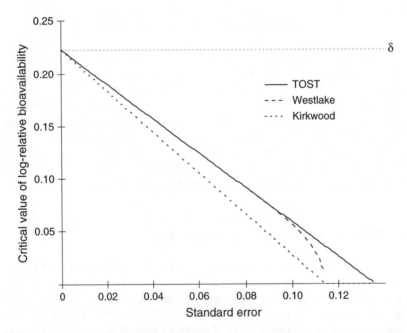

Figure 22.4 Kirkwood, Westlake and Shuirmann (TOST) critical boundaries for the point estimate for log relative bioavailability as a function of the standard error.

for three approaches – Kirkwood, Schuirmann (TOST) and Westlake – as a function of the standard error of estimated bioavailability. It can be seen that Kirkwood's is the most stringent, that Schuirmann's is the most liberal and that Westlake's lies between the two. This is because for sufficiently small standard error the Westlake approach can play off one boundary against the other. This means that under such circumstance it has nearly all of the 5% to devote to the most critical limit, but 5% is what Schuirmann's approach allocates for each limit. However, for high standard error there is no room to manouevre and 2.5% has to be devoted to each limit, which is the case with Kirkwood's approach.

One criticism of the symmetric interval approach is that we may wish to control two types of error independently. We may wish to know that the probability of committing a type I error is not more than some level when the new drug is less bioavailable than the standard and we may wish to have the same control when it is more bioavailable. The symmetric confidence interval approach trades off one kind of error against the other. Rightly or wrongly, it now seems that almost all commentators agree that conventional limits symmetrical about the point estimate should be employed. For reasons given in section 22.2.4, 90% limits are used. This is an example, therefore, of an 'issue' in drug development which (for the time being at least) has been resolved.

22.2.13   Other frequentist approaches

Various other approaches have been suggested. As we pointed out in Chapter 15, carrying out two one-sided tests at the 5% level does not quite lead to a type I error rate of 5%. Consider, for example, the case where the standard error is very large compared to the region of equivalence and suppose we test first of all the null hypothesis that the new treatment has an AUC which is 1.25 or more times that of the standard. Because of the large standard error, the critical value for the observed mean will be less than 1. Thus we can only ever reject this hypothesis of inequivalence if the observed ratio is less than 1. However, when we come to apply the second test, that which belongs to the null hypothesis that the ratio is less than 0.8, the critical value for the mean ratio will now be in excess of 1. Thus, if we reject the first hypothesis of inequality we *must* accept the second and vice versa. Hence, although the type I error rate for each of the two tests is 5%, our type I error rate for declaring equivalence is 0. (See also Chapter 15, section 15.2.1 and the technical appendix.)

As a consequence, various authors, following Hauck and Anderson (1984), have considered improvements to the one-sided testing procedure which are designed to produce tests of correct size. Schuirman points out, however, that the Anderson and Hauck procedure can be liberal (Schuirmann, 1987). The best analysis of this whole question is that provided by my former colleague the late Gunther Mehring (Mehring, 1993) who considered general interval testing for the Polya family of distributions. (See also Berger and Hsu (1996) and Brown *et al*. (1997).) These refinements of adjusting the tests to remove their conservatism are of theoretical interest only, however, and from other perspectives they are far from ideal (Perlman and Wu, 1999). They would really only ever be of interest if a decision *had* to be made on the basis of extremely limited data and one *had* to leave open the possibility of concluding equivalence (Senn, 2001). In practice this does not obtain, and wherever the confidence interval approach is conservative to any appreciable degree it simply means that the amount of evidence available is inadequate. This can be seen by considering what the ratio of likelihoods will be comparing the best-supported alternative hypothesis with the best-supported null hypothesis. As we pointed out in Chapter 13, for conventional trials designed to show significance, this ratio for a *P*-value of 0.05 two-sided is about 6. For tests which 'improve' on the confidence limit approach to equivalence testing and where this makes any appreciable difference (which is to say that the standard error will be large), this ratio will be close to 1.

22.2.14   Bayesian approaches

There are two aspects to any fully Bayesian approach. The first is the mechanics of producing a posterior distribution for the bioavailability ratio. Various approaches have been proposed (Fluehler *et al.*, 1983; Mandallaz and Mau, 1981; Racine *et al.*, 1986; Selwyn *et al.*, 1981; Selwyn and Hall, 1984). The second aspect is the practical decision rule which should link the posterior distribution to a declaration of equivalence or inequivalence as the case may be. To be fully Bayesian, the utilities associated with declaring equivalence or inequivalence should be established as a function of the true bioavailability ratio. For a given posterior distribution the declaration with maximum expected utility should be made.

In practice this second step is not generally taken because of the difficulty of establishing the utilities. (Presumably one should invite the FDA, HPB, MCA, EMEA or whatever to state their utilities.) However, in an interesting paper Lindley has investigated theoretical aspects of this (Lindley, 1998). What is particularly interesting is the extent to which the addition of a loss function changes the Bayesian solution in the presence of high variability, where Lindley's approach would lead to acceptance of bioequivalence more frequently (Senn, 2001). Figure 22.5 shows the critical

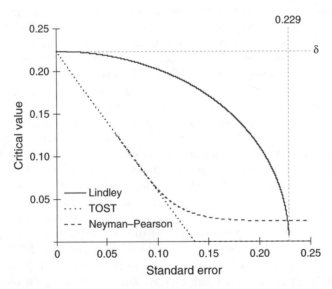

Figure 22.5 Schuirmann (TOST), Lindley and Neyman–Pearson crtical values for log-bioavailability as a function of the standard error.

boundary for Lindley's procedure together with the conventional TOST boundary and also the 'optimal' Neyman – Pearson (NP) boundary. The different behaviour of these three is striking. For low variability the NP approach is effectively identical to TOST, but as variability increases the type I error rate associated with TOST as a whole starts to drop markedly below 5% and, this being so, the NP procedure diverges as it makes good this loss. Except for the case of a zero standard error, Lindley's procedure is never close to TOST, being always more liberal. For very low precision it does cross the NP boundary. TOST will never allow equivalence if the standard error exceeds $\delta/\Phi^{-1}(0.95) = \ln(1.25)/1.645 = 0.136$, where $\Phi^{-1}(0.95)$ is the inverse cumulative density of the normal distribution. On the other hand, a declaration of equivalence is possible for Lindley's procedure provided that the standard error is less than 0.229. For the NP procedure a declaration is always possible and, indeed, the probability that it will be made is at least 5% whatever the standard error.

One explanation why Lindley's formulation is so liberal compared to the other two is that it is relevant to the two-valued decision problem: *accept* versus *reject for ever*. The second of these alternatives is not, however, what applies in practice: a sponsor is usually allowed to return with new evidence. Thus, the real choice is between *accept, require new evidence, reject for ever*. At the point of regulation, the relevant decision is between the first and the last two options and this would make the circumstances under which the drug was not accepted more common, especially if, as would be the case where variability was high, more information would be valuable (Senn, 2001).

In practice, neither Lindley's approach nor any of the other Bayesian suggestions is used. However, some standard frequentist approaches can be given a fiducial interpretation, which is very similar to a Bayesian one involving uninformative priors (O'Quigley and Baudoin, 1988). For example, if one requires that the probability that the true unknown bioavailability ratio lies within the limits of equivalence should be at least 95%, then this is approximately equivalent to Westlake's symmetrical confidence limit approach. Alternatively, if one requires that the probability of inferior bioavailability should be less than 5% and also that the probability of superior bioavailability should be less than 5%, then this is approximately equivalent to requiring that conventional 90% limits should lie within the ranges of equivalence.

22.2.15 The 75/75 rule

This is another historical curiosity. At one time it was proposed that, in addition to satisfying the requirement for average bioequivalence, the bioavailability of the test drug should be proved to be within 75% of that for the reference for 75% of the subjects. The intention of this, perhaps, was to address the issue of individual bioavailability. This sort of requirement suffers from the same difficulties covered by the requirement for 15% FEV_1 bronchodilation in Chapter 8.

Among these difficulties are that, even where the two formulations are absolutely identical, the probability of meeting this requirement cannot necessarily be increased to 100% simply by increasing the sample size. (One would have to increase the number of occasions a given individual was studied instead and compare the mean of the occasions under test to the mean under reference.) Because of inherent variability from occasion to occasion, certain drugs would fail to satisfy this requirement even when tested against themselves. For example, in an investigation of 19 pharmaceuticals, Fluehler *et al.* (1981) found coefficients of pure variation (residual within-patient standard deviation as a percentage of the mean reference result) ranging from 3.6% for isoniazid to 34.5% to hydralazine. The hydralazine results were based on four studies, the lowest of which had a value of 27%. Taking the lowest of these and working in terms of a standard mean of 1 and ignoring some distributional difficulties by treating ratios as if they could be handled symmetrically, this implies a standard deviation of the difference between two replicate measurements of about 0.38, which translates to there only being about a 50% probability that a given individual will have a test bioavailability within 0.25 of the reference. As a consequence, since this probability is actually less than 0.75, a study with a large number of subjects would almost certainly fail to 'demonstrate' bioequivalence, whereas a small one might (by luck) do so. For this and other reasons, this requirement has now been abandoned.

22.2.16   Blinding and bioequivalence

As with ACES, blinding is of little value in bioequivalence trials in protecting the conclusion we wish to assert (Senn, 1994). Any unscrupulous scientist could simply take the blood sample for a given subject for a given time point on the reference drug and mix it with the corresponding sample for the test drug and then divide the two samples arbitrarily in two. Given a large enough sample of subjects, bioequivalence is assured and no resort to the treatment code is needed. (I first heard Joachim Röhmel use this particularly vivid way of making a general point.) This example has to be thought about carefully. It is only one illustration of dozens of ways in which fraud or prejudice could bias results towards equivalence without knowledge of the treatment code. Any competent statistician, for example, could simulate data to 'prove' equivalence without having to know the randomization code. The same could not be done if the object were to prove difference from placebo.

I am not suggesting that this will happen, still less that it should! Blinding is valuable in bioequivalence studies because when we find a difference we are able to dismiss prejudice as a possible explanation. I am just making the point to reinforce the message given in Chapter 15: equivalence is different.

22.2.17   Adjusting for carry-over

The general undesirability of attempting to adjust for cross-over trial was dealt with in detail in Chapter 17. It applies *a fortiori* to bioequivalence studies, where it should be possible to check by taking baseline measurements that no carry-over has occurred (at least to the limit of detection) (Senn *et al.*, 2005). In general, there will be a not inconsiderable loss in efficiency in adjusting for carry-over (Senn *et al.*, 2004) and the strategy of testing fror carry-over and only adjusting if 'detected' is illogical.

Furthermore, there is empirical evidence that the issue of carry-over in bioequivalence studies is not important. In a study of more than 400 cross-over trials D'Angelo *et al.* (2001) found that significant carry-over effects occurred about as often as might be expected by chance and furthermore that the distribution of *P*-values was uniform (Senn *et al.*, 2004). For further discussion see Chapter 17.

References

Anderson S, Hauck WW (1990) Consideration of individual bioequivalence. *Journal of Pharmacokinetics and Biopharmaceutics* **18**: 259–273.

Berger RL, Hsu JC (1996) Bioequivalence trials, intersection-union tests and equivalence confidence sets. *Statistical Science* **11**: 283–302.

Brown LD, Hwang JTG, Munk A (1997) An unbiased test for the bioequivalence problem. *Annals of Statistics* **25**: 2345–2367.

Chow SC, Liu JP (2000) *Design and Analysis of Bioavailability and Bioequivalence Studies*. Marcel Dekker, New York.

Committee for Proprietary Medicinal Products (2001) Note for guidance on the investigation of bioavailability and bioequivalence. European Medicines Evaluation Agency, London, pp. 1–19.

D'Angelo G, Potvin D, Turgeon J (2001) Carryover effects in bioequivalence studies. *Journal of Biopharmaceutical Statistics* **11**: 27–36.

Division of Biopharmaceutics (1977) Bioavailability protocol guideline for ANDA and NDA submission. Food and Drug Administration, Rockville, MD.

Dragalin V, Fedorov V, Patterson S, Jones B (2003) Kullback – Leibler divergence for evaluating bioequivalence. *Statistics in Medicine* **22**: 913–930.

Fieller EC (1940) The biological standardization of insulin. *Journal of the Royal Statistical Society (Supplement)* **1**: 1–54.

Fieller EC (1944) A fundamental formula in the statistics of biological assay, and some applications. *Quarterly Journal of Pharmacology* **17**: 117–123.

Fluehler H, Hirtz J, Moser HA (1981) An aid to decision-making in bioequivalence assessment. *Journal of Pharmacokinetics and Biopharmaceutics* **9**: 223–243.

Fluehler H, Grieve AP, Mandallaz D, Mau J, Moser HA (1983) Bayesian approach to bioequivalence assessment: an example. *Journal of Pharmaceutical Sciences* **72**: 1178–1181.

Grieve AP (1998) Joint equivalence of means and variances of two populations. *Journal of Biopharmaceutical Statistics* **8**: 377–390.

Hauck WW, Anderson S (1984) A new statistical procedure for testing equivalence in two-group comparative bioavailability trials. *Journal of Pharmacokinetics and Biopharmaceutics* **12**: 83–91.

Hauschke D, Steinijans VW, Dlietti E (1990) A distribution-free procedure for the statistical analysis of bioequivalence studies. *International Journal of Clinical Pharmacology, Therapy and Toxicology* **28**: 72–78.

Hauschke D, Steinijans VW, Diletti E, Burke M (1992) Sample size determination for bioequivalence assessment using a multiplicative model. *Journal of Pharmacokinetics and Biopharmaceutics* **20**: 557–561.

Hauschke D, Steinijans VW, Hothorn LA (1996) A note on Welch's approximate t-solution to bioequivalence assessment. *Biometrika* **83**: 236–237.

Hauschke D, Kieser M, Diletti E, Burke M (1999) Sample size determination for proving equivalence based on the ratio of two means for normally distributed data. *Statistics in Medicine* **18**: 93–105.

Hauschke D, Steinijans V, Pigeot I (2007) *Bioequivalence Studies in Drug Development: Methods and Applications*. John Wiley & Sons, Ltd, Chichester.

Keene ON (1995) The log transformation is special. *Statistics in Medicine* **14**: 811–819.

Kirkwood TBL (1981) Bioequivalence testing – a need to rethink. *Biometrics* **37**: 589–591.

Kullback S, Leibler RA (1951) On information and sufficiency. *Annals of Mathematical Statistics* **22**: 79–86.

Lacey LF, Bye A, Keene ON (1996) Glaxo's experience of different absorption rate metrics of immediate release and extended release dosage forms. *Drug Information Journal* **29**: 821–840.

Lindley DV (1998) Decision analysis and bioequivalence trials. *Statistical Science* **13**: 136–141.

Liu JP, Weng CS (1992) Estimation of direct formulation effect under log-normal distribution in bioavailability/bioequivalence studies. *Statistics in Medicine* **11**: 881–896.

Locke CS (1984) An Exact Confidence-Interval from Untransformed Data for the Ratio of 2 Formulation Means. *Journal of Pharmacokinetics and Biopharmaceutics* **12**: 649–655

Longford NT (1999) Selection bias and treatment heterogeneity in clinical trials. *Statistics in Medicine* **18**: 1467–1474.

Longford NT, Nelder JA (1999) Statistics versus statistical science in the regulatory process. *Statistics in Medicine* **18**: 2311–2320.

Mandallaz D, Mau J (1981) Comparison of different methods for decision-making in bioequivalence assessment. *Biometrics* **37**: 213–222.

Medical Research Council Streptomycin in Tuberculosis Trials Committee (1948) Streptomycin treatment for pulmonary tuberculosis. *British Medical Journal* **ii**: 769–782.

Mehring G (1993) On optimal tests for general interval hypotheses. *Communications in Statistics: Theory and Methods* **22**: 1257–1297.

Miller CJ, Senn S, Mezznotte WS (2007) Bronchodilation of formoterol administered with budesonide: device and formulation effects. *Contemporary Clinical Trials*.

O'Quigley J, Baudoin C (1988) General approaches to the problem of bioequivalence. *The Statistician* **37**: 51–58.

Patterson S, Jones B (2005) *Bioequivalence and Statistics in Clinical Pharmacology* Chapman and Hall/CRC, Boca Raton, FL.

Pereira LM (2007) Bioequivalence testing by statistical shape analysis. *Journal of Pharmacokinetics and Pharmacodynamics* **34**: 451–484.

Perlman MD, Wu L (1999) The emperor's new tests. *Statistical Science* **14**: 355–369.

Polli JE, McLean AM (2001) Novel direct curve comparison metrics for bioequivalence. *Pharmaceutical Research* **18**: 734–741.

Racine A, Grieve AP, Fluhler H, Smith AFM (1986) Bayesian methods in practice – experiences in the pharmaceutical industry. *Journal of the Royal Statistical Society Series C – Applied Statistics* **35**: 93–150.

Rhodes C (1994) Bioequivalence evaluation – possible future development. *Clinical Research and Regulatory Affairs* **11**: 181–192.

Rowland M, Towzer TN (1995) *Clinical Pharmacokinetics: Concepts and Applications*. Williams and Wilkins, Baltimore.

Rubin DB (1980) Randomization analysis of experimental data – the Fisher randomization test – Comment. *Journal of the American Statistical Association* **75**: 591–593.

Schuirmann DJ (1987) A comparison of the two one-sided tests procedure and the power approach for assessing the equivalence of average bioavailability. *Journal of Pharmacokinetics and Biopharmaceutics* **15**: 657–680.

Selwyn MR, Hall NR (1984) On Bayesian methods for bioequivalence. *Biometrics* **40**: 1103–1108.

Selwyn MR, Dempster AP, Hall NR (1981) A Bayesian approach to bioequivalence for the 2×2 changeover design. *Biometrics* **37**: 11–21.

Senn SJ (1991) Falsificationism and clinical trials [see comments]. *Statistics in Medicine* **10**: 1679–1692. [Comment in *Statistics in Medicine* **11**(9): 1263–1265 (1992)].

Senn SJ (1993a) *Cross-over Trials in Clinical Research*. John Wiley & Sons, Ltd, Chichester.

Senn SJ (1993b) Inherent difficulties with active control equivalence studies. *Statistics in Medicine* **12**: 2367–2375.

Senn SJ (1994) Fisher's game with the devil. *Statistics in Medicine* **13**: 217–230.

Senn SJ (1998) In the blood: proposed new requirements for registering generic drugs. *Lancet* **352**: 85–86.

Senn SJ (2001) Statistical issues in bioequivalence. *Statistics in Medicine* **20**: 2785–2799.

Senn SJ (2002) *Cross-over Trials in Clinical Research* (2nd edition). John Wiley & Sons, Ltd, Chichester.

Senn SJ (2006) Cross-over trials in Statistics in Medicine: the first '25' years. *Statistics in Medicine* **25**: 3430–3442.

Senn SJ, Lillienthal J, Patalano F, Till MD (1997) An incomplete blocks cross-over in asthma: a case study in collaboration. In: Vollmar J, Hothorn LA (eds), *Cross-over Clinical Trials*. Fischer, Stuttgart, pp. 3–26.

Senn SJ, D'Angelo G, Potvin D (2004) Carry-over in cross-over trials in bioequivalence: theoretical concerns and empirical evidence. *Pharmaceutical Statistics* **3**: 133–142.

Senn SJ, D'Angelo G, Potvin D (2005) Rejoinder. *Pharmaceutical Statistics* **4**: 216–219.

Sheiner LB (1992) Bioequivalence revisited. *Statistics in Medicine* **11**: 1777–1788.

Steinijans VW, Hauschke D (1993) International harmonization of regulatory bioequivalence requirements. *Clinical Research and Regulatory Affairs* **10**: 203–220.

Steinijans VW, Hauschke D, Schall R (1995) International harmonization of regulatory bioequivalence requirements for average bioequivalence and current issues in individual bioequivalence. *Drug Information Journal* **29**: 1055–1062.

Wellek S (2002) *Testing Statistical Hypotheses of Equivalence*. Chapman and Hall/CRC, Boca Raton, FL.

Welling PG, Tse FLS, Dighe SV (eds) (1991) *Pharmaceutical Bioequivalence*. Marcel Dekker, New York.

Westlake WJ (1976) Symmetrical confidence intervals for bioequivalence trials. Biometrics, **32**: 741–744.

Westlake WJ (1979) Statistical aspects of comparitive bioavailability trials. Biometrics **35**: 273–280.

Westlake WJ (1981) Response to Kirkwood. *Biometrics*: **37**: 591–593.

23

Safety Data, Harms, Drug Monitoring and Pharmaco-epidemiology

I think it wrong, merely because a man's hat has been blown off his head, by chance, the first night he comes to Avignon – that he should therefore say 'Avignon is more subject to high winds than any town in all France'.

Laurence Sterne, *Tristram Shandy*

Met with Hadley, our Clerke, who upon my asking how the plague goes, he told me it increases much, and much in our parish: 'For', says he, 'there died nine this week, though I have returned but six' – which is a very ill practice and makes me think it is so in other places and therefore the plague much greater than people take it to be.

Samuel Pepys, *Diary, 30 August 1665*

23.1 BACKGROUND

It is a curious fact that whereas the original inspiration for much legislation covering drug development has its origin in concerns about the safety of pharmaceuticals (inspired in some cases by tragedies such as that involving the use of thalidomide by pregnant women in the 1960s), much of the statistical theory of planning clinical trials has to do with investigating efficacy rather than safety. In fact, the general assumption in all of the chapters of this book, apart from this one, has been that efficacy is being investigated.

There are a number of reasons for this. First, in developing a drug, the sponsor has intended benefits of the therapy in mind: the therapeutic need, together with a model of action for the pharmaceutical, are what defined the project in the first place. Thus the scientific focus will be in terms of benefit. Second, although there may be some idea, based on the mechanism of the treatment, what sort of adverse effects might arise, unexpected ones may also occur. It is, of course, difficult to plan for the unexpected. Third, such unexpected events may generally be rare and therefore difficult to detect.

Statistical Issues in Drug Development/2nd Edition   Stephen Senn
© 2007 John Wiley & Sons, Ltd

In this chapter, various statistical issues to do with safety of pharmaceuticals will be addressed. The field is extremely large and not all possible issues will be addressed. Instead, some typical problems will be covered. The subject is extremely important. Safety issues can cause drugs to be abandoned and companies to fail. If there are problems with a drug, then the sooner they are discovered the better. But it is also the case that some drugs have been lost through witch-hunts, and occasionally such persecutions have been justified by fraudulent research. Either way, the moral to the sponsor is 'know your drug'.

Because this chapter is less well served by the introductory chapters in Part 1 than are others in Part 2, various background technical matters will be covered before proceeding to the issues.

Safety is often concerned with establishing the presence or absence of **adverse drug reactions** (ADRs). These, of course, require a judgement of causality, so that, in order not to prejudge the issue, there is often value in initially recording ADEs (**adverse drug experiences** or **events**). The declared ADRs are then a subset of the ADEs. In addition to being able to classify ADEs by their probable relationship to treatment, they can also be classified by severity. Obviously the most severe sort of ADE is a death. Most regulatory agencies require sponsors to notify them of serious ADEs. For example, the FDA requires that for clinical trials conducted under their regulations they, and all participating investigators, shall be informed within 10 working days of any adverse experience which is serious and unexpected and has some reasonable possibility of being caused by the drug (Guess, 2000). (An unexpected ADE is, essentially, one whose nature, severity and frequency is not covered in the basic information provided to investigators.)

ADRs are often classified into two major sorts: so called Type A and Type B reactions. **Type A adverse reactions** are those which may be anticipated from the nature of the treatment (perhaps due to knowledge of class effects or mechanisms of action) and are dose-dependent. **Type B adverse reactions** are those which are unpredictable from background knowledge. They are usually a form of hypersensitivity or immunological reaction peculiar to the individual and may occur even with very small doses. They may be caused by the drug itself or by metabolites. Type B reactions are usually rarer and more serious than type A reactions.

Authors associated with the CONSORT statement on clinical trials (Altman *et al.*, 2001) have recently made ten recommendations as regards the reporting of what they refer to as **harms** (Ioannidis *et al.*, 2004). Indeed, part of the purpose of their recommendations is to promote the use of the term *harm*, or *harms*, since they believe that talk of drug safety gives an unrealistic impression of the inevitable risks associated with pharmaceutical therapy. As they put it, 'We encourage authors to use the term 'harms' instead of 'safety'(p. 781). The definition they offer for this term is

> *Harms*: The totality of possible adverse consequences of an intervention or therapy; they are the direct opposite of benefits, aainst which they must be compared.
>
> (p. 782)

Some of these recommendations are picked up later in this chapter under Issues

Laboratory data obtained in clinical trials may provide further information on safety. Patients have blood and perhaps urine samples measured prior to starting on trial medication, again at the end of the trial, and perhaps on various occasions in between. One of the purposes of such information can be simply to document the general physiological state of the patient at entry and exit of the trial for reasons more directly concerned with monitoring his or her health than with learning about the general effects of the treatment. However, such data can be useful for this latter purpose also. Because patients in different centres may have had such data measured by different laboratories, and because resulting differences from centre to centre may reflect not only differences in populations but also in assays, such data are usually interpreted by referring them to so-called **normal ranges**, specific to the given laboratory. These are sometimes used to construct so-called **shift tables**, which indicate how many patients have moved from being 'normal' to 'abnormal' and vice versa (Chuang-Stein, 1998, 2001).

General **tolerability data** are also commonly collected. For example, because beta-agonists (a class of drugs used in treating asthma) also can have cardiac side-effects, it is not uncommon to measure cardiovascular parameters such as pulse rate, blood pressure and QTc interval in trials of such drugs. Different sorts of tolerability measures tend to be obtained from single-dose and multidose trials. 'Harder', clinical-based measures are more usefully examined using the former and 'therapeutic' symptoms and self-reported measures using the latter.

Because serious ADRs are (one hopes) rare, but because it can be vital to know about even rare serious ADRs, important information about them is often obtained after the drug has been approved (Idanpaan-Heikkila, 1985). For example, usually fewer than 3000 patients will have been exposed to a drug by the time a regulatory dossier is prepared. It may, however, need 10 000 exposures to have a reasonable chance of detecting a rare serious side-effect (Strom, 2000a). Such post-marking surveillance can occur in a number of ways and there are a various different types of study upon which the pharmaco-epidemiologist may rely. First, the basic methodology of the clinical trial can be employed in so-called **phase IV** studies. These are usually much simpler in design and involve more patients than do phase III studies. For example, Glaxo (now GlaxoSmithKline) carried out a parallel-group trial in asthma to compare two of their own products, salbutamol and salmeterol in a study which involved 25 180 patients recruited by 3516 general practitioners and treated over 16 weeks (Castle *et al.*, 1993). At the other end of the scale, another common source of information is spontaneous reporting as provided by prescribing physicians and logged and analysed by the **drug monitoring** department of the sponsor.

The business of monitoring drug use with a view to detecting potential side-effects in order to identify possible harms, especially once drugs are marketed, is sometimes known as **pharmacovigilance** (Evans, 2000).

A form of study much loved of epidemiologists is the so-called **case–control study** (Breslow, 1996). This is a sort of back-to-front clinical trial. The purpose of the clinical trial may be described as being to establish the effects of causes. The case–control study tries to establish the causes of effects (Holland, 1986). This may be explained by an example. When Crane *et al.* (1989) wished to investigate a possible link between fenoterol and deaths among asthmatics in New Zealand, they collected information regarding use of fenoterol for a number of dead asthmatics (the cases). They also collected the same information for a number of non-deceased patients (the controls). The idea was to see whether there were more fenoterol users among the cases than the controls. This sort of study is sometimes referred to as **retrospective**. It should be noted that spontaneous ADE reporting does not lend itself to case–control work. This is because the cases reported to a sponsor will all have taken one of the sponsor's products. What is needed to find and demonstrate an association, however, is not only information on controls but to establish the number of cases which have *not* been exposed to the drug in question. Obviously, these will not be reported as a matter of course to the sponsor. Case–control studies tend to be initiated by sponsors once some other *prima facie* evidence of an association has been provided.

Unlike a clinical trial, a case control study is not **experimental**. The allocation of treatment is not under the control of the investigator. In that sense it is **observational**. Not all observational studies are retrospective, however; they can also be **prospective**. A **cohort study** is such an example. (*Cohort* originally meant the tenth part of a Roman legion, and came to be used by epidemiologists to mean a group of persons moving together through time.) In a cohort study, a number of patients would be followed through time and those taking a drug would be compared to those who did not. Because the investigator does not allocate the treatment (either at random or according to some other rule), this is not an experiment and hence not a clinical trial. Unlike clinical trials, therefore, it becomes crucial to deal with so-called **confounders**, variables which may be associated with the decision of the patient to take a treatment and also with the outcome being measured and which, unless controlled for, may distort the conclusions.

Much of the above discussion has centered on considering aggregates: a number of patients are studied in a clinical trial, or a cohort study or some other study, with the intention of using such numbers to establish causal relationships. In fact, given suitable information about timing, it is *sometimes* possible to assess causality for single cases. Such **single-case causality assessment** is one of the major functions of a drug monitoring department. Four methods are in common use: unstructured clinical judgement, structured decision algorithms, scoring methods, and Bayesian probabilistic assessment (Jones, 2000).

Pharmacovigilance: A game of hunt the thimble, in which you are not sure if it is a thimble you are looking for, you don't want to find it anyway and the only time anyone shouts 'warm' is when you have already burned your fingers.

When it comes to reporting various event rates, various sorts of probability statement are possible. Ordinary rates are meaningless unless referred to a time frame (see *Concerning time* under issues below).Thus, for example, epidemiologists, statisticians and actuaries commonly use death rates per year. Obviously, the figure would be different if quoted per month or per decade. It is important, however, to distinguish between instantaneous rates and rates per elapsed time. For example, there may be a 1 in 1500 chance that a one-hour rock-climb will result in a fatality. If you wish to compare this to other sporting activities there may be some value in expressing the figure as a rate per man-year of rock-climbing. This figure would then be about 6 deaths per man-year. This does not mean, however, that a man who clocked up two month's rock-climbing would be sure to die!

Much investigational work is comparative. For this purpose a **relative risk** is often used. This is the ratio of the probability in a treated group to that in a control group. Thus if P_t is the rate in the treated group and P_c is the rate in the control group and RR is the relative risk, then $RR = P_t/P_c$. This measure makes most sense if the event rate is low. There are often advantages in using **odds ratios** (OR) instead. The odds for the two groups are the ratios of events to 'non-events' and thus equal to $P_t/(1 - P_t)$ and $P_c/(1 - P_c)$ respectively. Their ratio is

$$OR = \left(\frac{P_t}{1 - P_t}\right) \Big/ \left(\frac{P_c}{1 - P_c}\right) = \frac{P_t(1 - P_c)}{P_c(1 - P_t)} \tag{23.1}$$

This ratio has the advantage of not depending arbitrarily on whether 'successes' or 'failures' are the focus of interest (since both the ratio of successes and the ratio of failures are used to calculate it). However, for small values of P_t and P_c, the relative risk is almost identical to it. For statistical modelling, there is often value in working with the logarithm of (23.1), the **log-odds ratio**. This has properties which make it valuable in regression modelling, for example that it can take on any negative or positive value.

The above methods are suitable when all patients have the same time exposure and where only a minority experience the event of interest. Where patients have differing exposures it is not meaningful to compare their experiences unless these have been standardized in some way. Similarly, where most patients suffer the event in question, valuable information is lost by comparing numbers rather than times to event. Actuaries and demographers have long been used to describing the mortality of populations over time based on techniques associated with the **life table** and these have now been adapted and extended by statisticians and epidemiologists. Although originally used for mortality, these techniques can readily be adapted for any unique event, and most events can be defined in a way which makes them unique, so that, for example, we may model time until first seizures in an epilepsy trial or time to first adverse reaction in any trial at all, using techniques originally adapted for mortality. (The theory can also be extended for multiple events.) Traditionally, a life table incorporates mortality information obtained from a population over a given time interval to calculate what would happen to a cohort (generation) of individuals (often assumed to number either 1000 or 100 000) who, if born now, would be subject at each future age of life to the mortality experience of the mixture of generations constituting the (current) population from which the mortality information has been obtained. From the original notional cohort of births, termed the **radix** of the table, the 'survivors' at each age are recorded as well as the intervening deaths. When calculating such a table for a large population, say the population of the United States in a given year, the demographer has an advantage not usually granted the trialist, in that for each age the mortality rates from which the probabilities are calculated will be based on large numbers. In a trial, not only are the numbers small but typically follow-up is limited, so that for many patients we know only that they survived for at least x months (or had no adverse reactions by month x). On the other hand, where a patient has an adverse reaction it may be useful to record the exact number of days on treatment or therapy. Where this mixture of exact and **censored** information is available, probabilities of adverse reaction-free survival can then be calculated using the so-called **Kaplan – Meier estimate** (Kaplan and Meier, 1958).

In describing disease, epidemiologists draw an important distinction between **incidence** and **prevalence**. The former relates to the number of new cases arising in a given time interval, the latter to the frequency (or relative frequency) of cases in the population. If we imagine an unplugged bath into which water is pouring vigorously, then incidence is the water pouring in, prevalence is the water in the bath, and deaths and cures are the waters exiting the plug-hole. For safety reporting in clinical trials, incidence is the more relevant concept and in defining this, time is important. For a thorough treatment of problems that arise in estimating various epidemiological measures of risk, the reader should consult the book in this series by Lui (2004). For coverage of many pharmaco-epidemiological issues, the book edited by Strom is recommended (Strom, 2000b). For a discussion of the role of pharmacovigilance in drug regulation, Evans (2000) is extremely useful.

A key concept in modelling events over time is the so-called **hazard rate**, which is the instantaneous probability of failure given survival to date. Since Cox's seminal paper (Cox, 1972), an enormous amount of developmental work on **survival analysis** in general and in particular on the so-called **proportional hazard** model (sometimes referred to as **Cox regression**) has been carried out and there are now more than forty books on survival analysis as well as at least one journal devoted entirely to it. This topic is extremely important in judging the efficacy of treatments, since in some indications survival is the major endpoint. (Although it is perhaps worth noting that survival analysis is more likely to be used by the medical statistician working in the public or semi-public sector on collaborative trials sponsored by organizations such as the National Institutes of Health in the USA or the Medical Research Council in Britain, than by the biopharmaceutical statistician.) However, such techniques can also be adapted for modelling adverse events, although this is perhaps not done as often as it ought to be (O'Neill, 1995). For a short but excellent introduction to survival analysis see Albert (1995). For more extensive treatment, the book by Marubini and Valsecchi (1995) in this series and that by Collett (2003) can be recommended.

An important demographic technique in comparing death rates is standardization. The most popular such technique is to calculate a **standardized mortality ratio**. This is the ratio of the deaths observed in the study population to those 'expected'. The expected deaths are those which would have been observed given the mortality experience of a standard population and the exposure by age and sex in the study population.

23.2 ISSUES

23.2.1 Formal analyses are irrelevant

It is often argued that formal analyses of safety data are inappropriate, usually because pre-specified hypotheses are not available. This raises the issues of multiplicity and intentions (in designing the experiment) for a frequentist analysis. For a Bayesian analysis the equivalent problem is raised of having to establish prior distributions after the data are in. Neither mode of inference deals well with carrying out 'post-hoc' analyses.

It seems to me highly questionable, however, to say that therefore all formal analyses should be ruled out. In the end some sort of decision may be required and it would be difficult to maintain that the problems which a formal analysis would have to face have gone away by virtue of their being ignored. I tend to the view that, on the contrary, whereas for many well-designed trials a description of the results may be adequate for making a judgement of efficacy, when it comes to analysing safety data it is often the case that only an extremely complex investigation can make any sense of them at all. This is a point of view with which many statisticians would disagree (but see O'Neill (1995, 1998) for the case for complex analysis of such data).

23.2.2   Treatment emergent signs and symptoms (TESS)

A popular way to present adverse events in a clinical trial is in terms of treatment emergent signs and symptoms (Nilsson and Koke, 2001). The idea behind this is that if an adverse event was being experienced by a patient before he or she took the treatment, then it cannot have been caused by the treatment. Thus, in order to compare a treatment with its control in terms of adverse events it is only necessary to record those adverse events which have either arisen since the beginning of the trial or become worse.

There is no question that concentrating on this subset of events will eliminate some which have no connection whatsoever to treatment. Thus, in many cases, by removing this clutter, the comparison will have been sharpened. However, the practice is not without dangers because, as we explained in Chapter 3, a useful way to think about causality is in terms of comparing that which has happened to that which would have happened. Now, it is at least conceivable that a particular problem from which a patient was suffering at the beginning of a trial would have cleared up but for the treatment given. If that is so, then even if the patient is in the same condition at the end of the trial as at the beginning, the adverse event that he or she continues to suffer will have been caused by the treatment.

Suppose, for example we design a clinical trial for a new ACE inhibitor (which is believed not to have the usual problem of giving some patients a cough) to be compared with a standard ACE inhibitor. We recruit to this trial patients currently receiving an ACE inhibitor and with cough. The TESS form of reporting will just lead us to report no events in either group and we shall fail to detect any improvement. However, by simply reporting the number of patients who have a cough at the end of the trial, without the TESS refinement, we would pick this up.

In my opinion TESS makes an inappropriate use of baseline information. If it is desired to use this information, then an alternative approach, which I recommend, is to stratify patients by presence or absence of symptoms at baseline and perform some suitable test, for example the Mantel–Haenszel procedure (Mantel and Haenszel, 1959). The basic situation is illustrated in Table 23.1.

23.2.3   Laboratory shift tables

The objection to reporting laboratory data using so-called shift tables is essentially the objection to dichotomization made in Chapter 8. The original continuous data on laboratory values may contain valuable information which is lost by simply classifying patients according to whether their values have moved from 'normal' to 'abnormal'. There are circumstances, for example, where calculating the mean value for all patients in the treatment group and comparing this to the mean value of the patients in the placebo group would actually give the better means of predicting under what future circumstances a patient would be caused to have an abnormal value.

Table 23.1 Illustration of treatment emergent signs and symptoms (TESS). In the cross-classification by baseline and outcome, patients with TESS number c for the experimental group and g for the control group. Thus c patients with TESS out of n_e on the one hand are compared with g patients out of n_c on the other. A more conventional analysis would compare $a + c$ patients with adverse events in the treatment group with $e + g$ in the control group. A more sophisticated analysis might stratify by baseline state and compare treatment and control using the Mantel–Haenszel procedure.

	Experimental Treatment		
	Outcome		Total
Baseline	Present	Not Present	
Present	a	b	$a + b$
Not Present	c	d	$c + d$
	$a + c$	$b + d$	$n_e = a + b + c + d$

	Control Treatment		
	Outcome		
Baseline	Present	Not Present	
Present	e	f	$e + f$
Not Present	g	h	$g + h$
	$e + g$	$f + h$	$n_c = e + f + g + h$

The practical difficulty in many trials in using raw laboratory values, however, is that various laboratories with different values may have been used. Although this may not quite amount to mixing apples and pears, it may at least be equivalent to mixing Worcesters and Granny Smiths. (More and more trials now are being handled by central laboratories, but this is not always so.) A possible technique for dealing with laboratory data is similar to one proposed by Glass for meta-analysis (Glass, 1976). An effect size of sorts is used, but calculated as the ratio of the actual recorded laboratory value to the width of the normal range, rather than using the observed standard deviation as denominator. This is a unit-free measure which may have better properties. There does not seem to be any general consensus on this issue, however, and the topic remains underdeveloped. However, see Chuang-Stein (1998, 2001) for further discussion.

23.2.4   Controls for cohort studies

As a product moves through phase III and is registered in some countries and is hoped to be registered in others, it is often the case that deaths start to accrue in important numbers. Often this information is of fairly high quality (compared with that which will come later) in that it is collected through studies with a proper protocol, but it is also often the case that information of a comparable quality on control patients is not available. For example, the studies concerned may be open-label long-term follow-up studies to randomized phase III trials. That is to say, patients who were originally randomized to either the experimental treatment or its control are all given the chance to try the experimental treatment in the follow-up. For example, in asthma many long-term randomized trials are of 3 months' duration and the open follow-up may last an additional year. If most patients agree to continue or to be switched to the experimental treatment at the end of the double-blind phase, then the information obtained in the follow-up relates to almost eight times the exposure (double the patients for four times as long) in the randomized trial.

Given enough exposure, deaths are inevitable. For example, if 1000 potato eaters chosen at random from the general population are followed for a year, it is quite likely that at least 10 will die. This does not mean that eating potatoes is dangerous. The challenge for any sponsor is to have the means in place of predicting what numbers of deaths would be seen in the ongoing studies given the amount of exposure.

There are two key elements to this. The first is to have accurate information by age and sex (and perhaps other relevant prognostic factors) of the total amount of exposure to treatment: so many 30–34-year-old women treated for six months, so many 70–74-year-old men treated for one year, and so forth. Given a good enough database, exact information can be obtained. The second is more difficult and that is to have mortality rates by age and sex for a suitable control population which, ideally, should be as similar to the treated population as possible.

In a sense, this is a technical matter and there is no disagreement among statisticians that information from such a control population is desirable. It may be considered, therefore, that its inclusion as a statistical issue in this book is inappropriate. It is included for the following reason. Recognizing that identification of an ideal control population is not possible, there is a tendency to do nothing at all. However, in my view, a sponsor is under an obligation to give this matter some thought. In many cases it will be a better policy to calculate an expected number of deaths from a 'standard' population (or set of standard populations), even though there may be many reasons why the population of patients will differ. (For many diseases life expectancy of patients will be lower than for the general population, but in some chronic diseases it is even conceivable that due to the entry criteria of clinical trials, there may be a 'healthy patient' effect.) The industry as a whole could also do more by collaborating to set up databases based on jointly funded cohort studies for given diseases in order to establish appropriate standard populations. (This need is met to some degree by commercial organizations who set up databases based on surveys of drug use and sell the information to the pharmaceutical industry.)

In fact, a similar recommendation regarding safety databases was made be the Royal Statistical Society (RSS) working party on first-in-human studies that I chaired and which reported in March 2007. This suggested that one of the problems in assessing the risk to healthy volunteers in entering first-in-human studies was that data regarding adverse events were not being collected in a coordinated way to cover the whole pharmaceutical industry. The RSS working party recommendation was that data collection should be coordinated by the regulators.

23.2.5   Reporting rates

Ideally the sponsor would include, in what used to be called in the company I worked for at one time the *basic drug information* (BDI), a list of all adverse *reactions* with the probability of their occurrence (as a function of some exposure) in such a way that this information was immediately relevant to the decisions to be made by a potential prescribing physician or her patient. There are various reasons why this is difficult, if not impossible. To know that an adverse event is an adverse reaction requires an unequivocal assessment of causality. Such assessment is rarely forthcoming. Causality may be established indirectly in a clinical trial by noting an excess of a given type of adverse event in the treated group compared with the control. The excess (given the usual qualifications regarding chance variation and so forth) may then be ascribed to the drug. This, however, would require reporting in the BDI not only ADEs under the treatment but also under the control. This is, indeed, sometimes done but may, in turn, raise further difficulties because controls are only controls within the context of the given trial, yet what is needed is a summary across all trials. Some of these may be uncontrolled, different controls may have been used in different trials, the trials will have been of differing durations and so forth. This makes the provision of a simple summary extremely difficult.

A further problem has to do with the nature of clinical trials. As has been explained elsewhere, these are comparative rather than representative and one of the tasks for analysis is to find a scale of measurement upon which the treatment effect is additive. If this can be found for adverse events, then even for quite different populations it may be applicable. Unfortunately, the sort of measure which, *a priori* at least is most likely to be additive is the log-odds scale and this is not easy for the amateur to interpret. The question then arises whether, in order to increase interpretability, the raw rates should be used, although possibly not applicable where we wish to apply them. This issue was also discussed in Chapter 8.

Nevertheless, despite the inherent difficulties involved in reporting rates of adverse events or harms, there is no question that this could generally be done better in clinical trials. The additional CONSORT recommendation on harms (Ioannidis *et al.*, 2004) referred to above includes the following amongst its list of recommendations:

> *Recommendation 7.* Provide the denominators for analyses on harms.
> *Recommendation 8.* Present the absolute risk of each adverse event (specifying type, grade, and seriousness per arm), and present appropriate metrics for recurrent events, continuous variables and scale variables, whenever pertinent.

23.2.6   Concerning time

For many years now, Robert O'Neill of the FDA has drawn attention to the subtle relationship between time and the pattern of reporting of ADEs and the inadequate way in which sponsors often summarize such occurrence in clinical trials (O'Neill, 1995, 1998). As already mentioned, a key concept in describing rates over time is the hazard rate. This can be explained with an example. Imagine that we roll a fair die until we first obtain a 6, at which point we stop. On any roll of the die, the probability of stopping, given that we have not stopped to date, is the hazard rate, and this is clearly equal to $\frac{1}{6}$. Apart from the first roll however, the probability of stopping at a given roll is not equal to $\frac{1}{6}$. For example, we shall only stop on the second roll if we do not stop on the first, so that the probability of stopping then is $\frac{5}{6} \times \frac{1}{6}$ In general the probability of stopping on the ith roll is $p(i) = \left(\frac{5}{6}\right)^{i-1}\left(\frac{1}{6}\right)$ and this failure probability declines all the time, whereas the hazard rate, $h(i)$ is constant. This may seem paradoxical but it simply reflects the trivial fact that once we have obtained our first 6 we can no longer obtain our first 6. The distribution, which describes the number of trials until the first failure (or success) is known as the **geometric distribution**. Its continuous time equivalent is the **exponential distribution** and for this we would define a **probability** density $f(t)$ as a function of continuous time t. Thus if the hazard rate of an adverse event is constant for a patient, then the probability density function $f(t)$ of the first adverse event over time for that patient is given by the exponential distribution. Also of interest are the survivor distribution, $S(t)$, the probability that the patient will be free of adverse events until a given moment, and the cumulative probability density function, $F(t) = 1 - S(t)$. These four functions are plotted in Figure 23.1 for a patient with a hazard rate of one per week.

Of course, the hazard rate does not have to be constant. It may be, for example, that the risk is dose related. This may mean that the patient is at greatest hazard when the treatment reaches steady state. This will usually happen after a few doses have been taken. Another possibility is that some relatively unimportant (in terms of quantity) but slowly accumulating metabolite may be the difficulty. This may then cause difficulties after a treatment has been taken for some time. Figure 23.2 illustrates the same four functions for a linearly increasing hazard rate. Note, that although the hazard rate increases steadily, the probability density does not. For this example the greatest number of cases would occur at 2 weeks, although the hazard would continue to increase thereafter. This is simply because most patients who were going to have an ADR would already have had one. The ones that remain are at increasing risk but there are fewer of them left. Of course, both of the examples are extreme. Except perhaps in cancer therapy, no drug would get to phase three with this sort of rate of ADRs.

Another case might be more complex. It could be possible, for example, that a minority of patients cannot tolerate the drug, but that the rest are at fairly constant but extremely low risk. This is perhaps about the only example where it is reasonable to report ADEs as a rate per patient only and without quoting time, for the reasons that if a patient is susceptible this susceptibility will be manifested whatever the length of the trial. In general, however, reporting the rates of ADEs without specifying the time scale is not meaningful. Even where the hazard rate is constant it is not appropriate to lump one-week, one-month, three-month and one-year studies together.

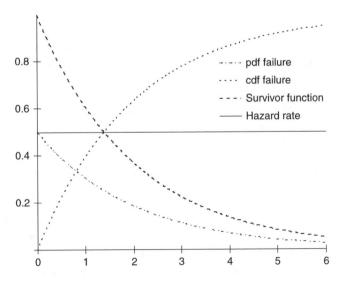

Figure 23.1 Various functions plotted against time for the case of a constant hazard rate for ADRs.

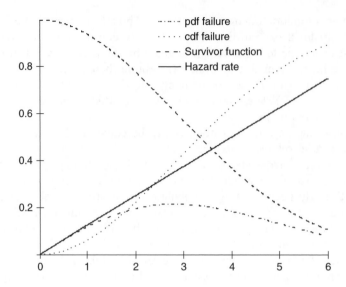

Figure 23.2 Various functions plotted against time for the case of an increasing hazard rate for ADRs.

This does not mean that the solutions are easy. Frequently tabular presentation will fail to capture the essence of what is going on and will have the potential to mislead. One may claim, indeed, that this is a problem which clearly shows that when describing safety issues descriptive statistics are often not enough. More complex methods, in this case those of survival analysis, may be needed. See Sünder and Peters (1994) for a discussion of some relevant issues.

23.2.7   Concerning numerators: under-reporting

The chapter quote from Pepys's diary shows that under-reporting of unpleasant medical events has been around for a long time. If our object in recording events is hypothesis testing, and if we stick to controlled experiments such as the clinical trial (in particular if they are double-blind), then this particular issue may not be so serious. We shall suffer some loss of power to detect adverse events, but where we find an important and significant difference, then it will usually be reasonable to conclude that this difference could not have occurred as a result of differential reporting rates alone but must reflect some genuine difference between treatments. (Of course, our estimate of the true difference will, on average, be too low.)

For spontaneous reporting of adverse events, however, the matter is quite different. Here any assessment of incidence is fraught with difficulty, since not only do we need some measure of exposure (see below) but we must make some sort of an assumption regarding reporting rates. This can work both ways as regards interpretation of results. For example, under-reporting can only lead to an underestimate of the rate of adverse events. Not all adverse events, however, are adverse reactions. Although some attempts may be made to establish whether an event is a reaction on the basis of the information attending it (see below) one basis upon which causality will be assessed in general is by comparison with what is known about other drugs. It is conceivable, however, that physician and patient awareness may be heightened with a new drug so that that there may be less under-reporting than for an established treatment. This can lead to difficulties in making comparisons.

23.2.8   Concerning numerators: patients or events

A serious ADE will often lead to the patient being withdrawn from the trial. (Almost invariably so if confirmed as a serious ADR.) For minor (presumed) side-effects this may not be the case and thus sometimes a number of these will be collected for one patient. The issues then arise in a clinical trial whether one should concentrate on the number of patients showing at least one side-effect or simply count the number of side-effects. (The former is, of course, less than or equal to the latter.)

The advantage in counting patients rather than side-effects is that the issue of non-independence is finessed. Two patients suffering one side-effect is generally more convincing evidence of a problem with a drug than one patient suffering the same side-effect twice. Conventional standard statistical analyses assume independence of the observations and cannot be used to analyse side-effects.

The argument against simply using patients is that some information is being thrown away. Ideally, a random-effects model would be applied and this would be able to take account of the repeated-measures nature of the data. In practice this hardly ever seems to be done.

23.2.9   Concerning denominators

A difficulty with making any sense at all of spontaneous reports of adverse events is to establish a denominator: the number of patients at risk and the time and dose for which they have been exposed. It is usually the case that only extremely crude estimates of this can be gained from sales figures. There are a number of reasons why these are not very good for calculating exposure. One problem is that the sort of time when it becomes most important to monitor the use of a drug is during the launch period. This is a time when sales are likely to rise rapidly, and not only may it take some time for accurate figures to come in but also it will be necessary to establish the appropriate time lag to be used when comparing events to sales. A further difficulty is that in many cases the dose on which a patient is put is independent of the unit dose (for example, a double dosage may simply involve twice as many pills per day of the same strength). Thus, for the purpose of investigating dose–response relationships (which are important for type A reactions), sales data are of little use.

There are certain commercial databases to which sponsors may turn, but these are also not without problems. One difficulty is that they may be limited in terms of markets and periods to which they apply so that they may not be relevant for all the ADEs which the sponsor has collected. The choice must then be made between disregarding certain ADEs when calculating the numerator or finding some way to scale up the denominator. However, see also sections 23.2.10 and 23.2.14 below.

23.2.10   Dose-response

My former colleague, Franco Spinelli, is an enthusiastic proponent of a method of analysing dose-response of ADEs that is rather similar to the case–control study. This is to calculate, for each dose, the ratio of a particular ADE which was suspected to be potentially dose-related to all other ADEs (or some suitable subset of other ADEs). The idea is that these can be taken as an index of usage of the various doses.

A number of criticisms can be made of this approach. First, it depends on the assumption that the ratio of the reporting rate for the ADE of interest to the rate for all other ADEs is the same at all doses. Second, a dose relationship may be indicative of such a relationship for other ADEs rather than in the category of interest. Third, it cannot be used to establish absolute risks.

All these criticisms are valid, but that does not mean that the method is without interest. For example, as regards the first criticism, any study of the effect of dose on ADEs, even a study using perfectly accurate population denominators, requires an assumption regarding reporting rates. As regards the second criticism, unless ADEs can show an inverse relationship with dose, then the method can only be conservative. Hence, there will usually be reasons for believing that a strong observed relationship is genuine. The third criticism is the most important, but, of course, any method which wishes to establish absolute risks would (among other requirements) need 100% reporting rates (or at least knowledge of what the rates were) and in practice these conditions will not obtain.

O'Neill (1995) draws attention to some difficulties in establishing dose relationship for ADEs, even where we have data from clinical trials. One problem is that dose as prescribed is not the same as dose as taken. (Of course, if we were to take an 'intention to treat' stand on the issue we would say that we are only interested in dose as prescribed.) For many drugs the peak plasma levels obtained will be most associated with ADEs rather than mean levels. This is clearly an issue where patients omit treatment and then make up the deficit by taking double doses. How serious this is depends on many factors. For example, if dosing is at half-life intervals, then the plasma concentration may be presumed to vary between that produced by one single unit dose (at foot-point) and two unit doses (just after treatment). Presumably the two-unit level will be safe as a single dose, or this regimen would not have been chosen. Omission of one dose reduces plasma concentration to half a unit dose and taking of a double dose raises it to two and a half. For many drugs this would not be serious. But of course more extreme patterns of patient behaviour are possible.

Another issue is what constitutes a given dose exposure. Is it unit dose, area under the curve achieved or total dosage taken? The last would not usually be a sensible measure of dosage as regards efficacy, although for antibiotics it might be, and one could conceive of cases, where the disease is acute and where accumulation of a metabolite is the problem, in which it could be relevant for side-effects.

23.2.11 Single-case causality assessment

It is an important duty of safety monitors working for a sponsor to make some sort of assessment of causal relationship between ADEs and treatment. Often a preliminary assessment has been made by the reporting physician. In the past such assessment was made by skilled judgement on the part of the physician and/or monitor. There has been some interesting work on applying Bayesian quantitative methods in order to provide numerical assessments of the probability that an ADE is really an ADR (Cowell *et al.*, 1993; Hutchinson *et al.*, 1991a,b). Such single-case causality assessment is, in fact, concerned with the causes-of-effects question rather than the effects-of-causes question. See section 23.2.15 for a discussion.

An issue that arises is how we should use such assessments and, in particular, how we should treat them in aggregate. Suppose that in a paediatric clinical trial in asthma comparing a beta-agonist with a placebo, a mother reports to a physician that her child wet his bed. If this is an isolated case the physician might well record 'probably unrelated to treatment'. Suppose, however, that this is a multicentre trial and that almost every physician can report one or two such cases and that hardly any of them are children who have been given placebo. We should then most probably disregard the individual assessments and conclude that this was, indeed, a side-effect of the drug. (And we might search for reasons. Perhaps the children sleep more deeply with the new treatment.) Suppose, on the other hand, that we are running a placebo-controlled trial in hypertension of a new ACE inhibitor. Since they expect this side-effect, physicians may record any case of cough as 'probably related to treatment'. However, if on decoding the results at the end we find that there are just as many of these cases of cough where placebo was being given as cases where the ACE inhibitor was given, we would tend to conclude that, after all, there was no relationship between treatment and this side-effect.

This seems to suggest that given high-quality information from a controlled clinical trial, we would usually disregard individual case assessment and that also we are likely to want to use the information from aggregates to re-assess judgements of causality on individuals. But this raises the issue whether this individual causal assessment is of any use in global assessment. Provided the assessments have been made by physicians blind to the treatment, then an obvious use to make of the data in a frequentist analysis is to code side-effects as an ordered categorical variable with levels 'unrelated', 'doubtful', 'possible', 'probable' and 'definite', or some such other scale. This may add a small amount of discriminatory power to simply recording the number of ADEs.

No doubt a better use could be made in a Bayesian approach, but there is a problem which is similar to the 'date of information problem' raised for meta-analysis. It is important to distinguish between a causal assessment as evidence and a causal assessment as judgement. The latter would depend on what else is known about the effect of the drug in other cases. In an open trial we might, for example, code the first bed-wetting case as doubtful but wish to re-code it, once we have 20 more, as probable. But this simply reflects that our 'posterior distribution' has changed in the meantime due to the addition of other evidence not directly related to this case. The evidential value of the case is, presumably, given by the likelihood ratio for the case itself, and this has not changed. There are various further complications to do with random effects and global and individual judgements which are too complicated to enter into here.

Yet another issue has to do with what we mean when we say that a drug 'caused' a side-effect. Suppose that a given hypertensive patient may safely take beta-blockers most of the year but is in danger of suffering severe bronchospasm if they are taken during the hay-fever season and that this sort of side-effect can occur for this patient with almost any beta-blocker. (I am just speculating that this is possible.) Suppose that in January and February he takes beta-blocker *oldanolol* dispensed by pharmacy A, in March and April, takes beta-blocker *neweranolol* dispensed by pharmacy A, and in May and June takes essentially identical neweranolol (produced by the same manufacturer) but dispensed by pharmacy B. On Friday 13 June the pollen count reaches a record high and the patient has a severe asthma attack. Now, one might say, of course, that the pollen caused the attack or that neweranolol caused the attack or that both together caused the attack. But which pharmacy was responsible for providing the dangerous medicine? Obviously not pharmacy A. One might say that it makes no sense whatsoever to attach any causal role to pharmacy B, since exactly the same would have happened had the patient continued to receive neweranol from pharmacy A. But by the same token one could take the argument further and say that it makes no sense to assign a causal role to neweranol since the attack would have happened with oldanolol anyway. One way out of this is to say that what is really relevant is the consequence of choices. It is more important to know what increased risk, if any, one runs by taking one treatment rather than another (if one must be taken) than to know what side-effects the treatment can cause.

23.2.12   Risk–benefit analysis

Most drugs have some side-effects and are not universally effective. An important task in evaluating whether, and under what circumstances, a drug should be licensed, is to weigh up the risk and benefit. This will, in fact, not be the same for all patients under all circumstances and, indeed, this is something which is explicitly taken account of in 'evidence-based medicine'.

An example may help. Suppose that it is the case that a particular modern antacid drug, say an H_2-agonist, will prove effective in 90% of ulcer cases but have an undesirable cardiac side-effect in 1% of the cases. Suppose, in fact, that 20% of all cases would show a spontaneous improvement. We may then argue that of 100 patients treated, 70 will receive a benefit they would not have had and one will have some harm as a result of treatment. Depending on the seriousness of this harm, this might make it an attractive proposition for treating someone with a diagnosed stomach ulcer. Suppose, however, that it is equally effective in prevention of ulcers and suppose that we believe that 5% of all patients suffering from osteoarthritis who are treated with a particular nonsteroidal anti-inflammatory drug (NSAID) will develop an ulcer unless preventive measures are taken. If we give all of these patients the H_2-agonist we shall expect to prevent 4 to 5 cases of ulcer per 100 treated patients at the expense of one cardiac side-effect. This is a much less attractive proposition.

This particular topic has the capacity to get the pharmaceutical industry into serious difficulties with consumer groups. It is not always appreciated that it could be quite logical to license a drug in some countries but not in others. All therapy has the potential to be harmful. Whether the benefit outweighs the risk depends on what might be termed the geographical-demographic context of the disease. A common model used in evidence-based medicine assumes that the benefit depends on the level of background risk but that side-effect probabilities are similar for most individuals. (An excellent discussion of this model and the issues is given by Glasziou and Irwig (1995).) For example, a treatment for malaria may have some side-effects, but malaria is an extremely unpleasant disease. Whether it is logical to take antimalarial tablets depends on what the risk is of an unprotected person developing malaria. There is no single simple answer to this question.

This does not mean, however, that the industry may wash its hands of the issue. On the contrary, it just goes to show that in order to prescribe medicines rationally, calculation and yet more calculation is needed. With the growth in demand for information, the increase through on-line databases and sophisticated statistical software of the means to supply it, and the modern development of evidence-based medicine (Sackett *et al.*, 2000) we can confidently predict that this topic will become more important.

23.2.13   The case series approach

In a series of papers, Paddy Farrington and co-workers have developed methodology for judging causal relationships by using the timing of adverse events relative to exposure (Farrington *et al.*, 1996; Farrington and Whitaker, 2006). This method uses cases only, which act as their own controls. Essentially, the idea is that there are certain periods in which events occur that are more indicative of causality than others. Most obviously, if an event occurs before exposure it cannot have been caused by it. A discussion of these highly technical papers will not be attempted here, but there is a close relationship to Bayesian causality approaches discussed in section 23.2.11. Other papers in which methods using the timing of events have played a key role include Feldmann (1993) and Maclure (1991); see also Glasziou *et al.* (2007).

One genuine issue with these methods is that they do not use information from controls that may be available and it is a moot point how such information could usefully be combined (Senn, 2006). Nevertheless, this is an extremely important development in epidemiology with no doubt many potential applications in assessing the safety or otherwise of medicines.

23.2.14   Data-mining in pharmacovigilence

An important paper by William DuMouchel considers data-mining of large frequency tables (DuMouchel, 1999). A particular application that he describes in detail is that of analysing the FDA's spontaneous reporting system. (Similar data sets are produced by other agencies. For example the UK system is called ADROIT, which stands for Adverse Drug On-line Information and Tracking System.) Data produced in this way can be regarded (conceptually at least) as consisting of series of frequencies stored in a large contingency table with rows (say) indexing treatments and columns (say) indexing adverse events. Many of the cells defined by such a cross-classification will be empty, but some will contain hundreds of observations. At the time of his paper (1999) DuMouchel was analysing 1398 drugs and 952 types of adverse event, leading to a table with $1398 \times 952 = 1\,330\,896$. (A further complication was that he had the data further classified by six reporting periods and three sexes of patient: male, female and unknown. This will be ignored in what follows.)

An inherent deficiency of such data is that they consist of numerators without denominators: there is no information on the number of patients taking the treatmements. This is the problem to which we drew attention in Section 23.2.9 and the solution here is similar to that in section 23.2.10, which is that whereas it is not possible to use such tables to establish absolute risk they may be used to examine drug and side-effect associations.

The first step is to calculate the 'expected' number of side-effects for each cell. If we denote the number of observations for treatment i and side-effect j as N_{ij} then (ignoring various possible complications) one might calculate the expected cell frequencies as

$$E_{ij} = \frac{N_{i.}N_{.j}}{N_{ij}}, \tag{23.2}$$

where $N_{i.} = \sum_j N_{ij}$ and $N_{.j} = \sum_i N_{ij}$.

Having established expected values for the cells, the next task is to identify those cells for which the observed frequencies are relevantly larger. Du Mouchel considers three possible general approaches: relative reporting rate, statistical significance and empirical Bayes. We shall consider these in turn. In the discussion that follows shall refer to adverse reactions as reactions.

The relative reporting rate for drug i and reaction j is defined as

$$RR_{ij} = \frac{N_{ij}}{E_{ij}}. \tag{23.3}$$

In his interesting article on pharmacovigilance, Stephen Evans describes a closely related measure, that of the proportional reporting ratio (PRR). In order to understand the relationship between the two, it will be helpful to look at expression (23.4):

$$\begin{array}{ccc} a & b & N_{i.} \\ c & d & N_{i'.} \\ N_{.j} & N_{.j'} & N_{..} \end{array} \tag{23.4}$$

Here, we assume that the contingency table has been sorted so that the particular cell representing the drug/reaction combination we are interested in appears in the top left-hand corner. All other cells in the original table have been collapsed and their frequencies totalled. Thus b is the total other reactions to drug i and c is the total of reactions of type j to drugs other than drug i. Finally, d is the total number of reactions involving neither drug i nor reaction j. The PRR is then defined as

$$PRR = \left(\frac{a}{a+b}\right) \bigg/ \left(\frac{c}{c+d}\right). \tag{23.5}$$

By substituting (23.2) in (23.3) and then using (23.4), we can redefine the RR as

$$RR = \left(\frac{a}{a+b}\right) \bigg/ \left(\frac{a+c}{a+b+c+d}\right). \tag{23.6}$$

However, the numerators of (23.5) and (23.6) are identical, and with a very large number of drugs we can expect that a and b will be small compared to c and d so that these two measures will be fairly similar.

Both the RR and PRR suffer from the fact that there is no adjustment for random variation, so that if numbers of events are small it is possible that they could be large just by chance. At the other extreme we have statistical significance measures. One example is what one might call the Poisson Z-score (PZ), commonly used in epidemiology. To calculate this we assume the null-hypothesis that $E[N_{ij}] = E_{ij}$; then under plausible assumptions, N_{ij} is approximately distributed as a Poisson variable. (Or at least it may plausibly be assumed to have at least the variability of a Poisson distribution.) That being so, the variance of N_{ij} will be E_{ij} and we can calculate

$$PZ = \frac{N_{ij} - E_{ij}}{\sqrt{E_{ij}}}. \tag{23.7}$$

Note that this treats E_{ij} as known and, among other matter, ignores some slight but in practice unimportant dependence of E_{ij} on N_{ij}. Many other measures of this sort are possible.

Measures like (23.7) suffer from the disadvantage that where the expected number of events is large, statistical significance can occur without there being much excess risk. Furthermore, since such spontaneous reporting systems are subject to various biases, the fear may be that all that has been detected is a reporting bias.

A third sort of measure is the empirical Bayes estimate. Here we assume that each N_{ij} is drawn from Poisson distribution with mean μ_{ij}. We are really interested in

$$\lambda_{ij} = \mu_{ij} / E_{ij}, \tag{23.8}$$

that is to say the ratio of 'true' mean to expected under the null rather than the ratio of observed to expected given by (23.3). However, if we had to estimate each μ_{ij} independently with no other information, nothing would be gained since we should simply substitute N_{ij} for μ_{ij} and we should be back to square one. It is here that the empirical Bayes approach makes a difference. We assume that the λ_{ij} are drawn from some hyperdistribution whose parameters we have to estimate. The trick is to choose one that, in addition to defining a distribution on a suitable scale (0 to ∞), is sufficiently flexible to be realistic (that is to say, with enough adjustable parameters) but not so flexible that shrinkage does not occur. DuMouchel discusses this approach in great detail.

This strikes me as being a very attractive approach. Of course it inherits all the problems of a spontaneous reporting system and really suffers *a fortiori* from the difficulties of case–control studies. For example, if a drug leads to equally elevated risks of all types of side-effects it will not be detected. This is analogous to the well-known problem of underestimating odds ratios in case–control studies when over-control occurs. For example, in the famous study of smoking in lung cancer by Doll and Hill, hospital controls for the lung cancer cases were chosen. We now know that smoking causes many illnesses apart from lung cancer and so smokers would be over-represented in the control compared to a healthy population, leading to an underestimate of the odds ratio.

However, this is not a reason for not analysing such data and this is an intelligent approach. Stephen Evans has described another attractive approach (Evans, 2000). This is to produce a bivariate plot in which each combination of drug and reaction is represented using one coordinate representing the PRR and another a standardized measure such as (23.7). (In fact, Evans uses a chi-square but the square of (23.7) will be approximately distributed as a chi-square with one degree of freedom.)

23.2.15 Causes of effects or effects of causes

In an important paper, Paul Holland drew attention to two different types of causal question (Holland, 1986). (See section 23.1.) In the first we consider what will happen if we make an intervention. We examine what the effect will be of a (putative) cause. In the second sort of question, we have observed an outcome and consider what the causal explanation of this outcome might be. We attempt to establish what the cause was of an observed effect.

The temporal logic of these two questions matches that of the clinical trial (or cohort study) on the one hand and the case – control study on the other. In the clinical trial we manipulate the conditions and observe the effects. In the cohort study no manipulation is involved, but the logic is the same. In the cohort study, on the other hand, sampling is by outcome (effects) and one then tries to work out the possible causes by comparing groups (cases and controls) that differ in terms of effects.

The causes-of-effects question is typically what a legal trial involving so-called toxic torts seeks to establish (Loue, 2000). A particular patient has had a side-effect and her lawyer will attempt to prove that the pharmaceutical she took caused it.

It is debatable, however, whether the causes-of-effect question ought to have any influence on the way we regard medicines. Particularly pernicious is the fact that in the legal setting it is often combined with a balance-of-probabilities argument, that is to say, it is sufficient to prove that it was more probable than not that the drug caused the side-effect but the damages awarded are not discounted to take the probability into account.

Suppose, for example, that a treatment for hypertension prevents 100 strokes per 1000 patient years of use in a particular population but causes one case of hypotensive stroke (Hankey and Gubbay, 1987). Suppose, furthermore, that where this happens it will be possible to establish this with high probability. In that case the manufacturer will face a regular series of successful suits despite the fact that the treatment has a considerable net beneficial effect. Of course, the patients who would have had a stroke but did not won't be identified. However, it might still be rational for any patient with hypertension to take the medicine (assuming that even better therapy was not available.) In short, it seems from the practical point of view that what should be considered is the effects of causes, and in his paper Holland described this as being the more important question generally (Holland, 1986).

23.2.16   First-in-human studies

An important step in investigating safety of any pharmaceutical is its first use in humans. Obviously this will have been preceded by background preclinical work including, but not restricted to, studies in animals. The dramatic events of 13 March 2006 in which, out of eight healthy volunteers involved in a placebo-controlled trial of TGN1412 at Parexel's clinical trial unit at Northwick Park Hospital, the six who had been given the active treatment suffered extremely serious rapidly developing side-effects with, in some cases, long-term consequences for their health, have caused such trials to come under extreme scrutiny. The Royal Statistical Society set up a working party to make recommendations regarding the conduct of such trial and this reported one year later on 12 March 2007 (Working Party on Statistical Issues in First-in-Man Studies, 2007).

The report made 21 recommendations regarding such trials, which it would be pointless to repeat here. However, some brief discussion of issues can be attempted. The first is that it was established that there was no global, easily interrogated central database recording serious adverse reactions in first in human studies. The recommendation was that regulatory agencies should facilitate the exchange of information between sponsors by maintaining such a database.

Much of the report dealt with the design of such studies and in particular the sequencing of treatments and the allocation of subjects to treatment and control. The issue is that of **veiled studies** discussed in Chapter 6. Of course, with such rapidly developing rare side-effects one does not need a control group to establish causality. This does not mean, however, that design should not be taken seriously since, when such trials proceed to planned conclusion, such serious events do not occur and, indeed, they are only to be contemplated if the probability of such events is rare.

A further recommendation was that prior to beginning first-in-human studies a document should be prepared outlining in some detail an assessment of risk based on preclinical studies and other general background information and that this should be available to all parties concerned: treating physicians, insurers, regulators and, of course human subjects.

References

Albert A (1995) Survival data analysis in clinical research. *Biocybernetics and Biomedical Engineering* **15**: 189–202.

Altman DG, Schulz KF, Moher D, *et al.* (2001) The revised CONSORT statement for reporting randomized trials: explanation and elaboration. *Annals of Internal Medicine* **134**: 663–694.

Breslow NE (1996) Statistics in epidemiology: the case – control study. *Journal of the American Statistical Association* **91**: 14–28.

Castle W, Fuller R, Hall J, Palmer J (1993) Serevent Nationwide Surveillance Study – comparison of salmeterol with salbutamol in asthmatic patients who require regular bronchodilator treatment. *British Medical Journal* **306**: 1034–1037.

Chuang-Stein C (1998) Laboratory data in clinical trials: a statistician's perspective. *Controlled Clinical Trials* **19**: 167–177.

Chuang-Stein C (2001) Some issues concerning the normalization of laboratory data based on reference ranges. *Drug Information Journal* **35**: 153–156.

Collett D (2003) *Modelling Survival Data in Medical Research.* Chapman & Hall/CRC, Boca Raton, FL.

Cowell RG, Dawid AP, Hutchinson TA, Roden S, Spiegelhalter DJ (1993) Bayesian networks for the analysis of drug safety. *Statistician* **42**: 369–384.

Cox DR (1972) Regression models and life-tables (with discussion). *Journal of the Royal Statistical Society Series B* **34**: 187–220.

Crane J, Pearce N, Flatt A, *et al.* (1989) Prescribed fenoterol and death from asthma in New Zealand, 1981–83 – case – control study. *Lancet* **1**: 917–922.

DuMouchel W (1999) Bayesian data mining in large frequency tables, with an application to the FDA spontaneous reporting system. *American Statistician* **53**: 177–190.

Evans SJ (2000) Pharmacovigilance: a science or fielding emergencies? *Statistics in Medicine* **19**: 3199–3209.

Farrington CP, Nash J, Miller E (1996) Case series analysis of adverse reactions to vaccines: a comparative evaluation. *American Journal of Epidemiology* **143**: 1165–1173.

Farrington CP, Whitaker HJ (2006) Semiparametric analysis of case series data (with discussion). *Journal of the Royal Statistical Society Series C – Applied Statistics* **55**: 1–28.

Feldmann U (1993) Epidemiologic assessment of risks of adverse reactions associated with intermittent exposure. *Biometrics* **49**: 419–428.

Glass GE (1976) Primary, secondary and meta-analysis of research. *Educational Research* **5**: 3–8.

Glasziou PP, Irwig LM (1995) An evidence based approach to individualising treatment. *British Medical Journal* **311**: 1356–1359.

Glasziou P, Chalmers I, Rawlins M, McCulloch P (2007) When are randomised trials unnecessary? Picking signal from noise. *British Medical Journal* **334**: 349–351.

Guess HA (2000) Premarketing applications of pharmacoepidemiology. In: Strom BL (ed.), *Pharmacoepidemiology*. John Wiley and Sons, Inc., Hoboken, pp. 391–400.

Hankey GJ, Gubbay SS (1987) Focal cerebral ischaemia and infarction due to antihypertensive therapy. *Med J Aust* **146**: 412–414.

Holland PW (1986) Statistics and causal inference. *Journal of the American Statistical Association* **81**: 945–960.

Hutchinson TA, Dawid AP, Spiegelhalter D, Cowell RG, Roden S (1991a) Computerized aids for probabilistic assessment of drug safety I; a spreadsheet program. *Drug Information Journal* **25**: 29–30.

Hutchinson TA, Dawid AP, Spiegelhalter D, Cowell RG, Roden S (1991b) Computerized aids for probabilistic assessment of drug safety II: an expert system. *Drug Information Journal* **25**: 41–48.

Idanpaan-Heikkila JE (1985) Adverse reactions. In: Burley D, Binns TB (eds), *Pharmaceutical Medicine*. Edward Arnold, London.

Ioannidis JPA, Evans SJW, Gotzsche PC, *et al.* (2004) Better reporting of harms in randomized trials: an extension of the CONSORT statement. *Annals of Internal Medicine* **141**: 781–788.

Jones JK (2000) Determining causation from case reports. In: Strom BL (ed.), *Pharmacoepidemiology*. John Wiley & Sons, Inc., New York, pp. 557–570.

Kaplan EL, Meier P (1958) Non parametric estimation from incomplete observations. *Journal of the American Statistical Association* **53**: 457–481.

Loue S (2000) Epidemiological causation in the legal context: substance and procedures. In: Gastwirth JL (ed.), *Statistical Science in the Courtroom*. Springer, New York, pp. 4430–4387, 98997–98998.

Lui K-J (2004) *Statistical Estimation of Epidemiological Risk*. John Wiley & Sons, Inc., Hoboken.

Maclure M (1991) The case-crossover design: a method for studying transient effects on the risk of acute events. *Am J Epidemiol* **133**: 144–153.

Mantel N, Haenszel W (1959) Statistical aspect of the analysis of data from retrospective studies of disease. *Journal of the National Cancer Institute* **22**: 719–748.

Marubini E, Valsecchi MG (1995) *Analysing Survival Data from Clinical Trials and Observational Studies*. John Wiley & Sons, Ltd, Chichester & New York.

Nilsson ME, Koke SC (2001) Defining treatment-emergent adverse events with the medical dictionary for regulatory activities (MedDRA). *Drug Information Journal* **35**: 1289–1299.

O'Neill RT (1995) Statistical concepts in the planning and evaluation of drug safety from clinical trials in drug development – issues of international harmonization. *Statistics in Medicine* **14**: 1117–1127.

O'Neill RT (1998) Biostatistical considerations in pharmacovigilance and pharmacoepidemiology: Linking quantitative risk assessment in pre-market licensure application safety data, post-market alert reports and formal epidemiological studies. *Statistics in Medicine* **17**: 1851–1858.

Sackett DL, Richardson WS, Rosenberg W, Haynes RB (2000) *Evidence-based Medicine: How to Practice and Teach EBM*. Churchill-Livingstone, New York.

Senn SJ (2006) Comment on Farrington and Whitaker: Semiparametric analysis of case series data. *Journal of the Royal Statistical Society Series C – Applied Statistics* **55**: 581–583.

Strom BL (2000a) Other approaches to pharmacoepidemiology studies. In: Strom BL (ed.), *Pharmacoepidemiology*. John Wiley and Sons, Inc., New York, pp. 349–362.

Strom BL (ed) (2000b) *Pharmacoepidemiology*. John Wiley and Sons, Inc., New York.

Sünder G, Peters TK (1994) Estimating incidence rates in the evaluation of pooled safety data. *Drug Information Journal* **28**: 797–803.

Working Party on Statistical Issues in First-in-Man Studies (2007) *Report of the Working Party on Statistical Issues in First-in-Man Studies*. Royal Statistical Society, London.

24

Pharmaco-economics and Portfolio Management

You that choose not by the view
Chance as fair and choose as true
Since this fortune falls to you.

William Shakespeare, *The Merchant of Venice*

My ventures are not in one bottom trusted,
Nor to one place; nor is my whole estate
Upon the fortune of this present year

William Shakespeare, *The Merchant of Venice*

He is the ferryman
To dead land
His price is everything

Ted Hughes, *The Bear, Wodwo*

24.1 BACKGROUND

In fact, those readers who have encountered that curious person, the pharmaco-economist, will know that it is not so much the case that his price is everything (although his advice is certainly not free) but rather that everything is in the price.

Resources are finite and competing demands are made upon them. This is true whether we talk about a national health budget or the research and development budget of a pharmaceutical company. In both cases it turns out that short-term costs are much easier to quantify than long-term benefits and the former are in any case usually more certain, whereas the latter are more speculative. In order to make rational decisions about a medicine, whether it be the price which should be paid for it or whether it is a decision whether it should be developed, complex calculations involving costs, probabilities and utilities are necessary. In the first edition, I wrote 'There is a growing realization that this is so and hence the science of pharmaco-economics is currently enjoying a terrific boom. By far the most remarkable fact associated with this development, however, is that it did not occur earlier.' In the ten years since,

Statistical Issues in Drug Development/2nd Edition   Stephen Senn
© 2007 John Wiley & Sons, Ltd

pharmaco-economics has become more important, certainly as regards the attention that pharmaceutical companies have to pay to reimbursers. For example, the United Kingdom's reimbursement recommending agency, if one may describe it thus, the National Institute for Clinical Excellence (NICE) was set up in 1999, two years after the first edition of this book, and has had a considerable influence on the fate of certain pharmaceuticals. In one case, that of the influenza treatment Relenza, where NICE refused reimbursement (Anderson, 2007), it probably had a considerable influence on its marketing success (or lack of it). However, the progress in using decision analysis for optimizing drug development has been less impressive.

A complication in applying economic thinking to this field is that the way in which health care is paid for means that there is no market for drugs in the same sense that there is a market, say, for television sets. The 'customer' does not pay directly for the product. Even in countries where there is no compulsory national insurance, individuals are covered by private insurance schemes. In the case of compulsory insurance, it becomes almost impossible to allow markets to determine prices, although in the United Kingdom an attempt has been made to do so by distinguishing between providing and purchasing authorities. In the case of private schemes, these policies are taken out by individuals who (1) hope that if they need to have recourse to the benefits it will be in the distant future, (2) do not know what treatments will be 'available' in the future, (3) may not even know what diseases will be most important in the future and (4) are generally offered package insurances anyway. Again, it seems difficult to harness markets to determine prices, but even where the attempt can be made it would appear that the rational choice of an individual consumer would have to involve much more complex calculation than as with most commodities.

Since markets are not available to determine prices, regulation seems to be stepping in to take its place. There has been some suggestion that value for money will become the fourth regulatory hurdle after quality, safety and efficacy. (In many cases the reimburser is not the same body as the official regulator, but this will not stop reimbursers from regulating the market.) In fact, Australia and Canada effectively require pharmaco-economic studies for registration.

This chapter is about statistical issues that are relevant to pharmaco-economics: whether that science be used to determine a 'fair price' for a drug or which projects to develop. Those issues which are mainly economic in nature will not be covered, but the choice as to which is which is, of course, partly arbitrary. A useful introduction to various economic issues is given by Luce and Simpson (1995) and a thorough account by the book in this series by Willan and Briggs (2006). Also valuable and relevant to this chapter are the sections on decision analysis and cost-effectiveness analysis in Petitti (2000). Bayesian approaches to health economics are certainly being discussed more frequently (although I suspect that the number of Bayesian evaluations is lagging behind somewhat). The little booklet by O'Hagan and Luce (2003) is a good introduction. Three excellent books in this series are also useful: Parmigiani (2002) covers decision analysis in some depth; Spiegelhalter *et al.* (2003) covers Bayesian synthesis of evidence; and for those who wish to elicit and specify prior probabilities, this is covered by O'Hagan *et al.* (2006).

Various types of economic evaluation are currently undertaken and the terminology is both confusing and somewhat variable. The basic task is to try to link monetary costs to health outcomes in a way which permits rational choices between therapies to be made. Torrance identifies five major types of study (Torrance, 1996).

Cost-minimization analysis compares costs for identical outcomes. **Cost-consequence analysis** establishes consequences and costs of a therapy but leaves the synthesis to the decision maker. **Cost-effectiveness analysis** uses natural medical units, such as life years gained, and costs them. **Cost-utility analysis** converts all effects into some common utility measure. **Cost-benefit analysis** converts everything, including medical outcomes, to a monetary equivalent.

An important decision to be made in development is between projects to develop. This requires some sort of economic assessment of candidate products: what may loosely be referred to as **project evaluation and prioritization**. It is a remarkable fact, however, that whereas the industry has developed an extensive theory, and what is largely a common code of practice, regarding all aspects of the clinical trial process, including, increasingly, economic evaluation, there is relatively little discussion about how the task of evaluating candidate drugs for development is to be approached. This statement is nearly as applicable now as it was at the time of the first edition. The potential link to economic evaluation of products is strong, for this is largely the economics appropriate to marketing (since the true value of a product must be an essential element in marketing) whereas the economic evaluation of projects is the economics of investment, but a rational approach to investment must, at the very least, involve speculation as to the eventual value of the product on the market.

This is not the place to go into a detailed exposé of the extremely complex theory of project evaluation and prioritization. The interested reader may find it useful to consult Senn (1996) for an introduction and also Burman *et al.* (2007), Burman and Senn (2003), Senn (1998a) and Senn and Rosati (2002). A good discussion of various approaches which have been used is given by Bergman and Gittins (1985) in chapter 4 of their book. An expert and important account of approaches to real investment under certainty is given in the book by Dixit and Pyndick (1994). Some relevant issues are picked up in due course below.

> **Pharmaco-economics**: Drug development's dismal science.

24.2 ISSUES

24.2.1 Economic evaluations should be carried out by using randomized clinical trials.

Of course, no pharmaco-economic evaluation is undertaken using the results from a clinical trial alone. Other inputs are necessary. The issue is whether the evaluation needs to be based on a randomized clinical trial (RCT). The arguments in favour of this point of view boil down to this: The RCT is generally accepted as being the single most powerful tool for investigating the effects of a treatment. If economic evaluations are to be credible, therefore, this 'best of tools' needs to be employed. Since the RCT provides a framework which enables the regulator to accept results produced by the sponsor, it is necessary that it be used for pharmaco-economic evaluations, since these are investigations where, above all others, the temptation for the sponsor to load the dice will be greatest. Only pharmaco-economic evaluations based on RCTs will be acceptable.

There are, however, several practical difficulties (Drummond, 1995), but also some philosophical ones. As has been argued elsewhere in this book, a clinical trial is better understood as an attempt to establish what a treatment *can* do rather than what it *will* do. For this purpose, it is not necessary to have representative patient populations and it is acceptable to concentrate on particular outcomes in a given trial. The interests of the reimburser, however, are likely to be more practical. What is needed is a prediction, for the population of patients who will actually use the drug, of the likely costs and benefits. What is important from the point of view of measurement is not only the sort of clinical outcomes, measured in a standard trial, but health and quality of life outcomes (utilities if possible) and costs (including all incidental costs) of the treatment in question.

For such outcomes it may be less easy to find additive scales for translating effects from trial population to target population and, to make up the deficit, further data and extensive modelling may be needed. That being the case, the RCT will be only one of a number of sources of information and it could be argued that the most efficient overall strategy for information gathering and use will be employed if the clinical trial is reserved for doing that which it does best: investigating the (medical) effects of treatment. For an interesting discussion of the way modelling approaches could be used, and will almost certainly be required, to supplement clinical trials in order to construct an economic evaluation, see Rittenhouse (1997).

With a question like this, a little empirical work is worth a mountain of speculation. In her comparison of methods of cost estimation in health care effectiveness in the field of perinatal care, Mugford found that there was little evidence that unit costs derived from simpler methods were very different from those derived from more costly research methods, including clinical trials (Mugford, 1996). General approaches to modelling costs appeared to have been more influential.

24.2.2 All RCTs with a therapeutic aim should include economic evaluation

This is a rather stronger view than that given above. There are three principle arguments in favour of this viewpoint. First, that if economic evaluation is to be done, it will be economic not to have to run extra trials to do it. Therefore, it will be appropriate to make sure that all trials which are potentially suitable for performing economic evaluations should be converted at relatively little extra cost to do so. (This point is also discussed under Section 24.2.5 below.) The second point is that it is unrealistic to think that any appropriate decision about therapy can be made without counting the cost. Either a given RCT will be superfluous, in which case it should not be run, or it will be answering a clinical question not answered elsewhere (perhaps the indication is different or the subpopulation of patients for the given indication is different) in which case the opportunity should be taken to find out about costs also, since these are essential for rational decision-making. The third point is that in some indications there will be no second opportunity to study economic issues, since it will be ethically impossible to run a further trial.

Whether these arguments are compelling or not depends partly upon whether one believes that the RCT is as valuable in answering economic questions as in answering clinical ones. Certainly, the cost of adding economic evaluation is not negligible, but obviously it is less than the cost of a further trial run with economic evaluation in mind. Whether the game is worth the candle, however, depends not only on the quality of information but on approaches to sequential decision making (Burman and Senn, 2003). For example, if a trial is run and turns out to be clinically very disappointing, there are few circumstances under which economic data can rescue it. Therefore, with hindsight, it may be seen that under those circumstances the economic assessment was a costly waste of time. If, however, the clinical evaluation had been carried out and the option to perform an economic evaluation only exercised if the clinical outcome made it worthwhile, then this exercise of foresight might prove valuable. As far as I am aware, although the economics of the clinical trial itself has been studied (for example, in the path-breaking work of Detsky (1985)), the economic case for economic evaluation alongside the RCT has not been made in formal terms. However, Ungar (1997a,b) considers this in terms of decision analysis. Using data for purely illustrative purposes, she shows that it can be advantageous to run a separate trial rather than using an add-on. This general point is picked up again in Section 24.2.5 below.

The ethical argument that the opportunity should be taken to study economic questions to avoid duplicating trials is, it must be conceded, a strong one. It is not valid for all indications, however and it also presupposes that it is appropriate to use the RCT to investigate economic questions. It should also be noted that economists have some difficulties in using such ethical arguments as imperative, since the very science of health economics requires that there be some trade-off between personal requirements for health and society's willingness to pay and that the latter must be accepted by decision-makers as an important factor to be considered. I do not dispute the validity of the economist's position here, which seems to me to be realistic and free of a lot of the moralizing cant which affects discussions of clinical trials. It does, however, imply that patients do not automatically have a right to receive what is currently believed to be the best treatment, and the fact that this is so also affects strategies for conducting clinical trials (Senn, 2001, 2002b).

24.2.3   Information or decisions?

This theme has come up in a number of places in this book. Should we measure how well a drug does what we should like it to do, or simply what it does? The former view has the advantage that we focus design on really important questions and may largely be able to finesse the issues attendant on multiplicity. It appears to be appropriate where global decisions have to be made. (Although even here it depends to what extent the target population is similar to the trial population.) The latter view recognizes that a treatment may have many different effects, that the patients in a trial are unrepresentative, but that given detailed knowledge of a treatment, then, with suitable models, we can make some attempt at predicting what will happen to a given patient and so attempt to make rational decisions for him or her. In fact, Hilden (1987) has gone even further and made the (in my view logical) suggestion that we should simply provide information for the patient to make his or her own decision.

However, pharmaco-economic studies seem to be nearly always entirely run along the first model. Of course, in many cases, a global decision of sorts is being sought since a price must be established for the drug, but even here it does not follow that individual decisions are irrelevant.

24.2.4   Price-determining or price-deriving?

The price of a finished product is one of the few things about it that can still be varied. The dose has been determined and at the determined dose the product will have particular effects and side-effects in the target population, and these in their turn will bring with them certain benefits and costs. To change the dose, for example, might require further studies to be run, and to change the formulation might need further work also. The price, however, could be other than envisaged without having to repeat or add further studies. It is rather surprising, therefore, that in many economic evaluations (in particular cost-efficiency studies) a pre-determined price is fed into the calculations. It is then established via a significance test on the overall costs whether the price is justified. The alternative, which seems to me more reasonable, would be not to take the price into account at all in the initial calculations but then see what range of prices are tolerable.

One reason for taking this point of view is that the choice of prices can impact considerably on the 'significance' of the result. (In making this point I am not endorsing significance testing as a suitable framework for carrying out economic evaluation but reflecting a reality.) Rittenhouse *et al.* (1999) have shown that 'depending on the relative prices used in an analysis, between-group differences in total costs per patient may be either statistically significant or insignificant, regardless of whether differences in utilization of the underlying resources are statistically significant' (p. 213). That being so, it would seem to make more sense to consider the effect of treatment in resource utilization and allow local decisions regarding reimbursement to be made taking prices into account. Indeed, price adjustment would seem logical.

Of course, from the reimburser's point of view, the fact that a new product at a price proposed by a sponsor is valuable doesn't mean that this is a desirable price. An even lower price would be more attractive! What is an appropriate price is then a very difficult question to answer. If it is set too low, innovation may be discouraged. If it is set too high, perhaps there is 'a producer surplus' which should be shared with the consumer. It is impossible to pursue this further without getting into very difficult economic waters involving, innovation, patents, knowledge and risk, and I shall not be taking the plunge. However, the reader who is interested for a brief discussion of issues may wish to consult Senn and Rosati (2003).

24.2.5   Choice of comparator and strategies for study

If it is decided to use a clinical trial for comparison, then it will have most direct relevance to economic evaluation if the comparator is an established treatment which is a true alternative to the experimental drug. There is a considerable tradition in the RCT, however, of using placebos instead. Of course, as was discussed in Chapter 6, even where the main purpose of the trial is to measure biological, not economic, outcomes, there are many who would argue on ethical or practical grounds, or both, that an active treatment should be used rather than a placebo. (Since all sorts of measurements, including economic ones, can be taken in a clinical trial, a qualifier is needed, apart from *clinical*, to cover the usual sort of noneconomic measurements taken in a clinical trial. In the discussion here the qualifier *biological* will be used.)

It is sometimes suggested that a 'gold standard' trial may be used in economic evaluations, whereby both an active treatment and a placebo are included as comparators. (As discussed in Chapter 15, such trials have also been strongly supported as being appropriate for equivalence studies.) In the context of economic evaluations, however, there are several disadvantages. For example, other things being equal, trials with economic evaluation as well as biological measurements have a heavier burden of measurement than either a biological trial alone or an economic trial alone. On the other hand, suppose that it were the case that n patients per treatment group would be needed whether an economic or biological question was being examined. In that case, the 'two-trials strategy' would require $4n$ patients and the 'one-trial strategy' $3n$. This appears to give the advantage to the one-trial strategy, especially since there will be a fixed cost element with a trial, but a further difficulty is that the economic trial will usually require more patients than the biological trial and if all treatments in the one trial are to have equal numbers of patients, this tilts the balance back in favour of the two-trials approach. (If equal numbers per arm are not required, however, then this is a flexibility which the one-trial strategy can exploit.)

Other disadvantages of the one-trial strategy are more serious, however. First, there may be other regulatory requirements on the total number of patients exposed to the new drug. If this is the case, and tolerability rather than efficacy considerations are sample-size-determining, then trials with three arms, only one of which is the experimental treatment, are unwelcome. Consider also a placebo-controlled trial of a new long-acting bronchodilator to be given twice daily. Blinding can be achieved by accommodating the placebo to the proposed dosing schedule. Suppose, however, that the standard active comparator would be given four times daily. Blinding must inevitably involve dummy loading: with certainly at least four administrations in each arm and maybe six (if the four-times-daily schedule does not mesh well with the twice daily schedule). This makes the administration of the trial complex. If it is decided to make the trial open-label as a result, *then there is no point in including the placebo*. However, there are number of practical questions with an impact on economics which it might be interesting to ask in an open-label trial. For example, do patients prefer a twice-daily administration to a four-times-daily one? Is compliance effected? Thus a two-trials strategy with one blind and the other open-label might have many attractions.

As explained above, a further potential advantage of the two-trials strategy is that it is more flexible in that it can be run sequentially. This means that if the first trial is unsuccessful, there is no need to run the second and unnecessary costs can be avoided. Of course, depending upon the position the trials occupy on the development path, the two-trial strategy may delay registration if it turns out that the drug is a success. This delay will be costly.

In conclusion, my opinion is that there are no hard and fast rules regarding choice of comparator and strategies for trials. Each case will need to be considered carefully and the appropriate calculations will have to be made before it can be decided whether an economic trial should be merged with a biological one. For further analysis of the advantages and disadvantages of parallel as opposed to sequential development see Burman and Senn (2003) and for specific discussion of the choice of type of study see Ungar (1997a,b).

24.2.6   Concerning the measurement of costs

We can think of at least three levels of costs. Direct treatment costs, which may be divided into drug acquisition costs and other health care costs, and other non-health care costs (for example costs of days lost through absence from work). Obviously, decisions as to which of these are to be included in costing a treatment can make a considerable difference. The standard errors associated with measuring costs become progressively larger as more items are included under the cost heading, and this is usually true even as a percentage of the cost measured. It is sometimes wrongly stated that direct costs per patient-day are not stochastic but determined, but this is not true under all pricing systems. For example, partial compliers may come back less frequently for repeat prescriptions. If this is so, and new prescriptions are written when needed, then partial compliers cost less to treat per day in direct treatment costs than do full compliers, and whether a patient complies or not and if not to what degree is a matter of chance. Thus daily treatment costs do become a stochastic variable. (See Urquhart (1996) for a discussion.)

It is perhaps also useful to mention the distinction between use data and unit costs (prices). The latter are largely determined by external economic factors and are not an intrinsic feature of the drug. For example, even if, as is in practice unlikely, the most important element in the price of a drug is the cost of manufacture, it is conceivable that this will reduce over time due to economies of scale, improved production methods, simpler syntheses and so forth. On the other hand, the speed with which a curative treatment will affect a cure, which also has an important effect on costs, is more likely to be a permanent quality of the treatment. In the discussion which follows we shall generally refer to costs without making this distinction, using the terms *use costs* and *unit costs* where such distinction is important.

The more extensive the cost measurements, the more the statistical problems. One problem has to do with follow-up. If one wishes to measure all costs of a treatment, then from one point of view it is necessary to measure all costs of health care downstream of the point of treatment. For some diseases, it may be presumed that when a patient stops a given treatment, the treatment originally given eventually becomes irrelevant to current costs. This is a similar point of view to that which permits us to run cross-over trials in some indications given a suitable washout. This mainly applies to chronic diseases. For acute diseases, however, it may be the case that the whole future course of the disease is affected by treatment (after all it is often in this hope that the treatment is given). Under such circumstances, follow up until death or cure or remission and perhaps relapse may be needed. Some patients, however, may be lost to follow-up. It will usually be more difficult to get data on costs than on survival.

Harrell points to a number of difficulties in estimating costs under such circumstances (Harrell, 1996, 1999). For example, the effect of death itself on costs may be difficult to account for. Where a patient has been followed up until death, should the costs be considered complete or not? From a hospital's point of view the costs of treating the patient stop with the patient's death thus costs are complete. On the other hand, consider a case where two intensive care units are compared. The unit with higher mortality has shorter lengths of stay and hence lower costs. A statistical model might actually fit better when cumulative costs at time of death are not considered complete (Dudley *et al.*, 1993). (This is an estimation issue. What is to be done with the cost estimates is another matter.) As Harrell (1996, 1999) points out, there are some technical difficulties in treating cumulative costs via survival analysis. A problem arises if time on therapy does not have a one-to-one mapping on cost because the censoring variable (true survival) is not on the same scale as the 'survival' variable (cost). Thus such outcomes have all the difficulties attendant on survival analysis: censoring, loss to follow-up and so forth, with the additional complications which changing costs over time can impose. (See also Fenn *et al.* (1995).)

> **Pharmaco-economist**: One who asks not only if the treatment for dysentery was effective but also after the price of toilet paper.

Even for 'simpler' approaches to the estimation of costs, not based on survival analysis, it can be difficult to calculate an individual cost for every patient. For example, if one only uses patients still in the trial to calculate costs and there are progressive drop-outs, the mean cost between visits will be based on progressively fewer patients. If one then uses these means to 'estimate' naively what the 'average' patient would consume in resources at each period in order to cumulate these, then one has a total cost which is not based on individual total costs and for which a measure of variability cannot be directly computed. On the other hand, if one were to use only those patients who provided cost information for the whole period – the 'completers' – one would be throwing away information. Ideally some sort of random effect model with suitable assumptions would be used but it is idle to pretend that this is easy and currently within the grasp of most investigators.

The distinction between use costs and unit costs raises an issue similar to that discussed in section 24.2.3 in connection with health outcomes: should we try to reduce to a single measure or keep our measurement multidimensional? The former approach makes any updating of the assessment extremely difficult if unit costs change. The problem is analogous to that encountered in constructing a price index. It is not generally possible to tell how increases in various prices over time affect the purchasing power of money unless one has some basis in terms of quantities. The use costs associated with a treatment are like the basket of goods used in constructing an index. We need to know their pattern in order to work out the overall effect on costs.

One further issue is raised by this analogy. A problem in constructing index numbers is the pattern of quantities of goods purchased over time varies and this makes the choice of weights difficult. As discussed above, many of the use costs associated with a treatment may be taken to be 'permanent' features of the drug. This will not be true for all of them, however. Approaches to managing the care of patients may change as unit costs change (or for other reasons) and this raises the prospect that economic evaluations would have to be repeated at regular intervals.

24.2.7 Concerning the measurement of outcomes

In cost-effectiveness analysis so-called 'natural units' are used for measuring outcomes. However, these measurements are not necessarily those which a clinician or a medical statistician would use. For example, in survival analysis, physicians might be interested in median survival and statisticians in log-hazard rates, but health economists might wish to use so called 'quality of life outcomes', arguing that one year without disability is worth more than one with and that this aspect of the quality of life must be taken into account. Already, an enormous amount has been published on the subject of so-called QALYs (quality-adjusted life years) and I will not add to this particular debate (see Petitti (2000) for an introduction). However, note that a QALY attempts to produce a single-dimensional answer from multidimensional data and so the issues discussed under Section 24.2.3 are relevant. Instead a specific example of a related measure sometimes used in chronic disease studies will be taken to illustrate some issues.

In an interesting comparison of a combination therapy in asthma with a monotherapy, Rutten-van Mölken *et al.* calculated the advantage of the combination therapy (bronchodilator + steroid) compared with the monotherapy (bronchodilator) for a number of measures (Rutten-van Mölken *et al.*, 1993). For all these measures, the combination therapy appeared to be more effective, in some cases significantly so. For example, the improvement in FEV_1 as a percentage of the predicted value was highly significant. When it came to costs, however, whether there was an advantage or not depended on the basis of calculation. For the most conservative cost approach, the combination therapy was at a disadvantage regarding direct health care costs and therefore it became relevant to calculate the cost per gain in a particular clinical outcome. These increased costs were estimated to be NLG (Dutch Gulders) 207. On the other hand the benefits were an 11.85% increase in the FEV_1 measure, an increase in the PD_{20} by a factor of 1.53 and an extra 38 symptom-free days. The cost-effectiveness ratios were then calculated as $(NLG273/11.85) \times 10 = NLG175$ per 10% FEV_1, $(NLG273/1.53) \times 2 = NLG270$ per doubling of PD_{20}, and $(NLG273/38) = NLG7$ per symptom-free day.

However, these measures have very different status. The FEV_1 benefit was 11.85%; therefore, if the uncertainty associated with this measure is ignored, one could say that 10% is an attainable benefit. On the other hand the PD_{20} was only raised by a factor of 1.53 on average and there is no guarantee that any patient could ever achieve a doubling using this therapy. The most serious problem, however, applies to the symptom-free day measure. This general approach is popular with health economists, who see it as a means of finessing the difficult problem of combining symptom information: symptoms may be of different sorts, wheezing tightening of chest, full attack and of different severity. However, all symptoms are alike when they are absent and so the absence of symptoms *seems* to be a useful way to combine them. The trouble is that the time period is entirely arbitrary and that potentially important information regarding events is suppressed by concentrating on nonevents. Why not use symptom-free weeks? But the number of symptom free weeks gained in the study will not have been 1/7 of the number of symptom free days, which in turn will not be 1/24 the number of symptom-free hours. Furthermore, two patients who do not experience a symptom-free day do not necessarily experience the same symptoms in that day. Thus, my opinion is that although cost-effectiveness studies appear to avoid the difficult issue of assigning utilities to outcome, to the extent that they attempt to reduce a multitude of clinical outcomes to a single measure, they only do so in a way which is, essentially, arbitrary.

24.2.8   Concerning precision

In Chapter 13 we discussed various approaches to determining the sample size in clinical trials. For trials in which there is an ethical imperative not to randomize patients to a known inferior treatment, we do not wish to make trials larger than is strictly necessary to prove superiority. Thus it is enough to show that the drug is better without establishing how much better. Unfortunately, when it comes to economic outcomes, not only may we require larger sample sizes to show significance in the purely economic variables but, in view of cost differences, it is not always enough to know that a drug has a better clinical outcome than another to make it prescribable; we may also need to know how much better. Hence, quite different standards of precision may be needed for economic analysis. This of course, affects the considerations of where, when and how to study the economic aspects of a treatment touched upon in various sections above.

However, the relationship cuts both ways. It is not enough to say that clinical requirements for sample sizes determine what is achievable for the measurement of economic outcomes and that therefore clinical requirements have priority over economic ones. As we pointed out in Chapter 13, practical requirements, which are in some sense at least economic, have an inevitable influence on the sample size. It is a severe criticism of conventional sample size calculations that no element of cost is included. Ideally costs should be, as they are in various Bayesian approaches (Burman *et al.*, 2007; Gittins and Pezeshk, 2000; Lindley, 1997). It is naive to regard the sample size as being the determined result of variability, power, type I error requirements and the clinically relevant difference. As Detsky has pointed out, the choice of a clinically relevant difference may be influenced by economic considerations of two kinds (Detsky, 1985). First, the smaller the difference, the larger and hence more costly the trial. Second, 'the difference you would not like to miss' depends on the costs and benefits associated with a disease. For a disease with high prevalence and high costs (whether monetary or in lost utility) it will be more attractive to look for a small clinically relevant difference. These economic considerations ought to impinge on the target precision adopted for a trial whether or not economic outcomes are measured within the trial.

24.2.9 Concerning cost-effectiveness ratios

Figure 24.1 is based on Grieve (1996) and plots the cost-effectiveness 'space' for a trial comparing an experimental treatment to a standard comparator. (See also Grieve (1998), Willan and Briggs (2006).) If we take the two dimensions of cost and effectiveness, the new treatment can prove to be either more expensive or cheaper and either more or less effective (if exact equality is excluded), thus giving four combinations corresponding to the four quadrants of the diagram. If the issue of random variation is set aside for the moment, then a position in two of the quadrants will lead to clear decisions. The south-east quadrant corresponds to a cheaper and more effective experimental treatment which is thus clearly superior to the standard. The north-west quadrant corresponds to a more expensive and less effective experimental treatment, to which the standard treatment will inevitably be preferred. In the other two quadrants, there is a cost–effectiveness trade-off and there is no immediate answer as to which treatment will be preferred.

We may imagine, however, that a health care purchaser has some sort of benefit–cost trade-off. This is represented by a diagonal line of slope R drawn on the diagram. (This has been drawn at 45 degrees for ease of presentation but in practice it could

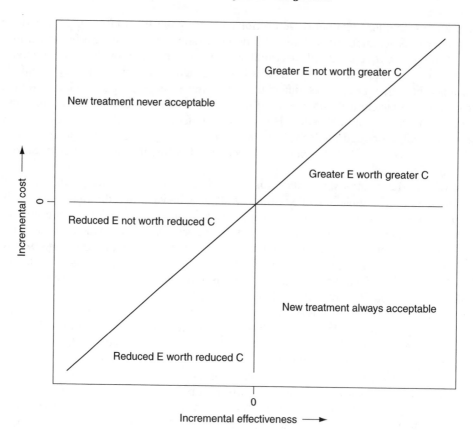

Figure 24.1   Plot of the cost-effectiveness for a trial comparing an experimental treatment with a standard comparator.

be either steeper or shallower than this.) Given that this represents the purchaser's trade-off, then positions to the left of the line correspond to the standard therapy being preferable and positions to the right of the line correspond to the new treatment being preferable.

This concept appears to make it useful to calculate a cost-effectiveness ratio, $R' = \Delta C / \Delta E$, in a comparative study, since a purchaser may then compare R' to the slope R of his trade-off line to see whether it is preferred. The value of R', however, will not be measured with perfect precision and the question then arises as to how the uncertainty attendant on its estimation should be expressed.

Where we have statistics which are estimable for individual patients, then the same simple general procedure can be used for calculating standard errors. To consider another important application where ratios are calculated, bioequivalence studies, we can calculate a ratio of areas under the curve for test and reference product for every subject and hence (working usually with the logarithms) calculate the standard deviation and hence the standard error. This method is less easy to apply where there is no natural zero because then individual estimates may show considerable instability as the denominator may cross zero. Therefore, what is usually done is to calculate a ratio of means rather than the mean (geometric or otherwise) of ratios. In order to calculate the variance of the estimate it is then necessary to apply a Taylor's expansion to obtain an approximation, with the added difficulty that cost and effectiveness are not necessarily independent so that some estimate of their covariance is needed. Alternatively, an extension of Fieller's theorem may permit calculation of the confidence limit for the ratio. An excellent discussion of various approaches to the calculation of confidence limits, including Taylor's expansions and Fieller's theorem is given by Chaudhary and Stearns (1996). See also chapter 4 of Willan and Briggs (2006).

24.2.10   The cost–effectiveness curve

As discussed by Grieve (1996, 1998), van Hout *et al.* (1994) propose that for a given value of R the probability be calculated that R' lies in the acceptable region. They define this probability in terms of the integral of the joint probability density of ΔC and ΔE, the differences in costs and effectiveness. The value of the integral varies with the region of integration and this is a function of R. Hence the probability of a new treatment being acceptable can be evaluated as a function $p(R)$ of the reimburser's trade-off limit between cost and effectiveness. It is then possible to plot $p(R)$ against R to give a useful representation of the probability of the new treatment being of interest without having to commit oneself, at the time of analysis, to a given value of R.

As Grieve (1996) points out, however, for a given study the sample ratio either does or does not lie in the acceptability region. Given the data obtained in the study, this is not a matter for probability. Therefore, the only way in which sense can be made of such an integral is if the probability density in question is that of the parameters in question (the 'true' average values of the difference in cost and effectiveness). A frequentist point of view would be that the parameters either do or do not lie in the region of interest and that this is not a matter for probability. A Bayesian interpretation is possible, however, if we interpret the probability as being a statement of belief. Hence, according to Grieve (1996), what is being presented by van Hout *et al.* (1994) only makes sense if a Bayesian interpretation is given. See O'Hagan and Stevens (2001) for further development of the Bayesian point of view.

In one sense, Grieve's claim must be correct. As discussed in Chapter 3, direct probability statements about parameters are not possible in a frequentist framework. Only probability statements about sample statistics given assumed parameter values are possible. If any mainstream frequentist interpretation of the C/E acceptability curve is possible, it would only be in the sense of a 'confidence' rather than a probability. (See Chaudhary and Stearns (1996).). Without giving the matter more thought than I am able to at this juncture, I cannot say whether such an interpretation is possible. Whether it is desirable is of course another matter altogether.

24.2.11   The standard gamble

In the more complex sort of economic evaluation, cost-utility and cost-benefit analysis, the task of evaluating outcomes on a utility or even monetary scale must be addressed. A device which is used to do this is known as the **standard gamble**, ably discussed by Spiegelhalter, (1982) and also by Petitti (2000). We wish to evaluate the utility of a certain outcome, C, and to do so we consider that the patient may be offered instead a gamble G whose result will be with probability p the best possible outcome,

B, which has utility 1, or will be with probability $(1-p)$ the worst outcome, W, which has utility 0. The expected value of the gamble is thus $p \times 1 + (1-p) \times 0 = p$. If the patient prefers the certain outcome C to G, it then follows that the value of C exceeds p. If, on the other hand, the patient prefers G, it thus follows that the value of C is less than p. By varying the value of p in the gamble offered, until the patient is indifferent between C and G, value of C on the 0 to 1 utility scale may be established. Petitti gives the example, for a patient with kidney failure, of choosing between staying on hospital dialysis or having renal transplant surgery, the outcome of which will either be health (with probability p) or death (with probability $(1-p)$). The value of p at which the patient is indifferent to dialysis or surgery defines the relative utility of dialysis.

A worrying feature about employing the standard gamble, however, is that it corresponds to finding a patient's answers to a hypothetical question and such answers are sometimes treated as being of more relevance than the answer to an actual question. Consider the case of dialysis above. If a given patient is to decide whether to take surgery, the gamble is irrelevant. Once the utility, p_u of hospital dialysis is known, the patient can only make a rational decision if he or she has (as many Bayesians would insist the patient must have) some assessment, however imperfect, of the probability of success p_s. But, given p_s, it is not necessary at all to establish p_u. It is only necessary to know whether the relative utility of hospital dialysis is greater or less than p_s. This is all that the patient needs to know to make the actual decision. Of course, if the patient had to pay for the operation, other considerations might come into play but, first, patients generally do not have to pay at the point of purchase and, second, it is doubtful whether, in deciding to pay for something, consumers do assess their consumer surplus. (This being the difference they would be prepared to pay and the amount they have paid.)

For an attempt to actually evaluate patient utilities in a clinical setting, the reader might be interested in Bass *et al.* (2004). The authors surveyed, '109 patients on hemodialysis therapy, 57 patients on continuous ambulatory peritoneal dialysis (CAPD), and 22 patients on continuous cycling peritoneal dialysis (CCPD)' (p. 695). They found that whereas many patients would be prepared to increase their dose to increase survival chances, few would be prepared to change the modality of treatment.

24.2.12   Who should perform the evaluation?

Not least among the many advantages of the randomized clinical trial is its ability to promote utmost good faith in drug regulation. A carefully designed 'fiduciary framework' Is provided. The analysis is pre-specified in the protocol. A report is produced in which the fate of each patient and each measurement on him or her is carefully recorded. Missing records can easily be identified and must be explained and so forth. In fact the documentation in the protocol is so explicit that in many cases different statisticians analysing the trial would come up with exactly the same answer (at least as regards the main outcome variable). In my opinion, this feature has been of considerable importance in the rise of contract research organizations providing external statistical services to the industry. It has meant that for *relatively* little additional in-house work, the analysis of a trial may be contracted out. In short, the randomized controlled trial has been a device which has permitted the regulator to mandate the sponsor to analyse the data.

There is a growing realization, however, that when it comes to economic evaluation, the clinical trial is not enough but must be supplemented by data from other sources and more complex modelling (Rittenhouse, 1997). But problems arise as soon as the RCT framework is left. The regulator/reimburser can no longer trust the sponsor to the same degree. This raises the issue of who should perform economic analysis. Of course, even if the reimburser requires to carry out this analysis himself, or nominates a third party to do so, the sponsor will still wish to undertake such evaluations himself at an earlier stage, if only to predict the likely result of the reimburser's evaluation. I think it is fair to say that the industry as a whole is still groping towards a solution to this difficult problem.

24.2.13   Concerning indices for project evaluation and prioritization

Almost everybody agrees that four factors which are important when assessing the potential of a product in development are costs, probability of success, time to develop, and eventual rewards if successful. The third of these, time to develop, may be dealt with to some extent by adjusting cost and reward calculations appropriately; for example by discounting costs and future rewards according to when they are due and by taking into account the possibility of pre-emption (i.e. that another company will get there first) when assessing rewards. (But see below for a discussion of discount rates.)

Project prioritization: A scientific means of continuously ranking drugs in development until the chief executive officer's favourite project comes out top.

Various companies have used simple indices using total costs, overall probability of success, time to develop, total expected reward if successful and so forth when comparing projects. For example, characteristics have been awarded some points on a suitable scale, and these have then been weighted and added up. Such indices cannot give a reasonable answer, since two projects with identical values for each of these constituent parts would have to be given the same evaluation. However, if one project is more likely to fail early if it fails, and the other is more likely to fail later if it fails, then, other things being equal, the former is more valuable than the latter. This shows that any simple index based on ranking *must* be wrong.

The problem can be illustrated with respect to a simple game of chance which I call 'coins' and which comes in two versions. In each version a fair coin is tossed three times and a Swiss franc is paid for each toss. A reward is paid if and only if all three tosses are successful. In the first version, the reward is Sfr 25.00 and in the second Sfr 20.00. However, for the first game the three francs must be paid up front. In the second they are only paid to see each toss and the player can stop any time he or she likes and start another game. Which of the two games is more valuable?

A summary comparing the two games would look like Table 24.1, from which it appears that game 1 is more valuable, since the games have nothing to distinguish them in terms of overall cost and probability of success. In fact, however, game 2 is six

Table 24.1 Naive Summary of two games.

	Game 1	Game 2
Cost to complete	Sfr 3	Sfr 3
Probability of success	1/8	1/8
Reward if successful	Sfr 25	Sfr 20

Table 24.2 Calculation of expected value for game 1.

Result	Net winnings
HHT HTH THH TTH THT HTT TTT	−3
HHH	22
On average	$1/8 = 0.125$

Table 24.3 Calculation of expected value for game 2.

Result	Net winnings
T(TT) T(TH) T(HT) T(TT)	−1
HT(T) HT(H)	−2
HHT	−3
HHH	17
On average	$6/8 = 0.75$

times as valuable as is shown by the calculations in Tables 24.2 and 24.3. There are eight possible sequences of results from tossing a fair coin. These are shown for game 1. One of them, 'three heads' leads to a *net* reward of Sfr 22.00, the others lead to a loss of Sfr 3.00. Hence the expected reward per 8 games is Sfr $22.00 - (7 \times Sfr\ 3.00) = 1$ Sfr or 1/8 Sfr per game. However, for game 2, the losses are not the same because some of the sequences will be suppressed by choice and never occur. For example, the sequence THH is one of four which will be suppressed after the first tail appears at the cost of Sfr 1.00 rather than proceeding to cost the player Sfr 3.00.

The lesson for the evaluation of projects in development is that detailed examination of the *cost and probability architecture* is necessary (Senn, 1996, 1998a). (See also Zipfel 2003.) It is not adequate to rely on total dimensions. A simple index which captures some of this is the Pearson index (Pearson, 1972). The position is illustrated in Figure 24.2, which shows the example of a three-stage project whose evolution is represented by movement along a two-dimensional path. It progresses through time from left to right and towards eventual success at the top or failure at the bottom. Each stage culminates in a chance node which is either passed successfully or (if failed) leads to termination of the project. If all stages are passed successfully, a reward is reached.

More generally, if we have a project in n stages and stage i has cost c_i and the probability of success in this stage, given that it has succeeded so far, is p_i, with $p_o = 1$, and the

The Pearson Index

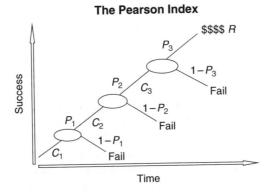

Figure 24.2 Diagrammatic representation of a three-stage project.

final reward is r (all costs and rewards being discounted), then the Pearson index (PI) ranks a project using

$$\text{PI} = \frac{p_1 p_2 \cdots p_n r - (c_1 + p_1 c_2 + p_1 p_2 c_3 \cdots)}{(c_1 + p_1 c_2 + p_1 p_2 c_3 \cdots)} = \frac{r \prod_{i=1}^{n} p_i - \sum_{i=1}^{n} c_i \prod_{j=0}^{i-1} p_j}{\sum_{i=1}^{n} c_i \prod_{j=0}^{i-1} p_j} \tag{24.1}$$

The top line of the index is an expected net present value which takes account of the sequential nature of the decision-making process and thus captures (unlike indices based on totals only) the value of the option to abandon given technical failure which the developer holds. (Note that this option is not held if the stages are done in parallel.) The bottom line is used to scale projects according to their investment requirements.

This index may be regarded as a crude first approximation as to what is necessary to evaluate projects. It captures one important aspect of option value but not others. For example, as a project proceeds, market uncertainties may be resolved and these too may lead to exercising the option to abandon. This is not reflected in the index (Senn, 1996, 1998a). The index will also require the use of a given rate of interest for discounting purposes and this will also not reflect the fact that the cost of capital will vary during the course of the project.

As Talias (2007) has pointed out, there is an interesting analogy between the Pearson Index and the Neyman–Pearson lemma. (The Pearsons in question are different. Alan Pearson is the author of the Pearson index and Egon Pearson, 1895–1980, was the son of Karl Pearson, 1857–1936 and the collaborator of Jerzey Neyman, 1894–1981, in developing hypothesis testing.) Both are relevant to optimizing a function subject to a constraint. In the case of the Pearson index this is profit subject to total cost, and for the Neyman–Pearson lemma it is power subject to the constraint of an overall type I error rate. In both cases a ratio plays a key role. For the Neyman–Pearson lemma this is the likelihood ratio and for the Pearson index the index itself is a ratio of expected profit to expected cost.

This raises an interesting inferential point. Because projects are not infinitely divisible for any given cost constraint, the solution of choosing projects with highest Pearson indices until there were no more funds available would not necessarily produce the portfolio of projects with the highest value given the cost restraints. This is well known in the operational research field, where the problem is usually dealt with by integer programming. Indeed, the more difficult problem of constructing portfolios with given return and risk combinations (albeit in the more conventional context of share portfolios) analogous to that discussed in Section 24.2.18 is dealt with also using this approach. See Corazza and Favaretto (2007), for example.

An analogous problem exists in inferential statistics, where discrete data lead to a sample space with finite number of points and hence in practice the situation that it is usually impossible to construct a rule for a hypothesis test with exactly the type I error rate required unless an auxiliary randomizing device is allowed. In consequence, if this is not allowed, the criterion of likelihood ratio does not produce an optimal test in the sense of having maximum power for given type I error rate. This issue was discussed in Chapter 12. This is often taken to mean that the likelihood ratio criterion is not appropriate. In my view the reverse is the case. There is no point in trying to 'improve' tests under such circumstances (Senn, 2007). The key paper is that of Pitman (1965) who shows that if a statistician wishes to go through life maximizing power for a certain type of problem while controlling the average type I error rate, it is the likelihood ratio criterion that should be kept constant from case to case.

The analogy for a capitalist should be that if, from time to time, investment opportunities arise, he should invest in projects with a given Pearson index, either borrowing money where current funds are inadequate or part investing if necessary by offering a share to others. It would be a mistake under such circumstances to use integer programming to turn what ought to be a continuous problem into a discrete one.

For further discussion of the Pearson index in project management see Burman *et al.* (2007), Burman and Senn (2003), Regan and Senn (1997), Senn (1996, 1998a) and Senn and Rosati, 2002); for its relation to the Neyman–Pearson lemma see Talias (2007) and for real option theory see Dixit and Pyndick (1994).

24.2.14   Is faster better?

When the importance of the option to abandon is fully grasped it can be seen that speeding up development can actually destroy value. It is true, of course, that the longer a development, the greater the danger of pre-preemption, and of course also the longer the wait for the eventual reward (a feature which high interest rates certainly make undesirable). However, by doing things in parallel, the structure of a development project turns from resembling the second of the 'coins' games towards resembling the first. Knowledge of failure in one stage no longer permits us to avoid the costs of another since the investment is already irreversibly committed (Burman and Senn, 2003). Thus, drug development is one of at least two things in life where faster is not necessarily better.

24.2.15   Concerning the assessment of probabilities

Project prioritization is a case where Bayesian statistics seems particularly appropriate. Every project is different and a *naive* frequentist view, defining probabilities in terms of limiting relative frequency of repeated events, seems both inappropriate and difficult. (But see below.) There is a considerable literature on eliciting subjective probabilities, including the classic text of O'Hagan (1988) and now, a companion volume in this series (O'Hagan *et al.*, 2006).

What is needed to apply (24.1) is to assess the probability of passing a given stage, given that the previous stages have been passed successfully. 'Divide and conquer' is a useful motto. For example, if the overall success objective of the given stage of a project depends on a number of targets, each of which must be hit, and success or failure for each target is independent, then the probability of overall success in the stage is the product of the individual probabilities for each target. In practice, however, these conditions are rarely met exactly and usually there is some dependence between targets.

A surprising feature of the way in which Bayesian statistics has been applied to the assessment of stage probabilities is that Bayes' theorem never seems to be involved. Prior probabilities of success for a given stage are estimated, but there is no formal updating using Bayes' theorem. In fact, in general, data hardly ever seem to be used at all in any formal way and I have even heard one practitioner describe probability as being, 'something inside the subject-matter expert's head which it is the decision analyst's job to extract'. It is perhaps worth mentioning at this stage that frequentist models *are* commonly used to assess single case probabilities. For example, a clinical trial in hypertension in which the outcome is whether the patient suffered a stroke or not and which, in addition to treatment given, covariates such as diastolic and systolic blood pressure at baseline and age are fitted may, in fact, have no two patients with exactly the same covariates. This would not prevent a model being fitted using logistic regression. In exactly the same way, given a large enough database, it would be possible to model success probabilities for projects given suitable 'covariate' information. It seems to me that there is a genuine opportunity for some more sophisticated Bayesian thinking here. We know how to assess probabilities when there are no data (everything is in the subjective prior) and we also know how when we have many data (the prior is largely irrelevant), but surprisingly little seems to have been done for the case where we have a few data from different sources, at least in the way of putting such models into practice. However, the companion book in this series by Spiegelhalter *et al.* (2003) does treat this seriously.

24.2.16   Concerning the assessment of the costs of development

Estimating costs should be the easiest aspect of evaluating projects, but more could be done. Clinical grant costs are available for a large number of trials on commercial databases. (For example, Fast Track's System's GrantSpace Trials Manager) Regression analysis makes it possible in principle, therefore, to estimate the fixed costs per centre as well as variable costs per patient (and possibly also, per page of the case record form) for a number of indications. More difficult is to establish the in-house costs associated with running clinical trials, although the increasing competition among contract research organizations to do such work as was previously done in-house makes some sort of estimate feasible.

24.2.17   Concerning the assessment of eventual rewards

This is also extremely difficult. A common approach is the demographic component method. Projections of future populations per region are made using current population figures and current death rates (and also birth rates if children are a relevant market). More difficult is the application of suitable incidence and/or prevalence figures in order to obtain numbers of potential clients. Most difficult of all is to assess market penetration since this is dependent not only on the as yet uncertain features of the drug but also on its yet unknown competitors.

> **Blockbuster**: Any product that treats mild, common, incurable and possibly asymptomatic disease in the developing world.

In any case, sales are effort dependent, so that strictly speaking a complex decision problem is involved. What is the ideal amount of money to spend on selling the product and, given that the ability to vary this sum is an option which the sponsor holds, at what value should this option be priced?

The option side of rewards is potentially extremely important, not least because new and unforeseen uses may be found for products which are developed. One might argue that if a product is not developed then this opportunity for future discovery still remains, but in practice this is not so. Undeveloped drugs are rarely revived subsequently. Thus, developing drugs has a serendipity option. The phenomenon of serendipitous scientific discovery is not, of course, restricted to the pharmaceutical industry. Nelson (1959) gives some interesting examples of cases where important discoveries were made by pursuing apparently unrelated lines of inquiry. For example, acetylene was discovered by a group attempting to develop a better way to extract aluminium from clay; W.H. Perkin discovered mauve, the first aniline dye, when trying to synthesize quinine. And of course the reverse relationship between dyestuffs and pharmaceuticals is well known: many of the early druggists experimented with dyes and this process has continued into this century as the story of Paul Ehrlich and the discovery of the treatment for syphilis, Salvarsan, shows, or that of Gelmo and Domagk's work which led to the development of sulphonamide (Youngson, 1994). Nelson also points out that it is doubtful whether X-ray analysis would ever have been developed by any group with the specific objective of trying to find a means for better medical diagnosis of maladies of internal organs (Nelson, 1959).

There are also many examples of more direct relevance, of drugs originally developed for one purpose which have actually proved more successful in other indications. The general message must be that options in rewards of development are potentially large but difficult to quantify.

24.2.18 Concerning risk and risk diversification

A portfolio is more than just the sum of its constituent projects. The Merchant of Venice, very wisely, did not convey all his trade goods in one ship. Similarly, the drug developer will generally have a number of projects in development and it is the riskiness of the total portfolio which is relevant rather than the individual projects. If the pharmaceutical company has some degree of risk aversion, it may not automatically prefer the portfolio with the largest expected return. It might, for example, prefer a portfolio for which the expected return was lower but more certain. The disadvantage of relying on an index

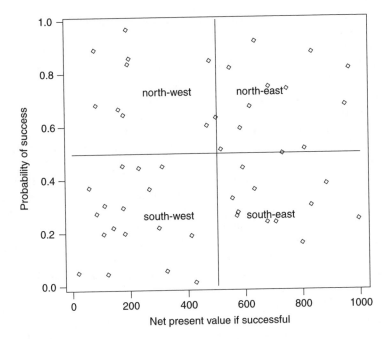

Figure 24.3   Candidates for a portfolio.

like the Pearson index to select individual projects is that it uses expected value as the criterion for selection. It has been suggested that a portfolio of appropriate projects might be selected by constructing what may be referred to as a risk–reward grid. Such a grid is illustrated in Figure 24.3, where a set of candidate projects in development are plotted according to the expected reward if successful and the estimated probability of success.

Management consultants: (1) Executioners disguised as judges. (2) Those who, having failed in drug development themselves, advise others how to do likewise.

It is implicit in the risk–reward grid that any project which lies either further 'north' or further 'east' or further in both directions than another must be more desirable to a developer. The best projects are those which lie in the north-east quadrant and the worst those which lie in the south-west. North-west projects are low in value but high in certainty and south-east projects are high-risk high-reward. The argument then goes that a wise developer will eliminate the south-western projects, obviously keep whatever few north-eastern projects he has and also hold a mix of south-eastern and north-western: the former as exciting speculations and the latter as dull but safe bets in order to diversify his risk.

This theory is wrong on a number of counts (Senn, 1998a). First, the probability of failure does not constitute an adequate index of the downside risk of a project, for reasons discussed earlier. Suppose that the project is highly speculative because it is unlikely to pass toxicological investigation but not otherwise expected to be problematic.

Its overall probability of success will be low but the sum which will have to be paid to find out whether it is successful or not will also be low. Thus the project is not, in fact, particularly risky. We do not consider that a person who holds one ticket in a national lottery is running a great risk, even though his chances of losing are considerable. On the other hand, a market trader who bets more than his merchant bank can afford on the Japanese stock market is following a risky strategy, even though his chances of success are many thousand times greater than the individual holding the lottery ticket. And a merchant is risking much when the collateral is a pound of flesh, however probable it may be that he can discharge his debt. In short, the important cost dimension is missing entirely from the risk–reward grid. In fact, for a number of cheap but speculative projects, the probability that at least one may be successful may exceed the probability that a single far less speculative project, whose expected development cost is equal to the overall cost of the speculative projects, will succeed. Thus, a portfolio consisting of such projects is actually relatively safe. Secondly, as our discussion of the Pearson index shows, even where costs are included, projects cannot be compared on the basis of total cost, reward if successful and overall probability of success. Thus, quite apart from the missing dimension, using *overall* probability of success and *overall* reward is not an appropriate way to compare projects.

An analysis in terms of means and variances of returns might be superior, as was famously considered in Nobel prize-winner Markowitz's much cited paper (Markowitz, 1952). Here portfolios can be compared in terms of both the expected return and variances. For given expected return one prefers a less risky (lower variance) portfolio. Similarly, for a given variance one prefers a higher expected return. The efficient frontier is the set of all portfolios that will give the highest expected return for a given variance. Note, however, that this is a theory that applies to portfolios, not projects, and this raises the issue whether it is possible to evaluate projects independently in order to establish the risk of a portfolio: for example, two of the drugs in consideration might have a similar mode of action.

24.2.19 The economic value of finding out more about treatments with possible application to pharmacogenetic subgrouping

Evidently, if patients respond differently to treatment, the value of a given treatment varies from patient to patient. If the information as to who would benefit and who would not were free, it would seem logical to acquire it. One of the great hopes (in fact for many it is more than a hope it is a firm belief) attending pharmacogenetics is that it will deliver tailor-made medicine (Mayor, 2007). From the pharmaceutical provider's point of view, of course, such testing is likely to result in a smaller market and in practice it is not free. Therefore the case for pharmacogenetic subgrouping is perhaps not so obvious for the drug developer (Smith, 2003), and since costs to the developer are passed on to the health care provider, perhaps not so obvious for society either. Pharmacogenetics is the subject of Chapter 25 and the economics of pharmacogenetics will also be treated briefly, but there the perspective will be mainly statistical and genetic rather economic. Here, I consider the issue briefly from a more economic perspective using the important but neglected paper of Kwerel (1980). There is not space for me to go into this paper in full detail and all I will attempt here is to convey some impression of its contents.

The paper treats the production of information by a monopoly pharmaceutical provider and shows that, despite the fact that a monopoly position is held, it can still be in the interest of the provider to test pharmaceuticals further than the minimum legally required amount provided that the price can be adjusted as a result of the test. Such a situation is referred to as *responsive pricing*. Actually, Kwerel (1980) is not specifically concerned with subgrouping, let alone pharmacogenetics; nevertheless, much of the argument carries over to this application. Specifically, Kwerel considers the case of testing for the frequency of a side-effect where the frequency is unknown for sure but something might be believed about it. This is easily described in a Bayesian framework. Suppose that at time 0, prior to carrying out testing, the expected value of the probability π of the side-effect is π_0 and that at time 1, after carrying out testing, its effect is π_1; then the martingale property of Bayesian forecasts (Senn, 2002a) requires that $E_0[\pi_1] = \pi_0$, where $E_0[.]$ is expectation at time zero. In other words, it is rational to believe that *on average* testing will leave the probability unchanged, although in practice it will increase or decrease. This is somewhat different from the case of pharmacogenetic subgrouping where one might believe that further testing will leave the average probability of a side-effect unchanged over time but resolve it into different values per subgroup. Nevertheless, Kwerel's model can be adapted to say something about this case also and, in any case, has importance for the economics of drug development more generally.

Further elements of the model used by Kwerel (1980) are b, the benefit of using the drug, L, the loss due to side-effects, and p, the price. It is assumed that all of these are measured in the same units on a scale from 0 to 1 and that a single decision maker takes them all into account. It is also assumed that the only decision made on behalf of any given patient (which may of course be made repeatedly at appropriate intervals) is whether or not to take one unit of the drug. Next, it is assumed that benefit is uniformly distributed over all patients in the interval 0 to β, $\beta > \pi L + p$. In that case, the probability that a given patient has a positive net benefit is

$$\int_{\pi_L+\beta}^{\beta} \frac{1}{\beta} \, db = 1 - \frac{\pi L + p}{\beta}. \tag{24.2}$$

If it is assumed that all patients who have a positive net benefit take the drug, then if C is the marginal cost of selling one drug, the marginal revenue per sale is $p - C$ and per potential prescription is proportional to

$$\left(1 - \frac{\pi L + p}{\beta}\right)(p - C). \tag{24.3}$$

For a market of (potentially) N (discounted) prescriptions, (24.3) would have to be multiplied by N in order to get the total marginal value. Note, however, that in (24.3), since sales depend on the patient or the patient's agent (let us use the word *consumer*), π is the consumer's perceived probability. The pharmaceutical sponsor (let us use the word *producer*) may have a different probability. Note that (24.3) attains its maximum when

$$p = \frac{C + \beta - \pi L}{2}, \tag{24.4}$$

at which value the marginal revenue is

$$\frac{(\beta - \pi L - C)^2}{4\beta}. \tag{24.5}$$

Kwerel (1980) shows, however, that unless the producer believes that the side-effect is rarer than does the consumer, there will be no benefit to the producer in carrying out any testing unless the producer can change the price. However, even if the producer believes that the side-effect is more common than does the consumer, there might be some value in testing if it will resolve uncertainty. In what follows, we shall use the basic marginal revenue model of Kwerel (1980) but adapt it for the case where genotyping divides patients into two groups of differing risk of a side-effect.

We suppose the following values apply: $\beta = 1$, $L = 2$, $C = 0.2$, $\pi = 0.08$, where π is the consumers' perceived risk. Actually, the manufacturer has carried out genotyping and knows that the patients can be divided into two groups, those who with probability $\phi = 0.86$ have a risk of $\pi_1 = 0.05$ of side-effect and those who with probability $(1 - \phi) = 0.14$ have a risk of $\pi_2 = 0.3$ of side-effect. Note that this implies that the producer knows that the average risk is $\phi\pi_1 + (1 - \phi)\pi_2 = 0.085$, which is actually higher than the value of 0.08 that the consumer perceives it to be. Despite this, it is in the producer's interest to release the information. Figure 24.4 illustrates why. The solid curve shows revenue as a function of price. The optimal price using (24.4) is 0.52 and the marginal revenue at this optimal price using (24.5) is 0.102. The dotted curve shows the situation that would apply were all patients low risk. The optimal price would be 0.55 and the revenue would be 0.122. The dashed curve shows the situation if the market consisted of high-risk patients only. The optimal price would be 0.3 and the return would only be 0.01. For any price above 0.4, no return can be made in such a market.

Given this combination, however, it is in the producer's interests to reveal the information, lose all the high-risk patients as potential customers, but shift the price to 0.55 gaining a marginal revenue of $0.86 \times 0.122 = 0.105$, from low risk patients only, which is slightly higher than before.

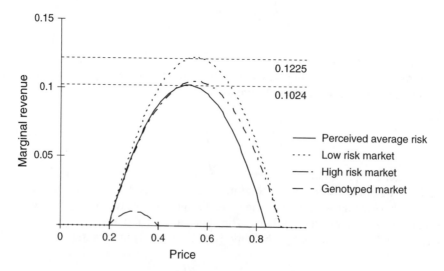

Figure 24.4 Illustration of value of genotyping patients. See text for explanation.

24.2.20   Concerning numbers needed to treat (NNTs)

This particular approach to summarizing the effects of treatment is, alas, all too common in pharmaco-economics. It was discussed in Chapter 8. Decision analysis does require the use of probabilities and NNTs are more closely related to these than are, for example, log-odds ratios. This is not an excuse, however, for reporting NNTs from clinical trials, even if they have a pharmaco-economic purpose. Summarizing results requires an additive scale and applying results may require more extensive modeling (Senn, 1998b, 2004). Thus, even if NNTs were useful at the point of application, they would not be useful in reporting individual trials. They are, for example, an unpromising scale for a meta-analysis (Smeeth *et al.*, 1999).

References

Anderson A (2007) Interview: Michael Rawlins. *Prospect* February (131), pp. 20–23.

Bass EB, Wills S, Fink NE, *et al.* (2004) How strong are patients' preferences in choices between dialysis modalities and doses? *American Journal of Kidney Diseases* **44**: 695–705.

Bergman SW, Gittins JC (1985) *Statistical Methods for Pharmaceutical Research Planning.* Marcel Dekker, New York.

Burman C-F, Senn SJ (2003) Examples of option value in drug development. *Pharmaceutical Statistics* **2**: 113–125.

Burman C-F, Grieve AP, Senn S (2007) Decision analysis in drug development. In: Dmitrienko A, Chuang-Stein C, Agostino R (eds), *Pharmaceutical Statistics Using SAS: A Practical Guide.* SAS Institute, Cary, NC, pp. 385–428.

Chaudhary MA, Stearns SC (1996) Estimating confidence intervals for cost-effectiveness ratios: An example from a randomized trial. *Statistics in Medicine* **15**: 1447–1458.

Corazza M, Favaretto D (2007) On the existence of solutions to the quadratic mixed-integer mean-variance portfolio selection problem. *European Journal of Operational Research* **176**: 1947–1960.

Detsky AS (1985) Using economic analysis to determine the resource consequences of choices made in planning clinical trials. *Journal of Chronic Diseases* **38**: 753–765.

Dixit AK, Pyndick RS (1994) *Investment under Uncertainty.* Princeton University Press, Princeton.

Drummond M (1995) Economic analysis alongside clinical trials – problems and potential. *Journal of Rheumatology* **22**: 1403–1407.

Dudley RA, Harrell FE Jr, Smith LR, *et al.* (1993) Comparison of analytic models for estimating the effect of clinical factors on the cost of coronary artery bypass graft surgery. *Journal of Clinical Epidemiology* **46**: 261–271.

Fenn P, McGuire A, Phillips V, Backhouse M, Jones D (1995) The analysis of censored treatment cost data in economic evaluation. *Medical Care* **33**: 851–863.

Gittins J, Pezeshk H (2000) A behavioral Bayes method for determining the size of a clinical trial. *Drug Information Journal* **34**: 355–363.

Grieve AP (1996) Bayesian statistics and the C/E-acceptability curve derived from clinical trials data. (Personal communication).

Grieve AP (1998) Issues for statisticians in pharmaco-economic evaluations. *Statistics in Medicine* **17**: 1715–1723; discussion 1741–1713.

Harrell F (1996) *Statistical Methods for the Evaluation of Health Care.* International Society for Clinical Biostatistics, Budapest. [Abstract].

Harrell F (1999) *Semiparametric Modeling of Health Care Cost and Resource Utilization.* Available at: http://biostat.mc.vanderbilt.edu/twiki/pub/Main/FHHandouts/slide.pdf.Accessed: 5 April 2007.

Hilden J (1987) Reporting clinical trials from the viewpoint of a patient's choice of treatment. *Statistics in Medicine* **6**: 745–752.

Kwerel ER (1980) Economic welfare and the production of information by a monopolist – the case of drug testing. *Bell Journal of Economics* **11**: 505–518.

Lindley DV (1997) The choice of sample size. *Statistician* **46**: 129–138.

Luce BR, Simpson K (1995) Methods of cost-effectiveness analysis – areas of consensus and debate. *Clinical Therapeutics* **17**: 109–125.

Markowitz HM (1952) Portfolio selection. *Journal of Finance* **7**: 77–91.

Mayor S (2007) Fitting the drug to the patient. *British Medical Journal* **334**: 452–453.

Mugford M (1996) *How does the method of cost estimation affect the assessment effectiveness in health care?* PhD, Oxford University, Oxford.

Nelson R (1959) The simple economics of basic scientific research. *Journal of Political Economy* June: 297–307.

O'Hagan A (1988) *Probability: Methods and Measurement.* Chapman and Hall, London.

O'Hagan A, Luce B (2003) *A Primer on Bayesian Statistics in Health Economics and Outcomes Research.* Medtap, Bethesda, NC.

O'Hagan A, Stevens JW (2001) A framework for cost-effectiveness analysis from clinical trial data. *Health Economics* **10**: 303–315.

O'Hagan A, Buck CE, Daneshkah A, *et al.* (2006) *Uncertain Judgements.* John Wiley & Sons, Inc., Hoboken.

Parmigiani G (2002) *Modeling in Medical Decision Making: A Bayesian Approach.* John Wiley & Sons, Ltd, Chichester.

Pearson AW (1972) The use of ranking formulae in R&D projects. *R&D Management* **2**: 69–73.

Petitti DB (2000) *Meta-Analysis, Decision Analysis and Cost-Effectiveness Analysis.* Oxford University Press, Oxford.

Pitman EJG (1965) Some remarks on statistical inference. In: *Proceedings of the International Research Seminar, Berkeley (Bernoulli-Bayes-Laplace Anniversary Volume).* Springer, New York, pp. 209–216.

Regan P, Senn SJ (1997) Project prioritisation in drug development: a case study in collaboration. In: French S, Smith JQ (eds), *Bayesian Decision Analysis.* Arnold, London.

Rittenhouse BE (1997) Exorcising protocol-induced spirits: making the clinical trial relevant for economics. *Medical Decision Making* **17**: 331–339.

Rittenhouse BE, Dulisse B, Stinnett AA (1999) At what price significance? The effect of price estimates on statistical inference in economic evaluation. *Health Economics* **8**: 213–219.

Rutten-van Mölken M, Vandoorslaer EKA, Jansen MCC, Vanessenzandvliet EE, Rutten FFH (1993) Cost-effectiveness of inhaled corticosteroid plus bronchodilator therapy versus bronchodilator monotherapy in children with asthma. *Pharmacoeconomics* **4**: 257–270.

Senn SJ (1996) Some statistical issues in project prioritization in the pharmaceutical industry. *Statistics in Medicine* **15**: 2689–2702.

Senn SJ (1998a) Further statistical issues in project prioritization in the pharmaceutical industry. *Drug Information Journal* **32**: 253–259.

Senn SJ (1998b) Odds ratios revisited. *Evidence-Based Medicine* **3**: 71.

Senn SJ (2001) The misunderstood placebo. *Applied Clinical Trials* **10**: 40–46.

Senn SJ (2002a) A comment on replication, p-values and evidence, S.N. Goodman, Statistics in Medicine 1992; 11: 875–879. *Statistics in Medicine* **21**: 2437–2444.

Senn SJ (2002b) Ethical considerations concerning treatment allocation in drug development trials. *Statistical Methods in Medical Research* **11**: 403–411.

Senn SJ (2004) Added values: controversies concerning randomization and additivity in clinical trials. *Statistics in Medicine* **23**: 3729–3753.

Senn SJ (2007) Drawbacks to noninteger scoring for ordered categorical data. *Biometrics* **63**: 296–299.

Senn SJ, Rosati N (2002) Project selection, decision analysis and profitability in the pharmaceutical industry. In: *Business Briefing: Pharmatech 2002.* World Markets Research Centre Ltd, London, pp. 18–21.

Senn SJ, Rosati N (2003) Editorial: Pharmaceuticals, patents and competition – some statistical issues. *Journal of the Royal Statistical Society Series A – Statistics in Society* **166**: 271–277.

Smeeth L, Haines A, Ebrahim S (1999) Numbers needed to treat derived from meta-analyses – sometimes informative, usually misleading [see comments]. *British Medical Journal* **318**: 1548–1551.

Smith R (2003) The drugs don't work. *British Medical Journal* **327**, http://www.bmj.com/cgi/content/full/327/7428/0-h, accessed online on 18 September 2007.

Spiegelhalter DJ (1982) Statistical aids in clinical decision making. *Statistician* **31**: 19–36.

Spiegelhalter DJ, Abrams KR, Myles JP (2003) *Bayesian Approaches to Clinical Trials and Health-Care Evaluation*. John Wiley & Sons, Ltd, Chichester.

Talias MA (2007) Optimal decision indices for R&D project evaluation in the pharmaceutical industry: Pearson index versus Gittins index. *European Journal of Operational Research* **177**: 1105–1112.

Torrance G (1996) Current experience with guidelines for economic evaluation in Canada. *Drug Information Journal* **30**: 507–511.

Ungar W (1997a) The choice of pharmacoeconomic study design during drug development – Part 1. *Pharmacoepidemiology and Drug Safety* **6**: 391–397.

Ungar W (1997b) The choice of pharmacoeconomic study design during drug development – Part 2. *Pharmacoepidemiology and Drug Safety* **6**: 399–407.

Urquhart J (1996) Pharmaco-economic evaluation – terms of reference. International Society for Clinical Biostatistics, Budapest. [Abstract].

van Hout BA, Al MJ, Gordon GS, Rutten FF (1994) Costs, effects and C/E-ratios alongside a clinical trial. *Health Economics* **3**: 309–319.

Willan AR, Briggs AH (2006) *Statistical Analysis of Cost-effectiveness Data*. John Wiley & Sons, Inc., Hoboken.

Youngson RM (1994) *Prescription Drugs*. Harper-Collins, Glasgow.

Zipfel A (2003) Modeling the probability-cost-profitability architecture of portfolio management in the pharmaceutical industry. *Drug Information Journal* **37**: 185–205.

Concerning Pharmacogenetics, Pharmacogenomics and Related Matters

'When I use a word,' Humpty Dumpty said, in a rather scornful tone, 'it means just what I choose it to mean – neither more nor less.'

Lewis Caroll, *Through the Looking Glass*

25.1 BACKGROUND

Many pharmaceutical companies seem to be pinning their faith on the 'omics', – genomics, transcriptomics, metabonomics, proteomics and other gnomic sciences – to provide the magic bullets that will cure the disease of spiralling cost and falling discovery rates from which the industry believes, rightly or wrongly, that it suffers. The spectacularly successful advances in *understanding* of molecular genetics that characterized the second half of the last century, and which continue in this, will surely, it is argued, deliver similar advances in *therapy*. Arising to deal with the wealth of data that molecular genetics delivers, we have computational developments, including the apparently new science of bioinformatics. Statisticians have also been busy in considering the implications for statistical analysis and design that these new forms of data deliver. In particular there has been much work on the design and analysis of experiments using so-called microarrays (Wit and McClure, 2004) and also on new approaches to handling multiplicity. In fact, developments in controlling the false-discovery rate (Benjamini and Hochberg, 1995) discussed in Chapter 10 have been very much associated with the sort of multiple testing problems that arise in genetics.

At this stage I feel the need of providing some penetrating insight as to what exactly the difference between pharmacogenetics and pharmacogenomics is. Alas, I cannot oblige. Nebert, in his informative and thought-provoking essay, despite having a subsection headed 'Pharmacogenetics and pharmacogenomics defined,' fails to do so (Nebert, 1999). He claims that pharmacogenetics is, 'the study of variability in drug response due to heredity' (p. 248) and then implies that pharmacogenomics is somehow to do with the development of novel drugs based on sequencing the whole **genome**. However, he admits that the two terms have been used interchangeably. For those who are interested in ephemeral sources, when I looked at *Wikipedia* on 6 March 2007 it said 'The terms pharmacogenomics and pharmacogenetics tend to be used interchangeably, and a precise, consensus definition of either remains elusive.' Of course, it may say something quite different when *you* look at it. In this chapter I shall take the Humpty Dumpty line on linguistics: words mean what I say they mean. That is, whatever the difference between pharmacogenetics and pharmacogenomics may or may not be, this chapter is about differences (presumed or real) in the effect of treatment due to genetic variation between patients, how to detect such differences and what to do with them. From now on I shall use the term *pharmacogenetics* to describe this field.

Many of the statistical issues that arise in connection with pharmacogenetics arise at the stage of drug discovery and research rather than of drug development. As such, they do not fall within the scope of this book. However, everything that survives drug research becomes the business of drug development and although many aspects of clinical trial design and analysis are not greatly altered because questions to do with genetic variability arise, some *are*. It is these aspects that form the subject matter of this chapter.

Some terminology of genetics will probably be helpful in understanding this chapter and the paragraphs that follow are particularly indebted to Robert Elston's excellent article (Elston, 2000) and the wonderful book by Ziegler and König (2006).

What makes human being differ genetically is that at particular positions or *loci* (singular **locus**) on the human genetic code, the code can vary, or present in various alternative **alleles**. The word *gene* has been used in various differing ways in genetics. Originally, it was more often used to mean allele and latterly it has often been more precisely used to mean locus. The former usage is analogous to the statistician's term level and the latter to factor (Elston, 2000). Medical statisticians, including myself, have also been similarly inconsistent in their terminology. For example, we often say treatment to mean *either* active treatment *or* placebo but often to mean active treatment *as opposed to* placebo. The former is using treatment as a *factor*, analogous to *locus* and the latter as a *level*, analogous to *allele*.

A further complication arises in genetics, however, and that is to do with the distinction between a gene and its effects. The human genetic code is contained in sequences known as chromosomes. There are 23 pairs of these sequences. For 22 pairs, known as autosomes, the two members of a pair are very similar. The remaining pair determines sex. Two so-called X chromosomes make a female, and an X and a Y a male. Because of this pairing it is usually the action of two paired alleles (except for some loci for males) that determines the physical consequences of genetic inheritance. In this connection the word *genotype* is used to indicate a particular variant in terms of genetic code and *phenotype* to indicate a particular variant in terms of physical expression. So, for example, two individuals might both have brown hair and so not vary in terms of phenotype. However, since an allele for brown hair is dominant over one for red hair, one of the individuals could have two alleles for brown hair and the other one brown and one red. They would thus differ in terms of genotype. Where the two alleles possessed by an individual at a given locus are the same then the individual is said to be *homozygous* (as regards that locus). Where the alleles are different, the individual is *heterozygous.* In general, sticking with a two-hair-colour system, there would be three genotypes: homozygous for brown (two brown alleles), homozygous for red (two red alleles) and heterozygous (one brown and one red allele).

If a characteristic is inherited by *autosomal dominant inheritance* (ADI) (Ziegler and König 2006) then it is sufficient for an individual to have inherited the relevant allele for the phenotypic characteristic associated with it to be expressed. Examples of diseases that are ADI are Huntington's chorea and myotonic dystrophy. Being autosomal, the relevant loci is on one of the 22 pairs of autosomes and hence males and females are equally affected. For *autosomal recessive inheritance* (ARI), it is necessary for two copies of the relevant alleles (one from each parent) to be inherited. An example of an ARI disease is cystic fibrosis. Other forms of inheritance, X-chromosomal both dominant and recessive (of which haemophilia is famously an example) and Y-chromosomal are discussed in Ziegler and König (2006) but will not be considered here.

Note, however, that in pharmacogenetics we are not just interested in diseases but also, for example, in genetic ability to metabolize drugs or, possibly, to respond to drugs in terms of receptors. Also, the simple scheme of dominant and recessive does not cover all situations. In that connection, consider an analogy to dose–response models and suppose that we consider inheritance of a particular allele at a given locus and classify each individual in a population as having zero, one or two *doses* (to use a term not normally used in genetics!), that is to say copies, of the allele. Obviously we could have very different possible 'dose–response' models. (Here response is either the probability of a particular phenotype occurring or even directly some quantitative phenotypic outcome, that is to say a phenotypic *degree*.) Consider the three curves in Figure 25.1. The curves are conceptual only because only observable at three points corresponding to 0, 1 or 2 on the *X* axis. They show three very different situations, dominant, recessive and *additive*. For all three there is full response at two copies and none at zero copies; for one copy there is (near) full response for dominant, (near) zero response with recessive and a response that is half-way between the two for 'additive'

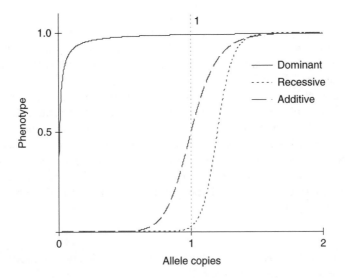

Figure 25.1 Phenotypic response to genotypic score.

(Elston *et al.*, 1999). However, the three curves concerned were actually produced using the same Hill equation (see Chapter 21), namely

$$Y = \frac{X^\gamma}{X^\gamma + \delta^\gamma}, \tag{25.1}$$

but with different settings for δ and γ. Where a dichotomous phenotype is being observed and the response in Figure 25.1 is the probability of this response, this probability is referred to as a *penetrance*.

Further complications to the above situation can arise because there can be more than two types of allele at one locus (the ABO human blood type system is a famous example) and also because genes may act together as regards some phenotypic manifestation but not always be inherited together. However, the above scheme is already sufficiently complicated for the purpose of discussing many issues that arise in clinical trials, so these further issues will not be considered here.

A further important concept in genetics is that of *Hardy–Weinberg equilibrium*. This is a statement about a relationship between allele and genotype frequencies that strictly speaking applies only to infinite, perfectly mixed populations with random mating and no evolutionary selection. The details of this are unimportant for the purposes of this chapter except that, as regards trial design, the relationship it implies between the homozygous and heterozygous groups for a locus with two alleles, A with probability p, and a with probability $1 - p$, are as follows:

Genotype	Alleles	Probability
Homozygous A	AA	p^2
Heterozygous	Aa	$2p(1 - p)$
Homozygous a	aa	$(1 - p)^2$

Figure 25.2 plots the probability of the three genotypes as a function of the frequency of allele a when Hardy–Weinberg (H-W) equilibrium applies. (Note, however, that there are reasons why the patients in a clinical trial might *not* exhibit H-W equilibrium, and this point is mentioned briefly below.)

Genetics is a fascinating field to which I am a very inexpert guide, although I do claim to know something about sources of variation and their identification in clinical trials (Senn, 2001, 2003). The reader who wishes to know more about genetic epidemiology is referred to the articles and book already cited. For specific issues of 'associating genes to drug response,' the paper by Katz with that title is recommended (Katz, 2002). Also extremely useful is the paper by Balding, although this is not specifically about pharmacogenetics (Balding, 2006). Papers by Elston (2000) and Kelly *et al.* (2005) are particularly useful for trial design.

Pharmacogenetics: A cutting-edge science that will start delivering miracle cures the year after next.

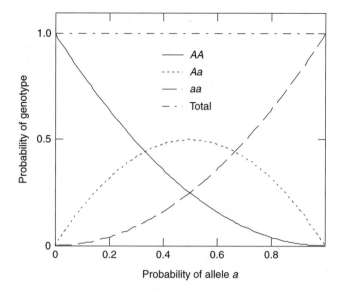

Figure 25.2 Illustration of Hardy–Weinberg equilibrium. Probability for each of three genotypes as a function of the probability of allele *a*.

In the rest of the chapter I shall be considering a very simple (perhaps unrealistically simple) model of drug–gene interaction. The interaction will be assumed to be moderated by a single locus for which it is assumed that there can be only two alleles. However, this will be sufficient to show that the search for genetic modifiers of treatment will be difficult. In practice it will be worse than this simplified case will suggest.

25.2 ISSUES

25.2.1 Due to genetic variability most treatments only work in a minority of patients

This claim is often made (Smith, 2003) and it may or may not be true, but for many treatments and diseases we simply do not know *whether* or not it is true. My position here is *not* that I *don't believe* in genetic variability but rather that I *do* believe in human gullability (or at least that many humans seem genetically disposed towards it).

Of course there are some proven gene-by-treatment interactions. However, as far as I am aware, most of them have been 'pharmacokinetic' rather than 'pharmacodynamic', that is to say that have been differences in what the body does to the drug not in what the drug does to the body. Thus, famously the cytochrome P450 2D6 enzyme is involved in metabolizing many drugs and also shows many genetic variants (Mayor, 2007; Nebert, 1999) and genetic factors affecting drug metabolism have been suspected at least since the early 1970s (Cascorbi *et al.*, 1970). Nevertheless, showing that there is genetic interaction for the elimination of some pharmaceuticals is far from demonstrating that genetic variation is an important treatment effect modifier in general.

Consider Table 25.1, which is based on Senn (2004). This shows results from a series of two trials involving the same patients. The patients have been identified according to whether they were a 'responder' or 'non-responder' not only in the first trial but also in the second. Their response has been determined by comparing the outcome when they were given active treatment with that when given placebo. And since they were treated in each of the two cross-overs with both active treatment and placebo their response can be estimated in a controlled fashion in each. The set of two trials clearly consists of 24 patients who respond and 8 who do not.

Now consider Table 25.2. This shows a very different situation. There are 18 patients who responded in both trials, a rather lower number than previously. On the positive side it appears that there are only 2 patients who responded in neither. We now have some intermediate results where 6 patients responded in the first trial and not the second and 6 who did not respond in the first trial did respond in the second. In fact in this (admittedly extreme) example we seem to have complete independence of response since $18/24 = 3/4$ of those who responded in the first trial responded in the second and $6/8 = 3/4$ of those who did not respond in the first trial responded in the second.

Now consider Table 25.3. This shows the result after the first trial *before the second has been conducted*. But to which of case 1 and case 2 does it apply? The answer is *either*; the data in the table apply equally well to either case. Thus, from having observed only one cross-over trial we do not know whether the observed response is permanent or transitory. In other words, Table 25.1 gives evidence for patient-by-treatment

Table 25.1   Patients in two cross-over trials: case 1.

First cross-over	Second cross-over		
	Responders	Non-responders	Total
Responders	24	0	24
Non-responders	0	8	8
Total	24	8	32

Table 25.2   Patients in two cross-over trials: case 2.

First cross-over	Second cross-over		
	Responders	Non-responders	Total
Responders	18	6	24
Non-responders	6	2	8
Total	24	8	32

Table 25.3   Patients in one cross-over trial: case 1 or 2.

First cross-over	Second cross-over		
	Responders	Non-responders	Total
Responders	?	?	24
Non-responders	?	?	8
Total			32

interaction, Table 25.2 gives evidence against it, and Table 25.3 says precisely nothing about it.

All of this is, in my opinion, extremely obvious. One can hardly complete a statistical education without encountering two-way analysis of variance and then learning the initially mysterious fact that unless there is replication, then although one can fit row and column effects one cannot fit their interaction. (I remember encountering this in the first year of my undergraduate course and still associate it in my mind with Freund's fine book (Freund, 1971), where it appears on pp. 409–412.) Replication is the key to detecting interaction, but hardly any trial provides it at the level of patient, at least if by replication we mean repeated random assignment as opposed to merely repeated measurement during one period of observation. Cross-over trials are rare enough, but repeated cross-overs are like hen's teeth. Random variation works strange wonders; it can throw up curious patterns across centres, as discussed in Chapter 14 and by Senn and Harrell (1997) and Senn and Hildebrand (1991), or between episodes of treatment for a given patient, as discussed in Chapters 2, 17 and 18 and by Senn (1998, 2003) and unless we calculate carefully, we are liable to mistake mere noise for a signal.

Yet, astonishingly, not only does this particular point regularly catch out trialists but even their statistical collaborators are not immune. Identifiability in clinical trials is treated in more detail in Section 25.2.2 below.

An example where individual response has received serious attention in clinical trials is actually one where ironically it is likely to be least important and of least consequence if detected, namely that of individual bioequivalence. This issue was discussed in Chapter 22. The key, as everybody has recognized, is replicated cross-overs. This is discussed in Section 25.2.3 below.

25.2.2   Identifiability in clinical trials

Table 25.4, which is based on table 1 of Senn (2001) is a crude classification of sources of variation seen in clinical trials.

Table 25.4   Sources of variation in clinical trials.

Label	Source	Description
A	Between treatments	The average difference between treatments over all randomizations (and hence over all patients). The 'true' mean difference between treatments.
B	Between patients	The average difference between patients. (Averaged over both experimental and control treatments.)
C	Patient-by-treatment interaction	The extent to which the difference between treatments differs from one patient to another. (Equivalently, the extent to which the difference between patients being given the same treatment depends on treatment given.) This source of variation reflect both gene-by-treatment interaction and interactive effects due to the patient's current and past environment and personal history
D	Within-patient error	The variability shown from treatments period to treatment period when the same patient is given the same treatment

Table 25.5 Identifiability and clinical trials.

Type of trial	Description	Identifiable effects	Error term
Parallel	Each patient receives one treatment	A	B+C+D
Cross-over	Each patient receives each treatments in one period only	A and B	C+D
Repeated period cross-overs (sets of n-of-1 trials)	Each patient receives each treatments in at least two periods	A and B and C	D

If we now look at the ability of various types of clinical trial to resolve total variation, then the situation is as illustrated in Table 25.5, which is also taken from Senn (2001). We can see that, as discussed above, a single cross-over trial is not capable of distinguishing between sources of variation C and D. This is the situation discussed in Section 25.2.1. A slight caveat must be entered here. If more than two treatments are being studied in a cross-over trial, then some partial identification of treatment-by-patient interaction is possible. This is because in a cross-over trial in n and t treatments in t periods the $nt - 1$ degrees of freedom resolve into $n - 1$ for patients and $t - 1$ for each of treatments and periods. This leaves $nt - n - 2t + 2$ for error. If $t = 2$ the degrees of freedom reduce to $n - 2$, which is fewer than the number of patients. However, if $t \geq 3$ then the residual degrees of freedom for even moderately sized trials exceed the number of patients and this means that some partial identification is possible (Senn, 2002; Senn and Hildebrand, 1991). Nevertheless, full identification requires full replication of patient–treatment combinations.

The classic parallel-group trial is not only incapable of distinguishing between C and D but also of distinguishing between B and C. What applies to cross-over trials applies *a fortiori* to parallel-group trials. However, most clinical trials are parallel-group trials. Hence, I repeat the claim I made in Section 25.2.1 that we simply do not know whether most variation seen in clinical trials is genetic because we have not done the studies to investigate this claim.

25.2.3   Cross-over studies for detecting gene-by-treatment interaction

Since patients differ by more than their genes, patient-by-treatment interaction provides an upper bound for gene-by treatment interaction (Senn, 2001). This has two implications. It means that if we find good evidence that the element of patient-by-treatment interaction is small, it suggests that there is not much point looking for gene-by-treatment interaction. On the other hand, it also means that although replication is the key to detecting interaction, as indicated in section 25.2.1, we do not have to have replication at the level of the patient; it would be sufficient to group patients by allele pairs at a particular locus to study the possible gene-by-treatment interaction.

Nevertheless, where repeated cross-over trials are feasible it suggests that a promising way to establish indication and treatment combinations with *potential* for pharmacogenetics would be to run such trials and see whether there is a genuine element of patient-by-treatment interaction. Repeated cross-over trials can also be regarded as sequences of n-of-1 trials (Senn, 2002) and this particular approach of looking for patient-by-treatment interaction was illustrated in Chapter 18.

Pharmacogenetics: A subject with great promise.

Kalow *et al.* have made a telling analogy to twin studies (Kalow *et al.*, 1998, 1999). Such studies have been beloved of psychologists studying heritability of mental traits, in particular intelligence. However, an even more perfect genetic match than a twin is the patient himself or herself, and such matching is provided by cross-over trials. In this way one can exclude that any variation from occasion to occasion when the same individual is repeatedly treated is genetic. This degree of variation within subjects is used to judge that between. That is to say, source D of Table 25.5 provides the means of judging the importance of C.

Of course, what the repeated cross-over achieves is whole-genome matching, since every patient is his or her own control. This has advantages and disadvantages. The advantage is that the residual variation (D) is completely purged of any gene-by-treatment interaction. The disadvantage is that C reflects the total genome-by-treatment interaction in the trial (and also further nongenetic interactions associated with patients). Obviously this means that having identified that patient-by-treatment interaction exists we still face the task of finding which, if any genes, are responsible or, at the least, of finding reliable markers of the response. What the repeated cross-over provides is the means of implementing a powerful omnibus test of gene-by-treatment variation. Such an omnibus test can be extremely useful because, if it is used wisely, many unsuitable indication–treatment combinations could be eliminated for further study.

Nevertheless, many treatments are not suitable for studying through cross-over trials. There is little choice then but to look at groupings of patients by genotype. That is to say, since replication at the level of patient becomes impossible, replication has to be achieved at the level of genotypic groupings. Inevitably, of course, patients deemed genetically similar for the particular grouping in mind will be genetically different as regards other possible groupings. This topic will be discussed further in section 25.2.5.

25.2.4 Genotypic score and phenotypic response

The essence of the discussion in this section applies to parallel-group as well as cross-over trials. However, the two arms of a parallel-group trial introduce certain largely irrelevant complications in discussion and to avoid being distracted by them it will be best if we have the following situation in mind. We have a two-period cross-over trial comparing active treatment with placebo, each patient receiving the two treatments in a completely random order. We suppose that period and carry-over effects can be ignored and for each patient we have calculated the difference between active and placebo, which we call Y. This is what I have referred to elsewhere as the *basic estimator* approach (Senn, 2002). The patients have been grouped by genotype and we now consider ways of establishing whether the treatment effect differs between genotypes.

In particular, consider a locus with two possible alleles and suppose we score patients according to the number of copies they have of one of the two alleles chosen. (We can, of course make the choice arbitrarily of which of the two we designate, but it would probably be more usual to choose the rarer one.) We can then give patients a genotypic score of 0, 1 or 2 depending on how many copies they have. In studying response we then have to make a choice how to analyse the response as a function of the score. There are two issues that have to be addressed. The first will be very familiar to most statisticians and is the choice of basic statistical framework (Balding, 2006). In generalized linear model terms, we need to choose the error–link function combination. For binary outcomes a Bernoulli error and logit link would be popular. If the outcome is continuous we may use Normal errors and an identity link. (This is the case we assume in the rest of this section.) However, there is another issue that is very important and that is implicit in Figure 25.1; that is that we need to decide whether the phenotypic response is dominant, recessive or somewhere in between.

The issue is closely related to that of dose-metameter discussed in Chapter 20 and indeed to that of analysing dose-response in general. Take the case where there are two alleles A or a at a locus, and we have equal numbers of patients for the three genotypes AA, Aa or aa. Actually, this is rather unlikely since if Hardy–Weinberg equilibrium applies and both alleles are equally frequent (and hence occur with probability 1/2), this implies that each of the homozygous genotypes has probability 1/4 of occurring and the heterozygous genotype has probability 1/2. However, although unlikely in a large population, the split 1/3, 1/3, 1/3 is possible in a given trial and it actually makes the discussion of what follows easier. So let use assume for the moment that we have $3n$ patients in total and n for each genotype. We shall return to the issue of genotypic frequencies in section 25.2.5.

Now suppose that we have a continuous response, which we will fit through a linear model with genotype as a factor with three levels, 0, 1 or 2 corresponding to the number of a alleles. The score is the number of copies of a for a given genotype and dominance will be discussed in terms of a. Table 25.6 gives weights for possible contrasts we could fit. We will consider the dominant and recessive contrasts in due course, but for the moment concentrate on the linear and quadratic ones.

Given the three mean responses from each of the three genotypic groups of patients, $\overline{Y}_0$, $\overline{Y}_1$, and $\overline{Y}_2$ we can construct linear contrasts by multiplying by the weights in the table. For the reader who is familiar with `proc glm` or `proc mixed` of SAS the weights in the table are the multipliers that can be used in connection with the `estimate` statement. We assume, however, that genotype will have been fitted as a factor with three levels, which is to say two degrees of freedom. The variance of any

Table 25.6 Possible contrasts for comparing genotype.

Genotype score	AA 0	Aa 1	aa 2	
Outcome	$\overline{Y}_0$	$\overline{Y}_1$	$\overline{Y}_2$	Variance multiplier
Linear	−1	0	1	2
Quadratic	−1	2	−1	6
Dominant	−2	1	1	6
Within a	0	−1	1	2
Recessive	−1	−1	2	6
Within A	−1	1	0	2

one of the contrasts used is estimated by taking the mean square error from the linear model, $\hat{\sigma}^2$, dividing this by n and multiplying by the appropriate variance multiplier term in the final column of the table.

The contrasts are grouped in orthogonal pairs: linear and quadratic, dominant and within a, recessive and within A. The first of any such pair of contrasts is inherently likely to be of more interest than the second and linear, dominant and recessive contrasts were specifically targeted for discussion in Elston *et al.* (1999) and Kelly *et al.* (2005). However, in order to make a connection between one-degree and two-degree-of-freedom tests, in what follows we shall concentrate on the linear and quadratic *pair*. Each of the two contrasts is formed by multiplying the $\overline{Y}_i$ values by the corresponding multiplier and adding. If we then square each of the two contrasts, weight inversely by the variance multiplier and add together, we find

$$\frac{\left(\overline{Y}_2 - \overline{Y}_0\right)^2}{2} + \frac{\left(2\overline{Y}_1 - \overline{Y}_0 - \overline{Y}_2\right)^2}{6}$$

$$= \frac{2}{3}\left(\overline{Y}_0^2 + \overline{Y}_1^2 + \overline{Y}_2^2 - \overline{Y}_0\overline{Y}_1 - \overline{Y}_0\overline{Y}_1 - \overline{Y}_1\overline{Y}_2\right) \tag{25.2}$$

$$= \sum_{i=0}^{2}\overline{Y}_i^2 - \frac{\left(\sum\limits_{i=0}^{2}\overline{Y}_i\right)^2}{3} = \sum_{i=0}^{2}(\overline{Y}_i - \overline{Y}_.)^2.$$

Finally, if from the sum of these two squared weighted contrasts we form the average by dividing by 2, then we obtain

$$\frac{\sum\limits_{i=0}^{2}(\overline{Y}_i - \overline{Y}_.)^2}{2}. \tag{25.3}$$

In other words, the average of the two weighted squared contrasts, being a mean sum of squares between genotypes, is the numerator of an F-statistic. In fact, if we divided each of the weighted squared contrasts by $\hat{\sigma}^2/n$, then each has an F-distribution with $\nu_1 = 1, \nu_2 = 3n - 3$ degrees of freedom and their average has an F-distribution with $\nu_2 = 2, \nu_2 = 3n - 3$.

Furthermore, the square of a t_{ν_2} variable is an F_{1,ν_2} so that we can represent one-degree-of-freedom t-tests involving the linear and quadratic contrasts and the two-degree-of-freedom F-tests in a simple diagram. This has been done in Figure 25.3, where, however the asymptotic case has been considered. This means that instead of t-statistics we can have standard Normal statistics and that we can replace the F-statistic by twice its value which, asymptotically, has a chi-square distribution with two degrees of freedom. The tests illustrated are at the 5% level.

In the figure, the areas outside the two dashed vertical lines (that is to say to the left of the leftmost and to the right of the rightmost) defines the critical region if we decide only to test the linear contrast. If we use the global two-degree-of-freedom chi-square test then the critical region is outside the circle. The point, however, is that this two-degree-of-freedom test is really a more efficient version of the two-degree-of-freedom test based on testing each of the linear and quadratic contrasts at a level designed to control the probability of making at least one type I error at 5%. (This means that each

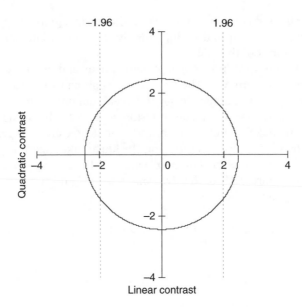

Figure 25.3 Comparison of single one-degree-of-freedom *t*-test and single two-degree-of-freedom *F*-test. The latter has a critical region outside the circle and the former outside the dashed lines.

test will be carried out at level α such that $0.05 = 1 - (1 - \alpha)^2$, which implies that $\alpha = 1 - \sqrt{1 - 0.05} \approx 0.025$.) This situation is illustrated in Figure 25.4. This alternative test is significant if either the linear or quadratic test is significant at the 2.5% level (two-sided), which means that the critical region is outside of the square defined by the horizontal and vertical dashed lines. Under the null hypothesis, the integral of the joint probability density function over the square is the same as over the circle.

The point is, however, that one of these dimensions is plausibly much less important than the other. We do not expect the quadratic contrast to be different from zero if the linear one is not. We do not expect a difference between the heterozygous genotype and the average of both homozygous genotypes if there is no difference between different homozygous genotypes. Thus the general approach represented in Figure 25.4, whether we implement a test using the two linear contrasts or more efficiently using the *F*-test with two degrees of freedom is not a good idea. The fact that the two-contrasts approach is not a good idea will seem obvious to most, since the quadratic contrast does not seem very sensible, but the fact that the *F*-test is closely related to it and hence also not a good idea may seem less obvious to some and is our excuse for having treated it at such length.

In other words, what we should use instead, rather than the two-degree-of-freedom test, is a one-degree-of-freedom test based on the linear contrast only. Similar arguments could be made for the other two pairs of contrasts. The first member of the pair is probably more interesting than the second. This raises the issue whether the particular contrast chosen is the best. This depends, of course on the true relationship between genotype and phenotypic response. We investigate the implication of this is the next section.

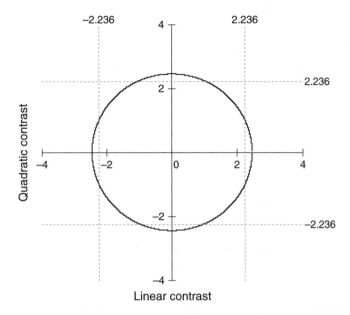

Figure 25.4 Illustration of two approaches to testing, each using two degrees of freedom. The dashed lines represent independent *t*-tests using linear and quadratic contrasts. The one critical boundary for the two-degree-of-freedom *F*-test is a circle.

25.2.5 The design of pharmacogenetic studies

Suppose now more generally that we have a more realistic model in which we expect, unless we take steps to do something about it, that the proportion of patients in our large trial should follow Hardy–Weinberg equilibrium (H-W) as regards the relationship between allele frequency and genotype frequency. Note that this implies that there is no direct relationship between chosen locus and probability of having the disease. It is a requirement of H-W that we do *not* have selection. Usually this refers to evolutionary selection but selection into a clinical trial is just as important. Suppose, in fact, that the genotype predicts presence or absence of disease with allele *a* dominant for disease. We then expect no *AA* patients in the trial and, since the proportion of patients in the population eligible for the trial is $2p(1-p)+(1-p)$ we have

$$P(Aa) = \frac{2p(1-p)}{2p(1-p)+(1-p)^2} = \frac{2p(1-p)}{(1+p)(1-p)} = \frac{2p}{1+p},$$

$$P(aa) = \frac{1-p}{1+p} = \frac{1-p}{1+p}.$$

(25.4)

However, we will assume that is *not* the case and that the three genotypes are present in H-W frequencies. This might be reasonable if the gene-by-treatment interaction is to do with drug metabolism rather than the disease process itself.

It now turns out that the least-squares estimate for both dominant and recessive cases is very simple. We just create two groups by pooling patients appropriately and then calculate the average treatment effect for the group. (Remember that in our simple

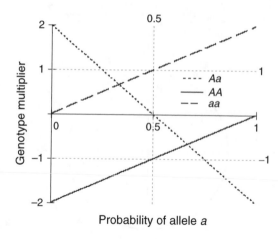

Figure 25.5 Multipliers for the three genotypic groups where a linear contrast is being applied as a function of the relative frequency of allele *a* and Hardy–Weinberg equilibrium applies.

example these means are calculated on pairwise differences patient by patient between treatments.) In other, words, we either compare the means of all the values in *AA* and *Aa* with the mean of all the values in *aa*, or the mean of all the values in *AA* with the mean of all the values in *Aa* and *aa*.

For the linear case, things are more complicated. It is only in the situation where the two homozygous genotypes are equally frequent that the weights we have in Section 25.2.4 apply. Otherwise the weights for *AA*, *Aa* and *aa* are $-2(1-p)$, $2(1-2p)$, $2p$ as illustrated in Figure 25.5, where the weights (multipliers) are represented by three lines as a function of the relative allele frequency (or probability) of *a*. The two associated with the homozygous genotypes *aa* and *AA* are increasing. The former starts at zero and rises to 2. The latter starts at -2 and rises to zero. For the heterozygous group *Aa*, the weights start at 2 and fall to -2. For any value of the probability of allele *a*, the sum of three weights, as must be the case for a true contrast, are zero. The reason for this behaviour is that, although in the additive model, for which the linear contrasts is appropriate, the stronger phenotypic response to *a* compared to *A* is given by the homozygous *aa* group, for low values of the probability of *a*, *Aa* is so much more common than *aa* that it becomes of value to use the *Aa* group to measure the effect of *a* relative to *AA*. However as the frequency of *a* rises and passes 0.5, the greater uncertainty is the effect of *A* and so the weight for the *Aa* group becomes negative. At the midpoint, where the probability of *a* is 0.5, there is no point using the *Aa* group at all. The justification of the weights is given in the technical appendix.

Associated with each of the three schemes of contrasts one can calculate the variance of the resulting estimates. Figure 25.6 gives the factor by which σ^2/N would have to be multiplied to obtain the variance for each of the three ordinary least-squares estimators of phenotypic response. A fourth 'universal' contrast has been added. This does not correspond to any least-squares solution, except the linear one when $p(a) = 0.5$. It is, however, universally unbiased for any of the three models of inheritance being considered here: dominant, recessive, additive (linear). This is because it uses the contrast $(-1, 1)$ and hence does not use the heterozygous group at all. In fact, it is

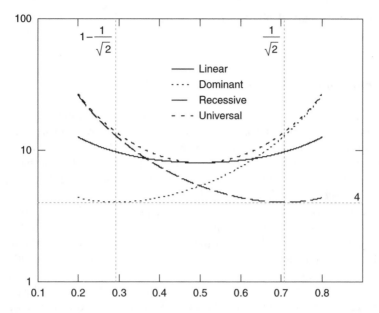

Figure 25.6 Variances of four possible estimators of phenotypic response. The graph shows the factor by which σ^2 / N must be multiplied to obtain the variance of the given contrast.

the vexed question of how to treat the heterozygous group that governs the choice of contrast, and if this is ignored altogether then unbiased estimation follows.

Bioinformatics: A science devoted to finding wonderful patterns in databases.

However, as the figure shows, this comes at a cost since the variance of the universal contrast is always at least as great as that from any of the other three. Furthermore, the figure also shows that even if one is able to choose the correct model, unless the allele relative frequency of a, $p(a)$, is favourable for the particular model, then a very high price will be paid in variance. For the recessive model the optimal value can be shown to be $p(a) = 1/\sqrt{2}$. The reason this is the optimal value is not hard to explain: it is the value for which $p(aa) = p^2 = \left(1/\sqrt{2}\right)^2 = 1/2$. This is thus the value that makes the two phenotypes to be compared equally frequent. By argument of symmetry, the optimal value for the dominant case is $p(a) = 1 - (1/\sqrt{2})$.

In short, the variances of contrasts to estimate gene-by-treatment interactions are likely to be high. The lowest values achievable are $4/N$, these being the values corresponding to the recessive and dominant case for $p(a) = 1/\sqrt{2}$ or $1 - (1/\sqrt{2})$ respectively. Note, however, that the vertical scale on Figure 25.6 is logarithmic and the situation can be very much worse than this. In other words, the problems described in Chapter 9 regarding subgroup analysis are likely to be particularly acute for pharmacogenetic trials. Not only are we likely to have inefficient contrasts, we are also unlikely to know for sure which one to use.

For further discussion of pharmacogenetic trials see Elston *et al.* (1999) and Kelly *et al.* (2005).

25.2.6   Enrichment studies

The problems outlined Section in 25.2.5 suggest that one possible strategy would be to over-sample from particular genotypes. If a particularly rare allele were suspected to be relevant, this might seem an attractive strategy. The trial would be enriched by recruiting a higher number from the relevant genotypes. The problem with this approach, as was discussed in Chapter 9, is that sampling unequally from presenting patients in a clinical trial delays the time until some total target number has been recruited. This generally makes it an unattractive proposition. There is the added difficulty with a genetic characteristic that prospective patients will have to be genotyped before the decision to recruit has been made. In my view, the practical difficulties are considerable. Targeted trials are discussed by Maitournam and Simon (2005).

There is some relationship also to the literature on screening patients for compliance using run-ins prior to randomization. The idea behind this is to increase the proportion of patients in a clinical trial who will benefit because taking the medicine, and this is clearly similar to increasing the proportion of patients who will benefit because genetically suitable. The screening-for-compliance literature, however, is far from unanimous that this is a good idea. For sceptical views see Brittain and Wittes (1990) and Schechtman and Gordon (1993).

25.2.7   The economic case for gene-based therapy is obvious

It is not so obvious and depends rather on circumstances. Tailor-made therapy implies the use of what has been referred to as *theranostics*, although it could just as well have been called *diapeutics*, that is to say, strategies involving diagnostic tests and therapeutic interventions. Such combinations are not confined to genetics. For example, receptor status is regarded as being an important determinant of therapy in breast cancer, and indeed there is no medical intervention that does not require diagnosis of condition in the first place. The real issue as regards this chapter is whether additional genotype testing is valuable in most indications.

I am rather sceptical about this and often explain my scepticism as follows. Suppose we could divide patients into two groups, approximately equally frequent, and that the genetic difference between them was enormous, one group suffering a huge chromosomal deficiency which was reflected by a much worse prognosis, and that the diagnostic procedure for identifying patients as one group or the other was free and easily implemented. These are more or less the best possible conditions for providing scope for studying gene-by-treatment and theranostic strategies. Well, this situation exists. The two groups are males and females, with life expectancy at birth for males being some 4–5 years less in the USA and UK compared to females. Yet remarkably few medicines are prescribed differently for males and females.

Nevertheless, there are cases where, in principle at least, theranostic strategies would be beneficial for the patient. But the condition is not just that the diagnostic part of the strategy has the potential to bring good news or bad, it has to have the potential for changing choice of therapy. If all that happens is that prognosis changes but no different strategy is indicated, then genotyping of the patient brings no advantage.

Pharmacogenetics: A mysterious science by which marketing expect to increase profits while reducing the scope for drugs.

This issue was also considered in Chapter 24 by adapting an economic model of Kwerel (1980) and the interested reader may wish to consult section 24.2.19. Here it will be investigated again from scratch using a somewhat different approach.

A simple, if unrealistic case may help fix ideas. Suppose that we have a drug D_1 for which the treatment effect is modulated by a single locus with two alleles, one of which shows complete dominance. Phenotype is then determined by presence or absence of this allele. We assume that the phenotype, Pt_1, occurs with probability θ and has the greater benefit from the treatment being investigated. Without loss of generality we can transform the scale of benefit so that the benefit associated with the common phenotype is 1 and that with the other phenotype, Pt_0 is 0. Hence the expected benefit of a patient who has not been genotyped in taking the treatment is

$$B_n = (1 - \theta) \times 0 + \theta \times 1 = \theta. \tag{25.5}$$

We now suppose that there is an alternative treatment, D_2 whose benefit is not modulated by phenotype. We suppose that the benefit associated with this treatment is ϕ. Now, for there to be any point in testing we must have

$$0 < \phi < 1, \tag{25.6}$$

because if $\phi > 1$ we would always choose D_2 in preference to D_1, irrespective of phenotype, and if $\phi < 0$, we would always choose D_1 in preference to D_2. Now suppose that we can assign individuals with perfect discrimination to phenotype. Then with probability $1 - \theta$ the individual will be diagnosed as Pt_0, we shall choose D_2 and the benefit will be ϕ, whereas with probability θ he or she will be diagnosed as Pt_1, we shall choose D_1 and the benefit will be 1. Hence the benefit of the strategy of testing and treating is

$$B_t = (1 - \theta) \phi + \theta. \tag{25.7}$$

Since the difference between (25.7) and (25.5) is

$$B_t - B_n = (1 - \theta) \phi, \tag{25.8}$$

which is always positive, there is value in carrying out the test.

However, this simple example somewhat overstates the case. First, there are great difficulties in developing any treatment that does not show adequate efficacy on average. One is unlikely to get far enough down the road of drug exploration to investigate gene-by-treatment interaction, especially with so many genes to look for, without some satisfactory efficacy on average. This implies that if ϕ is the standard set by D_2, then D_1 does not reach it on average unless $\phi \leq \theta$. Hence in practice we may have something like

$$B_t - B_n \leq (1 - \theta)\,\theta. \tag{25.9}$$

Now consider the rewards that the sponsor has to seek to bring in the same revenue (net of all costs except the cost of diagnosis) with a theranostic strategy, rather than 'one size fits all'. If previously the net revenue per patient was R it now has to become R/θ. To the price, must be added a not inconsiderable sum to pay for the extra development, and somebody has to pay for the diagnostic procedure. See Danzon and Towse (2002) for discussion of the economic difficulties and also Kwerel (1980) for a general discussion of the economics of testing.

Of course this does not mean that the case for theranostic strategies cannot be made. In fact, the issues are very similar to those affecting use of any diagnostic procedure. There are some cases where we take auxiliary information into account; warfarin is an example where relatively sophisticated treatment strategies have been used for a long time now (Holford, 1986; Sheiner, 1969). By the same token, however, there are also grounds for some scepticism. We could dose patients by body weight, but usually don't; or with greater difficulty but more value, even by clearance, but usually don't. The general aversion that the marketing departments of the pharmaceutical industry show for diagnosis using bathroom scales contrasts strangely with their love of pharmacogenetics. Perhaps, however, far from being part of the cure for increasing costs of development, pharmacogenetics is part of the problem.

References

Balding DJ (2006) A tutorial on statistical methods for population association studies. *Nature Reviews. Genetics* **7**: 781–791.

Benjamini Y, Hochberg Y (1995) Controlling the false discovery rate – a practical and powerful approach to multiple testing. *Journal of the Royal Statistical Society Series B – Methodological* **57**: 289–300.

Brittain E, Wittes J (1990) The run-in period in clinical trials. The effect of misclassification on efficiency. *Controlled Clinical Trials* **11**: 327–338.

Cascorbi HF, Blake DA, Helrich M (1970) Differences in biotransformation of halothane in man. *Anesthesiology* **32**: 119.

Danzon P, Towse A (2002) The economics of gene therapy and of pharmacogenetics. *Value Health* **5**: 5–13.

Elston RC (2000) Introduction and overview: statistical methods in genetic epidemiology. *Statistical Methods in Medical Research* **9**: 527–541.

Elston RC, Idury RM, Cardon LR, Lichter JB (1999) The study of candidate genes in drug trials: Sample size considerations. *Statistics in Medicine* **18**: 741–751.

Freund JE (1971) *Mathematical Statistics*, 2nd edition. Prentice-Hall, Englewood Cliffs. NJ.

Holford NH (1986) Clinical pharmacokinetics and pharmacodynamics of warfarin. Understanding the dose – effect relationship. *Clinical Pharmacokinetics* **11**: 483–504.

Kalow W, Tang BK, Endrenyi L (1998) Hypothesis: comparisons of inter- and intra-individual variations can substitute for twin studies in drug research. *Pharmacogenetics* **8**: 283–289.

Kalow W, Ozdemir V, Tang BK, Tothfalusi L, Endrenyi L (1999) The science of pharmacological variability: an essay. *Clinical Pharmacology and Therapeutics* **66**: 445–447.

Katz DA (2002) Associating genes to drug response. *Drug Information Journal* **36**: 751–761.

Kelly PJ, Stallard N, Whittaker JC (2005) Statistical design and analysis of pharmacogenetic trials. *Statistics in Medicine* **24**: 1495–1508.

Kwerel ER (1980) Economic welfare and the production of information by a monopolist – the case of drug testing. *Bell Journal of Economics* **11**: 505–518.

Maitournam A, Simon R (2005) On the efficiency of targeted clinical trials. *Statistics in Medicine* **24**: 329–339.

Mayor S (2007) Fitting the drug to the patient. *British Medical Journal* **334**: 452–453.

Nebert DW (1999) Pharmacogenetics and pharmacogenomics: why is this relevant to the clinical geneticist? *Clinical Genetics* **56**: 247–258.

Schechtman KB, Gordon ME (1993) A comprehensive algorithm for determining whether a run-in strategy will be a cost-effective design modification in a randomized clinical trial. *Statistics in Medicine* **12**: 111–128.

Senn SJ (1998) Applying results of randomised trials to patients. N of 1 trials are needed [letter; comment]. *British Medical Journal* **317**: 537–538.

Senn SJ (2001) Individual therapy: new dawn or false dawn. *Drug Information Journal* **35**: 1479–1494.

Senn SJ (2002) *Cross-over Trials in Clinical Research* (2nd edition). John Wiley & Sons, Ltd, Chichester.

Senn SJ (2003) Author's reply to Walter and Guyatt. *Drug Information Journal* **37**: 7–10.

Senn SJ (2004) Individual response to treatment: is it a valid assumption? *British Medical Journal* **329**: 966–968.

Senn SJ, Harrell F (1997) On wisdom after the event [comment] [see comments]. *Journal of Clinical Epidemiology* **50**: 749–751. [Comment in *Journal of Clinical Epidemiology* **50**(7): 753–755 (1997); **51**(4): 301–303 (1998)].

Senn SJ, Hildebrand H (1991) Crossover trials, degrees of freedom, the carryover problem and its dual. *Statistics in Medicine* **10**: 1361–1374.

Sheiner LB (1969) Computer-aided long-term anticoagulation therapy. *Computers and Biomedical Research* **2**: 507–518.

Smith R (2003) The drugs don't work. *British Medical Journal* **327**. Available at: http://www.bmj.com/cgi/content/full/327/7242/0-h.

Wit E, McClure J (2004) *Statistics for Microarrays*. John Wiley & Sons, Inc., Hoboken.

Ziegler A, König F (2006) *A Statistical Approach to Genetic Epidemiology*. Wiley-VCH, Weinheim.

25.A   TECHNICAL APPENDIX

25.A.1   Ordinary least-squares weights for linear contrasts

We take the score for allele copies and divide by 2 so that they become 1/2, 1. We do this is in order to define the rate of change (linear slope) in terms of moving from lowest to highest number of copies, which is then comparable to dominant and recessive models. Call this new score X. We then have that

$$E[X] = (1-p)^2 \times 0 + 2p(1-p) \times \frac{1}{2} + p^2 \times 1 = p,$$

$$E[X^2] = (1-p)^2 \times 0 + 2p(1-p) \times \frac{1}{4} + p^2 \times 1 = \frac{p(1+p)}{2}, \qquad (25.10)$$

$$V[X] = E[X^2] - \{E[X]\}^2 = \frac{p(1+p)}{2} - p^2 = \frac{p(1-p)}{2}.$$

Now, in general the formula for a regression of a response Y on a predictor X is

$$\hat{\beta} = \frac{\text{cov}(X, Y)}{\text{var}(X)} = \frac{E[\{X - E(X)\}Y]}{\text{var}(X)} = \frac{\sum \theta_i \{X_i - \overline{X}\} Y_i}{\text{var}(X)}$$

$$= \sum w_i Y_i, \quad \text{where} \quad w_i = \frac{\theta_i \{X_i - \overline{X}\}}{\text{var}(X)}. \tag{25.11}$$

Where θ_i is the probability with which a given pair (X_i, Y_i) occur

The three possible genotypes yield three possible values of θ_i and correspondingly of X_i. Hence, the three possible values of the numerator for W_i in (25.11) are

$$(1-p)^2 \times (0-p) = -p(1-p)^2,$$

$$2p(1-p) \times (\tfrac{1}{2} - p) = p(1-p)(1-2p), \tag{25.12}$$

$$\text{and} \quad p^2 \times (1-p) = p^2(1-p).$$

and from (25.10) the denominator is $\{p(1-p)\}/2$ from which we have weights for the regression of

$$
\begin{array}{ll}
AA & -2(1-p) \\
Aa & 2(1-2p). \\
aa & 2p
\end{array}
\tag{25.13}
$$

Note that only when $p = \tfrac{1}{2}$ does (25.13) reduce to weights of -1, 0, 1.

Glossary

Definitions and Explanations of Some Commonly Encountered Terms

Lexicographer, n. *A pestilent fellow, who, under the pretense of recording some particular stage of a language, does what he can to arrest its growth, stiffen its flexibility and mechanize its methods.'*

Ambrose Bierce

Statistician, n. *A mathematician manqué who has abandoned the provable in favour of the probable. A being with the brain of an accountant and the soul of a philatelist. A charmless drudge.*

Guernsey McPearson

INTRODUCTION

In this glossary will be found various terms in common use in drug development and in pharmaceutical statistics. Further help may be obtained in the dictionaries and other useful works of reference listed at the end (Abercrombie *et al.*, 1990; Bannock *et al.*, 1992; Borowski and Borewin, 1989; Day, 1999; Dodge, 1993, 2006; Evans *et al.*, 1993; Everitt, 1995; Henry, 1994; Last, 1995; Martin, 1990; Nahler, 1994; Sharp, 1990; Vesey and Foulkes, 1990; Winslade and Hutchinson, 1992; Youngson, 1994). The book on subjective probability assessments in this series (O'Hagan *et al.*, 2006) also has a very useful glossary. These are the some of the various reference books I consulted while writing this one. The definitions here, however, have not been taken from these dictionaries. They thus have the value of originality, with the attendant drawback that where they are wrong, there is no quotable precedent for their being so.

Definitions

Absorption. In pharmacokinetics, the process by which treatments which are not given intravenously enter the blood stream. This process is important for the bioavailability of the product.

Statistical Issues in Drug Development/2nd Edition   Stephen Senn
© 2007 John Wiley & Sons, Ltd

ACE inhibitor. Angiotensin-converting enzyme inhibitor. A treatment for hypertension. The ace of hearts in drug development's game of poker.

Active control equivalence study. A trial with the purpose of attempting to demonstrate that an experimental treatment is similar in effects to a standard therapy.

Adaptive designs. Clinical trials in which the probability that a patient receives a given treatment is, to some extent at least, determined by the results on patients who have been treated so far. Examples are *play the winner designs* and *bandits*.

Add-on trial. A trial in which an experimental treatment is compared with a control treatment (often a placebo) in the presence of at least one other treatment. So, for example, one might compare a bronchodilator with placebo in a group of patients all of whom are receiving steroids. From one point of view all conventional clinical trials are add-on trials is some sense, since all patients will receive some element of standard care even if this only consists of nursing care, food, drink, etc.

Addition rule of probability. If A and B are two events and $A \cup B$ is the event 'A or B' and $A \cap B$ is the event 'A and B' and $P(X)$ is the probability of any event X, then the general addition rule of probability is that $P(A \cup B) = P(A) + P(B) - P(A \cap B)$. For mutually exclusive events, $P(A \cap B) = 0$, so that the rule simplifies to the *special* addition rule of probability, $P(A \cup B) = P(A) + P(B)$.

Adverse experience (or event). A putative adverse drug reaction. Any unwanted medical event obtained during treatment with a drug.

Adverse drug reactions. 'Proven' unwanted side-effects due to treatment with a drug. They are conventionally classified into two sorts. **Type A**, which are due to a 'predictable' pharmacological effect of the drug and are usually dose-dependent, and **Type B**, which are 'unpredictable' (perhaps allergic) and are usually more serious and rarer.

Allele. A variant of the genetic code at a particular **locus**. It is a more precise term for one of the two variant meanings, one is tempted to say 'alleles', of the word or logos *gene*, namely gene in the sense of levels of a factor. At each locus a single allele is inherited from each parent.

Alpha-spending approach. One of a number of frequentist approaches to sequential trials. It controls the type I error rate by proposing a time path for spending the type I error rate allowed for the trial. This avoids having to specify in advance the exact time points at which analysis must take place.

Alternative hypothesis. In the context of hypothesis testing, a hypothesis which will be 'accepted' if the null hypothesis is rejected. In drug development, the alternative hypothesis usually represents a state of nature that the sponsor would like to be able to assert as true. For example, the alternative hypothesis might correspond to the sponsor's treatment being superior to placebo.

Analysis of covariance. In the context of clinical trials, a statistical technique used for taking account of the effect of various prognostic factors on the outcome observed, with a view to obtaining a more precise estimate of the effect of the treatment itself or in order to account for accidental bias. It is more general than post-stratification and can be used, for example, for continuous prognostic covariates without having to form arbitrary groupings of patients.

Analysis of variance. A statistical technique, originally developed by R.A Fisher in connection with agricultural experiments, and used for dividing the total variability in results into various sources in order to assess the contribution of various factors, in particular that of treatment.

Area under the curve (AUC). A summary statistic calculated on repeated measures often, but not exclusively, of serum concentration in pharmacokinetic studies (where it is more properly referred to as the *area under the concentration – time curve*). But for a constant of proportionality, it is a weighted sum of individual measures, the weights being determined by the intervals between measurements and (to a certain extent) by the method of estimation used. (The trapezoidal rule is common.) Where the measurement intervals are regular, AUC gives very similar results to using the mean.

Assurance. A sort of chimeric probability in which a frequentist power is averaged using a Bayesian prior distribution. It is thus the unconditional expected probability of a significant result as opposed to the conditional probability given a particular clinically relevant difference.

Bandit design. An adaptive allocation design based on ideas of sequential decision-making with the following features. (1) Results to date are used to determine which treatment a patient will receive. (2) The patient does not necessarily receive whatever treatment is currently believed to be the best because it is recognized that there may be value in studying less-studied treatments. (3) The allocation rule attempts to maximize the (discounted) totality of future patients on the better treatment (including the one about to be treated).

Baseline comparison. A common activity which comes in two different but usually futile forms. (1) A comparison of treatment groups in terms of baseline characteristics in order to justify ignoring prognostic information in the analysis. (2) A comparison of outcomes and baselines as a means of establishing effects.

Bayes' theorem. A theorem due to Thomas Bayes (1701–1761) relating conditional probabilities of the sort $P(X|Y)$, where this is the probability X given Y, and which can be expressed in many forms. A simple form is

$$P(A|B) = \frac{P(A)P(B|A)}{P(B)}.$$

The theorem itself is uncontroversial and follows directly from the **multiplication rule of probability** but its application to providing probability statements about hypotheses has two difficulties. Suppose we have a particular hypothesis H_i in mind and have obtained some evidence E. If we wish to use the theorem to obtain $P(H_i|E)$ then we must substitute H_i for A and E for B in the equation of the theorem as given above. The first difficulty is that this requires us to evaluate a so called *prior probability* of the hypothesis $P(H_i)$. The second difficulty is even more severe. We have to evaluate $P(E)$, which is the unconditional probability of the evidence. If there are k possible hypotheses then mathematically we have the relationship

$$P(E) = \sum_{j=1}^{k} P(H_j) P(E|H_j),$$

which then involves further prior probabilities and which also in more complex cases may be difficult to evaluate.

This second difficulty can be avoided if we are only interested in the odds of one hypothesis H_i compared to another H_j. We can then evaluate expressions of the form

$$\frac{P(H_i|E)}{P(H_j|E)} = \frac{P(H_i)}{P(H_j)} \times \frac{P(E|H_i)}{P(E|H_j)}.$$

Here the ratio on the left-hand side is the posterior odds, the first ratio on the right-hand side is the prior odds and the last ratio is the ratio of likelihoods. In this form Bayes' theorem can be expressed as, 'posterior odds equal prior odds times ratio of likelihoods'.

Bayesian statistics. An approach to statistics named for Thomas Bayes (1701–1761) and which has the following features. (1) A subjective interpretation is given to probability. (2) It is accepted that one may talk of the probability of hypotheses being true and of parameters having particular values. (3) *Prior probabilities* are assigned on a personal basis to hypotheses or to parameter values. (4) These probabilities are updated in the light of evidence to become *posterior probabilities* in a way which is described by Bayes' theorem. (5) Only the prior probability and the data actually obtained are directly relevant to the assessment of the posterior probability. (Data which might have been obtained but weren't play no direct role.) (6) As a consequence of point (3), the resulting answer is valid only for the person for whom it is calculated.

Bernoulli trials. Independent trials of constant probability with binary outcomes. Repeated coin tossing is often used as an example.

Bias. A term that in statistical usage has a technical meaning as the difference between the average value in probability of an estimate and the parameter of which it is an estimate. Put formally, if θ is a parameter to be estimated and $\hat{\theta}$ is an estimate of the parameter, then $B(\hat{\theta}) = E[\hat{\theta}] - \theta$ is the bias of $\hat{\theta}$. The term has unfortunate connotations because, although in everyday speech it is taken as self-evident that unbiasedness is a good thing, a biased statistical estimator can often out-perform an unbiased one. The old statistical joke, that a statistician is one who with one foot in ice and the other in boiling water says that on average he's comfortable, is apposite.

Bias–variance trade-off. A situation in which a choice must be made between two statistics (or two statistical designs that will produce different statistics) whereby one has the lesser bias but greater variance and the other has the greater bias but lesser variance. A logical choice would be to use the statistic (or approach or design) with the lower **mean square error**. Unfortunately, the exact magnitude of the biases will not in general be known (else one could correct for them), so that there may be a dilemma in making a choice. An example is between choosing a cross-over design and a parallel-group design with the same number of observations. The former will produce an estimate with a lower variance but perhaps some bias due to carry-over. The latter will be unbiased but with a higher variance.

Binary outcome. In the context of a clinical trial, a measurement on a patient which can take one of two possible values such as 'success' or 'failure', 'alive' or 'dead', '0' or '1'.

Binomial distribution. The simplest common probability model used for binary outcomes from a series of independent trials. (Where *trial* is to be understood in the sense of the first meaning of the definition.) If n is the number of trials, θ is the probability of success in an individual trial and X is the number of successes, then the probability mass function of the binomial distribution is

$$P(X=x) = \frac{n!}{x!(n-x)!}\theta^x(1-\theta)^{n-x}$$

(where x must be an integer between 0 and n). The binomial distribution is sometimes referred to as the *Bernoulli* distribution, although this use is often reserved for the case $n = 1$.

Bioavailability. The fraction (or sometimes absolute amount) of a dose absorbed by the subject. Also sometimes the rate at which it is absorbed.

Bioequivalence study. A study usually carried out on healthy volunteers, and often as a single-dose cross-over, in which, by repeated sampling (usually of blood), it is attempted to show that the pharmacokinetic profile of an experimental treatment is very similar to that of a reference product with the same chemical structure. Such a demonstration is usually taken to mean that there is no need to carry out a full development programme on the experimental treatment, as results which are valid for the reference treatment may be presumed valid for the experimental treatment. By enabling generic companies to avoid the costs of development borne by the major pharmaceutical companies, bioequivalence studies, depending on your view, can either be seen as being a 'free lunch' for the parasites of drug development, or the weapon by which the double dragons of exclusivity and excess profit may be slain by the shining knights of competition.

Biometrics. An alternative name for statistics (and more than one hundred years old), especially if applied, intended to be applied or supposed (sometimes falsely) that it might be applied to the life sciences. In the first edition of this book I then wrote, 'The advantage of the name compared to statistics is that the general public does not understand what it means, whereas with statistics it thinks it understands what it means.' This is, however, no longer true as the general public now thinks that biometrics is the identification of human beings by fingerprints, iris-scans and DNA profiling. In this they have been misled by a group of 'scientists' who, having made unique and correct identification their sole *raison d'etre*, could not uniquely identify a correct name for what they do

Biostatistics. A term which ought to mean statistics for biology (see biometrics) but is now increasingly reserved for medical statistics.

Biostatistician. One who has neither the intellect for mathematics nor the commitment for medicine but likes to dabble in both.

Block. A term taken over from agriculture where it originally meant a group of plots in a field whose fertility might be presumed to be similar. In general in statistics a block is a group of experimental units presumed similar. In a clinical trial, for example, it might be a group of patients at a given centre. Where such blocks of similar patients exist, there are good reasons for doing the randomization within the blocks so that the treatment numbers are balanced at this level also. By extension, therefore, the word block has come also to mean any group of experimental units handled together for the purposes of randomization and treatment allocation. This second meaning is the one most commonly employed in clinical trials, where it is not unusual to find quite small block sizes used. Quite frequently the block size is smaller than is strictly necessary for the purpose of balancing treatments among patients. For example, in a trial comparing a verum (V) to a placebo (P) in which there are 12 patients per centre, a block size of 12 would be adequate for balancing treatments per centre. However, patients might be randomized to blocks of size 4. This would mean that for every set of 4 patients one of the following series of treatments would be used at random:

$$V\,V\,P\,P$$
$$V\,P\,V\,P$$
$$V\,P\,P\,V$$
$$P\,P\,V\,V$$
$$P\,V\,P\,V$$
$$P\,V\,V\,P.$$

Boundary approach. An approach to running and analysing sequential trials whereby a statistic describing the cumulative difference between treatments is plotted against a statistic which describes the amount of evidence accumulated to date and the trial is stopped if one of the pre-specified boundaries of the design is crossed.

Carry-over. The persistence (whether physically or in terms of effect) in a later period of treatment of a treatment applied in an earlier period.

Case–control study. A sort of back-to-front clinical trial, in which the primary classification is by outcome and the secondary by treatment rather than vice versa (as in a clinical trial proper). In contradistinction to a clinical trial, however, there is no assignment of treatment by an experimenter. In drug development, the case–control study is not used to learn about treatment efficacy. Its use is in epidemiological post-market surveillance for the purpose of looking at side-effects. For example, having obtained a number of cases of hepatitis for which it was known whether or not a particular type of drug had been taken, one might also deliberately choose a number of comparable controls (persons not suffering from hepatitis) with a view to establishing whether the use of the drug was independent of the status 'case' or 'control'. An established lack of such independence (together with an excess use of the drug in question among hepatitis cases) would then be considered to be an indicator that the drug may cause hepatitis.

Censored. An adjective applied to a value which is imprecisely measured due to some feature of the observation process. In medical statistics, the more usual form of censoring occurs where the true value is known to be no less than some given value (right censoring); less commonly it is known that it is no more than some given value (left censoring). If a clinical trial finishes 4 years and 3 months after a patient entered it and she is still alive, then her survival time is right-censored at 4 years and 3 months.

Change-over design. An old-fashioned and minority term for cross-over trial. If you use it you should consider a change-over to *cross-over*.

Classical statistics. See *frequentist statistics*.

Clearance. The rate of elimination of a drug divided by its concentration. The units of clearance are volume per time (for example litres per hour). Its importance as a pharmacokinetic parameter arises from the fact that although rate of elimination increases with concentration, clearance usually remains constant.

Clinically relevant difference. A somewhat nebulous concept with various conventions used by statisticians in their power calculations and incidentally, therefore, a means by which they drive their medical colleagues to distraction. It is sometimes defined as, 'the difference one would not like to miss', and where this definition is used, the trial is usually powered to make fairly small the probability of failing to conclude that there is a difference between treatments when there is in fact a clinically relevant difference. This does not imply that if the trial *does* conclude there is a difference, that this difference is clinically relevant. However, where a statistically significant difference is found, it is usually the case that the drug will continue to be studied further and a more precise evaluation of its effects will be possible. Where no statistically significant difference is found, there is a danger that development of the drug will stop altogether. Hence, the importance of, 'the difference you would not like to miss'.

Closed test procedure. A structured approach to multiple comparisons and controlling the type I error rate, whereby all higher-level hypotheses in which lower-level hypotheses are implicated must be rejected before rejection of the lower-level hypotheses themselves.

C_{max}. Concentration maximum. The maximum plasma concentration achieved (in practice, the maximum *observed*) for a drug. A term used in pharmacokinetics and bioequivalence.

Cohort study. An observational study in which the evolution of a population over time is followed in order to see which characteristics or *exposures* appear to predispose to given outcomes. Such studies are often performed prospectively. A clinical trial can be regarded as a special case of a cohort study in which patients are randomized to exposure.

Concurrent controls. Patients recruited into a trial over the same period of time over which the patients to be given the experimental treatment are to be recruited but allocated to a control treatment, with the object of providing data which, with the exception of factors under the trialist's presumed control, has been subject to the same influences as that from the experimental group.

Confidence interval. An interval associated with an estimate of an effect and loosely supposed to give an impression of the uncertainty associated with it. For example, if the 95% confidence interval for the difference between an active treatment and a placebo in a trial of asthma is 27 ml to 345 ml of FEV_1, this implies that, were we to adopt as our null hypothesis any value of the true treatment effect less than 27 ml or greater than 345 ml, we would reject this hypothesis using a conventional two-sided hypothesis test at the 5% level. Thus the values between the limits are values that would *not* be rejected. A further property is that, under repeated sampling, 95% of all 95% confidence limits for a true treatment effect will include the true treatment effect. This does not, of itself, justify the conclusion that for any *given* sample the limits produced will contain the true treatment effect with the given probability. We might, for example, know from other information that the sample standard deviation was unusually small. In that case the inclusion probability would be less than the confidence level.

Conditional probability. Used to describe the probability that an event has occurred given that another has occurred. The symbol $P(A/B)$ is conventionally used to denote the conditional probability of A given B.

Confounders. A term used in connection with observational studies in epidemiology for factors (covariates) that, while not of direct interest in themselves, are presumed to be related to the outcome of interest and which may also be associated (either positively or negatively) with a putative causal factor under study.

Conjunctive power. The probability that a number of endpoints will be jointly significant as a function of a set of presumed clinically relevant differences.

CONSORT. Consolidated Statement of Reporting Trials. Guidelines with the object of improving clinical trial reporting in the journals. See http://www.consort-statement.org/. They are extremely useful as far as they go but far less ambitious in scope or detailed than the ICH guidelines.

Cost–benefit analysis. In the context of drug development, an investigation in which a therapy is evaluated by measuring all consequences of the therapy (effects, side-effects and costs), converting them into a monetary value, discounting them and adding them.

Cost–consequence analysis. An evaluation in which costs and therapeutic effects of a therapy are measured but no decision synthesis is attempted by the evaluator, this being left, instead, to the potential user(s).

Cost–effectiveness analysis. A pharmaco-economic term for an evaluation in which a therapy is assessed in terms of the cost to achieve a given therapeutic result. The result is usually expressed as a cost per increment of effect.

Cost-minimization analysis. A study in which therapies are standardized in terms of outcome and compared in terms of cost. For example, a new treatment might be shown to be no worse therapeutically than a standard but cheaper.

Cost utility analysis. A form of cost–effectiveness analysis in which all therapeutic benefits are transferred to a common utility scale.

Continuous observations. Values such as height, weight, blood pressure and so forth which arise from a process of measurement. They are not restricted to integer values and are represented by real numbers.

Continuous reassessment method (O'Quigley design.) An approach used in phase I trials in cancer for choosing the dose of the next patient, using results from the patients treated to date, in such a way that the probability of toxicity is at some pre-specified target level.

Contrast. The difference between two effects (or some weighted combination of differences between effects).

Control. A term which can be used in a number of ways in clinical trials but which is always related to the idea of controlling for various sources of bias. In a controlled (parallel) clinical trial, the control group is a group of patients otherwise presumed similar to the patients given the experimental treatment, but who are given an alternative treatment (for example, a placebo) in order to provide a standard of comparison for the experimental treatment.

Cox regression. Another name for the proportional hazards model originally proposed by Sir David Cox in 1972.

Credible interval. A Bayesian term. An interval based on a posterior probability distribution which has been calculated by updating an uninformative prior using the likelihood according to Bayes theorem.

CRF. Case record (or report) form. The form or recording schedule on which the trial data are recorded. These are nearly always maintained on a patient-by-patient basis. See *patient diary*.

Cross-over trial. A trial in which patients are allocated to sequences of treatments with the purpose of studying differences between individual treatments. The simplest common example is of a placebo controlled trial of an active treatment in which patients are allocated at random either the sequence 'placebo followed by active' or to the sequence 'active followed by placebo'.

CTA. Clinical Trial Authorization. In the UK this is the MHRA document for authorizing clinical trials of medicinal products, replacing the older system of clinical trial certificates (CTCs) and exemptions (CTXs) on 1 May 2004.

Cumulative probability density function. A mathematical function giving the probability that a continuous random variable is less than or equal to a given value. The integral of the probability density function from minus infinity to the given value. A special name for the *distribution function* where the random variable is continuous.

Database. The graveyard of clinical research. A rubbish dump built like a library.

Data cleaning. The means by which databases are purified so that they are fit for analysis. In double-blind trials this will usually take place before the treatment code is broken. An activity which ensures that through automatic error checking, vetting and queries the database will contain only uninteresting truths and plausible lies.

Discrete observations. Values which arise from counting events and (usually) which can be represented using integer values. An example would be the number of seizures suffered in a given time interval by epileptic patients.

Disjunctive power. The probability that at least one endpoint is significant given a particular set of alternative hypotheses. (That is to say, the probability that Y_1 or Y_2 or Y_3 etc is significant: hence disjunctive.)

Distribution. In pharmacokinetics, the processes which control the transfer of the drug to and from from site of measurement to target and other tissues.

Distribution function. In probability and statistics the function giving the probability that a random variable is less than or equal to some value.

Dose escalation study. A dose-finding study in which doses are gradually increased (usually for each individual within the study but sometimes group by group) until a satisfactory response has been observed, or until unacceptable tolerability has been observed, or until there are no more doses to study.

Dose metameter. A transformation of the original scale on which a dose is measured to a scale which is presumed to permit a more simple expression of the dose-response.

Double dummy technique. A means of achieving blinding (masking) in clinical trials where two active treatments are being compared and when (as is nearly always the case) they cannot be matched. A placebo to each is then employed and patients are allocated to receive either A and placebo to B or B and placebo to A.

Drug monitoring. A regular activity carried out by pharmaceutical companies which consists of studying reports of adverse experiences, as well as other relevant data, in order to become and remain informed about the safety profile of the drug.

Dummy loading. A technique of masking (blinding) treatments where the treatments being compared have different dosing schedules. Patients being treated with treatment A, according to its schedule, are also given placebos to treatment B, administered according to its schedule, and vice versa.

Duration of action. An important, if ill-defined, concept in establishing treatment regimes. It is the length of time for which a treatment is deemed to be effective. This is often investigated in single-dose pharmacodynamic trials, although it does not necessarily follow that an appropriate dosing interval is fixed by the length of time for which the single-dose is effective.

Effect size. A measure used by meta-analysts to combine information from studies for which the original scales of measurement were different. It is the ratio of the estimated treatment effect from a study to the estimate of the standard deviation (note: *not* the standard error). Since both treatment effect and standard deviation are measured on the same scale it is 'unit free'. Its expected value is more or less independent of the size of the study but it does depend on the study population as well as on the treatment effect. Since sponsors have access to raw data and the ability to plan drug development programmes, they should have little need of this measure.

Elimination. In pharmacokinetics, the process by which the drug is permanently disposed, either specifically from the site of measurement or more generally from the body. This contrasts with distribution, which is reversible.

Elimination rate constant. Once absorption of a drug has finished, the rate at which many drugs are eliminated from the body can often be adequately expressed in terms of the equation

$$C_{\tau+t} = C_\tau e^{-kt}, \quad \tau > 0, \ t > 0, \ k > 0,$$

where $C_{\tau+t}$ is the plasma concentration at time $\tau + t$, C_τ is the concentration at some time τ after absorption has finished and k is the *elimination rate constant*. The time it takes for the concentration to reduce to a half, the so called half-life, can be calculated as $t_{\text{half}} = (\log 2)/k$

EMEA. Formerly the European Medicines Evaluation Agency, now the European Medicines Agency (but the acronym survived unchanged). The drug regulatory agency of the European Union. A statistician-free zone.

Epidemiologist. One who thinks that an odds ratio is an approximation to a relative risk as opposed to a statistician who knows the opposite.

Exploratory data analysis. The practice of studying data without preconceived notions as a means of obtaining ill-conceived ones. The art of seeing a Rembrandt in a Jackson Pollock.

Exponential distribution. This simplest of probability distributions used to describe time, t, until an event. It is sometimes also called the negative exponential distribution because its probability density function

$$f(t) = \frac{1}{\theta} e^{-t/\theta}, \quad \theta > 0, \ t > 0,$$

where θ is the expected value of t, involves a negative exponent. If the number of events arising in a given interval of time is described by the *Poisson distribution*, the time between events is described by the exponential distribution. It is the continuous analogue of the *geometric distribution*.

Factorial design. A design used for assessing the individual contribution of treatments given in combination as well as any interactive effect they may have. For example, a factorial design to assess a combination therapy of a beta blocker and a diuretic might use four treatment groups: a group which receives the two treatments together; one which receives the beta-blocker and a placebo to the diuretic; one which receives the diuretic and a placebo to the beta-blocker; and one which receives both placebos.

FDA. Food and Drugs Administration. The body, which among other things, is responsible for drug regulation in the USA. The single most important body influencing drug development and which has been responsible for many innovations and current practices in pharmaceutical statistics.

Fixed combination therapy. A combination of two or more treatments combined in one pharmaceutical formulation so that they are delivered together.

Footpoint. The point in the response cycle in a multidose study at which therapeutic effect is presumed to be at a minimum. Since this is the point of minimum protection, it is especially important to measure effect at this point when comparing drugs with different dosing schedules. Sometimes referred to as *trough*.

Free combination therapy (or drug). A therapy consisting in combining two or more individual treatments but without physically incorporating them into one formulation so that, unlike a *fixed combination*, each constituent treatment could still, in principle, be given alone.

Frequentist statistics (Also frequently and classically referred to as classical statistics.) An approach to statistics commonly encountered in the analysis of clinical trials and having the following features. (1) An interpretation of probabilities is made which relates them to the long-run relative frequency of events in a series of (hypothetical) trials is made. (2) It is denied that hypotheses or parameters can have a probability: the former are either true or false and the latter are either equal to some value or not. (3) A decision to accept or reject a hypothesis (or presumed parameter value) is made indirectly using the probability of the evidence given the hypothesis (or presumed parameter value) rather than vice versa. (4) The probability of more extreme evidence must also be taken into account. (5) The experimenter's intentions in designing the trial have a bearing on the interpretation of the results.

Futility. The probability of a trial failing to reach a significant result as calculated at some interim stage. The calculation may either assume that the original clinically relevant difference obtains or use a Bayesian approach. In the former case it is only the effect that current results have on the eventual statistic that is taken into account. In the latter case their effect on current belief is also reflected.

Geometric distribution. A probability distribution for the number of independent trials until the first success. It is a special (simple) case of the negative binomial distribution and is a discrete analogue of the exponential distribution. If X is the number of trials before the first successful trial and p is the probability of success in an individual trial, then its probability mass function is

$$P(X=x) = p(1-p)^x, \quad x = 0, 1, 2, \ldots .$$

Alternatively, if X is the number of trials, including the first successful trial, then

$$P(X=x) = p(1-p)^{x-1}, \quad x = 1, 2, \ldots ,$$

Glossary. A sort of short-commons dictionary in which the omissions are more significant than the entries.

Good Clinical Practice. Ethical and scientific standards for the conduct of clinical trials in order to protect the rights of subject and patients entered in such trials and to ensure that the results are trustworthy and useful.

Group sequential method. A frequentist approach to running and analysing sequential trials whereby hypothesis tests are carried out at agreed intervals in such a way as to ensure that the probability, for the trial as a whole, of making a type I error, given that the null hypothesis is true, does not exceed some nominal level chosen

Half-life. In pharmacokinetics, the time it takes for the concentration of a drug to be reduced to a half. It is related to the *elimination rate constant*.

Harms. A term which is being promoted by the authors of the CONSORT statement to describe any undesirable consequences of treatment.

Hazard rate. The probability of failure (usually instantaneous) given survival to date: for example, the probability that you will stop reading this book this instant having got so far. This is obviously greater than the unconditional probability of failure that you will stop this instant since you may not have got this far. (However, since you *are* reading this, it is the hazard rate and not the unconditional failure which is important.) An important concept in survival analysis. Like a probability density (see below), a hazard rate has to be defined with respect to some unit interval (in this case of time).

Historical controls. Patients who have been treated prior to the study being initiated and whose data will provide the yardstick against which current experimental results will be applied. It is often difficult to find patients who are sufficiently comparable to those being studied to make such controls useful. There is also the further problem that coincidental conditions and concomitant treatments will have changed in the meantime.

HPB. Health Protection Branch. The Canadian regulatory agency. Part of Health Canada.

Hypothesis test. A statistical procedure designed to determine whether to reject or not a null hypothesis on the basis of observed data. A procedure which, apart from the subjective choice of statistical model, alternative hypothesis and type I error rate, is completely objective.

ICH. International Conference on Harmonisation. An international forum for regulatory authorities in the European Union, Japan and the United States established in 1990. The ICH has issued more than 60 documents of regulatory guidance divided into the major areas of Quality (Q), Safety (S), Efficacy (E) and Multidisciplinary (M). Many of these are relevant to this book but the most relevant is ICH E9: Statistical Principles for Clinical Trials.

Incidence. The rate at which new cases of a disease occur in a population. Incidence must be defined with respect to a time window. (Often per year.)

IND. Investigation New Drug application. The application to the FDA, based on pre-clinical results, for permission to begin testing a pharmaceutical in humans.

Independence. The condition applying to events such that knowledge of the occurrence or nonoccurrence of one has no bearing on the probability of occurrence or nonoccurrence of the other.

Informed consent. A subject's or patient's documented agreement to participate in a clinical trial as a result of having all risks and benefit frankly and honestly explained to him or her.

Joint probability. The probability of events occurring together.

Kaplan–Meier estimator. A term from survival analysis. A statistic which was developed to estimate survival probabilities as a function of time for populations in which some observations have been *censored*.

Kaplan–Meier procedure. A method of estimating survival probabilities from data on survival times for individuals in a cohort which can handle the case where a number of the individuals are still alive, so that their eventual survival times are *censored*.

Koseisho (Ministry of health and welfare.) Japanese regulatory agency.

Label invariance. A term used in this book to designate forms of analysis which lead to essentially the same conclusions if the labels of the treatments are switched.

Latin square. Objects (for example a selection of letters from the alphabet) arranged in a square in such a way that each appears once and once only in each row and column as, for example:

$$Q U A D$$
$$U Q D A$$
$$A D Q U$$
$$D A U Q.$$

The finding of such squares is an old problem in mathematics and was, for example, studied by Euler. In statistics they find use in experimental design as a means of balancing the effects of various factors. Cross-over trials, for example, are often arranged according to Latin square designs with columns as periods, rows as patients (or group of patients) and treatments taking the place of letters.

Life table. An actuarial device for illustrating the mortality of a population by tabulating year by year the number of individuals still surviving (as well as other associated numbers such as deaths in each year, years of life lived and so forth) from an original fictional cohort of (say) 100 000 individuals subject at each year of life to the current age specific mortality of the given population. Usually life tables are calculated separately for males and females.

Likelihood. The probability of the data observed given a particular hypothesis postulated or parameter value assumed. When talking about likelihood, the statistician considers how this probability varies as the parameter value is varied. The likelihood does not in general sum to 1 over the possible parameter values. A probability distribution, on the other hand, takes the parameter (rather than the data) as being given and considers how the probability varies according to different values of the data. This summation of the probability over all possible data sets (the so called *sample space*) does sum to 1.

Likelihood principle. Roughly, the idea that inferences about unknown parameters given a sample of data should depend only on the likelihood and not, say, on any particular sampling scheme.

Linear kinetics. Used to describe the pharmacokinetics of a drug for which absorption, distribution and elimination are all proportional to the dose.

Loading dose. A nonstandard and larger than usual dose given at the beginning of a course of regular treatment in order to shorten the time until the concentration is within the therapeutic window.

Locus. A position, or sometimes a region, on the genetic code sometimes restricted to regions that are expressed or have significance in terms of *phenotype*. Roughly corresponds to the use of the word *gene* as the factor (in the sense for example of the gene for eye colour) rather than as the levels of the factor (as say in the gene for blue eyes).

Log-odds ratio. The logarithm of the *odds ratio*. A transformation very frequently used for modelling binary data. See *logistic regression*.

Logistic regression. One of many techniques which enables regression-type models to be applied to binary data. For example, a treatment may increase the probability of a cure but in practice we will only observe a cure or a failure. A regression model, if naively applied, may occasionally produce nonsensical results such as negative probabilities of a cure or probabilities in excess of 1. One way to handle this is to model on the log-odds scale, is a scale which, although unambiguously related to probability, lies between plus and minus infinity. Logistic regression is a technique for fitting models on this scale.

Marginal probability. A term used to describe the probability of a given event occurring without reference to (that is to say, unconditional upon) the occurrence of other events, in a context in which, however, certain events are being considered together. So called because in a table of bivariate (or joint) probabilities such marginal probabilities may be calculated as the marginal totals (row or column as the case may be).

Maximum likelihood. A technique for estimating unknown parameters whereby the likelihood is expressed as a function of them and the set of parameter values is chosen which makes this a maximum.

Maximum tolerated dose. The dark doppelgänger of the minimum effective dose. In practice, a dose for which there is good evidence that it is too high to be usable without there being conclusive proof that it is safe.

Mean. Unless otherwise qualified, 'mean' means 'arithmetic mean'. The sum of all the values, divided by the number of values. A precise term for what is often meant by 'average' in everyday English.

Mean square error. A term with two meanings: (1) The residual sum of squares from a regression or analysis of variance divided by the degrees of freedom which belong to it. (These degrees of freedom are generally equal to the number of observations minus the number of parameters fitted.) (2) The sum of the square of the bias of an estimator and its variance. This is a quantity that can be used to compare estimators. The smaller the mean square error is, the more useful the estimator.

Median. Any value which will divide a set of ordered values in to two. If there is an odd number of values, it is the middle value. If there is an even number of values it is conventionally taken to be half-way between the middle two values.

Meta-analysis. Also called *overview*. A term which has been introduced to cover the process of summarizing, through formal statistical means, the results from a number of trials. The usual general approach is to weight the results from individual studies inversely proportionally to their variances, so that more precise studies get more weight. If the variance that is used for weighting a given is based purely on the internal evidence from that study, this leads to a so-called fixed-effects approach. If the extent to which effects vary from study to study also contributes to constructing the study weight, this leads to a so-called random-effects approach.

MHRA. Medicines and Healthcare products Regulatory Agency. The executive body charged with drug regulation in the United Kingdom

Minimization. A procedure for allocating patients sequentially to clinical trials taking account of the demographic characteristics of the given patient and of those already entered on the trial in such a way as to attempt to deliberately balance the groups. In practice this achieves a higher degree of balance than for randomization, although the difference for even moderately sized trials is small.

Minimum effective dose. A term which combines the tricks of being both self-explanatory and difficult to define. In practice it is usually the minimum dose which has been 'proved' to have a nonzero effect, but this neither means that it is the lowest dose which has any effect nor that it is a dose which has a useful effect.

Multiple-dose study. A (usually) therapeutic trial in which repeated administrations of a treatment are given (usually in the way in which it is intended that the treatment will eventually be prescribed). The main purpose of a multiple-dose study is to examine the steady-state effects of a treatment.

Multiplication rule of probability. If A and B are two events and $A \cap B$ is the event 'A and B' and $B|A$ is the event 'B given A' and $P(X)$ is the probability of any event X, then the multiplication rule of probability states that

$$P(A \cap B) = P(A)P(B|A) = P(B)P(A|B).$$

If A and B are independent, then since $P(A|B) = P(B)$ and $P(B|A) = P(B)$ the rule simplifies to

$$P(A \cap B) = P(A)P(B).$$

Mutually exclusive events. Events which stand in that relationship to each other whereby one or other may occur separately but both cannot occur together. For such events the *addition rule* of probability is simpler than otherwise.

n-of-1 study. A trial in a single patient using repeated administrations of a treatment over a number of episodes in order to establish its effect for that patient. In a well-conducted study a control treatment will be employed and the order of administration for repeated treating with experimental and control treatments will be randomized.

Named patient basis A mode of supplying an unlicensed drug for use by a physician for a given named patient usually for compassionate grounds where the drug would not otherwise be available. Sometimes patients are allowed to continue at the end of a trial on this basis. Various regulations cover such use. Also known as *treatment IND* is the USA.

NDA. New Drug Application. The dossier submitted to the FDA at the end of a phase III programme if the sponsor deems it successful in order to see whether the FDA agrees.

Nonparametric analysis A term used rather loosely with various meanings but which may be defined here as a method of analysis which makes rather fewer assumptions about the shape and form of the data than are 'required' for a parametric analysis.

Normal distribution. Sometimes called the Gaussian distribution, which term, however, while honouring the work of Gauss, inadequately recognizes the contribution of De Moivre and Laplace. A probability distribution whose frequency density is given by

$$f(X=x) = \frac{1}{\sigma\sqrt{2\pi}} e^{-\frac{1}{2}[(x-\mu)/\sigma]^2}, \quad -\infty < x < \infty, \ \sigma > 0,$$

a definition which will leave anyone in need of a glossary like this one no wiser than before.

The Normal distribution is a probabilistic model which often approximates continuous biological data *fairly* well, especially if these are suitably transformed. (For many measurements a log-transformation is appropriate.) Its importance, however, derives largely from the fact that it approximates the *sampling distribution* of various *statistics* even better. The Normal distribution is also the limiting distribution for a number of others. For example, as the degrees of freedom for the t-distribution increase, the t-distribution approaches the Normal. The curve given by the equation above is bell-shaped, and symmetrical, achieves its maximum at μ, the mean of the distribution, and has points of inflection at $\mu - \sigma$ and $\mu + \sigma$. (σ is the standard deviation of the Normal distribution.) If the frequencies of a very large sample of blood pressures from a general population were represented by a histogram, the curve joining the tops of the bars would *fairly* closely resemble that given by the formula above. In drug development, the Normal distribution is often used to model continuous measurement data such as blood pressure, lung function and so forth, either on the original scale or, as mentioned above, after some suitable transformation.

Normal ranges. Limits to the laboratory values usually seen by a given laboratory and which are then used to interpret values actually obtained. They are supposed to reflect differences in local assays and also (sometimes) local populations.

Number needed to treat (NNT) The number of patients you would need to treat with one treatment rather than another in order to see one extra positive outcome. It is the reciprocal of the absolute risk reduction.

Null hypothesis. A term used in frequentist statistics in connection with hypothesis testing. The null hypothesis is a hypothesis which is assumed (for formal testing purposes) to hold true until evidence has been accrued which leads to its rejection. For example, one might assume, for the time being, that a drug was ineffective but attempt to show that this 'null hypothesis' was untrue.

Odds. A means of expressing probabilities often used by gamblers and sometimes by statisticians in certain contexts. If the probability of something occurring is 1/5 (or 0.2) then the odds against it occurring are 4 to 1, representing the ratio of the probability of nonoccurrence, 4/5 (or 0.8) to the probability of occurrence, 1/5 (or 0.2). The concept is sometimes claimed to be too complex for physicians to understand, although gambler and readers of popular newspapers appear to have no difficulty with it.

Odds ratio. In a clinical trial, the ratio of the odds in the experimental group to the odds in the control group. Similar ratios can be used in cohort and case–control studies.

Option. A right without an obligation. For example, the right to buy a share at a nominated price on a given day with no obligation to do so or the right to continue to develop a drug with no obligation to do so.

Ordered categorical variable. A variable which may be used to classify observations onto an ordered scale. An example is where patients are asked to rate the control of asthma using the scale 'poor', 'fair', 'moderate' and 'good'. If we accept that moderate is better than fair (there is some ambiguity in the English language regarding this) then we can allocate scores 1, 2, 3 and 4 to these four categories. A score of 4 is then better than one of 3, but is not twice as good as one with 2. Such scores used to be analysed using methods developed for (unordered) categorical data, but this is inefficient and special techniques for ordered categorical data are now often used.

Ordinary least squares. A technique for fitting models to data which minimizes the sum of the squares of the deviations between the observed values and those predicted from the model. For example, the arithmetic mean is the ordinary least-squares estimator from a set of data values, $x_1, x_2, \cdots x_n$ since the function

$$\sum_{i=1}^{n} (x_i - a)^2$$

is minimized when a is set equal to the arithmetic mean. It is a commonly used and easily applied fitting technique which has 'optimal' properties under certain cases. In some case it gives the same results as applying the method of maximum likelihood. For example, in the case above, if $x_1, x_2, \ldots, x_n$ is a sample of observations drawn at random from a Normal distribution with mean, μ, then the maximum-likelihood estimator for μ is the sample mean.

P-value. In significance testing, the probability of obtaining a result as extreme or more extreme than that actually observed given that the null hypothesis is true.

Parallel assay. A dose-finding trial in which the potency of a new treatment is established by comparing its dose-response to the dose-response of a standard treatment.

Parallel group trial. A trial in which patients are allocated to a treatment (or sometimes a combination or sequence of treatments) with the purpose of studying differences between these treatments (or combination or sequence of treatments).

Parameter. In mathematics, a constant which affects the particular value of an equation but not its nature, so that (for example) the gradient is a parameter of the straight line: change the gradient and you still have a straight line; set the gradient and you have a particular line. In statistics a parameter is used in connection with an underlying (usually hypothetical and infinite) population and is a function of the values of this population which defines their distribution. So that, for example, the population mean and the population variance are parameters. (A similar function calculated for a sample is a *statistic*.) The word parameter is increasingly misunderstood and misused in modern psycho-babble and socio-speak to mean a constraint – probably because of the superficial similarity to 'perimeter'.

Patient diary. A record of symptoms and occasionally other measurements maintained by a patient in a therapeutic trial. Sometimes this is regarded as being part of the *CRF*. In other usages CRF is used only for that portion of the patient's data which is recorded by the investigator.

Pharmaco-economics. Drug development's dismal science.

Pharmacodynamics. The study of biochemical, physiological or therapeutic responses to a pharmaceutical as a function of dose and time. 'What the drug does to the body.'

Pharmacogenetics. The science of gene-by-treatment interaction. The study of the modification of treatment effects in consequence of genetic inheritance. Not to be confused with pharmacogenomics.

Pharmacogenomics. See pharmacogenetics.

Pharmacokinetics. The study of the absorption, distribution and elimination of a pharmaceutical in the body as a function of dose and time. 'What the body does to the drug.'

Pharmacovigilance. A branch of pharmacoepidemiology concerned with monitoring drug use in patients (whether in clinical trials or more generally) with the purpose of detecting possible harms and eventually establishing the risks (if any) attendant on taking particular treatments.

Phase I studies. The first studies in humans. Often, but not exclusively carried out in healthy volunteers. Pharmacokinetics of the drug and basic tolerability information are often obtained from these studies.

Phase II studies. The first attempts to prove efficacy of a treatment. These are often the first studies in patients. Dose-finding is a common objective of such studies.

Phase III studies. Large-scale 'definitive' studies carried out once probable effective and tolerated doses of the drug have been established with the object of proving that the drug is suitable for registration.

Phase IV studies. Studies undertaken either after registration or during registration with the purpose of discovering more about the drug, often with respect to safety but sometimes to look at efficacy in different populations. Such studies are often larger and simpler than regulatory studies and may lack a control group.

Phenotype. A classification of individuals in terms of their physical differences as a consequence of differences in their genetic code rather than in terms of differences in the code itself.

Play-the-winner design. An adaptive allocation design in which the next patient is allocated the last successful treatment.

Poisson distribution. The simplest probability distribution which may be used to model the number of events occurring during a given time interval. (Named after the

19th-century French mathematician Simeon-Denis Poisson, 1781–1840, who, however had little to do with its development.) Its probability mass function is

$$P(X=x) = \frac{\lambda^x e^{-\lambda}}{x!}, \quad x = 0, 1, 2, \ldots, \lambda > 0,$$

where λ is the mean number of events per interval. (The variance of this distribution is also equal to λ.) A distribution which stands somewhat in relationship to discrete observations as the Normal does to continuous ones. In drug development it is often used to model 'count data' of the form: number of epileptic attacks, number of asthma attacks and so forth.

Population. A largely theoretical concept which refers to a (sometimes infinite or undefined) totality of observations of interest. For example, a population might be all potential patients who might in future be treated with a drug. (This would be an example of a rather poorly defined population.) The word population as used in statistics does not, however, have necessarily to do with people. In the context of randomized clinical trials, a population of potential *randomizations* of the patients actually recruited to the trial might be considered, as being the 'population' of interest.

Post-stratification. The formation of relatively homogeneous groups of patients after the trial is completed for the purpose of providing a fair basis of comparison for the treatments. Treatment effects are established for each stratum by comparing like with like and are then combined in some appropriate way across strata. See also *analysis of covariance*.

Posterior probability. See discussion under *prior probability*. The hindsight which results from adding experience to foresight.

Power. The power is the probability of concluding that the alternative hypothesis is true given that it is in fact true. It depends on the statistical test being employed, the 'size' of that test, the nature and variability of the observations obtained and the size of the trial. It also depends on the alternative hypothesis. In practice there is no single alternative hypothesis, so a reference alternative based on a *clinically relevant difference* is usually employed. The power of a trial is a useful concept when planning the trial but has little relevance to the interpretation of its results. (**Caution**: not all statisticians agree with this last statement.)

Prevalence. The number of cases of a disease in a population, expressed as a proportion of the population.

Prior probability. In Bayesian statistics, a subjective probability assigned to a hypothesis (or statement or prediction) before seeing evidence. This is then updated after evidence is obtained, using Bayes' theorem, in order to obtain a further subjective probability known as a *posterior probability*. The terms *prior* and *posterior* are relative to a given set of evidence. Once a posterior probability has been calculated it becomes available as a prior probability to be used in connection with future evidence.

Pro drug. A drug for which the molecule delivered into the body is not directly effective but which metabolizes into an effective treatment.

Probability. A word about whose meaning whole books have been written including at least one which claims that the concept is meaningless. A number between 0 and 1 used to describe uncertain events – the higher the number the greater the certainty. There are at least four standard interpretations. (1) The so called 'classical' definition, which works by counting 'equally likely outcomes'. (Since a die has 6 faces and 3 correspond to odd numbers, the probability of obtaining an odd number on a single role is 3/6 or 1/2.) (2) The subjective interpretation. (If you are prepared to offer odds of 1 to 1 that the number will be odd then the probability of its being odd for *you* is 1/2.) (3) The frequency interpretation. (The probability of the number being odd is unknown but it is a limit which the relative frequency of odd numbers to throws obtained will probably approach given a large number of throws.) (4) The propensity interpretation. (The probability of an odd number on rolling the die is an inherent characteristic of the die and the manner in which it is rolled, which may find expression in a number of ways including betting odds and relative frequencies.)

Probability density. That which is to probability what velocity is to distance. In describing the instantaneous velocity at a given moment of an accelerating car as being 40 miles per hour, we readily accept the fact that there is no real 'hour' in question in which the car is observed to travel 40 miles. The velocity represents some sort of ideal limit of the actual distance travelled in a very small instant of time and scaled up to the arbitrary standard of one hour. Similarly, if we wish to describe the probability that a given individual sampled at random from a population has a given blood pressure, the answer would depend strongly upon the precision to which blood pressure was measured, the probability decreasing with increasing precision. This phenomenon can be avoided by dealing with a probability per standard interval. Such a probability is a probability density.

Probability density function. A function which assigns a probability density to values of a random variable. An example is given in the entry under *Normal distribution*.

Probability distribution. A mathematical model which, for a range of values, associates a probability (or probability density) with a given value. Common examples are the *Normal, binomial, t, F,* chi-square, *exponential* (or negative exponential) and *Poisson* distributions.

Probability mass function. A function which assigns a probability to values of a random variable. Used for discrete variables as opposed to *probability density function*, which is used for continuous ones. An example is given in the entry under *Poisson distribution*.

Project evaluation and prioritization. The business of valuing potential additions to the portfolio, to select a portfolio which will be an addition to the potential value of the business.

Proportional hazards model. Generally, a regression model used in survival analysis whereby it is assumed that the hazard functions of individuals under study are proportional to each other over time. (This is equivalent to assuming that the log-hazard functions differ by a constant.) More specifically, and in the form originally proposed by Cox (1972), no further definite assumption is made about the hazard functions themselves. One of the most commonly used statistical techniques in survival analysis.

Prospective study. A rather loose term which may, perhaps, be defined as a study in which the measurement of the presumed causal factors is both temporally and logically prior to the measurement of the outcomes of interest (the presumed 'effect'). In this sense the term applies to clinical trials and also to many cohort studies.

Protein binding. The reversible process by which the drug reacts with proteins in the body to form drug–protein complexes.

Racemate. A pharmaceutical which is a mixture of optical isomers. Many pharmaceuticals exhibit optical isomerism and most of these are marketed as racemates. Since effects and side-effects are not usually the same for different optical isomers of the same molecule, an optically pure form could show a higher therapeutic ratio. Difficulties in obtaining such forms, however, usually prohibit this from being a practical possibility.

Radix. The original number assumed alive at age 0 (typically 1000 or 100 000) for the purpose of presenting a life table. The root at which time and mortality will gnaw.

Random-effect model. A term which is used in at least two rather different senses by statisticians in the context of drug development. (1) A model for which more than one term is assumed random but the treatment effect is assumed fixed. (All statistical models, including so-called fixed ones have at least one 'error term' which is random.) (2) A model in which the treatment effect itself is assumed to vary randomly from unit to unit. For balanced designs, random-effect models of the first sort can lead to identical inferences to fixed-effect models. Even for balanced designs, random-effect models of the second sort will not.

Random variable. A term which has been given many variable, if not entirely random, definitions. Broadly and loosely for our purposes, some measurement which takes on given values with given probabilities.

Randomization. A means by which an element of chance is allowed to enter the allocation of patients to treatment. In clinical trials (and for that matter other experiments) several restrictions are usually imposed on the randomization, for example the requirement that equal numbers shall be assigned to each treatment in each centre. The allocation of patients to treatment according to chance as opposed to other methods which use either whim or prejudice.

Rank test. A statistical test, such as the Mann–Whitney–Wilcoxon test, carried out on the ranks of the data rather than on the original data. Thus, the statistic used in the test, the rank statistic, is calculated from ranks of the data. Usually such tests are associated with randomization. Given knowledge of the randomization procedure, the distribution of the rank statistic is perfectly general under the null hypothesis. *The rank is but the guinea stamp. The Mann's the gowd for a' that* (Burns).

Regression to the mean. A statistical phenomenon and an important (and often unrecognized) source of bias in uncontrolled studies which may be explained by example. If a large group of stable individuals chosen at random have their systolic blood pressure measured at two different times, then the mean of the blood pressure on the two occasions may well be similar and so may the variances. Because of variability within individuals, however, the correlation between repeat measures will not be perfect. The only way in which all these three statistical results (regarding mean, variance and correlation) can be satisfied will be if on average there is an increase for those individuals with the lowest blood pressure to start with and a decrease for those with the highest to start with. This phenomenon is **regression to the mean**. The consequence is that if an entry requirement for a clinical trial is that patients should have high blood pressure, then a spontaneous improvement is to be expected on purely statistical grounds.

Regulator's risk. The probability of registering a drug given that it is, in fact, either useless or worse than useless.

Relative risk. A term commonly used in epidemiology. The probability of an outcome in the 'exposed' group as a ratio to the probability in the 'unexposed' group.

Repeated-measures design. In the context of clinical trials, a trial in which patients are measured repeatedly as a means of determining the efficacy of treatment. Usually the term refers to repeated measurement at different time points of the same outcome variable. Almost all clinical trials in which survival is not the outcome fall into this category. The analysis of such measures can be a delicate matter. The term is also used by psychologists for *cross-over design*, although this use is potentially confusing and best avoided.

Residual sum of squares. Also known as error sum of squares. The sum of the variability not explained by the fitted model. It is the sum of the squares of the differences between the observed values and those which would be predicted by the model using the known values of the various factors and covariates incorporated in it.

Response surface design. A dose-finding design involving two or more treatments with doses chosen in such a way as to have a reasonable chance of establishing the general form of response as a function of the doses of the two or more treatments being studied.

Retrospective study. A term which has been given different meanings by different persons and which, although often used, is not sufficiently precise to be useful. Broadly, any study in which information regarding exposure to a potential causative factor is obtained after the information regarding an outcome of interest has been obtained. Sometimes used as a synonym for case–control study, although a cohort study can also be retrospective.

Robust statistics. Statistics which are less vulnerable to the presence of outliers and dirty data but which are generally slightly less efficient than the standard alternatives where the data are well behaved. The median, for example, is a robust statistic, whereas the mean is not. The mountain-bikes of the statistical world as opposed to its road-racers. A means to drink salt-water as if it were sweet.

Root mean square error. The square root of the mean square error. A sort of generalized standard deviation which can be used not only when observations are being compared to the mean value of them all but also where they are compared to predicted values under more complex models.

Sample. A set of observations.

Sample space. An important concept in frequentist statistics but one with no (or little) relevance in Bayesian statistics. The sample space is the set of all possible samples which *could* be obtained and must therefore be defined with respect to a particular sampling rule. For a sequential trial, for example, in which the sample size could differ from trial to trial, the sample space will be different than from an otherwise similar fixed-size trial. In frequentist statistics the distribution of the test statistic is established by considering how it would vary over the sample space.

SAS®. Statistical Analysis System. The most commonly used statistical analysis package within the pharmaceutical industry.

Sequential trial. (A somewhat unfortunate term since nearly all patients are recruited sequentially and in this sense nearly all trials would be sequential.) A clinical trial in which the results are analysed at various intervals with the intention of stopping the trial when a 'conclusive result' has been reached. A stopping rule is usually defined in advance. In frequentist statistics it is necessary to make an adjustment to the results of an otherwise standard analysis to take the stopping rule into account. Such an adjustment is not necessary in Bayesian statistics, although the stopping rule itself ought to be at least partly dependent on the prior distribution so that, for this reason alone, the posterior distribution *will* vary with the stopping rule.

Shift tables. Tables used to summarize and interpret laboratory (or similar) data showing, by treatment, the numbers of patients who have shifted from having 'normal' to having 'abnormal' values during the trial and so forth.

Significance level. See *size*.

Significance testing. An approach to statistical testing in which, rather than making (as in hypothesis testing) a formal decision to reject or not reject (as the case may be) the *null hypothesis*, an exact *P-value* is quoted instead. Since by comparing the P-value with a target significance level and by deciding to reject the null hypothesis where the P-value is lower, the significance test behaves like a hypothesis test, the term is frequently used interchangeably with *hypothesis test*.

Simple carry-over. Carry-over for simple minds. A form of carry-over which lasts for exactly one period and depends on the engendering but not the perturbed treatment and which ought to be spelled 'karry-over' to draw attention to its eccentricity, rarity and unnatural nature. An improbable fantasy in which mathematics triumphs over biology.

Simple random sampling. A form of sampling in which every sample of the given size chosen is equally likely to occur. An important theoretical concept in much of statistics but of little practical relevance in the context of clinical trials and hence, in my opinion, an irrelevant and potentially misleading notion.

Single-dose study. A trial in which the effect of a single administration of a treatment is studied. Rather confusingly, a single-dose study can still compare the effect of a number of doses provided only that each is given as a single administration. Compare *multiple-dose study*.

Size (of a test). When used in connection with hypothesis testing, the size of a test is the probability of rejecting the null hypothesis given that the null hypothesis is true. (In other words, it is the probability of committing a type I error when the null hypothesis is true.) Conventionally in clinical trials a size of 5% is used. Also called *significance level*.

Sponsors' risk. The probability of concluding that a drug is useless given that it is, in fact, useful.

Standard deviation. A measure of the variability of a set of data. It is the square root of the *variance* and has the advantage of being expressed in the units of the original data.

Standard error. A measure of the variability of a *statistic* from sample to sample. (As opposed to *standard deviation* which is a measure of variability for original observations.) Since repeated samples are not usually obtained, standard errors cannot be calculated directly. They can be calculated on the basis of a single sample using an appropriate model and the assumptions it requires. For example, on the assumption that a sample has been obtained by *simple random sampling*, the standard error of the mean will equal the standard deviation divided by the square root of the sample size. This particular assumption, which implies that variability between samples can be simply estimated with the help of variability within samples, is rarely valid, however, and this formula is often inappropriately used in clinical trials. In fact, it is a standard error to use it.

Standard gamble. A means of evaluating a subject's utility of a given outcome by establishing at what value of a probability, p, the subject would be indifferent to trading the given outcome for the best possible outcome with probability p or the worst possible outcome with probability $(1 - p)$. An aid to making decisions favoured by those who prefer hypothetical questions to real ones.

Standardized mortality ratio. Generally, the ratio of the observed deaths in a given population to those 'expected' given that some external standard of mortality applies. Suppose, for example, that the proportion of elderly persons in the town of Altdorf (A) is much higher than in the village of Kindhausen (K). Other things being equal, the death rate in A will be higher than in K. Given age- and sex-specific annual mortality rates for Switzerland, and given the population of A by age and sex, by applying the rates in Switzerland to the numbers in A, we can tell how many persons should have died during the year in each of these places if average Swiss mortality applied. The ratio of the observed number of deaths in A to the expected deaths for A is the ***standardized mortality ratio***. (This is often multiplied by 100.) A similar calculation can be made for K and the two places can then be compared on an equal basis.

Statistic. A function of the sample data. A summary which captures some general feature of interest of the sample.

Statistics. (1) A subject which most statisticians find difficult but which many physicians find easy. (2) A sort of elementary form of mathematics which consists of adding things together and occasionally squaring them.

Steady-state concentration. The concentration achieved in the limit by regular dosing with a pharmaceutical. In practice it varies throughout the dosing cycle, achieving a minimum just before (or shortly after) a dose is administered and a maximum some time later.

Stochastic curtailment. An approach to the conduct and analysis of sequential trials whereby trials may be terminated early on the basis of the conclusion predicted if run to the end.

Stratification. (1) In the context of the design of clinical trials, a means of carrying out the randomization within demographic strata of the trial population. For example, a separate randomization list may be maintained for male and female patients in order to ensure that there is a balance of sexes within the treatment groups. (2) In the context of the analysis of clinical trials, a means of analysis which first compares the effects of treatment within demographic strata before combining these results into an overall summary. It is usually considered necessary to stratify at analysis if one has stratified at randomization. However, it is generally accepted that one may (and under certain circumstances should) stratify at analysis even if one has not been able to do so at randomization.

Student's t-distribution. A distribution originally proposed in its modern form by R.A. Fisher in 1925 (Fisher, 1925) but related to a distribution derived by Student in 1908 (Student, 1908). It is a probability distribution for a variable which, like the standard Normal, is unbounded and symmetric about zero. It has a single parameter, the so-called degrees of freedom. As this parameter approaches infinity, the distribution approaches that of the standard Normal. Its main use is in testing hypotheses using statistics (for example the difference between two means) calculated from measurements of the continuous type, where the variance of these measurements has to be estimated and is, therefore, itself uncertain.

Summary measures approach. A means of analysing repeated-measures designs which proceeds in two stages. In the first, the repeated measures on each subject are reduced to a summary statistic. In the second stage, these statistics are treated as the data of the problem and analysed conventionally. The advantage is that whereas the original data will not all be independent, the summary measures are. The issue of correlation between the repeated measures is thus finessed. The problem resurfaces to some extent, however, if more than one summary measure is required per subject to capture the essence of the effect of treatment. The main disadvantage of the approach is that it can be inefficient if there are unequal amounts of information per subject.

Superposition principle. This is useful for calculating concentration for multiple doses for drugs with linear kinetics. It says that the concentration at any time is the sum of the concentrations which would be observed from the individual doses had they be given alone.

Survival analysis. The analysis of 'time to event' data in particular, but not exclusively, where the event is death. A common feature of such data is that they are very skewed and that there are many censored values. Survival analysis is one of the single most important topics in medical statistics, although its importance to pharmaceutical statistics is, because of the nature of the trials usually run in drug development, *relatively* less important than the contents of standard textbooks on medical statistics might suggest.

Swissmedic. The Swiss Agency for Therapeutic Products. The Swiss regulatory agency.

t-distribution. See *Student's t-distribution*.

Test statistic. A statistic defined and used for the purpose of carrying out a hypothesis test.

Therapeutic window. The prescribable dose range in which the treatment's benefits may outweigh its side-effects. Generally no wider than the range defined by the minimum effective dose and the maximum tolerated dose and sometimes considerably narrower.

Time trends. Any temporal changes in the outcome being measured which are independent of treatment. Such trends may arise as a result of changes in patients being recruited, changes in assays, observers and methods of measurement, treatment-independent progression of disease, alterations in concomitant therapies available, aging and so forth.

T_{max}. The time after dosing at which the C_{max} occurs.

Tolerability data. Any data collected with an eye on potential side-effects, and in order to profile the safety of a treatment, rather than to measure anticipated benefits of the drug. Measures which the trialist hopes will be irrelevant but fears may not be. They are context dependent, so that blood pressures are not tolerability data in a trial of hypertension (they are efficacy data) but might be in a trial in asthma.

Treatment IND. See *named patient basis*.

Trial. (1) An action whose outcome is uncertain but is presumed to reflect an underlying probability. Thus, treating a single patient constitutes a trial. (2) A clinical experiment usually involving many patients and therefore a set of trials in the sense of (1) above.

Triangular test. A common form of the *boundary approach* to analysing *sequential trials*.

Type I error. A concept used in *frequentist statistics*. It is an error committed in rejecting the *null hypothesis* when it is, in fact, true.

Type II error. A concept used in *frequentist statistics*. It is an error committed in rejecting the alternative hypothesis when it is, in fact, true.

Type III error. Sometimes used to designate the error committed in deciding that the less effective treatment is the more effective one.

Type I–III sums of squares. These labels are used within *SAS*(R) for describing various sums of squares which may be calculated in connection with analysis of variance, analysis of covariance and regression. Because the use of *SAS*(R) is so widespread within the industry, statisticians working there commonly refer to these terms when discussing analysis and models. Type I sums of squares generally depend on the order in which effects are fitted and for a given factor describe how much further variation (beyond that associated with all previously specified factors) is associated with a given term in the model. Other sums of squares are particular cases of type I sums of squares. If a factor is fitted after all other factors in a model (except any interaction terms in which it itself is implicated) and the resulting type I sum of squares is calculated, this is then a type II sum of squares. If a factor is adjusted for all other terms including interactions in which it is implicated, the resulting type I sum of squares may be referred to as type III sum of squares. (See Chapter 14 for a discussion.)

Uncontrolled study. A study without a control group. A means of using prejudice and regression to prove effectiveness. A study where faith must supply what evidence cannot deliver.

Uninformative prior. A term in Bayesian statistics. Some sort of diffuse distribution which does not enable one to distinguish the probable from the possible. Roughly, the sort of prior distribution which allows the posterior to be determined largely by the likelihood (that is to say the data acting on the basic model). Priors which are uninformative on one scale are not necessarily uninformative on another. For example if, using the $\log_{10}$ scale, it is just as likely that a number will fall between 0 and 1 as between 1 and 2, then, on the original scale, numbers between 1 and 10 are as likely as those between 10 and 100.

Utmost good faith. The truth, the whole truth and nothing but the truth. Deception-free dealing. The necessary basis for fair trade. The frank and willing provision of all information relevant to an exchange. The opposite of insider dealing. A virtue which is essential to drug development.

Variance. A measure of variability which is defined unambiguously on a population of values as the mean of the squared deviations of the observations from the mean. (The term is due to R.A. Fisher.) For a sample variance, however, two different conventions are observed. One is to take the sum of the squared deviations from the mean and divide by the number of observations; the other is to divide the same sum by one less than the number of observations. The variance is a statistic of considerable theoretical importance. For a sample of observations from a Normal distribution, when taken together with the mean, it provides a complete summary of all relevant features of the data. As a statistic, however, it is rather vulnerable to 'bad values' and various alternative measures of spread are sometimes used.

Veiled trial. A trial in which it is not possible to identify positively which treatment a patient is getting, although it can be definitely determined that he or she is not getting one or more of the treatments being compared. An example is a four-group parallel trial comparing two distinguishable active treatments in which a placebo to each is provided but the double dummy technique is not used. It is then possible to tell that a patient has not been allocated treatment B (say), although one cannot tell whether the patient has been allocated treatment A or placebo to A. Such trials raise particular problems in analysis.

Volume of distribution. The ratio of the amount of a drug in the body to its concentration in the plasma. Since the concentration is a mass/volume measurement and the amount of drug is a mass measurement, this ratio is a 'volume'. Hence this term for what is, in fact, an important pharmacokinetic parameter.

Wash-out. A period during which the influence of a previous treatment is eliminated (or is presumed to be eliminated) through the natural decay of effects over time. Often employed between periods of treatment and measurement in cross-over trials.

Z. (1) The symbol for a standardized value of a Normal variable. (2) The symbol for the test statistic in Whitehead's boundary approach to sequential clinical trials (see Chapter 19). (3) The symbol which R.A. Fisher used to designate half the difference of the natural logarithms of two independent estimates of variances when comparing them. (Nowadays we tend to use the ratio instead, which we compare to the F-distribution.) (4) The last entry in this glossary.

References

Abercrombie M, Hickman CJ, Johnson ML (eds) (1990) *Dictionary of Biology*. Penguin, London.

Bannock G, Baxter RE, Davis D (eds) (1992) *Dictionary of Economics*. Penguin, London.

Borowski EJ, Borewin JM (eds) (1989) *Dictionary of Mathematics*. Collins, Glasgow.

Cox DR (1972) Regression models and life-tables (with discussion). *Journal of the Royal Statistical Society Series B* **34**:187–220.

Day S (1999) *Dictionary for Clinical Trials*. John Wiley & Sons, Ltd, Chichester.

Dodge Y (1993) *Statistique: Dictionnaire Encyclopedique*. Dunod, Paris

Dodge Y (2006) *The Oxford Dictionary of Statistical Terms*. Oxford University Press, Oxford.

Evans M, Hastings N, Peacock B (1993) *Statistical Distributions*. John Wiley & Sons, Chichester and New York.

Everitt BS (1995) *The Cambridge Dictionary of Statistics in the Medical Sciences*. Cambridge University Press, Cambridge.

Fisher RA (1925) Applications of 'Student's' distribution. *Metron* **5**: 90–104.

Henry J (ed.) (1994) *British Medical Association: New Guide to Medicines and Drugs*. Dorling Kindersley, London.

Last JM (1995) *A Dictionary of Epidemiology*. Oxford University Press, New York and Oxford.

Martin EA (ed.) (1990) *Concise Medical Dictionary*. Oxford University Press, Oxford.

Nahler G (1994) *Dictionary of Pharmaceutical Medicine*. Springer, Vienna.

O'Hagan A, Buck CE, Daneshkah A, *et al.* (2006) *Uncertain Judgements*. John Wiley & Sons, Inc., Hoboken.

Sharp DWA (ed.) (1990) *Dictionary of Chemistry*. Penguin, London.

Student (1908) The probable error of a mean. *Biometrika* **6**: 1–25.

Vesey G, Foulkes P (eds) (1990) *Collins Dictionary of Philosophy*. Collins, Glasgow.

Winslade J, Hutchinson TA (1992) *Dictionary of Clinical Research*. Brookwood, Surrey.

Youngson RM (1994) *Prescription Drugs*. Harper-Collins, Glasgow.

Index

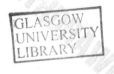

Statistics in Practice

Human and Biological Sciences

Berger – Selection Bias and Covariate Imbalances in Randomized Clinical Trials
Brown and Prescott – Applied Mixed Models in Medicine, Second Edition
Chevret (Ed) – Statistical Methods for Dose-Finding Experiments
Ellenberg, Fleming and DeMets – Data Monitoring Committees in Clinical Trials: A Practical Perspective
Hauschke, Steinijans and Pigeot – Bioequivalence Studies in Drug Development: Methods and Applications
Lawson, Browne and Vidal Rodeiro – Disease Mapping with WinBUGS and MLwiN
Lui – Statistical Estimation of Epidemiological Risk
Marubini and Valsecchi – Analysing Survival Data from Clinical Trials and Observation Studies
Molenberghs and Kenward – Missing Data in Clinical Studies
O'Hagan, Buck, Daneshkhah, Eiser, Garthwaite, Jenkinson, Oakley and Rakow – Uncertain Judgements: Eliciting Expert's Probabilities
Parmigiani – Modeling in Medical Decision Making: A Bayesian Approach
Pintilie – Competing Risks: A Practical Perspective
Senn – Cross-over Trials in Clinical Research, Second Edition
Senn – Statistical Issues in Drug Development, Second Edition
Spiegelhalter, Abrams and Myles – Bayesian Approaches to Clinical Trials and Health-Care Evaluation
Whitehead – Design and Analysis of Sequential Clinical Trials, Revised Second Edition
Whitehead – Meta-Analysis of Controlled Clinical Trials
Willan and Briggs – Statistical Analysis of Cost Effectiveness Data
Winkel and Zhang – Statistical Development of Quality in Medicine

Earth and Environmental Sciences

Buck, Cavanagh and Litton – Bayesian Approach to Interpreting Archaeological Data
Glasbey and Horgan – Image Analysis in the Biological Sciences
Helsel – Nondetects and Data Analysis: Statistics for Censored Environmental Data
Illian, Penttinen, Stoyan and Stoyan – Statistical Analysis and Modelling of Spatial Point Patterns
McBride – Using Statistical Methods for Water Quality Management
Webster and Oliver – Geostatistics for Environmental Scientists, Second Edition
Wymer (Ed) – Statistical Framework for Recreational Quality Criteria and Monitoring

Industry, Commerce and Finance

Aitken – Statistics and the Evaluation of Evidence for Forensic Scientists, Second Edition
Balding – Weight-of-evidence for Forensic DNA Profiles
Brandimarte – Numerical Methods in Finance and Economics: A MATLAB-Based Introduction, Second Edition

Brandimarte and Zotteri – Introduction to Distribution Logistics

Chan – Simulation Techniques in Financial Risk Management

Coleman, Greenfield, Stewardson and Montgomery (Eds) – Statistical Practice in Business and Industry

Frisén (Ed) – Financial Surveillance

Lehtonen and Pahkinen – Practical Methods for Design and Analysis of Complex Surveys, Second Edition

Ohser and Mücklich – Statistical Analysis of Microstructures in Materials Science

Taroni, Aitken, Garbolino and Biedermann – Bayesian Networks and Probabilistic Inference in Forensic Science